Hydrotherapy
for Bodyworkers

DEDICATION

This book is dedicated with my utmost appreciation to two groups of people.

First, to the medical visionaries whose work has so greatly informed and inspired me: the healers, authors and outside-the-box thinkers William H. Bates, John Sarno, and Agatha Thrash, along with writer and medical historian Edward Shorter PhD.

Second, to all the smart, hardworking, and committed massage therapist healers I have met over the years – this book is for you!

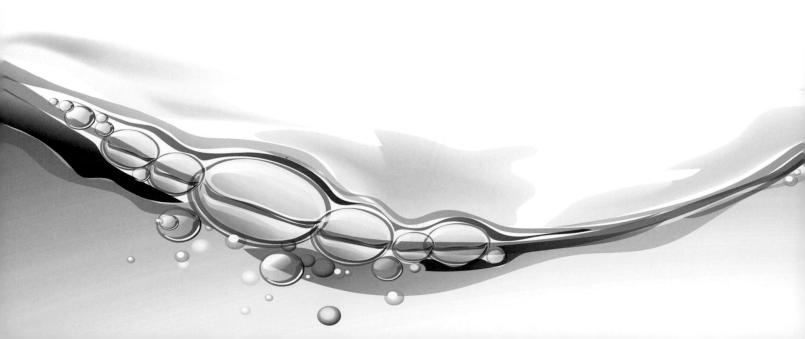

Second edition

Hydrotherapy for Bodyworkers

Improving outcomes with water therapies

MaryBetts Sinclair

Foreword by Almut Hatfield

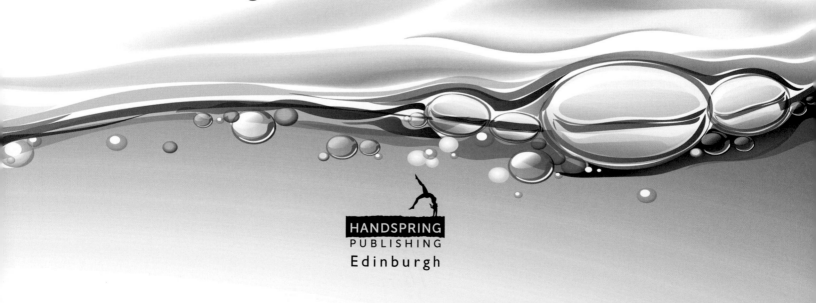

HANDSPRING
PUBLISHING
Edinburgh

HANDSPRING PUBLISHING LIMITED
The Old Manse, Fountainhall,
Pencaitland, East Lothian
EH34 5EY, Scotland
Tel: +44 1875 341 859
Website: www.handspringpublishing.com

Originally published in 2008 as *Modern Hydrotherapy for the Massage Therapist* by Lippincott Williams & Wilkins

First published 2020 in the United Kingdom by Handspring Publishing
Copyright © Handspring Publishing 2020

ISBN 978-1-912085-52-1
ISBN (Kindle eBook) 978-1-912085-53-8

British Library Cataloguing in Publication Data
A catalogue record for this book is available from the British Library

Library of Congress Cataloguing in Publication Data
A catalog record for this book is available from the Library of Congress

Notice
Neither the Publisher nor the Authors assume any responsibility for any loss or injury and/or damage to persons or property arising out of or relating to any use of the material contained in this book. It is the responsibility of the treating practitioner, relying on independent expertise and knowledge of the patient, to determine the best treatment and method of application for the patient.

All reasonable efforts have been made to obtain copyright clearance for illustrations in the book for which the authors or publishers do not own the rights. If you believe that one of your illustrations has been used without such clearance please contact the publishers and we will ensure that appropriate credit is given in the next reprint.

Commissioning Editor Mary Law
Project Manager Morven Dean
Copyeditor Jane Dingwall
Proofreader Andrew Nash
Designer Bruce Hogarth
Indexer Aptara, India
Typesetter Amnet, India
Printer Replika, India

The
Publisher's
policy is to use
paper manufactured
from sustainable forests

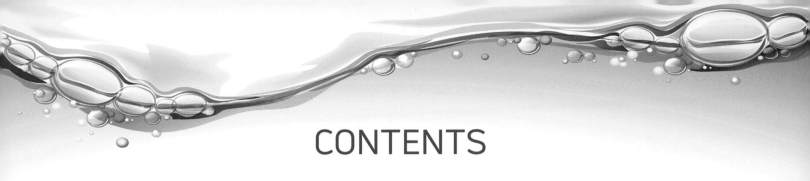

CONTENTS

Foreword   vii
Preface   ix
Acknowledgements   xi
Permissions   xiii
Glossary   xv

1 Introduction to hydrotherapy   1

2 Effects of hydrotherapy   23

3 Preparing to give hydrotherapy treatments   53

4 Fomentations, hot packs, compresses, and other local heat treatments   87

5 Cold packs, compresses, and ice massage: local cold applications   119

6 Immersion baths   141

7 Hot air baths   179

8 Showers   195

9 Body wraps   217

10 Friction treatments   231

11 Hydrotherapy self-treatments for health and wellness   243

12 Hydrotherapy and massage for musculoskeletal injuries   267

13 Hydrotherapy and massage for non-injury conditions   311

Appendices

   A Simple hydrotherapy record and self-treatment handouts   369
   B Pool therapy   375
   C Pyrotherapy (treatment of disease with artificial fever)   377
   D Answers to review questions   381

Index   387

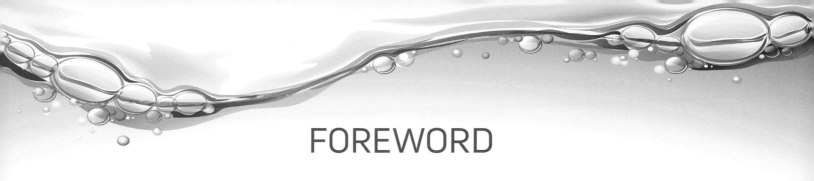

FOREWORD

Author MaryBetts Sinclair has poured her very extensive research as well as her considerable professional experience into this comprehensive and remarkable work, *Hydrotherapy for Bodyworkers*: documenting historical data and methods, presenting wellness traditions as well as new treatment techniques from around the globe, and doing so with a fresh and practical approach offering pathways to easily integrate hydrotherapy with modern bodywork practices.

I grew up in Europe, where water-based health treatments were commonly employed as part of the medical system. When opening Body Wisdom Massage Therapy School in Iowa in the late 1990s, I was surprised how difficult it was to find a hydrotherapy instructor and suitable textbooks and resources that focused on the science and medical benefits of hydrotherapy. Thankfully a search led me to Sinclair's book. *Hydrotherapy for Bodyworkers* will inspire anyone to explore hydrotherapy, whether as a client, to enhance self-care and home use, or for professional study; it will be a delight for each vocational instructor and a great resource for any business or facility where these techniques are offered.

Well written, structured and sequenced, and full of useful images, *Hydrotherapy for Bodyworkers* presents a vast store of information about hydrotherapy in relationship to the functions, needs, and wellness of the human body and its individual physiological systems. Medical aspects, as they relate to any part of the body, are taken into consideration with indications and contraindications. Applications are clearly laid out and detailed, with their benefits and effects, as well as up-to-date scientific findings. Further detailed are basics and specifics on water and temperature itself, and the array of conducting materials, tools, and methods. Different populations and their unique needs are considered alongside specific health or pathology conditions, injuries, and many other important factors. Treatment background information, purpose, logistics, practicalities, case histories, discussion points, references, summaries, review quizzes, and resource information add to the thorough content and practical teaching of each hydrotherapy modality (in view of COVID-19), together with step-by-step instructions for preparation, application, and careful sanitary clean-up.

Practitioners will find answers and assessment options to choose the best techniques for their unique practice and specific clientele, how to effectively incorporate hydrotherapy with other common and specific bodywork modalities, how to create a session menu, and how to combine multiple treatments to successfully market these skills. The author demonstrates how modern hydrotherapy is possible within any professional setting: private practice, assisted living, nursing home, health spa, in-home care, and more.

Hydrotherapy for Bodyworkers is a wonderful and highly valuable teaching tool and resource especially for massage and bodywork. I am grateful to MaryBetts Sinclair and everyone who has supported her studies, including Handspring Publishing, for recognizing the power and significance of hydrotherapy in today's wellness education and care.

Almut Hatfield
Owner, Body Wisdom School
Davenport, Iowa, USA
June 2020

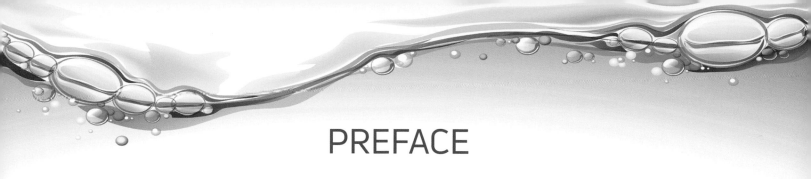

PREFACE

Hydrotherapy for Bodyworkers has been written to fill a significant gap in the education of the modern massage therapist, who has typically taken only one short course in hydrotherapy during school. There are almost no continuing education classes in this subject area, and few books which inspire therapists to go further. Without more background in hydrotherapy, today's new massage therapists have only the most basic information, and are thus in danger of losing this important adjunct to their hands-on methods. The purpose of this book, then, is to excite students about hydrotherapy and give them the knowledge to use it with ease. This will enhance their practices, allow them to better meet their clients' needs, and create unique treatments that combine their massage and hydrotherapy skills.

APPROACH TO HYDROTHERAPY

When I was licensed as a massage therapist in 1975, my study of hydrotherapy had been confined to one short class. The book that was used in the course was very old and its language antiquated, making the topic seem irrelevant and boring. Moreover, hydrotherapy, like massage, was little used in mainstream medicine at the time.

What convinced me of the effectiveness of hydrotherapy, therefore, was not what I learned in my formal education but my own personal experience. When I was younger and had a serious injury from a fall, I visited an old-school physical therapist who would treat me with a relaxing soak in a warm whirlpool bath followed by a rest period, massage, and therapeutic exercises. I found this treatment very healing, and later also witnessed the effectiveness of hydrotherapy in my professional life.

My first job as a massage therapist was at a health club with a sauna and a swimming pool: I learned that both helped extend the relaxing effects of my treatments, while the physical therapist who worked there used hot silica gel packs extensively to help his patients with their aches and pains. It became obvious to me that hydrotherapy had a great deal more potential than I had understood. I took more hydrotherapy classes, visited clinics where hydrotherapy was used in a medical context, spent time in pools with aquatic therapists, and did extensive research. When I began teaching hydrotherapy for a massage school, however, the available curriculum was just as outdated as the teaching I had encountered on my own. Students struggled with outdated terminology, and treatments that had been given by hospital nurses a half-century ago were mostly seen as irrelevant to today's massage therapist. Students needed a textbook that would help them learn not only about the fascinating past of hydrotherapy but also its potential for massage practice today; I wrote the first edition of *Hydrotherapy for Bodyworkers* to fill that need. It explained in today's language how hydrotherapy works, and gave the massage therapist the information he or she needs to use it safely and appropriately.

In the 13 years since the first edition was published, I have taught hundreds of massage therapists in the USA and abroad. At the same time my own massage practice has expanded to include patients at physical therapy clinics, hospice patients, homeless people, guests at up-scale spas, and loyal clients I have treated for decades. All were willing to try hydrotherapy treatments, and they taught me much more about how to incorporate such treatments into a practice. This edition features much of what I have learned in that time: it also benefits from up-dated medical research on the anatomy and physiology of hydrotherapy, which scientifically validates a great many treatments. Cautions, contraindications, and notes on proper scope of practice are included throughout to ensure the safety of both client and therapist.

ORGANIZATION AND FEATURES

The first three chapters of the book provide a theoretical foundation for the study of hydrotherapy: Chapter 1 introduces the reader to the field of hydrotherapy and provides a brief history of the therapeutic use of water; Chapter 2 explains its effects on the body; Chapter 3

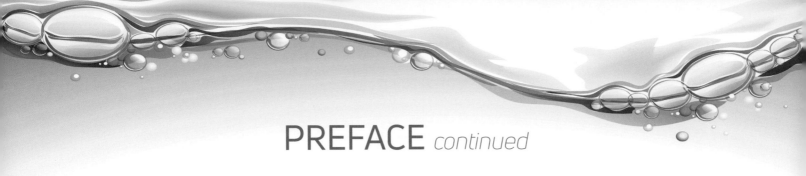

covers a variety of practical information that the reader needs to know, including guidelines for buying equipment, cautions and contraindications, and general instructions.

Chapters 4–10 each present an overview and step-by-step instructions for a variety of treatments; these include local hot and cold applications, water baths, hot air baths, showers, body wraps, and friction treatments. The last three chapters demonstrate how hydrotherapy treatments may be applied to many specific situations: Chapter 11 covers how hydrotherapy may be used by the client and the massage therapist as regular self-care treatments for detoxification, tonifying, and prevention of repetitive stress injuries; Chapters 12 and 13 describe how and why massage and hydrotherapy may be combined to address many new injuries and conditions, as well as those discussed in the previous edition. Finally, the appendices provide hydrotherapy handouts that therapists can give to their clients, as well as information on pool therapy and fever therapy, and answers to all the review questions in the book.

The following features are included in the book as learning aids:

- *Quotations* from experts in a variety of fields and time periods, at the start of each chapter, give additional perspectives.

- *Chapter objectives* clarify the goals of the chapter.

- *Key terms*, bold-faced in the main text and explained in the Glossary, help readers to understand important terminology.

- *Introductions* to chapters usher in the ideas presented in the chapter.

- *Treatment* overviews and step-by-step instructions are highlighted in the text for easy referencing.

- *Points of interest* deepen the student's understanding of hydrotherapy by highlighting interesting aspects and concepts.

- *Case histories* put concepts presented in the text into action, with all examples drawn from actual massage therapists and their clients.

- *Chapter summaries* give a concise overview of the content of each chapter.

- *Review questions* at the end of each chapter allow students to review the information they have just read.

FINAL NOTE

Because water has positive effects on human beings in both Mind–body and mechanical ways, water treatments have been paired with massage since time out of mind. Without contact with the earth through creeks, rivers, oceans, and other natural bodies of water, our emotional and spiritual health is at risk. Let us all work toward the health not only of our clients but of our natural environment, which nurtures and sustains us all.

MaryBetts Sinclair, LMT

State Licensed Massage Therapist (OR);
Certified Vocational Instructor (OR); Certified
Natural Vision Instructor; Member, Massage
Therapy Hall of Fame (USA)

Oregon, USA, June 2020

ACKNOWLEDGEMENTS

This book, labor of love as it has been, would have been impossible without the generosity and expertise of a host of fellow massage therapists, health professionals in many other fields, historians, researchers, librarians, and wordsmiths.

I cannot adequately thank all those who took the time out of their busy days to answer obscure and not-so-obscure questions and strange requests for information, and especially my clients, who cheerfully let me experiment on them, and otherwise encouraged, aided and abetted me. I deeply appreciate the work of Laurie Garrett, whose prescient book *The Coming Plague* began my interest in hydrotherapy as a healing modality. The reference librarians at the Corvallis Public Library continued, as they have for decades, to give consistently helpful, insightful and friendly service. Helena Tolis, RN, Agatha Thrash, MD, and physical therapists Pam Davidson, Jean Yzer and Frank Hahn all offered their years of perspective. Author Ruth Werner's book, *A Massage Therapist's Guide to Pathology*, continues to support and inform my writing and I often read sections out loud to my clients – that's how good it is! Over the years, a great many of my students have asked excellent questions, which spurred further research and led to many insights.

The good people of Uchee Pines Institute continue to impress me with their outstanding faith, compassion, dedication and smarts. A huge thank you goes to Fifi Lim, humanitarian and entrepreneur, for inviting me to teach her spa therapists in Indonesia multiple times.

Many thanks to Handspring Publishing for everything! I especially wish to give a shout-out to Jane Dingwall, whose super-sharp eyes and meticulous editing have vastly improved the organization and focus of both new material and old. Wonderful helpers at the second edition photoshoot included the staff of the Epic Spa of Corvallis, Oregon, and models Jill Beuter, Mari Hernadez, Craig Hanson, Krisa Gigon and Oscar Gigon. Special thanks to April Robinson for helping me organize all the hydro equipment.

And finally, a last heartfelt thank you to my dear Corvallis community – you know who you are – your love and support has been my rock through good times and bad, and I couldn't have done it without you all!

Mil gracias / terima kasih / tusind tak / thanks ever so much.

MaryBetts Sinclair

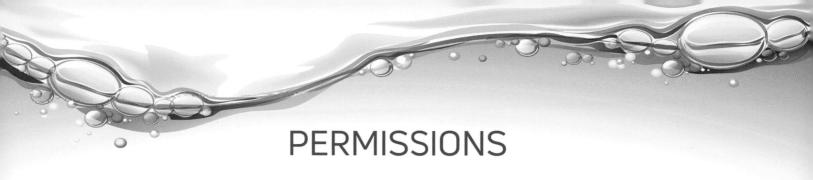

PERMISSIONS

Figure 1.1 (A) – Photo by Trinette Reed, courtesy of Stocksy images

Figure 1.1 (B) – Courtesy of Alamy Limited

Figure 1.2 (A) – Permission: Bath in Time

Figure 1.2 (B) – Permission: British Museum

Figure 1.2 (C) – Photograph courtesy of Thermae Bath Spa

Figure 1.5 – Painting by William Hoare, courtesy of Bath in Time

Figures 1.6, 1.8 – Photos with kind permission of National College of Naturopathic Medicine, Portland, Oregon

Figures 1.9, 1.10, 1.12 (B) – Photos from Rational Hydrotherapy, by John Harvey Kellogg, 1923

Figure 1.11 – Reprinted with permission from Willard Library, Battle Creek, Michigan

Figure 1.12 (A) – Illustration courtesy of Kunsstmuseum, Basel

Figure 1.13 – Reprinted with permission from Franklin Delano Roosevelt National Library, Hyde Park, New York

Figure 1.14 – Photo courtesy of SaunaRay Sauna Company

Box 1.4, Figure 4 – Reprinted with permission from Joey Banegas and Walter Reed Army Medical Center, Washington DC

Figure 2.1 – Photo courtesy of Rich Roberts

Figure 2.13 – Photo by Heidi Bradner, reprinted with permission from Panos Pictures, London, England

Box 3.5, Figure 1 – Photo courtesy of Earl Qualls, PT, and Wildwood Hospital, Wildwood, Georgia

Figures 4.10, 13.2, 13.6 – With permission from Fomentek company, Fayetteville, AR

Box 4.2 – Photos courtesy of The Dermatologist, East Windsor, New Jersey

Box 4.3, Figure 1 – Photograph courtesy of March of Dimes Birth Defects Foundation

Figure 5.2 – Photo courtesy of Whitehall Mfg Company

Figure 6.3 – Courtesy of Charcoal House, Crawford, Nebraska

Figure 6.6 – Photo courtesy of HEAT Spa Kur Therapy Development, Inc., Bonita, California

Figure 6.19 – Photo courtesy of Jeff Bisbee

Box 6.1, Figure 1 – Porcelain sitz bath, manufactured in 1905 by Standard Sanitary Manufacturing Company of Pittsburg, Pennsylvania

Figure 7.3 (B) – Courtesy of Natural Health Technologies, Fairfield, Iowa

Figure 7.4 – Photo courtesy of Promolife, Fayetteville, AZ

Figure 7.5 – Photo: Peter Rubens, courtesy of Breitenbush Hot Springs, Breitenbush, Oregon

Box 7.1, Figure A – Photo courtesy of SaunaRay

Box 8.2, Figures B, C, D – Photos courtesy of HEAT Spa Kur Therapy Development, Inc., Bonita, California

Figure 11.1 – Photo courtesy Mark Wexler

Figures 11.2, 11.3 – Photos courtesy of New York City Rescue Workers Detoxification Project

Box 11.1, Figure 1 – Photograph courtesy of Bob Madden

Box 11.1, Figure 2 – Photo: Rodney Palmer, courtesy of SaunaRay

Figure 12.1 – Reprinted with permission from Bucholz RW, Heckman JD. Rockwood and Green's Fractures in Adults, 5th ed. Baltimore, MD: Lippincott, Williams and Wilkins; 2001

Figure 12.2 – Reprinted with permission from Archer M. Therapeutic Massage in Athletics, page 104. Baltimore, MD: Lippincott, Williams and Wilkins; 2004, Figure 6.4

Figure 12.5 – Courtesy MaryBetts Sinclair

Figure 12.6 – Reprinted with permission from Yochum TR, Rowe LJ. Essentials of Skeletal Radiology, 2nd ed. Baltimore, MD: Lippincott, Williams and Wilkins; 1996, 1:398, Figure 6.38

Figure 13.1 – Reprinted with permission from Strickland JW, Graham TJ. Master Techniques in Orthopedic Surgery: The Hand, 2nd edn. Philadelphia: Lippincott, Williams and Wilkins; 2005, Figure 5.5

Images from History of Medicine, National Library of Medicine, Bethesda, Maryland. Sourced from ihm.nlm.nih.gov/images

Figure 1.3: A030070; Figure 1.4: A029447; Figure 1.7: 101393239; Box 1.4, Figure 1: A011823; Box 1.4, Figure 2: 101396512; Box 1.4, Figure 3: A09297; Figure 4.11: 101449253; Figure 6.17: 101395644; Box 8.2, Figure 1 (A): 101447290

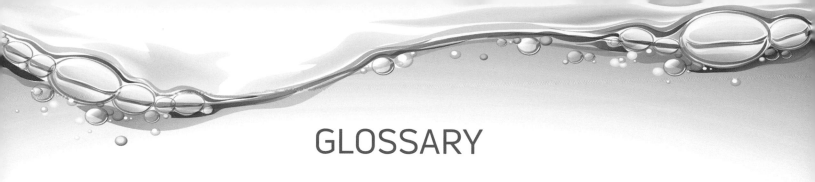

GLOSSARY

Activated charcoal
A substance made from heating or burning wood or other organic matter in the absence of air. Charcoal is used for its absorbent ability: it can absorb many times its weight in liquids or gases.

Acute
Sudden onset and not prolonged.

Adhesive capsulitis
Extreme stiffness caused by adhesions between a bone and its joint capsule, often painful.

Adrenalin
A hormone produced by the adrenal glands that increases the heart rate and has many other effects as well.

Arthritis
Inflammation of joints, usually accompanied by joint pain. The two most common types are rheumatoid arthritis, an immune system disorder, and osteoarthritis, which is more directly related to overuse of joints.

Ascites
An abnormal accumulation of fluid in the abdomen, caused when scarring of the liver damages its blood vessels and fluid is forced into the abdominal cavity.

Banya
Russian sauna, similar to a Scandinavian sauna: a heated room with water poured on the stove to make steam.

Baroreceptors
Sensory nerve endings, found in the walls of the heart, vena cava, aortic arch, and carotid sinuses. These nerve endings are very sensitive to stretching of the wall from increased pressure from inside the walls, so they can monitor blood pressure. They report this information back to the central nervous system

Bladder stones
Stones in the bladder made of crystallized uric acid, caused by problems such as urinary tract infections or prostatic hypertrophy or chronic dehydration.

Bronchospasm
The muscles that line the airways of the lungs constrict or tighten, reducing airflow. Bronchospasms may be caused by respiratory conditions such as asthma or bronchitis.

Buerger's disease (thromboangitis obliterans)
Inflammation of the entire wall and connective tissue surrounding medium-sized arteries and veins, especially of the legs of young and middle-aged men: associated with thrombotic occlusion and commonly resulting in gangrene.

Buoyancy
The upthrust which is equal to the weight of the fluid displaced when a body is partially or wholly immersed in water.

Bursa
Closed sac filled with synovial fluid, found over exposed or prominent body parts or where a tendon passes over a bone.

Carpal tunnel syndrome
Chronic entrapment of the median nerve at the wrist, accompanied by tingling, pain and numbness in the distribution of the nerve in the hand.

Cholesterol
A fat-like substance made by the body, with many important functions.

Chronic
Lasting longer than three months, and showing virtually no change.

Cirrhosis
Scarring of the liver, most often caused by alcohol consumption or viral hepatitis.

Claudication
From the Latin word *claudicare*, to limp. An ischemia of the calf muscles, causing lameness and pain when the patient tries to walk, because the blood supply to the calf muscles is insufficient to meet the increased blood demand during exercise. The pain caused by this ischemia stops as soon as the person rests, but then returns when he or she starts walking again, leading to the term to the term **Intermittent claudication**.

Cold mitten friction
A whole-body friction performed with a terrycloth mitt or washcloth which has been dipped in cold water.

Cold wet sheet wrap
A body wrap in which the client is wrapped in a cold wet sheet and two blankets: initially cold, the client gradually becomes warm and then hot.

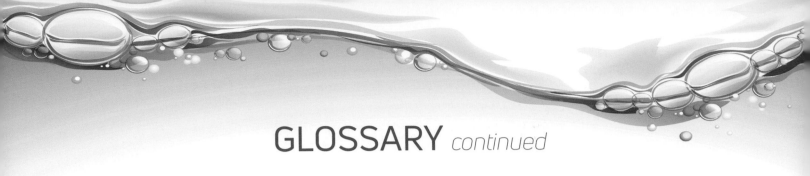

GLOSSARY *continued*

Complex regional pain syndrome
A chronic pain disorder which can develop after a traumatic injury or a period of immobilization. Patients often have edema, skin sensitivity, limited range of motion, and difficulty bearing weight on the injured limb.

Compress
A folded cloth dipped in water, with or without additives such as essential oils or mineral salts, which is applied to the body.

Concussion
An injury to a soft structure caused by a blow or violent shaking.

Conduction
The transfer of heat by direct contact between one heated or cooled substance and another.

Constipation
Reduced or difficult bowel movements.

Continuous bath
A bath in which the patient is placed on a hammock which is suspended in a bathtub. The tub with the patient in it is then covered with a canvas sheet which has a hole for his or her head; then warm or neutral water is run continuously, often for extended periods of time.

Contracture
Myofascial shortening due to tonic spasm or paralysis of antagonist muscles, leading to fibrosis and loss of motion in related joints. Contractures in early stages may be reversed with bodywork and stretching.

Contralateral reflex effect
Heat applied to one limb causes vasodilation in the other limb as well.

Contrast treatment
Alternating hot and cold, using either hot and cold baths, or hot and cold applications to the skin, such as hot packs followed by ice packs.

Convection
The giving off of heat by moving currents of liquid or gas.

Costochondritis
Inflammation of cartilage, usually at ribs 4–6, with tenderness and swelling. It can be caused by activities that stress the ribcage, such as plunging a toilet, performing planks in Pilates, or lifting heavy loads.

Counter-irritant
A substance that stimulates nerve endings on the skin and distracts the central nervous system from deeper-seated pain.

Cryokinetics
Combining cold applications with light therapeutic exercise. The idea behind cryokinetics is that muscles can atrophy after injuries such as joint sprains, because pain prevents the client from using the injured part. A typical method is to apply ice or immerse the part in very cold water – 34°F (1°C) – in order to numb it. Then the client performs light exercises—such as range of motion which would otherwise be too painful – for 2–3 minutes or until the part becomes painful again. The cold–exercise combination is repeated a few times.

Depletion
Decrease in blood flow to one area, caused by a reduction in the size of local blood vessels.

Derivation
From the Latin words *derivo* (to draw off) and *rivus* (stream), derivation is the decreased flow of blood and lymph to one particular part of the body created by increasing the flow of blood and lymph to another part. When less blood is flowing into an area, local blood pressure is lowered and then fluid (congestion) can be drawn into the blood vessels again, thus pulling it out of the congested area.

Detoxification
Removal of toxic materials from the body.

Diabetes
A disease characterized by glucose intolerance, excess discharge of urine containing glucose, and disturbances in the metabolism of fat, protein, and carbohydrates.

Dialysis
An artificial method of purifying the blood, which is used to substitute for normal kidney function.

Douche
A spray of water directed against some portion of the body. Douches may be of different temperatures, different

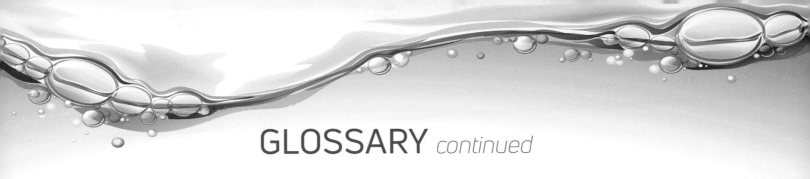

GLOSSARY *continued*

directions (horizontal or vertical), and applied locally or to the whole body.

Dry brushing
A friction technique using a dry brush applied to the skin surface.

Dry sheet wrap
A body wrap consisting of two blankets and one sheet, with external warming devices placed on top of the client's wrapped body.

Embolism
The plugging of a blood vessel by an embolus that has broken loose and traveled through the bloodstream. The embolus then cuts off the flow of blood to the part of the body supplied by the blood vessel.

Embolus
A blood clot formed inside a vein.

Emetic
An agent that causes vomiting.

Encephalitis
Inflammation of the brain.

Endorphin
A brain chemical which interacts with the opiate receptors in the brain to reduce our perception of pain and which can act similarly to drugs such as morphine – that is, it relieves pain and gives a sense of well-being. Endorphins can be released during activities such as hard exercise, laughter, and some hydrotherapy treatments.

Endothelium
The inner lining of blood vessels.

Evaporation
The process of changing water, a liquid, into water vapor, a gas.

Fibrin
A protein made up of long, sticky fibers.

Fibromyalgia
A musculoskeletal pain and fatigue disorder, with these symptoms: chronic pain in muscles and the soft tissue surrounding joints, tenderness to pressure at specific sites in the body, stiffness after rest, low pain tolerance, sensitivity to cold, non-restful sleep and chronic fatigue.

Fomentation
Any warm moist application which delivers heat to the body for healing. In this book, we refer to fomentations as the large pads, made for moist heat applications, which comprise many layers of thick laundry flannel or toweling.

Fracture
A break in a bone.

Frostbite
A cold injury caused by the freezing of body tissues, and occurs most often in the hands and feet. When a person's body temperature is decreasing due to cold exposure, constriction of the blood vessels of the arms and legs keeps warm blood in the body core, and if necessary sacrifices the extremities to maintain the internal organs and brain.

Glabral tear
The glabrum is a cup-shaped rim of cartilage that lines and reinforces the socket (glenoid fossa) of the ball and socket shoulder joint. A tear in this firm white structure can be caused by direct injury to the shoulder, or from overuse. Eventually the soft glabral tissue gets caught between the glenoid and the humerus, the shoulder tissue cannot hold the joint together as well, and the joint becomes less stable.

Gout
A disease of the joints, primarily of the toes, ankles, and knees, triggered when sodium urate crystals collect in the fluid around the joints. This causes inflammation, irritability, and attacks of excruciating pain. Gout is primarily an inherited disorder, but lead exposure can induce it in susceptible people.

Heatstroke
A condition produced by exposure to excessively high temperatures, especially when the person is exercising vigorously: symptoms include a rise in body temperature, hot dry skin, headache, confusion and vertigo. In extreme cases, when the person's body temperature rises very high, there can be vascular collapse, coma, and death.

Hematoma
A localized mass of blood which has leaked out of broken blood vessels, usually clotted or partially clotted.

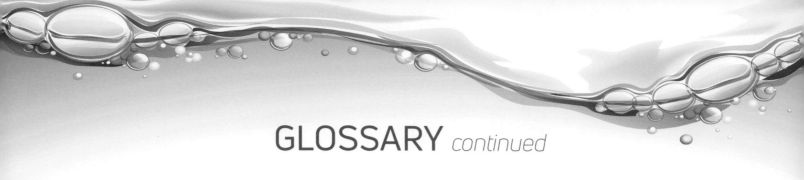

GLOSSARY *continued*

Homeostasis
The ability or tendency of a living organism to keep the conditions inside it the same, despite outside conditions: a state of internal balance. Warm-blooded animals achieve temperature homeostasis by adjustments of the nervous and circulatory systems.

Hydropathy
The treatment of all disease by the internal and external application of water. Formerly known as the "water-cure."

Hydrostatic (synonym: derivative)
Hydrostatic effects cause blood to either migrate towards one area of the body from another area, or to shift away from one area of the body to another.

Hydrostatic pressure
The force which water exerts on a submerged body: the deeper you go, the higher the pressure.

Hydrotherapy
The therapeutic application of water for the treatment of musculoskeletal disorders and promotion of general wellness.

Hypermobility
Some or all of a person's joints have an unusually large range of movement, sometimes leading to sprains, dislocations, muscle aches, and arthritis, and often to chronic pain. Considered a genetic connective tissue condition, ligaments and tendons are longer (lax) and do not hold joints together well. Prolotherapy may be helpful.

Hypothalamus
A small part of the brain, located in the lower front brain, that is considered the central controller of the autonomic nervous system. It monitors many visceral functions, such as skin temperature, blood temperature, and the amount of water in the blood.

Ice massage
A method of cooling tissues by applying an ice cube or ice cup over an area with a rotating motion.

Ice stroking
Stroking the length of a muscle with ice in order to temporarily release muscle tension and suppress pain.

Iced compress
A wet towel which has been placed in a resealable plastic bag and then frozen; when removed from the freezer and placed on the client's body, it remains cold for as long as 20 minutes.

Intermittent claudication
See **Claudication**.

Kidney stone
Small stones caused when certain natural chemicals, such as uric acid, crystallize in the kidney. Kidney stones may have a variety of causes.

Lateral epicondylitis
Inflammation of the wrist flexor tendons at their insertion on the lateral epicondyle of the humerus.

Lower leg compartment syndrome
Increased pressure within a muscle compartment resulting from bleeding or edema, the pressure being high enough to damage the nerves in the area. Mainly caused by leg injuries.

Lymph
Lymph, or lymphatic fluid, takes its name from the Latin word *lympha*, which means clear spring water. Lymphatic fluid is a largely clear liquid which carries white blood cells (leukocytes); a few red blood cells (erythrocytes) may give it a slight yellow tinge. Lymph is carried in the vein-like vessels of the lymphatic system.

Lymphedema
The accumulation of lymph in subcutaneous tissue which results when certain lymphatic vessels or nodes are obstructed. People with this condition suffer chronic swelling in at least one arm or leg. The most common cause of lymphedema is mastectomy surgery for breast cancer, when the surgeon removes numerous surrounding lymph nodes. Less commonly, lymphedema can be caused by trauma, radiation therapy, mechanical constraint (such as a tightly fitting cast), and some types of tumors.

Macrophage
A type of white blood cell.

Mechanical treatments
Friction treatments such as salt glows and percussion treatments such as sprays or jets of water.

Medial epicondylitis
Inflammation of the wrist flexor tendons at their insertion on the medial epicondyle of the humerus.

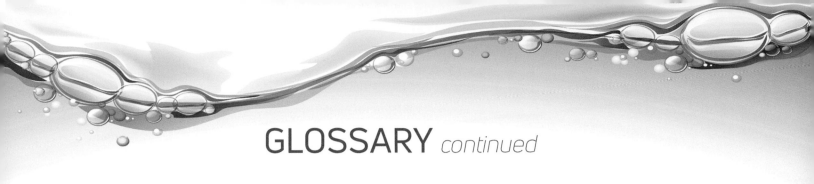

GLOSSARY *continued*

Migraine headache
A severely painful headache, usually limited to one side of the head and often accompanied by vertigo, nausea, and hypersensitivity to light, a perception of flashing lights, or other visual disorders. Migraine headaches begin with an extreme vasoconstriction of the blood vessels of the brain on the affected side of the head.

Moist blanket wrap
A body wrap in which the client is wrapped in a cotton blanket which is wrung out in 110°F (43°C) water and two additional blankets; external warming devices are then applied on the outside of the wrap.

Multiple sclerosis (MS)
A progressive autoimmune disease which causes the body to attack the myelin in the brain and spinal cord, resulting in a variety of symptoms including fatigue, muscle weakness, spasticity, bladder abnormalities, visual loss, and mood alterations. Some people with MS may have all these symptoms, and others just a few of them.

Muscle cramp
Strong, painful, short-lived involuntary contraction of skeletal muscle.

Muscle spasm
Low-grade, long-lasting involuntary contraction of skeletal muscle.

Neurocognitive disease
A disease that involves a reduction in thinking skills such as learning, memory and attention, including Alzheimer's disease and vascular dementia (brain damage caused by repeated small strokes).

Neurofibromatosis
A genetic disorder that causes non-cancerous tumors to form on nerve tissue.

Neuropathy
Damage, disease, or dysfunction of one or more nerves, with numbness, tingling, pain, or other uncomfortable sensations.

Noradrenaline
A neurotransmitter which has stimulating effects on many parts of the body. It plays a big part in the body's fight-or-flight response.

NSAIDS
Non-steroidal anti-inflammatory drugs. They are the world's most widely used kinds of pain medication.

Occipital migraine
A migraine "headache" that may have visual symptoms such as flashing lights or zigzag patterns and no pain. It is not completely understood but many scientists believe it can be linked to inflammation of peripheral nerves caused by chronic compression from surrounding structures (such as muscles or blood vessels) Raposio E et al. Occipital Migraine: A Vascular Approach 2017; 5 (9 Suppl): 78.

Palsy
A term that refers to various types of paralysis or muscle weakness.

PCB (polychlorinated biphenyl)
Industrial compound(s) produced by chlorination of biphenyls, which when accumulated in animal tissue can have pathenogenic effects, as well as causing abnormal prenatal development.

Percussion douche
A very strong spray of water, generally applied to either the entire front or the entire back of the body.

Peripheral neuropathy
A condition of damage to peripheral nerves, caused by poor circulation, chemical imbalances, or trauma. Symptoms may include burning, itching, numbness, and excessive sweating of the hands and feet. Burning or tingling pain will eventually be replaced by numbness. Most cases of peripheral neuropathy are caused by diabetes, when high blood sugar levels damage the capillary circulation in the hands and feet.

Phlebitis
Inflammation of a vein.

Plantar fasciitis
An inflammation of the plantar fascia which causes pain on the underside of the foot, most often in the heels or arches.

Plaster
A paste-like mixture made of ground herbs mixed with water, spread upon a cloth and applied to the body.

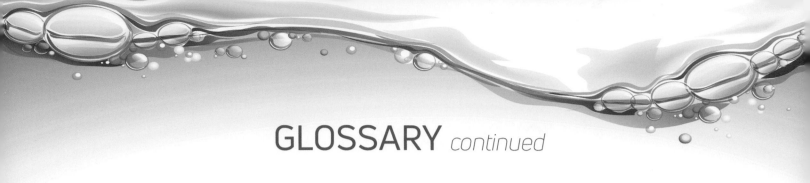

GLOSSARY *continued*

Polio (short term for poliomyelitis)
An acute infectious viral disease affecting the central nervous system, which can cause paralysis and muscle wasting. Compensatory movement patterns – having to overuse some parts of the body to compensate for paralyzed or weak muscles – can cause severe musculoskeletal pain, discomfort and deformity.

Pre-eclampsia
In a pregnant woman, hypertension occurring along with protein in the urine, or edema, or both. This condition usually develops after the 20th week of pregnancy, and occurs in only 4% of pregnant women. Blood pressure often rises dangerously high. Pre-eclampsia is associated with retarded fetal growth and dramatically increases the risk of death for both the pregnant woman and her baby.

Prolotherapy
The injection of natural substances at the exact site of a ligament injury. It stimulates the person's immune system to repair damaged ligaments, and can significantly increase ligament mass, thickness, and strength.

Psoriatic arthritis
A painful form of *arthritis* that affects some people who have *psoriasis*, an inherited condition that features red patches of skin topped with silvery scales. Most sufferers develop *psoriasis* first and are later diagnosed with *psoriatic arthritis*.

Psychosomatic
Describing the interplay between mind and body, often used when physical symptoms are caused or aggravated by a mental factor or emotional disturbance. Same as Somato-emotional.

Pyrogens
Substances that can produce a fever, typically produced by bacteria such as *E. coli*, but sometimes made by the body. They inhibit heat-sensing neurons in the hypothalamus and stimulate cold-sensing neurons, and thus stimulate heat production.

Radiation
The giving off of heat, such as when a part of the body which is not insulated is exposed to very cold air.

Raynaud's syndrome
A condition involving spasm of the arterioles in the extremities. Episodes of vasospasm can be triggered by exposure to cold or emotional stress. Tissues, especially in the hands and feet, can be damaged by lack of oxygen.

Reflex
An involuntary reaction to a stimulus, generally a body action or movement that happens rapidly and automatically in response to possible danger.

Repetitive strain injury (RSI)
A gradual build-up of damage to muscles, tendons and nerves, resulting in conditions such as chronic tendonitis or carpal tunnel syndrome. RSIs are caused by repetitive tasks or by exerting great force with small muscles.

Restless leg syndrome
A feeling of uneasiness, twitching, or restlessness after getting into bed, which can be mild to extreme and often leads to insomnia.

Revulsive
From the Latin *revulsio*, to pluck or pull away. The drawing away of blood and lymph from one particular part of the body by increasing the flow of blood and lymph to another part.

Rheumatism
A poorly defined term which has been applied in the past to various chronic conditions of pain in the soft tissues, and/or swelling of the joints.

Rheumatoid arthritis
An autoimmune disease which primarily affects connective tissue, and causes inflammation or the synovial membranes, leading to pain and stiffness in many joints, especially those of the hands and feet.

Rosacea
A chronic, inflammatory skin condition that most often affects the face. It causes redness and visible blood vessels in the face. It is often mistaken for acne, eczema, or a skin allergy. The person's skin may be very sensitive.

Russian steam bath
A steam bath given in a tiled room with a circular hole in one wall so that the client can lie on a bench inside the room while his or her head protrudes out of the hole. Sometimes applied to any head-out steam bath.

Salt glow
A friction treatment performed on the bare skin by rubbing it with moistened salt.

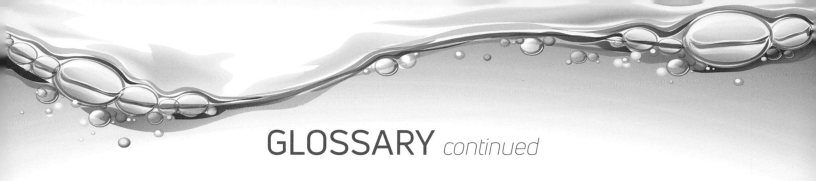

GLOSSARY *continued*

Sauna
A heated room used for sweating. Dry saunas can be changed into wet saunas by pouring water on the woodstove or electric heater or sometimes on rocks that are atop the stove.

Scar tissue
Tissue made of collagen fibers that replaces tissue that is damaged or killed by an injury or a disease.

Scotch hose or spray douche
A small pressurized hose designed to blast areas of pain and tension with a strong stream or water. The spray is under high pressure and is applied to the client from a distance of 6 feet or more.

Scrofulous
Relating to tuberculosis bacteria.

Shin splints
A catch-all term for a variety of lower leg problems that are characterized by aching pain along the medial border of the tibia.

Shower
A stream or streams of water from a showerhead, directed upon one or more parts of the body.

Silica gel hot pack
A pack made from canvas material, filled with a silica gel, and heated in hot water in special metal tanks that have electrical heating elements inside.

Sinus headache
A headache caused by sinus inflammation or congestion.

Skin pressure vegetative reflex
Activated by deep pressure on both sides of the body, this reflex normally results in a slower pulse, slower metabolism, decreased muscle tone, and fewer signs of an overly active sympathetic nervous system such as startling in response to loud noises.

Solvents
Industrial chemicals frequently used as paints, degreasers, varnishes, adhesives and for many other uses. They can be carcinogenic and neurotoxic.

Somato-emotional
Describing the interplay between mind and body, often used when physical symptoms are caused or aggravated by a mental factor or emotional disturbance. Same as Psychosomatic.

Spinal cord injury
Damage to some or all of the fibers which make up the spinal cord, if it is torn, bruised, or severed by mechanical force.

Steam cabinet
A small outer case or box with a door. It contains a seat for the client, a hole for his or her head to protrude, and a port through which steam can enter.

Steam canopy
A body-length canopy made of sturdy water-resistant fabric placed over a supine client. The canopy is filled with steam made in a crockpot at the foot of the massage table.

Stroke or cerebrovascular accident
The sudden death of brain cells that occurs when a blood vessel that carries oxygen and nutrients to the brain is either blocked by a clot or bursts. When that happens, part of the brain cannot get the blood (and oxygen) it needs and brain cells die.

Sweat lodge
Native American version of a steam bath. A low dome-shaped structure, constructed of willow branches covered by animal skins, and heated by bringing hot rocks inside it, then pouring water over them to create steam. In Central and South America, they are called temescals, and are constructed from mud or volcanic rock.

Swiss shower
A shower with many showerheads at different levels which sprays the whole body from head to toe.
The shower uses multiple showerheads (anywhere from 9 to 12) with varying pressures. There can be pipes in all four corners of the shower, with 8–16 water heads coming off each pipe.

Toxin
A chemical substance that can cause illness or poor health. Toxins from the external environment may be inhaled, swallowed, or absorbed through the skin.

Vascular dementia
Dementia caused by a lack of blood flow to the brain, often from strokes or other interruption of the blood supply to the brain.

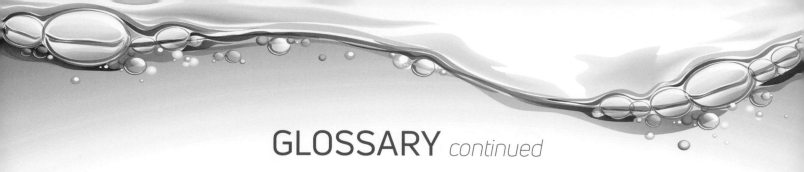

GLOSSARY *continued*

Vasoconstriction
Narrowing of a blood vessel caused by muscle contraction.

Vasodilation
Widening of a blood vessel caused by muscle contraction.

Venules
Minute veins which connect capillaries to larger systemic veins.

Vichy shower
A horizontal shower given with the person lying on a table. Water showers down from a swinging arm which contains about 7 jets and is positioned at a height of about 4 feet.

Watsu
A water massage therapy, invented by massage therapist Harold Dull, which is based upon traditional Shiatsu techniques but is performed in a swimming pool of warm water.

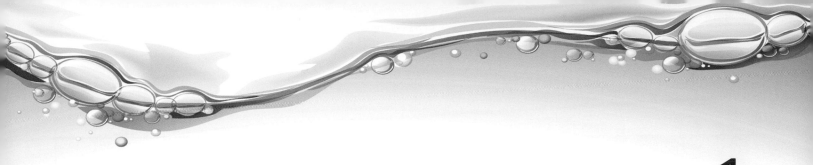

Introduction to hydrotherapy 1

"I firmly believe that there is more to a thermal spring than heat, and that warm waters are conducive to more than plant growth … It may well be that water extracts a subtle energy from deep within the earth and transmits it to truthseekers. Or perhaps the relaxation of the body while immersed in soothing warm water creates a new and enlightened ecology of the mind, allowing quantum leaps in understanding.

Bill Kaysing, *Great Hot Springs of the West*

CHAPTER OBJECTIVES

After completing this chapter, the student will be able to:

1. Explain several ways in which hydrotherapy can enhance and support the practice of massage
2. Explain the historical development of hydrotherapy in Europe and the United States
3. Describe the appeal of whole-body hydrotherapy such as baths, saunas and swimming
4. Give specific examples of both local and whole-body hydrotherapy treatments that have been used in the past
5. Explain how hydrotherapy treatments have changed in different times and cultures
6. Give examples of appropriate hydrotherapy treatments for somato-emotional issues
7. Describe how hydrotherapy can be used by massage therapists to treat different clients.

Skilled touch and water treatments are among the most ancient and revered of all healing modalities. From the great Roman baths, Russian saunas, and Indian herbal steams, to Turkish baths, sweat lodges of the Americas, and Japanese hot springs, hot waters are beloved because they both quiet the nervous system (Figure 1.1A) and soothe musculoskeletal pain (Figure 1.1B).

Injury, pain and nervous tension have long inspired healers to use compassionate touch and a wide variety of treatments that use water. This chapter introduces you to the history of hydrotherapy, which clearly demonstrates the benefits of incorporating it into your massage practice. In later chapters you will learn exactly how to perform treatments. We focus on the history and traditions of western hydrotherapy, but many other cultures also have well-developed hydrotherapy practices.

BENEFITS OF USING HYDROTHERAPY IN YOUR MASSAGE PRACTICE

As a massage therapy student or practitioner, you may be wondering how adding hydrotherapy to your massage practice could benefit your clients. Here are some important benefits:

- Hydrotherapy is relaxing and stress-reducing.

- Hydrotherapy can relieve discomfort and pain, stimulate the flow of blood and lymph, make connective tissue easier to stretch, and help soothe many aches, pains, injuries, and muscle problems.

- If your clients are uncomfortably hot or cold, you can use hydrotherapy treatments to make them more comfortable during a session.

- Hydrotherapy is an excellent adjunct to any kind of bodywork done for rehabilitation. Cold treatments such as local baths, ice packs, and ice massage can stimulate circulation and reduce spasm and pain,

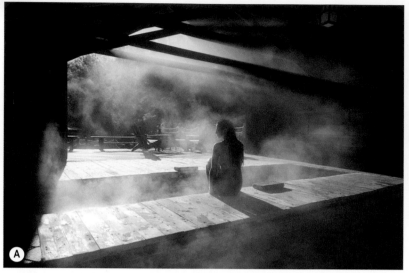
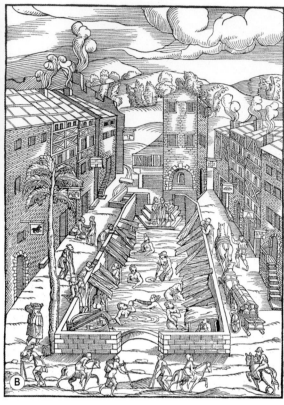

FIGURE 1.1
(**A**) Woman in hot springs, deeply relaxed after a hot soak. Photo by Trinette Reed, courtesy of Stocksy images. (**B**) Old Roman bath at Plombieres, France, 1565. Throughout history, hot water is like a magnet for those with injuries, arthritis, or other painful conditions. Courtesy of Alamy Limited.

while heat treatments soften scar tissue and make muscle tissues easier to stretch.

- Hydrotherapy treatments can provide different types of skin stimulation. Examples include the "body-hugging" sensation of being surrounded by water, the thermal sensations ranging from hot to cold, and the scratchy sensation of a salt glow, dry brush, or cold mitten friction.

- Hot applications can reduce stress on your hard-working hands by replacing the initial massage strokes needed to warm tissues, relax superficial muscles, and increase local blood flow.

- By combining the most appropriate massage techniques and most suitable water treatments, you can fine-tune your sessions to individual clients.

- Many treatments can be performed by clients at home to help them make faster progress in between sessions.

BRIEF HISTORY OF WESTERN HYDROTHERAPY

Among ancient civilizations, water was sanctified as the source of life, the seminal fluid, the juice of the earth's womb …

people everywhere feared, revered, or worshipped water deities, who differed in some ways but shared the fundamental creative and destructive substance of water.
Alexis Croutier, *Taking the Waters: Spirit, Art, Sensuality*

Medicine is an ever-changing combination of practices, featuring medical fads, bold experiments, changing belief systems, and ultimately, a few successful remedies that have been painstakingly worked out. Because water is plentiful, easy to obtain, and generally safe, some kind of water treatment is usually among the first remedies to be tried whenever a new health problem emerges.

Hydrotherapy in Ancient Greece and other early cultures

Thermal and mineral waters have been popular for thousands of years: the combination of warming and cleansing properties, combined with the opportunity to float free of gravity, has been almost irresistible. The waters of Baden-Baden, Germany, have been used for over 8000 years, and the waters in Bath, England, for 10,000 years (see Figure 1.2). Hot air baths have had wide appeal as

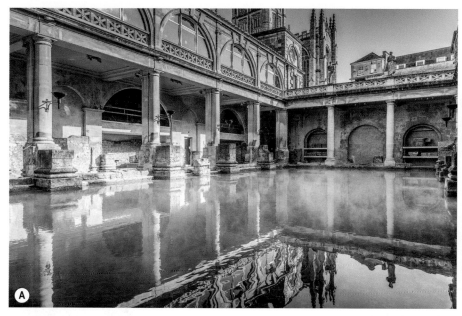

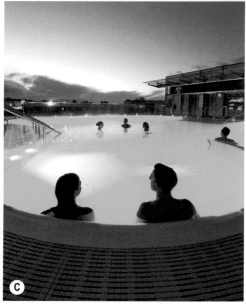

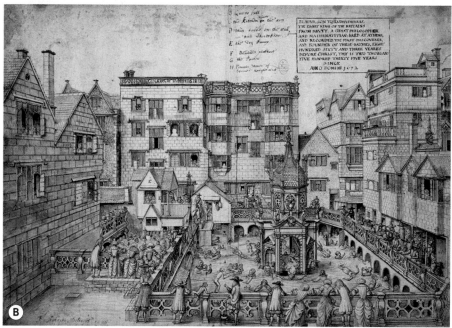

FIGURE 1.2
Bath through the centuries. The springs at Bath, England, originally flowed into a shrine sacred to the Celtic goddess Sulis. Later they supplied a Roman bathing complex, dedicated to the Roman goddess Minerva; later still, a medieval Catholic Church facility; and after that a city hospital. Today a privately operated spa makes use of water from the same springs. (**A**) The Great Bath, 60 AD. Permission: Bath in Time. (**B**) The King's Bath, Thomas Johnson, 1672. Sufferers spent 1–2 hours in the water daily: bath employees helped move paralyzed limbs and stretch contractures in the water. Permission: British Museum. (**C**) Rooftop pool at Thermae Bath Spa, 2019. Photograph courtesy of Thermae Bath Spa.

well: as early as the 8th century BC, Irish sweat houses made of sod and stone were used for **rheumatism**, while in the Americas, sweat lodges (see Box 1.1) were an important religious and physical ritual (Bruchac, 1993). Partial-body hydrotherapy treatments are also found in the most ancient of medical traditions: water has been used for its warming or cooling effect and as a carrier for herbs and minerals in baths, compresses, plasters, and other preparations. In medieval Spain, for example, a patient with gout might be treated with an herbal foot soak, a hot poultice to draw inflammation, and finally a cold foot soak with mineral salts to relieve pain (Roe, 2003).

Spiritual and religious function of water

Many primitive peoples worshipped water deities. Religious leaders were often physical healers as well, and performed water rituals such as baptisms, foot washing,

NATIVE AMERICAN HYDROTHERAPY

Hydrotherapy was part of the culture of indigenous peoples of the Americas long before the arrival of European colonists. Natural thermal springs were used for recuperation by warriors and for various ailments, and many Native American tribes used sweat lodges to perform religious ceremonies, to stay clean and warm, and to treat illnesses such as rheumatism, colds and fevers. Steamy air was created by heating rocks outside the lodge, then carrying them inside and pouring water over them. Herbs for decongesting the lungs or easing sore muscles were often added to the water. The sweat lodge ended with a plunge in a cold stream (Bruchac, 1993; Walker, 1966). European settlers adopted a variety of Native American medical practices such as steam treatments and herbal remedies. For example, the Lewis and Clark expedition of 1806 used a modified sweat lodge to treat a sick soldier they could not cure with their medicines (Vogel, 1970).

baths before sacred events, and washing the dead to prepare them for the afterlife. In the Bible, baths were used for skin diseases, gonorrhea, leprosy and other problems. The temple of Dendera in Egypt housed an extensive hydrotherapy center with stone tanks, where the sick bathed in the hope of being cured with the help of the goddess Hathor (Halioua, 2005). In the Greco-Roman tradition, pilgrimages to springs were often made in order to ask for help from a deity associated with healing, such as the Greek god of medicine Aesculapius, or the Roman goddess Minerva. Some deities oversaw specific ailments or parts of the body: for example, at one Roman temple, foot and hand disorders were the special concern of the goddess Nona, and visitors to her spring hoped to find relief from problems such as fallen arches, torn ligaments, ulcerations, arthritis and clubfoot (Phillips, 1973).

Doctrine of humors

In addition to the religious aspects of health, the Greeks also explained sickness and health using the "doctrine of humors," a theory that had come to them from Egyptian medicine. Health and disease were absolutely predictable depending upon the balance of four crucial vitality-sustaining bodily fluids: yellow bile (digestive juice), phlegm (colorless secretions), black bile (made by the kidneys and spleen) and blood accounted for all of the body's various and otherwise bewildering phenomena. The body was made hot and wet by blood, hot and dry by yellow bile, cold and wet by phlegm, and cold and dry by black bile. All was well when the vital fluids coexisted in a proper balance, but imbalance caused illness and only treatments that put the humors back in balance could heal (Porter, 1997).

The famous Greek physician and medical writer Hippocrates (460–377 BC), used hot and cold baths to balance humors: "baths in fresh water moisten and cool; salt baths warm and dry; hot baths taken on an empty stomach reduce and cool; cold baths dry the body." Thermal baths were used to cure headaches, relax joints, and relieve chest and back pains during bouts of pneumonia. Neutral baths were prescribed to combat insomnia, and cold plunges to stimulate circulation. Local treatments were used as well: for example, cold sitz baths were used for uterine hemorrhage; cold douches relieved swollen and painful joints; animal bladders filled with hot oil reduced menstrual and labor pain. Hippocrates also recommended massage to tone and normalize the body (Temkin, 1956). We now understand that many other humoral treatments did not benefit patients: for example, inducing vomiting and diarrhea, blistering the skin, and bleeding were common methods of eliminating "excess humors." Perhaps some of the heroic treatments had a helpful placebo effect: after all, a doctor with a good bedside manner and a dose of something specific, even if it was nasty, reassured the patient that something was being done and he or she was not being ignored. Humoral theory, despite its rather dismal record of success, would organize Western medical thinking for at least the next thousand years.

Specific treatments to balance the humors aside, the ancient Greeks believed that the ideal health regimen was strenuous gymnasium workouts followed by baths, saunas, and massage. Warriors bathed to reduce fatigue and promote wound healing, and warm baths relieved "dejection and low spirits" (Porter, 1997). Today we know body heating treatments can have a strong antidepressant effect (Koltyn, 1992; Beever, 2010; Janssen, 2016).

Humoral pathology or mind–body dynamics?

The Greek medical belief system was all about humors, so even joint pain might be thought of as a "falling of a humor into a joint." However, even as Hippocrates and other Greek doctors worked with that belief system, they also understood that emotions could speak through the body and affect health: one writer described an Athenian warrior who was so frightened during a battle that he became blind and never regained his vision (Roberts, 2013). Every culture has had to find a way to cope with somato-emotional issues using their belief system (see Box 1.2).

Hydrotherapy in the Roman Empire (510 BC–478 AD)

At its height, the Roman Empire was the political master of almost the entire western world. After conquering Greece, Rome adopted much of its culture, learning, and medical knowledge. For example, Galen of Pergamon (b. 130AD) was a surgeon, medical writer, and physician to several Roman emperors, and a staunch believer in humoral theory: his theories would dominate Western medical practice for more than 1300 years. As the Romans' technology and wealth increased over the centuries, their bathing practices continually became more elaborate and consumed more resources. The largest baths ever built in Rome, the Baths of Diocletian, covered 32 acres and could accommodate as many as three thousand bathers at a time. Public baths featured hot and cold pools, saunas and exercise areas. Being a typical Roman meant taking public, two-hour soaks in pools of various temperatures, having the body scraped off with a curved metal blade, and then receiving a massage.

Water treatments were also used for many medical problems: for example, cold water was used therapeutically for hemorrhages, fevers, skin complaints, gout, wounds, paralysis, and convalescence after surgery. Bathing in therapeutic waters was recommended for difficult menstruation and other uterine disorders, and for the painful wounds, tired muscles and general exhaustion of injured Roman soldiers. Seawater was thought to have a tonic effect on nervous and arthritic people (Porter, 1990; Temkin, 1956).

As the Roman Empire spread through Europe, the Romans' bathing culture went with it. Naturally occurring springs were taken over and developed wherever they were found, and local water deities were re-figured into Roman ones. Sulphur springs were recommended for their ability to heat and burn poisonous humors from the body; alum springs were helpful for paralysis; drinking water from acid springs could dissolve **bladder stones**; and alkaline springs could treat **scrofulous** tumors (bacterially-infected masses in the neck which started with inflamed lymph nodes; Phillips, 1973). Sciatica, psoriasis, rheumatic fever, gout, jaundice and edema all had their mineral bath prescriptions. The hot sulphur springs of Baiae in Northern Italy, which featured hot and cold baths, saunas, exercise rooms, massage and more, drew convalescents from across the empire. Rome's highly developed bathing practices finally ended for good in 537AD, when Gothic invaders cut off aqueducts and destroyed many baths. Those baths that were not destroyed outright gradually fell into ruins.

Hydrotherapy in the Middle Ages

Europe's water technology now deteriorated to a very primitive level. Gone were the days when hot water could be easily obtained to ease injured or arthritic joints: water was heavy, required precious fuel, and had to be hauled inside and then out again. Although many old Roman baths were now in disrepair, warm water was still irresistible and local people used them anyway (Porter, 1990). Medieval medicine was now based almost entirely upon the writings of the Greek physician Galen, who the reader may remember was a staunch believer in the doctrine of humors. Although he had frequently prescribed baths featuring different temperatures and additives, this was no longer practical.

The Catholic church was scandalized at the idea of public baths where both sexes might bathe together, but bathing still had its symbolic role in religious rituals, and natural springs attracted visitors regardless of church policy. Well-to-do people, of course, could bathe in the comfort of their own homes, with water carried indoors by servants and then heated. While general cleanliness and

Chapter one

SOMATO-EMOTIONAL ISSUES AND HYDROTHERAPY

We have all experienced the intimate correlation between our mental states and muscular tenseness: stress-induced vomiting is just as real as the vomiting due to pyloric obstruction, and so-called "tension headaches" may be as painful as if they were due to a brain tumor (Sarno, 1991). Stressful or traumatic childhoods may set the stage for long-lasting somato-emotional issues, including depression, anxiety disorders, increased muscle tension, muscle spasms, fatigue, poor sleep and painful medical conditions (Felitti, 1988; Harris, 2018; Sachs-Ericcson, 2017). Almost half of all adults with fibromyalgia suffered sexual abuse as children (Goldberg, 1999; Dube, 2003). This is relevant to massage therapists because many people who seek bodywork for pain relief are unconsciously presenting us with emotional pain that is manifesting physically. Add those who have had great stress or trauma during adulthood, and this is likely a sizeable percentage of our clients.

As a practicing doctor, Roy Porter voiced this same concern decades ago: "The open secret of general medical practice, its strength and weakness, is that many patients do not have a disease; they are sick, sad or solitary; they need solace" (Porter, 1997). Without a structural cause to their complaints, those clients do best when we can help them calm their nervous systems and relax under our touch.

In his book *From Paralysis to Fatigue,* medical historian Edward Shorter shares hundreds of case histories written by Western doctors from the 1600s through to the 21st century. Many had patients with **somato-emotional** issues which manifested as insomnia, muscle spasm, problems with digestion, vision and other body functions, and, above all, chronic pain.

Doctors were frequently aware that their patients had mood disorders, depression, high stress levels or a history of post-traumatic stress, but still found symptoms difficult to treat (Shorter, 1992 and 1997). One modern example is that of an American soldier who developed PTSD (post-traumatic stress disorder) during the Iraq War. This man visited a hospital emergency department 17 times, for chest pain that was found to be noncardiac, before receiving counseling, which ultimately helped eliminate his stress-caused pain for good (Jimenez, 2018).

This topic relates to hydrotherapy and bodywork because recent research has shown that heat applications can create deeply positive emotions. According to cognitive psychologist John Bargh, physical feelings of warmth are linked early in life to feelings of safety, and we subconsciously associate physical warmth with emotional warmth. "Especially with animals that breastfeed their infants, the experience of being fed and held and protected goes hand in glove with feelings of warmth and closeness ... the positive response to heat is hardwired into our brains" (Bargh, 2017). This helps to explain the deep enjoyment and relaxation our clients experience when we use any warm treatment before or during a session. A warm moist pack over the spine, warm compresses over the face, a heat lamp or heating pad over a painful knee, a paraffin bath for a scarred hand, and many more local heat treatments can help the client feel safe and relaxed, which will deepen the effectiveness of our bodywork (see Case history 12.3). Whole-body heating activates specific brain areas that are important for the regulation of mood and body temperature, and thus has antidepressant effects: this means that a steam bath, a sauna, or even a warm shower before a session will help the client calm and settle before the bodywork begins (Koltyn, 1992; Hanusch, 2013; Beever, 2010; Janssen, 2016).

personal hygiene remained poor, the late Middle Ages in Europe was a period of active and growing interest in the therapeutic use of waters. In some locations, new baths that had been rebuilt over the old Roman ones became centers of healing for those suffering from depression, musculoskeletal problems, infectious diseases such as leprosy and many other conditions. In Bath, England, a Catholic bishop repaired the old baths in 1200 AD, and diseased people from all over England came for healing. Bath was known as the "aching man's city" (Rolls, 2013).

Local hydrotherapy treatments with non-mineral water were used as well (Figure 1.3), and the circulatory effects of whole-body treatments were well understood (Figure 1.4).

Hydrotherapy during the Renaissance and the Industrial Revolution

As the Renaissance wore on in Europe, medicine was gradually transformed into a scientific practice based on rationalism. It would be well into the 1800s, however, before the humoral model was completely given up. For example, in 1685 King Charles II of England had a minor stroke. His physicians administered many humoral treatments, including removing over one quart (one liter) of blood through cutting and cupping; administering various substances designed to induce retching, vomiting, sneezing, diarrhea and scalp blisters; and finally cauterizing him with a red-hot iron. Despite his stroke's minor nature, he finally died from loss of blood and sheer misery. This misadventure forms a stark contrast to modern therapies for recovery from a stroke: see *Stroke recovery* on page 356 for an example of how hydrotherapy and massage can be important elements in a healing program. Some felt that the scientific method led to a mistaken focus on the individual parts of a system rather than on the organic whole, since it portrayed the body as

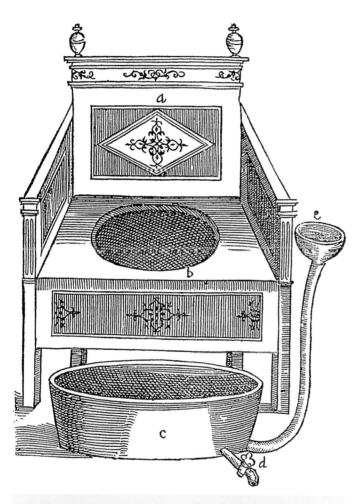

FIGURE 1.3
Steam Bath chair, 1564. This chair had an opening in the seat; the user's pelvic area was bathed in steam to alleviate the pain of bladder stones, a common condition of the time linked to chronic dehydration. Similar pelvic steams are used in many cultures for female problems and digestive issues, and often use herbal tea to create herbal steam. Image from History of Medicine, National Library of Medicine, Bethesda, Maryland. Sourced from ihm.nlm.nih.gov/images A030070.

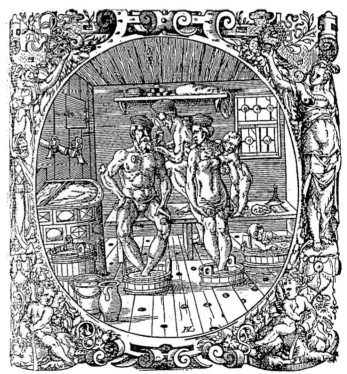

FIGURE 1.4
Sauna and footbath, 1565. While taking a sauna, patients also have a footbath and undergo cupping while supervised by a doctor. Engraving from the book *Opus Chyrugicum*. Image from History of Medicine, National Library of Medicine, Bethesda, Maryland. Sourced from ihm.nlm.nih.gov/images A029447.

nothing more than a machine (Porter, 1997). However, doctors were also aware that somato-emotional issues affected patients' health. For example, in 1662, while one doctor listed infectious diseases as the leading causes of deaths in London, he also reported cases where grief and fright had led to death (Gaunt, 1662). An English clergyman who worked with many depressed women noted that their melancholia typically began with the loss of a child, family troubles, a difficult childbirth, or financial worries (Shorter, 1992).

During this time period, the use of mineral springs became even more popular. European nobility often visited spas when they had health issues, including sufferers from psychiatric illness who patronized spas which had a reputation for curing "insane persons" (Porter, 1990). The healing springs of Bath, England, which provided the greatest supply of hot water in Europe, continued to be used year-round for a variety of complaints. In Figure 1.5, the child has a chronic skin disorder such as psoriasis; the man has wrist drop, a common sign of lead poisoning; and the woman's metacarpal-phalangeal joints are swollen, probably with a form of rheumatism or arthritis. All three conditions were known to benefit from regular bathing in Bath waters.

The explanation for the healing properties of baths and springs was now given in the language of science.

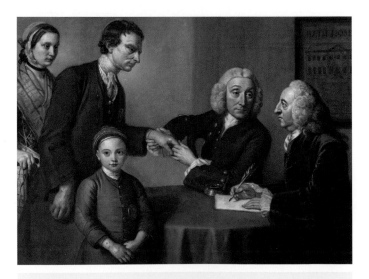

FIGURE 1.5
Bath Hospital doctors examining patients, 1762. Painting by William Hoare, courtesy of Bath in Time.

In 1697, one doctor said anyone who attributed cures at wells with "healing waters" to the blessing of Christian saints was deceiving common people. Curative effects were now attributed to the chemicals in the water or "chemical reactions" set in motion by heat. Many spas which had existed for hundreds of years renamed themselves "mineral water hospitals."

Hydrotherapy in the 19th century

As the century began, despite the continuing advances in medical knowledge and public health, Western medical practice was still not very effective. In fact, before the twentieth century, most of contemporary medicine would still consist of ancient remedies including bleeding, blistering and violent purges, plus administering opium and drugs containing lead and mercury. Surgery was still very risky. The average patient seeking help from the average doctor had less than a 50–50 chance of benefiting and actually ran a significant risk of getting worse! Doctors were often aware that some of their patients had primarily somato-emotional issues (Shorter, 1992 and 1997). When symptoms such as fatigue, digestive distress, fainting spells, headaches, backaches or other chronic pain had not responded to their standard treatments, doctors might well send patients for a spa-cure where the waters were supposedly helpful for their specific ailment. Often, patients with chronic somato-emotional complaints would jump at the chance to try something new.

Preissnitz, Kneipp, and the hydropathy movement

The environment was now ripe for a new "miracle" method of healing, and an Austrian peasant named Vincent Priessnitz (1801–1851) was in the right place at the right time. He was convinced that all illness was caused by "morbid humors" stemming from an unhealthy lifestyle, and developed a collection of water treatments called **hydropathy** (Figure 1.6). Exercise, diet, fresh air, vigorous massage, and above all water were used to expel bad humors and diseases. Virtually any illness or chronic disability could be addressed with this regimen of partial-body baths, showers, sweating treatments and cold baths. Probably Preissnitz's greatest contribution was convincing patients to adopt a healthier lifestyle in

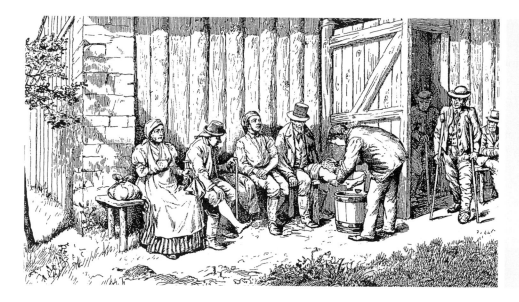

FIGURE 1.6
The beginnings of the water cure: Vincent Preissnitz treating patients with cold water sponging, 1816. From Philo vom Walde: Vincent Preissneitz: His Life and his Works, Published on his One Hundredth Birthday. Berlin: Vilhelm Moller, 1898. Illustration with kind permission of National College of Naturopathic Medicine, Portland, Oregon.

place of the popular remedies for pain (such as opiates) and mainstream concoctions which continued to contain heavy metals and other toxic ingredients. His fame quickly spread, and in 1840 Preissnitz treated 1600 patients from all over the world. He also mentored physicians from many countries, who then established their own "water-cures" back home, while an American health reform movement which began in the 1820s readily incorporated Preissnitz's methods along with herbal and homeopathic remedies (Legan, 1971).

Whether they were folk healers or trained doctors, hydropaths treated a wide variety of medical problems. Massage and exercise were an indispensable part of their programs, but they were most known for water treatments. Baths, steam inhalations, compresses, gargles, douches, sprays and fomentations were employed, while body "toughening" was achieved by cold showers, baths and walking barefoot in cold water, snow or dew. Patients were sponged, wrapped, "cooked" in saunas, scrubbed, hosed inside and out, sprayed, dunked, bathed and steamed – there seemed no end to the inventive ways that water could be applied to the body! These Spartan measures worked well on their overfed and stressed-out patients, who were accustomed to binging on harmful sedatives, tonics and narcotics, all washed down with brandy and various stimulants (Porter, 1990). With hydropathy the health fad of the moment, people on both sides of the Atlantic would satirize the movement (Figure 1.7). Twenty years after Priessnitz, Bavarian

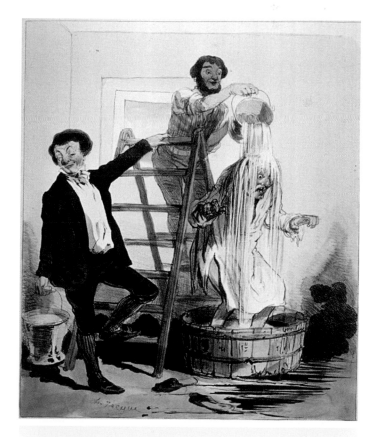

FIGURE 1.7
Hydrotherapy-Immersion, Submersion, and Contortion by C. Jaque, 1843. Image from the History of Medicine, National Library of Medicine. Sourced from ihm.nlm.nih.gov/images 101393239.

priest Sebastian Kneipp (1821–1897) established an-other influential water-cure center in Bad Worschofen, Germany, with similar methods and results (Figure 1.8).

Hydropathy in the United States

Back in America, some of those who had been healed in European water-cures would go on to found alterna-tive colleges, rename themselves "naturopaths," and give intense competition to orthodox doctors. Between 1840 and 1900 there were hundreds of American water-cure

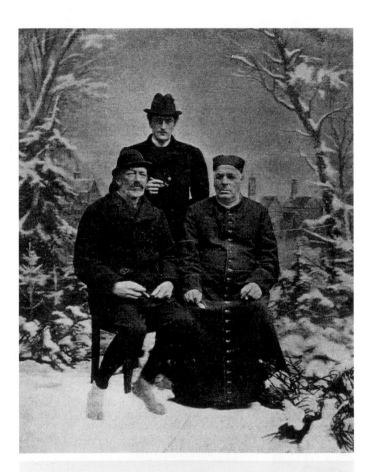

FIGURE 1.8
Sebastian Kneipp with Joseph and Francis Ferdinand, grand dukes of Austria, walking barefoot in the new fallen snow. Francis's 1914 assassination set off World War One. Photograph reproduced from Father Kneipp's Teachings by Paul Wendel, published by Paul Wendel, Brooklyn, New York, 1947. Reprinted with kind permission from National College of Naturopathic Medicine, Portland, Oregon.

hospitals treating patients with regular massage and hydrotherapy treatments. Water treatments were said to strengthen the nervous and circulatory systems, restore the body's secretions, and fill the patient's system with healthy new blood. Conventional doctors sometimes adopted cold-water treatments for ailments such as rheu-matism and dropsy (edema), high fevers, mania, hysteria, and other "nervous disorders."

One of the main movers in the American hydropathy movement was the Seventh Day Adventist Church. Ad-ventists abstained from meat, dairy products, alcohol, and tobacco, and performed medical missionary work which featured extensive use of hydrotherapy and mas-sage. The first Adventist health institution was built in 1866 and later became the Battle Creek Sanitarium, a 1200-bed institution that used water-cure methods. "The San" was the leading center for natural healing in the Western world, with a thousand patients in treatment there at any given time. Medical director John Harvey Kellogg was committed to incorporating "water-cure" methods and other natural remedies into legitimate med-ical practice. The San's hydrotherapy facilities consisted of two three-story buildings, and patients were expected in the bath department for treatment 40 minutes a day, six days a week (Figures 1.9, 1.10, and 1.11). The San would close soon after the Great Depression put it out of the financial reach of most people.

The resurgence of European spas

In the late 1800s, Europe's upper classes had both the wealth and the leisure time to retreat to spas for extend-ed periods, where a water-cure could last 24 weeks and required immersion up to the neck for many hours each day. Historian Janet Oppheim has noted that many wealthy and fashionable Victorians who suffered from depression spent their lives travelling from spa to spa in hope of a cure (Oppheim, 1991). Despite little or no scien-tific evidence to back up their claims, many spas still had a reputation for healing specific complaints. In Germa-ny, the waters of Baden-Baden were thought to be ideal for obesity, arthritis, rheumatism, circulatory problems and respiratory disorders, while in France, Bagnoles de l'Orne had hot radium-impregnated waters beneficial for blood vessel problems. As seen in Figure 1.12, the former public bath at Leukerbad, Switzerland, had become a

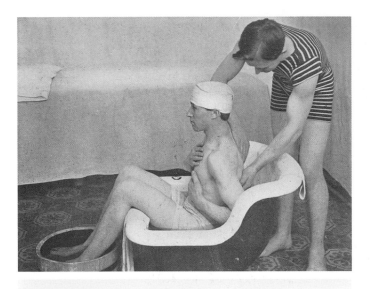

FIGURE 1.9
The cold sitz bath was combined with a hot footbath and vigorous rubbing to reduce pelvic pain, sciatica, menstrual cramps, constipation, and prostate problems, and to speed up slow labor. Photo from Rational Hydrotherapy, by John Harvey Kellogg, 1900.

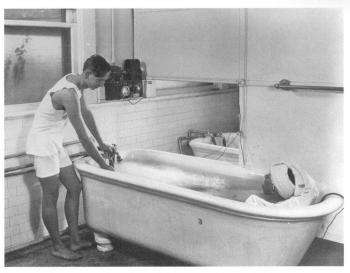

FIGURE 1.11
Patient receiving hydrotherapy treatment, Battle Creek Sanitarium. Note the cold compress on the patient's head. The inlets for hot and cold water, combined with the drain for outflow, allowed the water to be kept at a constant temperature. Reprinted with permission from Willard Library, Battle Creek, Michigan.

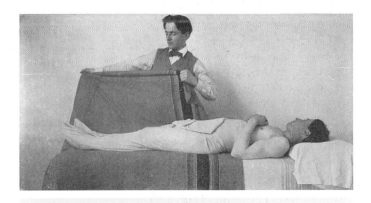

FIGURE 1.10
The leg wrap was used to improve circulation in legs and feet that were chronically cold, inflamed or painful, and as a derivative measure to stop migraines. Photo from Rational Hydrotherapy, by John Harvey Kellogg, 1900.

water-cure: the slightly warm mineral-water baths were used by patients suffering from nervous disorders, rheumatism and skin conditions. In 1883, the typical treatment consisted of 6–8 hours in the 97–104°F (36–40°C) water, followed by a thorough cold hosing from a large high-pressure jet, while being vigorously massaged with a horsehair mitt. Eventually, people went not only for the healing of ailments such as rheumatism, gout and depression, but also for the social life. Well-to-do invalids flocked to try the water and massage treatments and also enjoyed balls, theatre, gambling, chocolate-drinking houses and horse races. Spa therapies could have a strong placebo effect for those suffering from somato-emotional illnesses and "nerves": there are many reports of patients, especially young women, recovering completely after years of being bed ridden or paralyzed (Shorter, 1992).

Decline of the water-cure

Towards the end of the 19th century, hydropathy's popularity finally began to decline. Not only was there strong opposition from most of the orthodox medical profession, but bland diets, vigorous exercise, cold wet sheets, frequent enemas and ice-cold sitz baths had limited appeal to followers of fashion. And finally, not all of patients had

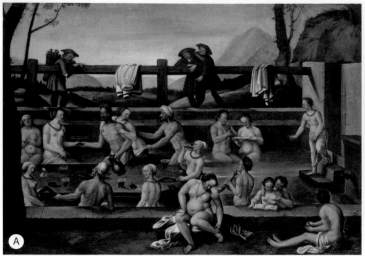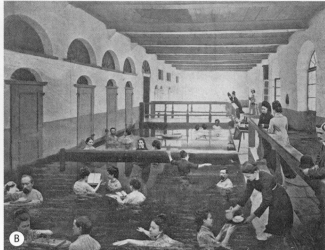

FIGURE 1.12
(**A**) Public baths at Leuk, Switzerland 1597, by Hans Bock the Elder. Illustration courtesy of Kunsstmuseum, Basel. (**B**) Neutral bath treatment, at Leuk, Switzerland, 1883. Photo from Rational Hydrotherapy, by John Harvey Kellogg, 1900.

ailments that spas or water-cures could address. Many people would find improvements short-lived if they returned from the spa to the same stressful home environment or continued to harbor deep-seated, unresolved emotional issues. However, some of the unorthodox figures who ran hydropathic establishments continued to challenge orthodox medicine by combining hydropathy with chiropractic, massage and lifestyle changes. In America, naturopaths Henry Lindlahr (1852–1925), Otis Carroll (1879–1962) and G. K. Abbot (1880–1959) treated tens of thousands of patients during their careers. Hydrotherapy also became a standard treatment for mental illness for half a century (see Box 1.3).

Hydrotherapy in the 20th century

Although the water-cure might have lost its trendiness, that did not reduce the appeal of natural waters, and eventually many spas became elegant watering places designed for pampering. At the same time, war injuries presented a distinct challenge to the medical profession. Massage was widely used, and in 1918 a new invention, the whirlpool bath, would be used to deepen its effectiveness. In 1919, the director of physiotherapy at a US Army hospital stated, "We have found the whirlpool bath is one of the most valuable modalities of this hospital in the treatment of war wounds. Its soothing warmth changes the cold purple of the swollen and painful hand or foot, leg or arm into a warm red, softening the parts for massage and passive exercise. Pain is reduced, and the circulation and nutrition of the part increased … we have found that the duration of massage is reduced from thirty to ten minutes. The actual process is easier and less laborious, while the results are in every way superior to those which could be obtained previously" (Numbers, 1976). The whirlpool would later be used for many other conditions, including sprains, fractures, lymphedema and frostbite (see Box 1.4, *Hydrotherapy for soldiers*).

The early 20th century also saw the beginning of pool therapy: in 1919 the Los Angeles Orthopedic Hospital turned their lily pond into a therapeutic pool so that patients with cerebral palsy could perform "hydrogymnastics." In 1927, Franklin Delano Roosevelt founded the Warm Springs Institute for Rehabilitation, which became a haven for polio survivors. FDR had been left paralyzed from the waist down by polio, and the spring's warm, highly mineralized water relieved much of his muscular spasm and discomfort, while its buoyancy allowed exercising for longer periods of time. As seen in Figure 1.13, polio patients did daily pool exercises, followed by rest periods in the warm sun. Other treatments

HYDROTHERAPY TREATMENTS FOR PSYCHIATRIC PROBLEMS

Psychiatric problems have always presented a distinct challenge to the medical profession, which usually tries whatever remedies go along with its current medical theories. Hippocrates recommended baths as a kind of soothing humoral treatment; in medieval Europe, being forcibly immersed in cold waters dedicated to Christian saints was thought to drive out the demons which caused mental illness (Shorter, 1992). Then, during the heyday of the hydropathic movement, the waters of certain spas were said to be good for psychiatric complaints. The first mental asylums were introduced around 1700, and managing disruptive or difficult patients always presented a dilemma. Calming and sedating medications such as morphine were common, but they were often addictive and toxic and did nothing to cure mental problems (Braslow, 1997). In the modern era, doctors came to believe mental problems were faults which resided in the body; however, they also realized stress had an influence, and patients might be forced into their mental state by troubles such as "too much studying, business failure, hunger, hard work,

poverty and dissipation" (Goeres-Gardner, 2013). Theories aside, because warm baths are so deeply soothing and relaxing, they almost always seemed a natural fit. The founder of modern psychiatry, Philippe Pinel, recommended warm baths to calm "overwrought nerves." For the first half of the 20th century, hydrotherapy was a mainstream treatment in mental institutions, complete with bathtubs, steam baths and fomentation stations. Treatments were intended to make mentally-ill patients more comfortable and compliant, and thus less likely to be violent. Fomentations were soothing, while hours-long neutral baths calmed restless or agitated patients. For patients who were combative or otherwise unmanageable, the wet sheet pack often not only restrained them but also had a sedative effect (Wright, 1940). These were also labor-intensive treatments: in 1936, a severely depressed patient at one mental hospital had two hydrotherapy sessions per week, each of which included a hot foot soak followed by a session in a heat cabinet, bath, massage and a scotch hose treatment to the back (Goeres-Gardner, 2013). In the late 1950s, these treatments were replaced by psychiatric medications, perhaps primarily as a labor-saving strategy.

---

used there included hot packs, paraffin dips, and therapeutic massage.

Although the Battle Creek Sanitarium and similar institutions shut down during the Great Depression, water treatments were still used by some in mainstream medicine. Nursing schools taught hydrotherapy techniques and massage until the 1950s, and every nurse learned how to perform the nightly back rub to help patients sleep without medication. Both naturopathic and some regular doctors used hydrotherapy treatments to treat infectious diseases and post-surgical infections. Cold-water treatments to cool feverish patients were popular, contrast treatments of the chest were routinely given after surgery to prevent pneumonia, and hyperthermia treatments were used for infectious illnesses. Even though the American Medical Association still affirmed the value of spa therapy for chronic disabling conditions including

rheumatic disorders, ailments of the digestive system, nervous conditions, certain skin problems, and some metabolic diseases, the introduction of penicillin in 1943 put an end to labor-intensive treatments (Thrash and Thrash, 1981).

Hydrotherapy in the late 20th century

The trend towards less labor-intensive therapies continued, leading to a reduction in hands-on treatments and personal attention from healthcare providers. Physical therapists were no longer trained to spend as much time with patients, and insurance did not reimburse for therapies that required them to do so. In many cases bodywork was replaced with therapies that could be applied with equipment, such as diathermy, ultrasound, TENS units, and exercise. Water treatments are now limited to

HYDROTHERAPY FOR SOLDIERS

In all wars, wounded soldiers outnumber those killed, and a sizeable number of veterans will need rehabilitation to ensure complete healing. Common injuries include:

- wounds from foreign objects such as bullets and shrapnel
- musculoskeletal injuries such as fractures, amputations and overuse injuries
- brain, spinal cord and nerve injuries
- post-traumatic stress syndrome (PTSD), known in the past as "soldier's heart," "shell shock," or "battle fatigue" – after World War I, psychiatrist Sigmund Freud noted that some veterans had "hysterical" symptoms such as complete paralysis or loss of sight, speech or hearing (Porter, 1997).

From the ancient Greeks to Native Americans, wounded warriors have found hot waters therapeutic. The springs in Bath, England, were used 2000 years ago by soldiers of the Roman Empire, and for centuries by veterans of English armed conflicts. Like many spas in Europe and the United States, Bath became a military hospital after World War I. Neutral baths were used to treat septic wounds, and therapeutic massage was combined with whirlpool baths, paraffin dips, and heat lamps (see Figures 1 and 3; and also Figure 4.11).

Whirlpools were still used after the Second World War (Figure 3) and pool therapy began to grow in popularity (Rolls, 2013; see Figure 4). Soldiers continue to receive massage and hydrotherapy for healing and rehabilitation. At Walter Reed National Army Hospital in Washington DC, the physical therapy department currently treats wounded soldiers from the Afghanistan and Iraq wars. The great majority of these veterans have orthopedic problems. In addition to exercise and manual therapies such as myofascial release and joint mobilization, water therapies are poplar. Immersion reduces pain and inflammation, and at the same time water exercise restores strength and joint range of motion. In Figure 4, Private First Class Joey Banegas, who lost his right leg in a bomb blast in Afghanistan,

is shown working on core stabilization in a hospital therapy pool, four months post-injury (Springer, 2004).

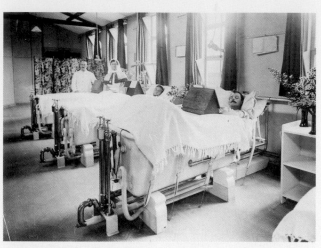

FIGURE 1

American soldiers being treated for septic wounds, using continuous neutral baths, 1919. Note the inlet for hot water and the outlet to drain cooling water, allowing the water temperature to remain at 98.6°F (37°C). Bathtub ward, British Red Cross Society Hospital, Richmond, South Africa. Image from History of Medicine, National Library of Medicine. Sourced from ihm.nlm.nih.gov/images A011823.

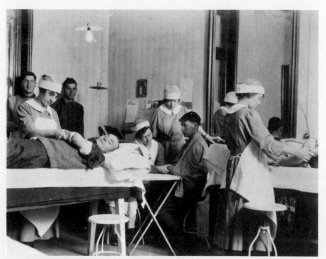

FIGURE 2

Reconstruction aides massage injured soldiers at a US Army Hospital, 1921. Image from History of Medicine, National Library of Medicine. Sourced from ihm.nlm.nih.gov/images 101396512.

BOX 1.4 *continued*

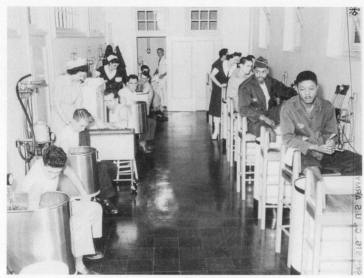

FIGURE 3
Whirlpool treatments for soldiers with injured arms and legs, US Army Hospital, 1945. Image from History of Medicine, National Library of Medicine. Sourced from ihm.nlm.nih.gov/images A09297.

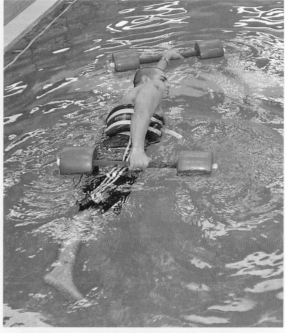

FIGURE 4
Pool therapy for an American soldier, Walter Reed Hospital, 2004. Reprinted with permission from Joey Banegas and Walter Reed Army Medical Center, Washington DC.

little more than hot packs and applications of ice, if that, and only small amounts of massage are given. Only a few physical therapists are trained to perform pool therapy with patients.

At the same time that hydrotherapy and massage techniques were steadily decreasing in physical therapy, a similar dynamic took place in nursing. Busy nurses had no time for labor-intensive treatments, and massage was given little or no support. According to Robert Calvert, author of *The History of Massage*, "The hands-on, general type of practice that had held out hope for massage and water treatments becoming more widely accepted as a medical treatment for disease gradually disappeared" (Calvert, 2002). The last holdouts were the few hardy iconoclasts who were outside of the medical mainstream, including naturopathic physicians and the allopathic physicians of the Seventh Day Adventist Church. These two small groups used

hydrotherapy not only for musculoskeletal ailments but also for difficult and challenging diseases. For example, a patient with hypertension could be treated by using neutral baths and massage to temporarily lower her blood pressure, and then weight loss, healthy diet and exercise would help keep her blood pressure normal. A patient with a diabetic foot ulcer might be treated with contrast leg baths and antimicrobial herbs, while being taught how to prevent ulcers in the future with exercise, regular massage and leg baths. Adventist physicians Agatha and Calvin Thrash's 1981 book *Home Remedies: Hydrotherapy, Massage, Charcoal and Other Simple Treatments*, summed up their approach to treating a wide variety of health problems. Based on their combined fifty years of experience, both doctors agreed that hydrotherapy was a highly effective part of a holistic approach to illness and musculoskeletal pain (Thrash and Thrash, 1981).

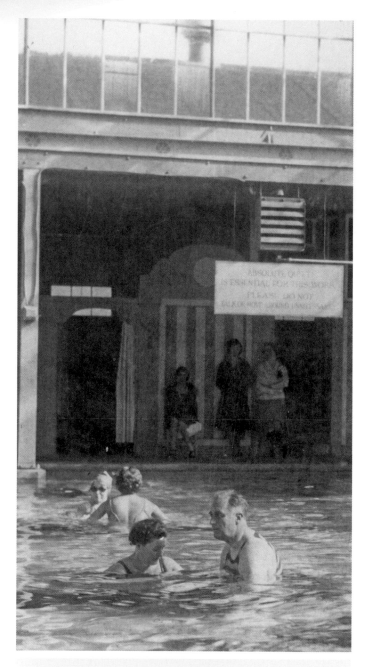

FIGURE 1.13
Franklin Delano Roosevelt and other patients with polio exercising in a warm pool, Warm Springs Georgia, 1924. FDR is in the center, being assisted by a physical therapist. Reprinted with permission from Franklin Delano Roosevelt National Library, Hyde Park, New York.

MODERN HYDROTHERAPY AND THE MASSAGE THERAPIST

Regardless of whether massage and water treatments are part of mainstream medicine or not, there has continued to be a demand for them by the public. In the heyday of hydropathy, water treatments and massage flourished. Later, even while massage was being relegated to the lowest rung of the healthcare ladder, it was still being taught and practiced outside medical circles. Health clubs featuring steam baths, saunas and massage have been popular wherever they have been introduced. The soothing warm waters of natural hot springs have continued to attract both sick people and healthy vacationers alike. Unfortunately, unlike in Europe, where therapeutic spa regimens were considered legitimate therapies paid for by health insurance (Forestier, 2017), few people in the United States took them seriously, and health insurance did not cover them.

However, change was afoot: in the 1970s, the growth of the human potential movement, a disenchantment with increasingly impersonal mainstream medicine, and a renewed interest in holistic health, contributed to a revival of massage and hydrotherapy. Bodywork now emerged as an independent, stand-alone therapy performed by professional massage therapists, who now worked in athletic clubs, chiropractic offices, physical therapy clinics,

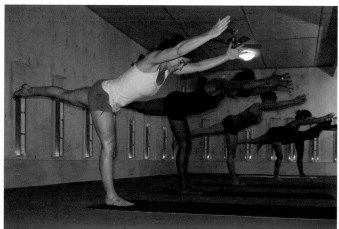

FIGURE 1.14
Hot yoga performed in a custom sauna. Photo courtesy of SaunaRay Sauna Company.

private offices, hospitals and hospices. Many innovative bodywork methods emerged, and spas of all kinds began to spring up. This growth in spas has been especially marked in the United States as the US did not already have a strong spa tradition. Spas became a "must have" amenity at resorts and large hotels, which offered exotic and ever-changing menus of bodywork and water treatments. Hospital-based spas began offering massage targeted to specific conditions such as lymphedema, cancer, pregnancy, arthritis and chronic pain. New hydrotherapy treatments were created as well, including flotation therapy for chronic pain, innovative products for applying local heat and cold, **Watsu** for relaxation, special saunas for performing "hot yoga," water exercise baths for tiny hospitalized premies, and hyperthermia treatments for depression (see Figure 1.14) (Bood, 2005; Edebol, 2008; Kjellgren, 2001; Tobinaga, 2016). In the 21st century, all of these new developments continue to keep the various combinations of massage and hydrotherapy both relevant and popular.

CHAPTER SUMMARY

This chapter has given an introduction to the multiple ways in which healers have combined water and massage therapies, and the benefits of using both in massage practice. Today's massage therapist can specialize in many types of massage therapies and work with clients with a wide variety of specific needs, and can use water treatments to enhance and complement the massage experience. In later chapters you will learn exactly how to perform such treatments. Much more is in store! Massage practitioners who are knowledgeable about the effects and benefits of these treatments have a powerful, versatile tool to complement and enhance their expertise in touch.

Chapter one

REVIEW QUESTIONS

Short answer

1. List five ways in which using hydrotherapy can enhance the practice of massage therapy.

2. Describe several different ways in which different cultures have explained the healing power of water.

3. Explain how a typical bather would progress through a Roman bath.

4. Name several hydrotherapy treatments developed in recent years.

Multiple choice

5. The Romans derived much of their medicine and many of their bathing practices from:

   A. Egyptians

   B. Ancient Greeks

   C. Invading Goths

   D. Celtic peoples

6. The water-cure methods of Vincent Preissnitz had popular appeal for three of the four reasons below. Which is the exception?

   A. Actively promoted healthy lifestyle

   B. Novel and different from standard medical practice

   C. Retained concept of humors

   D. Advocated toxic remedies

7. Whole-body baths have been prescribed for all but one of the following. Which is the exception?

   A. Thermal effects

   B. Strengthening effects

   C. Tonic effects

   D. Soothing effects

8. Massage has been used along with water treatments in all but one of the following. Which is the exception?

   A. Roman baths

   B. Preissnitz water-cure

   C. Modern nursing training

   D. Greek gymnasium

   E. Seventh-Day Adventist health facilities

True/False

9. True/False   Historically, heat stimulates and cold relaxes the body.

10. True/False   Warm springs have benefited soldiers recuperating from war injuries.

11. True/False   Spas were permanent cures for psychosomatic illnesses.

12. True/False   The sweat lodge was an ancient version of today's flotation therapy.

Matching

13.

1. Herbal baths   A. Used for mental disorders

2. Cold applications   B. Used for polio

3. Continuous baths   C. Used for swelling

4. Pool therapy   D. Used for chemical application

REVIEW QUESTIONS *continued*

14.

1. John Harvey Kellogg
2. Hippocrates
3. Franklin Delano Roosevelt
4. Galen

A. Physician to Roman emperors, whose ideas were the basis of medieval medicine
B. Pool exercise for polio
C. Greek physician, father of modern medicine
D. American physician, hydrotherapist and sanitarium director

15.

1. Alkaline springs
2. Sulphur springs
3. Alum springs
4. Acid drinking water

A. Bladder stones
B. Scrofulous tumors
C. Poisonous humors
D. Paralysis

16.

1. Control body temperature
2. Injury rehabilitation
3. Reduce stress on therapist's hands
4. Stimulate skin
5. Relaxation and stress reduction

A. Relaxes superficial muscles
B. Soothing effects
C. Mechanical and thermal sensations
D. Makes soft tissues more stretchable
E. Warm or cool client

17.

1. Fomentations
2. Body steam treatment
3. Whirlpool
4. Flotation therapy
5. Watsu

A. Chronic pain
B. Deep relaxation
C. War wounds
D. Infectious illness
E. Polio

Chapter one

References

Bargh J. Before You Know it: The Unconscious Reasons We Do What We Do. New York: Simon and Schuster, 2017

Beever R. The effects of repeated thermal therapy on quality of life in patients with type II diabetes mellitus. J Altern Complement Med 2010; 16(6): 677–81

Bood SA, Sundequist U, Kjellgren A et al. Effects of flotation-restricted environmental stimulation technique on stress-related muscle pain: what makes the difference in therapy – attention-placebo or the relaxation response? Pain Res Manag 2005; 10(4): 201–9

Braslow J. Mental Ills and Bodily Cures: Psychiatric Treatment in the First Half of the Twentieth Century. Berkeley: University of California Press, 1997

Bruchac J. The Native American Sweat Lodge: History and Legends. Freedom, CA: Crossing Press, 1993

Calvert R. The History of Massage: An Illustrated Survey from Around the World. Rochester, VT: Healing Arts Press, 2002, p. 180

Croutier A. *Taking the Waters: Spirit, Art, Sensuality.* New York, NY: Abbeville Press, 1992

Dube SR. et al. Childhood abuse, neglect and household dysfunction and the risk of illicit drug use: the adverse childhood experiences study. Pediatrics, 2003; 111: 564

Edebol H, Ake Bood S, Norlander T. Chronic whiplash-associated disorders and their treatment using flotation-REST (restricted environmental stimulation technique). Qual Health Res 2008; 18(4): 480–8

Felitti V et al. Relationship of childhood abuse and household dysfunction to many of the leading causes of death in adults: The Adverse Childhood Experiences (ACE) Study. American Journal of Preventive Medicine 1988; 14(4): 245–58

Forestier R. Current role for spa therapy in rheumatoid arthritis: mud packs, water walking, whirlpool, affusion massage, underwater shower. Joint Bone Spine, Jan 2017

Gaunt J. Natural and Political Observations made upon the Bills of Mortality. London, 1662

Goeres-Gardner D. Inside Oregon State Hospital: a History of Tragedy and Triumph. Charleston, SC: History Press, 2013

Goldberg R et al. Relationship between traumatic events in childhood and chronic pain. Disability and Rehabilitation 1999; 21: 23–30

Halioua B, Ziskind B. Medicine in the Days of the Pharaohs. Cambridge, MA: Harvard University Press, 2005, p. 31

Hanusch K et al. Whole-body hyperthermia for the treatment of major depression: association with thermoregulatory cooling. Am J Psychiatry 2013; 170: 7

Harris N. The Deepest Well: Healing the Long-Term Effects of Childhood Adversity. New York: Simon and Schuster, 2018

Janssen C et al. Whole-body hyperthermia for the treatment of major depressive disorder: a randomized clinical trial. JAMA Psychiatry 2016; 73(8): 789–95

Jimenez X. Severe noncardiac chest pain responds to interdisiplinary chronic pain rehabilitation. Psychosomatics 2018; 59(2): 204–6

Kaysing B. Great Hot Springs of the West. Santa Barbara, CA: Capra Press, 1994

Kellogg J. Rational Hydrotherapy. Battle Creek, Michigan: Modern Medicine Publishing Company, 1923, p. 381

Kjellgren A et al. Effects of floatation-REST on muscle tension pain, Pain Res Manag 2001; 6(4): 181–9.

Koltyn K, Robins H, Schmitt C et al. Changes in mood state following whole-body hyperthermia. Int J Hyperthermia 1992; 8(3): 305–7

Legan M. Hydropathy in America: a nineteenth century panacea. Bulletin of the History of Medicine 1971; 45: 267

Numbers R. Prophetess of Health: A Study of Ellen G. White. New York, NY: Harper and Row, 1976, p. 22

Oppheim J. Shattered Nerves: Doctors, Patients and Depression in Victorian England. Oxford: Oxford University Press, 1991

Phillips E. Aspects of Greek Medicine. New York, NY: St. Martin's Press, 1973, p. 119

Porter R. The Greatest Benefit to Mankind: A Medical History of Humanity. New York: WW Norton, 1997

Porter R. The Medical History of Waters and Spas. London: Wellcome Institute for the History of Medicine, 1990

Roberts J. Herodotus: The Histories: The Complete Translation, Backgrounds, Commentaries. New York: W. W. Norton, 2013

Roe C. Poultice for A Healer. New York: Penguin, 2003 [Set in medieval Spain in 1354]

Rolls R. Diseased, Douched and Doctored: Thermal Springs, Spa Doctors and Rheumatic Diseases. London: London Publishing Partnership, 2013

Sachs-Ericsson N. et al. When Emotional Pain Becomes Physical: Adverse Childhood Experiences, Pain, and the Role of Mood and Anxicty Disorders. J Clin Psychology 2017; 73(10): 1403–28

Sarno J. Healing Back Pain: The Mind-Body Connection. New York: Warner Books, 1991

Shorter E. A History of Psychiatry: from the Era of the Asylum to the Age of Prozac. New York: John Wiley and Sons, 1997

Shorter E. From Paralysis to Fatigue: a History of Psychosomatic Inness in the Modern Era. New York: Simon and Schuster, 1992

Springer B, Dunlavey K. Personal communication with author, telephone interview. November 2004

Temkin O. Soranus' Gynecology. Baltimore: Johns Hopkins Press, 1956

Thrash A, Thrash C. Home Remedies: Hydrotherapy, Massage, Charcoal, and Other Simple Treatments. Seale, AL: Thrash Publications, 1981

Tobinaga O et al. Short term effects of hydrokinesiotherapy in hospitalized preterm newborns. Rehabil Res Pract. 2016; Sept 08

Vogel V. American Indian Medicine. Norman, OK: The University of Oklahoma Press, 1970

Walker D. The Nez Perce Sweat Bath Complex: An Acculturational Analysis. Southwestern Journal of Anthropology 1966; 22: 133–71

Wright R. Hydrotherapy in Psychiatric Hospital. Boston, MA: Tudor Press, 1940

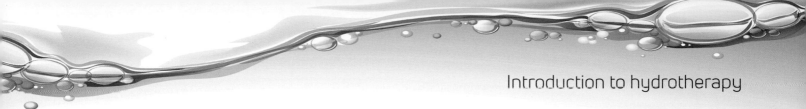

Recommended resources

Barclay J. In Good Hands: The History of the Chartered Society of Physiotherapists, 1894–1994. Oxford: Butterworth-Heinmann, 1994

Bender T et al. Evidence-based hydro- and balneotherapy in Hungary – a systematic review and meta-analysis. Int J Biometeorol 2014; 58(3): 311–23

Boyle W, Saine A. Lectures in Naturopathic Hydrotherapy. Sandy, Oregon: Eclectic Medical Publications, 1988, pp. 9, 24

Hembry P. The English Spa, 1560–1815: A Social History. London: The Athone Press, 1990

Millard O. Under My Thumb. London: Christopher Johnson, 1952, p.20

Moor F. et al. Manual of Hydrotherapy and Massage. Hagerstown, MD: Review and Herald Publishers, 1964

Wright L. Clean and Decent: The Fascinating History of the Bathroom and Water Closet. New York: Viking Press, 1960

Yegul F. Baths and Bathing in Classical Antiquity. Cambridge: MIT Press, 1992

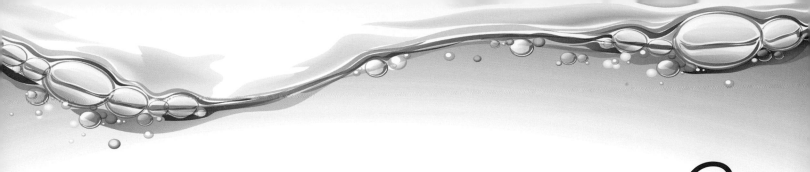

Effects of hydrotherapy 2

Humans must fiercely protect their internal temperature, for it holds the key to all their life functions. The human body is a mass of millions of exquisitely sequenced chemical reactions, … the timing, and thus the temperature of these reactions is so critical that if body temperature varies by more than 4°F from 98.6°F … the body's formidable defenses begin to crumble.

Kamler, *Surviving the Extremes: A Doctor's Journey to the Limits of Human Endurance*

CHAPTER OBJECTIVES

After completing this chapter, the student will be able to:

1. Describe the basic structures and functions of the circulatory system, the skin, and the nervous system
2. Explain various ways that the circulatory system responds to environmental threats
3. Explain how water and heat can increase skin absorption and why this is relevant to hydrotherapy
4. Explain the importance of keeping the core temperature at 98.6°F (37°C)
5. Explain the physiological effects of local and whole-body heating treatments
6. Discuss the reflex effects of local heat applications
7. Describe the physiological effects of local and whole-body cooling treatments
8. Explain the reflex effects of local cold applications
9. Describe the effects of mechanical hydrotherapy treatments
10. Describe the effects of chemical hydrotherapy treatments.

The human body is very skilled at detecting and responding to changes in its environment. A vast network of feedback mechanisms makes the body aware of threats to its stability, such as extreme heat or cold, physical danger, injuries and emotional stress, and the body can respond in many ingenious ways. Figure 2.1 shows a dramatic example of clever responses to extreme cold, a swimmer immersed in very cold water (see also Case history 2.1). In this chapter, you will learn how hydrotherapy treatments can improve massage outcomes by taking advantage of these **homeostatic** responses.

Depending on which treatments you choose and how you perform them, a wide range of physiological effects can be created. Various treatments can warm, cool, soothe, stimulate, relieve inflammation, soften connective tissue, numb painful areas, increase or decrease muscle tone, or detoxify.

However, in order to choose the right hydrotherapy treatment, it is important to understand how each one affects the body and when it can or cannot be properly used. For example, a client with a migraine headache who comes in for massage treatment could also be treated using a hot foot soak and an ice pack to the back of the neck, but not if that person is diabetic. A client who has a severely strained calf muscle could benefit from local ice massage before hands-on treatment, but not if that person has **Raynaud's syndrome**. Should you have a sauna or steam bath at your facility, understanding the effects of a whole-body heating treatment can help you assess whether or not this could be beneficial for your clients. Box 2.1 lists some of the basic principles of hydrotherapy to keep in mind as you choose treatments for your clients. These principles are covered in detail later in the chapter.

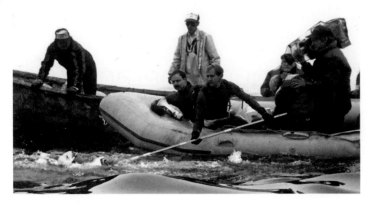

FIGURE 2.1
Scientists monitor Lynne Cox's circulatory system as she swims in the Bering Strait, 1987. Photo courtesy of Rich Roberts.

This chapter also explains how three of the body systems most affected in hydrotherapy, namely the circulatory, skin and nervous systems, can be manipulated to enhance the practice of massage. Because the body works as a whole, other systems play a part as well, but here we emphasize those most relevant to the practice of massage therapy. Hydrotherapy treatments are applied to the skin and sensed by the nerves, which communicate that information to the brain: then, taking orders from the nervous system, the skin and circulatory systems respond. First we briefly review the three systems, and then we will consider the thermal, mechanical and chemical effects of hydrotherapy on the body.

SURVIVING IN FRIGID WATERS	CASE HISTORY 2.1

BACKGROUND

In water colder than about 49°F (10°C), most people quickly lose body heat and go into hypothermic shock. Water sucks the air out of a body 25 times faster than air at the same temperature. However, Lynn Cox, a conditioned long-distance swimmer with an unusual percentage of body fat for natural insulation, has an extraordinary ability to survive cold.

RESEARCH

Researchers have monitored Cox's skin temperature, heart rate and core temperature on many cold-water swims, and found her core temperature can actually rise during immersion. Cox once swam across the Bering Strait, spending 2 hours in 37°F (2.8°C) water. Muscle contractions produce copious quantities of heat – for example, running generates ten times as much heat as walking – so as long as she kept moving, her circulatory system continued to function well, closing off some small arterioles in her extremities in order to limit blood flow there while keeping her vital organs full of warm blood. (Normal blood temperature is 100.4°F, 38°C.)

However, even though Cox was immediately wrapped in warm layers, the moment she came on land and stopped generating body heat her core temperature began to dip, reaching a dangerously low 94°F (34.4°C degrees). During another swim in even colder Antarctic waters (33°F; 0.5°C), Cox's circulatory system kept her alive by diverting blood away from exposed extremities. Her hands became splotchy, bluish white and had a "bone deep ache". They were so numb she could barely tell if she was moving forward. If Cox had stopped moving and her tissues had cooled any further, her blood would have lost even more heat, and thus lowered her core temperature when it flowed back to her heart. Muscles and nerve fibers don't work well when very cold, but Cox, in order not to freeze or become incapacitated, forced herself harder than ever before. When she exited the water, her core temperature was 97.7°F (36.5°C), showing that her constant movements had been enough to keep her core temperature up to survivable levels; soon, however, her temperature dropped to 95.5°F (35.5°C), despite her being indoors, surrounded by warm bodies and drinking warm beverages. Peripheral vessels in her arms and legs dilated as they were rewarmed, and then very cold, stagnated blood began to flow from her

CASE HISTORY 2.1 *continued*

periphery to her core. Cox shivered violently for many minutes and was not out of danger until she finally put on a track suit with heat packs placed over her arteries – at the neck for the carotid, at the armpits for the brachial, at the groin for the femoral, and at the palms of the hands for the palmar arterial arch. This quickly did the trick (Nyboer, 1989; Cox, 2004).

DISCUSSION QUESTIONS

1. Name three factors that enabled Cox to survive extreme cold-water immersion.
2. Why did Cox's temperature drop when she got out of the cold water?
3. What other warming devices could have been safely used?

BOX 2.1	POINT OF INTEREST

BASIC PRINCIPLES OF HYDROTHERAPY

Hydrotherapy treatments use the body's own defensive mechanisms to promote healing

For example, when a person steps into a short cold shower, the body reacts against the threat of a reduced core temperature by increasing many of its metabolic functions. When the cold shower is over, the person experiences an increased flow in surface blood vessels, increased muscle and tissue tone, increased function in the endocrine system, and a prolonged feeling of warmth.

Water plays a different role in different kinds of hydrotherapy treatments

For example, hot or cold treatments (such as hot or cold packs) affect the body primarily through temperature, and water's role in them is simply to transmit hot or cold. Mechanical treatments such as frictions, sprays or whirlpool jets, however, affect the body primarily by using water to apply pressure to the skin in different ways. Finally, chemical treatments (which mix substances such as herbs, salts and essential oils with water) affect the body primarily through the chemicals which are absorbed into the skin. Here, water is simply the medium which carries the chemical solution onto the skin. By using hot water, warming of the skin leads to an increase in local blood flow, which speeds absorption of the chemicals.

Many hydrotherapy treatments have multiple effects

For example, an application of moist heat may be appreciated mainly because it gives the client a sensation of warmth, but it can also be used for its fluid-shifting (derivative) effect or for its ability to reduce local muscle spasm.

Hydrotherapy treatments affect more than one body system at the same time

Any treatment that is applied to the skin also affects the nervous system through the sensory receptors of the skin, and any hot or cold treatment that touches the skin immediately affects not only the nervous system but the circulatory system as well. Clever use of reflex relationships can impact other parts of the body.

Hot and cold treatments may be performed specifically to change tissue temperature

For example, when an overheated client takes a cold shower before receiving a massage on a very hot day, the direct cooling of his or her tissues is the desired effect.

Hot or cold treatments and mechanical treatments can redistribute blood or lymph within the circulatory system

For example, a person with a sub-acute ankle sprain can be given a contrast leg bath before massage to reduce edema. Repeatedly dilating and constricting the blood vessels of the foot and lower leg pulls blood flow into and out of the tissues around the ankle, creating a pumping action that ultimately shifts edema out of the area.

Mechanical hydrotherapy treatments stimulate not only the skin, but the nerve endings, blood vessels, lymph vessels and muscles it contains

Treatments such as salt glows, showers, whirlpool jets, percussion douches, brushing and frictions have

BOX 2.1 *continued*

an intensely stimulating effect that is similar to such massage strokes as tapotement and vibration.

Hydrotherapy treatments can promote the absorption of chemicals through the skin

Herbs, salts, oils, minerals, and other substances containing beneficial chemicals can be dissolved in water and then applied to the skin through compresses, poultices, packs, steam inhalation, local baths or whole-body baths. For example, Epsom salts, which contain magnesium sulfate, have a muscle-relaxing and detoxifying effect, a moisture-drawing effect due to the salt content, and a detoxifying effect due to the action of the sulfate.

Some hydrotherapy treatments produce their results mainly through their effect upon the nervous system

For example, ice stroking can deactivate trigger points and release muscle tension long enough for individual muscles to be gently but thoroughly stretched. Application of intense cold is not intended to cause tissue chilling or the fluid-shifting effect of vasoconstriction—instead, the desired effect, of numbing the area, is a nervous system effect.

ANATOMY AND PHYSIOLOGY REVIEW: THE CIRCULATORY SYSTEM, SKIN, AND NERVOUS SYSTEM

Circulatory system

The human circulatory system consists of the heart, blood and lymphatic vessels, and the fluids they contain. Because hydrotherapy treatments have a strong effect on blood vessels and can shift blood flow from one part of the body to another, it is especially important for anyone using them to understand the circulatory system. Blood is rich in nutrients cells need, and they can die if they don't get enough blood, for example where an artery is damaged or blocked. (Blood not only supplies our cells with nutrients but carries away metabolic wastes such as lactic acid).

In this context it useful to picture the circulatory system as what physiologist Stephen Vogel has called "a serial arrangement of pipes and pumps" (Vogel, 1992). The "pipes" of the circulatory system are: (1) the heart and all the branching hollow tubes (arteries down to capillaries) that carry blood away from the center to the periphery; and (2) the vessels that return blood and lymphatic fluid from the tissues back to the heart (large veins down to tiny venules and lymphatic vessels of varying sizes). Arteries supply all major organs and areas in the body, while veins and lymphatic vessels drain blood and tissue fluid away from them (Figures 2.2 and 2.3).

Each type of vessel in the circulatory system is unique. For example, both small and larger arteries are similar, but larger ones are constructed to handle not only more blood, but blood that is under higher pressure and moving faster. Their walls are quite thick and contain both muscle and elastic fibers. By contrast, the blood and lymphatic fluids that are returning to the heart are under less pressure and flow more slowly; the walls of veins and lymphatic vessels are much thinner and contain no muscle and little or no elastic tissue (Figure 2.4).

Exchange of oxygen, nutrients, and wastes actually takes place in the very smallest vessels, the capillaries. Our bodies contain so many capillaries that there is one close to almost every one of our cells. The "pumps" of the circulatory system force blood from the center of the body to the extremities, and venous blood and lymphatic fluid back to the heart, mostly against gravity. These pumps include the heart, large arteries, skeletal muscles, and smooth muscle found in larger lymphatic vessels. The most powerful pump is the muscular four-chambered heart, which contracts hard enough to raise the pressure of the blood and force it towards the lungs or aorta. This delicate and durable organ pumps an incredible 100,000 times every day. The heart is extremely responsive to the needs of the body: normally, each heartbeat pushes out about half of all the blood that flows back in during **diastole**, the interval between two contractions. During strenuous exercise, however, it pumps out three quarters of all the blood that flows in during diastole.

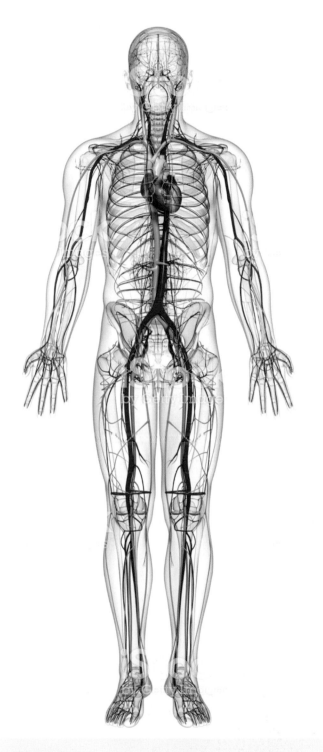

FIGURE 2.2
Arteries and veins of the circulatory system. An average-sized adult has 5 quarts (5.7 liters) of blood and 2 quarts (2.3 liters) of lymph in their body. Without nutrients, brain cells die in 4–6 minutes, 1.5 quarts (1.4 liters) of blood are pumped to the brain each minute.

Because they are made up of both elastic and muscular tissue, the largest arteries can also act as pumps: with each surge of blood from the heart, the arteries stretch and then recoil, like a rubber band snapping back. This action channels the intermittent waves of blood into one continuous stream, and gives the blood another push onward (loss of elasticity in these vessels is one sign of aging).

Skeletal muscles also function as pumps: for example, when a calf muscle contracts, its veins and lymphatic vessels are squeezed shut, and then, when the muscle relaxes and the pressure is off the vessels, capillary blood pours in. This creates a suction effect which propels venous blood and lymph forward, speeding up the flow and preventing them from pooling in the vessels. Meanwhile, valves in the veins and lymphatic vessels prevent back flow (Figure 2.5). Without this mechanism, much of the blood pumped to the legs would never get back to the heart. (For this reason, patients with muscle weakness from conditions such as spinal cord injuries, muscular dystrophy, and multiple sclerosis often have poor circulation in their legs). Fluids are also helped along by the movements of the respiratory muscles and the smooth muscle in the walls of larger lymphatic vessels.

Blood itself is composed of water, red and white blood cells, platelets, proteins, nutrients, antibodies, oxygen, and carbon dioxide. It feeds cells with oxygen, water, fats, electrolytes, vitamins, salts, glucose, proteins and carbohydrates: no wonder it is so nourishing that some animals (including insects such as mosquitoes) can actually use it for their food! The blood also carries urea, lactic acid and other wastes back to the kidneys, liver, lungs, or skin for elimination. The blood's temperature is very important to the proper functioning of tissues and organs, so it is carefully maintained at 102°F (39°C).

Lymph makes up about 2% of our body weight. When blood flows through our capillaries, hydrostatic pressure drives some of the water it contains into the spaces around our cells. This fluid eventually becomes lymph and carries bacteria, viruses, metabolic wastes, dead blood cells, large fat molecules and leukocytes. Good lymphatic flow prevents accumulation of fluid in the tissues. Eventually, once it returns to the bloodstream, the water which escaped from capillaries helps to maintain normal blood volume and pressure.

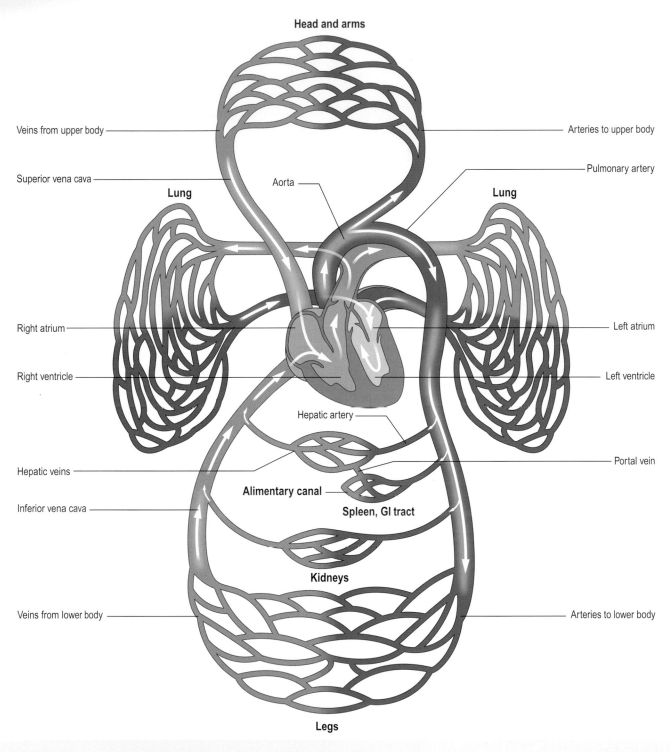

Head and arms

Veins from upper body

Arteries to upper body

Superior vena cava

Pulmonary artery

Aorta

Lung

Lung

Right atrium

Left atrium

Right ventricle

Left ventricle

Hepatic artery

Hepatic veins

Portal vein

Alimentary canal

Inferior vena cava

Spleen, GI tract

Kidneys

Veins from lower body

Arteries to lower body

Legs

FIGURE 2.3
Schematic plan of circulatory system.

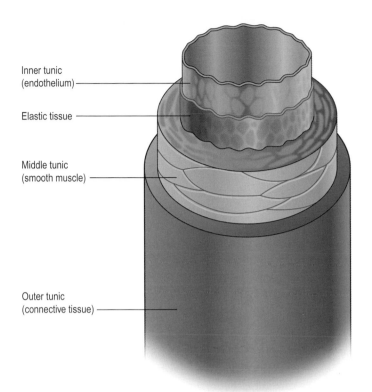

Inner tunic
(endothelium)

Elastic tissue

Middle tunic
(smooth muscle)

Outer tunic
(connective tissue)

FIGURE 2.4
Typical artery, showing layers of its wall

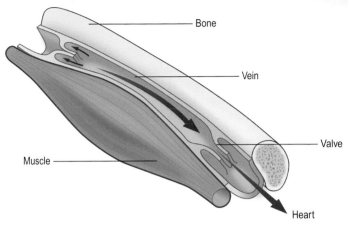

Bone

Vein

Valve

Muscle

Heart

FIGURE 2.5
Skeletal muscle pump. Venous flow towards the heart is increased by muscle contractions, while valves prevent backflow away from the heart.

As you can see, the entire circulatory system is exquisitely sensitive and capable of rapid responses to changing conditions. For more on how the circulatory system can respond to changes and threats, see Box 2.2.

Skin

Anyone fighting disease who will stimulate, cleanse, warm and protect the skin will have millions of robust allies in its versatile and talented structures.

Agatha and Calvin Thrash, *Home Remedies: Hydrotherapy, Massage, Charcoal and Other Simple Treatments*

Human skin is a complex organ with many important functions. Because hydrotherapy treatments are performed on the skin and call forth powerful reactions, it is especially important for us to understand these functions.

BOX 2.2	POINT OF INTEREST

THE CIRCULATORY SYSTEM'S AMAZING RESPONSES

The circulatory system not only responds to environmental threats such as heat and cold, but also fine-tunes many of its functions to protect the body. The nervous system senses danger and then communicates with the circulatory system, which can change the action of the heart or the diameter of blood vessels, or even adjust the actual composition of the blood. Here are some ingenious responses.

Shifting blood flow after a meal
Digestion is a complicated job that requires precise coordination between the digestive, nervous, and

BOX 2.2 *continued*

circulatory systems. After we have eaten, arteries in the stomach and intestines dilate and intestinal blood flow increases, while blood vessels in the skeletal muscles narrow and the heart beats faster and more forcefully. These two actions maintain blood pressure and blood flow to the brain, legs, and everywhere in between. Sleepiness after a meal is directly related to the shift of blood to the stomach and away from the brain (Guyton, 2010).

Shifting blood flow in response to mental activities

Thoughts can also change our circulatory system: for example, three practitioners of a Tibetan Buddhist meditation practice known as *heat yoga* were able to consciously increase the temperature of their fingers and toes by as much as 17°F (10°C). Meditators used mental imagery focusing on fire, and blood vessels in their fingers and toes dilated to increase blood flow there (Benson, 1982). In a similar fashion, people with Raynaud's syndrome have successfully used biofeedback to warm their extremities and stop vasospastic attacks there (Taub, 1976 and 1978). Intense mental activity also changes the circulatory system. Because the brain uses at least 20% of the body's supply of oxygen and glucose but cannot store nutrients, it is completely dependent upon blood flow for its moment-to-moment nutrition. Normally blood is supplied to the brain via the carotid and vertebral arteries, and oxygen and nutrients diffuse through a dense network of smaller arteries and capillaries. During intense mental activity such as doing a difficult mathematics problem, however, cerebral arteries dilate, and blood flow increases to the neurons involved in the activity (Ozturk, 2018).

Reacting to emotional stress

Psychologist James Lynch studied stress and the cardiovascular system by monitoring skin temperature, heart rate and blood pressure during counseling sessions. He found that talking about emotionally upsetting situations caused patients' hearts to beat harder and, at the same time, their peripheral arteries to constrict. Some people would literally get "cold feet" as their peripheral arteries contracted! These changes led to higher blood pressure. The body's purpose, of course, is to increase metabolism and prepare the body to fight danger or to run away (Lynch, 1995). About 15–20% of patients who visit a doctor's office find it a stressful experience, and their blood pressure may rise to unusual heights. Resting in a quiet room for a few minutes usually helps them to relax, and their blood pressure goes down as they do (Cobos, 2015). The chemistry of the circulatory system also adapts to stress: plasma volume is decreased and hematocrit, blood pressure, norepinephrine levels and platelets increase, so blood clots faster – a distinct advantage if you are injured and bleeding. For example, researchers gave a group of healthy men a stressful task of doing complex mental arithmetic. (Other healthy men who had no such stressful task were the controls). At the beginning, blood was drawn to get hematocrit and hemoglobin levels, and then blood pressure and heart rate were measured every 2 minutes. Data showed that after 20 minutes performing the stressful task, increases in blood pressure, heart rate, levels of cholesterol and stress hormones, the proportion of red blood cells per unit of blood, and activation of platelets were seen only in the men who did the task (Allen, 1995; Patterson, 1995; Muldoon, 1995).

Compensating for blockages in blood vessels that could starve cells

During fetal development, if nerves and blood vessels sense low levels of oxygen, this stimulates the sprouting of new capillaries. In adults, low levels of oxygen from heart attacks, strokes or narrowing of a vessel can also stimulate the growth of new arteries. To compensate for poor blood flow, in just a few days or weeks new blood vessels may grow around the area of blockage, making expanded connections between large arteries and their branches, and ultimately blood flow is restored to normal (Andreone, 2015). If intensive exercise is begun after a heart attack, new vessels will grow and become functional even sooner (Mobius-Winkler 2016).

Human skin is made up of three layers: the epidermis on the surface, the dermis under that, and superficial fascia deep to the dermis (Figure 2.6). It is tough yet supple, is thinner in infants and children, reaches its full maturity in adulthood, and undergoes a number of degenerative changes in old age.

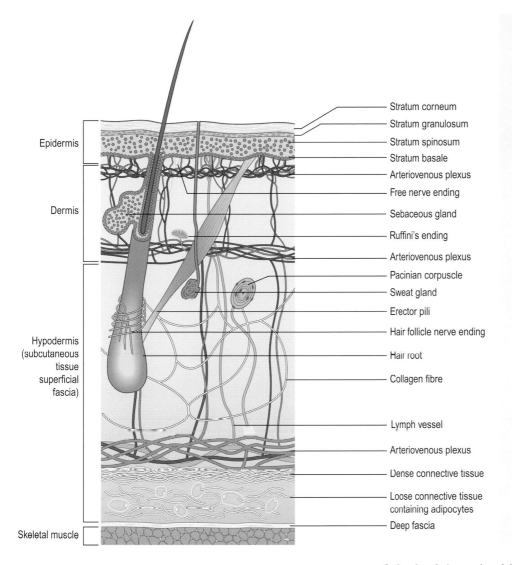

FIGURE 2.6
Anatomy of the skin.

Epidermis

Dermis

Hypodermis
(subcutaneous
tissue
superficial
fascia)

Skeletal muscle

Stratum corneum
Stratum granulosum
Stratum spinosum
Stratum basale
Arteriovenous plexus
Free nerve ending
Sebaceous gland
Ruffini's ending
Arteriovenous plexus
Pacinian corpuscle
Sweat gland
Erector pili
Hair follicle nerve ending
Hair root
Collagen fibre
Lymph vessel
Arteriovenous plexus
Dense connective tissue
Loose connective tissue
containing adipocytes
Deep fascia

The epidermis is made up mainly of dead cells which have moved from the dermis to the surface. The topmost layer of the epidermis, the *stratum corneum*, is constantly sloughing off dead cells as well as bacteria and other pathogens, while sweat and sebum form a fine acidic film which is a barrier to bacteria and viruses. Underneath lies the dermis, which is a hundred times as thick as the epidermis and contains skin cells, hair follicles, blood vessels, sweat glands, various types of nerve receptors, many lymphatic vessels, nerve endings, and over 50% of the immune system's killer T-cells. The nerve endings and hair follicles in the skin are fed by their own capillaries. The dermis contains many blood vessels (Figure 2.7). There are so many, in fact, that if they are all dilated during a sauna, hot tub or other heating treatment, they may hold up to a third

of the body's entire blood supply. Deep to the dermis is the superficial fascia: nerves and blood vessels from the skin pass through this loose connective tissue, and tiny ligaments anchor the skin firmly to the soft tissues beneath.

The structures of the skin form a dynamic interface between our inner universe and the outer world. The skin, just by being intact, protects the delicate tissues of the body from extremes of hot and cold, sharp objects, moisture loss and some harmful chemicals. With its profusion of immune system cells, the skin is the first line of defense against many invading organisms. Skin also plays a vital role in controlling body temperature, insulating the interior of the body while providing a surface from which heat can be lost through vasodilation

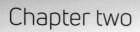
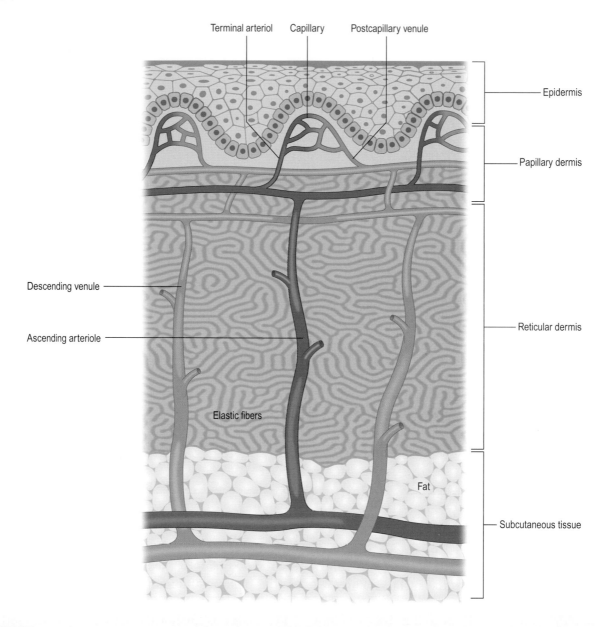

Terminal arteriol   Capillary   Postcapillary venule

Epidermis

Papillary dermis

Descending venule

Ascending arteriole

Reticular dermis

Elastic fibers

Fat

Subcutaneous tissue

FIGURE 2.7
Blood supply to the skin.

or conserved through vasoconstriction (see page 39). Body temperature can be raised one to two degrees through goosebumps and shivering, while it can be lowered through vasodilation and evaporation of sweat. (Profuse sweating can remove twenty times as much heat as can be lost through vasodilation of the skin alone.) The body contains about 3 million sweat glands, which are innervated by sympathetic nerve fibers: these are concentrated in areas that have greater amounts of blood just beneath the skin, such as the face, neck, chest, palms, back, groin, and soles of the feet. In general, the liver, colon and kidneys are the organs most responsible for eliminating wastes, but when these organs are not functioning, some wastes can be eliminated through sweat and sebum. For example, during: during intense heating, the sweat glands become very active, and toxins and metabolic wastes accumulated in the fatty layers under the skin can be metabolized and released.

In certain diseases some toxic waste products are more readily handled by the skin than by the kidneys. Solvents, nicotine, heavy metals, amphetamines, lead and other toxins have been detected in sweat. For more on this topic, see page 243, *Detoxification treatments.*

Just as some substances can pass out of the body through the skin, so some substances can pass in the other direction: many fat- or water-soluble substances on the skin can diffuse through it and into small capillaries. Here are some examples:

1. *Fat-soluble materials* (vitamins A, D, E).

2. *Chemicals absorbed by handling plants,* such as nicotine from tobacco leaves, methyl-butenol from hops, and sulfur from onions and garlic: tobacco pickers may experience nausea, vomiting and weakness, hop pickers may become sleepy, and onion pickers may have onion-scented sweat!.

3. *Industrial chemicals* such as solvents, lead, acetone, paint thinner, dry cleaning fluid, pesticides, chlorine and heavy metals. In 1944, the *Journal of Industrial Medicine* reported 20 cases of breast enlargement in men who worked at a plant that manufactured synthetic estrogen: the powder had gotten onto their skin, and was then absorbed into their bloodstreams (Fitzsimmons, 1944).

4. *Some minerals,* especially if dissolved in water first. For example, bathers have higher levels of magnesium in their blood and urine after taking Epsom salts baths. (For more on this topic, see Chapter 6.)

5. *A variety of medications now given by wearing skin patches,* including nicotine, estrogen, synthetic opiates, lidocaine, NSAIDS, dopamine antagonists, blood pressure medications, migraine medications, and nitroglycerine.

6. *Herbal preparations and essential oils.*

For more on this topic, see Box 2.3.

One of the skin's most critically important functions is monitor the external environment. Because it contains many specialized types of nerve endings, the skin can detect a greater variety of sensations than any other body tissue, from the tiny pressure of one raindrop striking the face to the forceful application of water with a high-pressure spray. Sensory receptors are located about the thickness of a piece of paper beneath the surface of the skin. When stimulated they send nerve impulses along sensory nerves to the brain's touch center in the somatosensory cortex.

There are many other receptors for light touch, deep pressure, and vibration. Thermal receptors register anything that is hotter or colder than skin temperature. They tend to react most strongly to changes in temperatures. (Box 2.4). Receptors can detect rapid changes of just one-fiftieth of a degree Fahrenheit, which helps us to avoid injuries such as burns from hot surfaces or contact with freezing-cold water. Heat-pain and cold-pain receptors kick in when temperatures rise above 113°F (45°C) or below 50°F (10°C).

Each type of sensory receptor is highly sensitive to only one type of stimulation. (For example, a tactile receptor will not respond to heat, and a pressure receptor will not respond to heat or cold.) Many of our sensations involve more than one type of receptor–for example, if you touch something that is cold and sharp, both cold and pain receptors will respond. Or if someone touches you with something that is hot and smooth, both heat and pressure receptors will respond. Thus, many hydrotherapy treatments stimulate multiple types of receptors: for example, a salt glow gives a mild thermal sensation from the water's temperature and a mechanical sensation as sharp-edged salt crystals are moved across the skin. A cold whirlpool gives a thermal sensation from the coldness of the water and a mechanical sensation as the whirlpool jets strike the skin.

Nervous system

The nervous system is sometimes likened to a control center for the body (Figure 2.8). It receives thousands of bits of information from the different sensory organs, then processes them in such a way that the appropriate motor response is made. For example, when a hand is first put in hot water, information from heat receptors is relayed to the brain, which determines whether the water is comfortably or dangerously hot, and whether pulling the hand out of the water is the appropriate response. After that, the brain signals the muscles to respond.

TO ABSORB OR NOT TO ABSORB? THAT IS THE SKIN'S QUESTION

In many hydrotherapy treatments, we combine water, heat and various substances that we hope are absorbed through the skin. Just how effective is this method? For thousands of years, healers have water and heat to apply various substances in baths, plasters, poultices and compresses (Pastore, 2015; Schendlein, 2004). For example, in medieval Spain, a hot herbal poultice and salt footbath would be used locally for a painful gouty foot; and for sciatica, a plaster would be applied right over the painful area (Roe, 2003). When a person was too sick to take anything by mouth, poultices, plasters, soaks and compresses were sometimes used to get substances into an affected organ via the skin.

The skin's ability to absorb substances was probably first noted when plant gatherers and farmers had physical side-effects just from picking certain plants, but industrial exposures were also noted from ancient times in workers whose trades used lead, mercury, arsenic or other toxic substances that were absorbed through the skin. Ancient doctors and herbalists then realized through trial and error that moisture and heat helped substances penetrate. Today skin absorption can be tested using the patient's blood, urine or feces to see how much of a certain chemical has entered the body through the skin. For example, researchers

investigating the penetration of solvents through the skin had subjects put their hands in water contaminated with solvents for 1–3 hours, then found the solvents in the subjects' urine (Brown, 1984).

Today, using drug patches to administer medication through the skin is increasingly common, and researchers have learned much about how the skin absorbs substances and when patches are better than medication by mouth. By getting medication into the body through the skin's blood vessels rather than by mouth, patches can bypass any loss of drug by its absorption in the gastrointestinal (GI) tract and prevent any damage the drug might do to the GI tract.

How do moisture and heat help with absorption? The wetter the skin, the greater the absorption, as the water enables molecules which are carried to the stratum corneum to diffuse through it into the capillaries, which are just 0.2mm underneath the skin surface. Hydrated skin is three times more likely to absorb substances in a drug patch. Warmer skin also absorbs more medication, because when the capillaries of the skin are dilated substances are absorbed into the blood vessels of the dermis and, from there, into deeper tissues. One study found people who wore drug patches in a sauna absorbed more of the drug (Hao, 2016). A hot Epsom salts bath or a mustard plaster combines moisture and heat in much the same way.

Dangerously hot water can prompt a withdrawal reflex (yanking the hand out out of the water) before the signal even gets as far as the brain. Our bodies are constantly reporting how the circulatory system is functioning, and, based upon that information, the brain monitors and adjusts how hard and fast the heart is beating, which vessels are open or closed, what the blood pressure is, and even the chemical makeup of our blood. These corrections are sometimes achieved with direct nerve impulses to change the activity in an area, but the brain often directs a hormone to be secreted which will cause the desired changes. For example, norepinephrine and epinephrine are two stress hormones that affect the circulatory system: the first causes vasoconstriction, and the second dilates

blood vessels in skeletal muscles. Both ready the body to run from an enemy or to stand and fight.

Central nervous system

The brain and the spinal cord make up the central nervous system. The spinal cord extends from the base of the brain to the bottom of the spine, and consists of grey matter (the cell bodies of nerve cells and their millions of dendrites) and white matter (nerve fibers that carry nerve impulses up and down the cord). Cranial nerves also bring the brain sensory information about touch, sound, taste, sight and smell. Although the brain makes up only a small fraction of our total body weight, it has very high

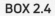

BOX 2.4	POINT OF INTEREST

TEMPERATURE RECEPTORS CAN BE FOOLED

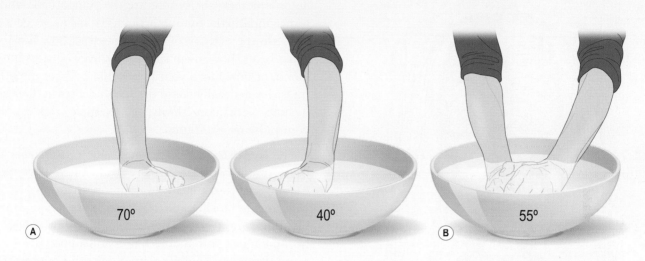

FIGURE 1
Figures **A** and **B** Temperature receptors can be fooled.

Put a bowl of 70°F water and a bowl of 40°F water on a table. Put a hand in each. After about one minute, put both hands in a bowl of 55°F water. The hand that was in the 70°F water will perceive that the 55°F water is cold, and the hand that was in the 40°F water will feel that the 55°F water is warm. This experiment shows that the receptors in the skin which sense temperature are better at sensing *changes* in temperature than absolute temperatures. The receptors that were in the hot water got used to that temperature, so the neutral water felt cold; and the receptors that were in the cold water got used to that temperature, so the neutral water felt hot! This explains why, when a person first gets into a moderately hot bath it feels burning hot at first, but soon feels comfortably warm—and why when a person first jumps into a cool (not cold) swimming pool, the water feels freezing cold, but soon feels comfortably cool.

metabolic needs and actually uses 20% of all the body's oxygen and other nutrients. The brain receives first priority when it comes to available blood supply.

Peripheral nervous system

The peripheral nervous system is a network of smaller nerves that branch out from the brain and spinal cord and reach every part of the body. Each spinal nerve has both a sensory and a motor tract: sensory information is carried to the brain, and motor signals are carried from the brain back out to the muscles. Sensations such as hot and cold,

pressure or injury can travel at about 300 feet per second. In a six- foot tall person, this means a message can travel from the feet to the brain in one-fiftieth of a second!

Autonomic nervous system

The autonomic nervous system controls the visceral functions of the body and is made up of various parts within the brain, spinal cord, and peripheral nerves. It continually checks and adjusts conditions inside the body such as blood chemistry, temperature and water balance. It helps control functions such as breathing, movement,

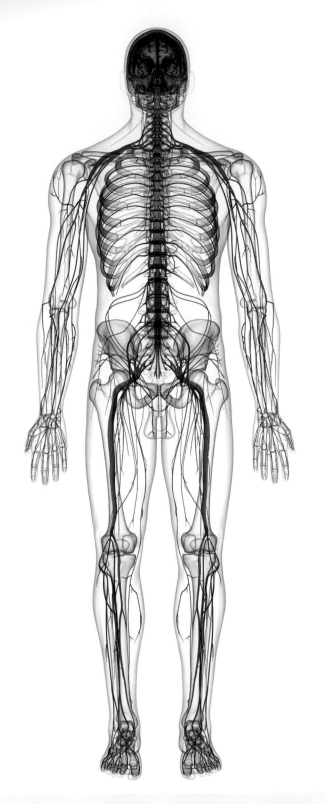

FIGURE 2.8
The nervous system.

digestion, vision, heart action, and making energy available for life processes. Adjustments can be made very quickly by this system: for example, if you suddenly need to run away from an angry tiger, your heart rate can double and your systolic blood pressure rise dramatically in as little as 5 seconds! The two major subdivisions of the autonomic nervous system are the sympathetic and the parasympathetic. Sympathetic nerve messages generally increase the activity of organs, such as how hard your heart beats, how much sugar your liver releases into the blood, or how much your pupils dilate. Parasympathetic messages generally cause organs to decrease their activity and work more slowly, for example, slowing down your pulse or respirations.

The **hypothalamus**, a small part of the lower front brain that is considered the central controller of the autonomic nervous system, contains an area that is specialized for monitoring and adjusting body temperature. If blood flowing through this area is hotter or cooler than normal, the hypothalamus senses and adjusts the temperature through a combination of defensive actions. If the core temperature increases by 0.5°F (-0.17°C), the hypothalamus initiates dilation of surface blood vessels. If this does not raise temperature enough, its next instructions activate glands. If the core temperature falls by 32.9°F (0.5°C), shivering begins. There is also a "thirst center" that monitors the amount of water in the blood and acts to correct it if necessary.

Reflexes

Using reflexes to affect different areas of the body is a fascinating aspect of hydrotherapy. Over many years of careful observation, old-time hydrotherapists learned how to take advantage of the body's reflex responses to enhance healing. **Reflexes** are simple nerve circuits between muscles and the spinal cord in response to sensory stimuli: as a result, body movements occur rapidly that may help to avert possible danger. Reflexes are involuntary and cannot be learned (Figure 2.9). For example, if something touches your eyeball, sensory nerve impulses speed into the spinal cord, then motor nerve impulses go directly back to nearby muscles and cause your eye to blink, and the entire process takes only a split second. Other impulses also travel up the cord to the brain, making the mind aware of what just happened, but these are too late to stop the reflex from taking place. Many of our

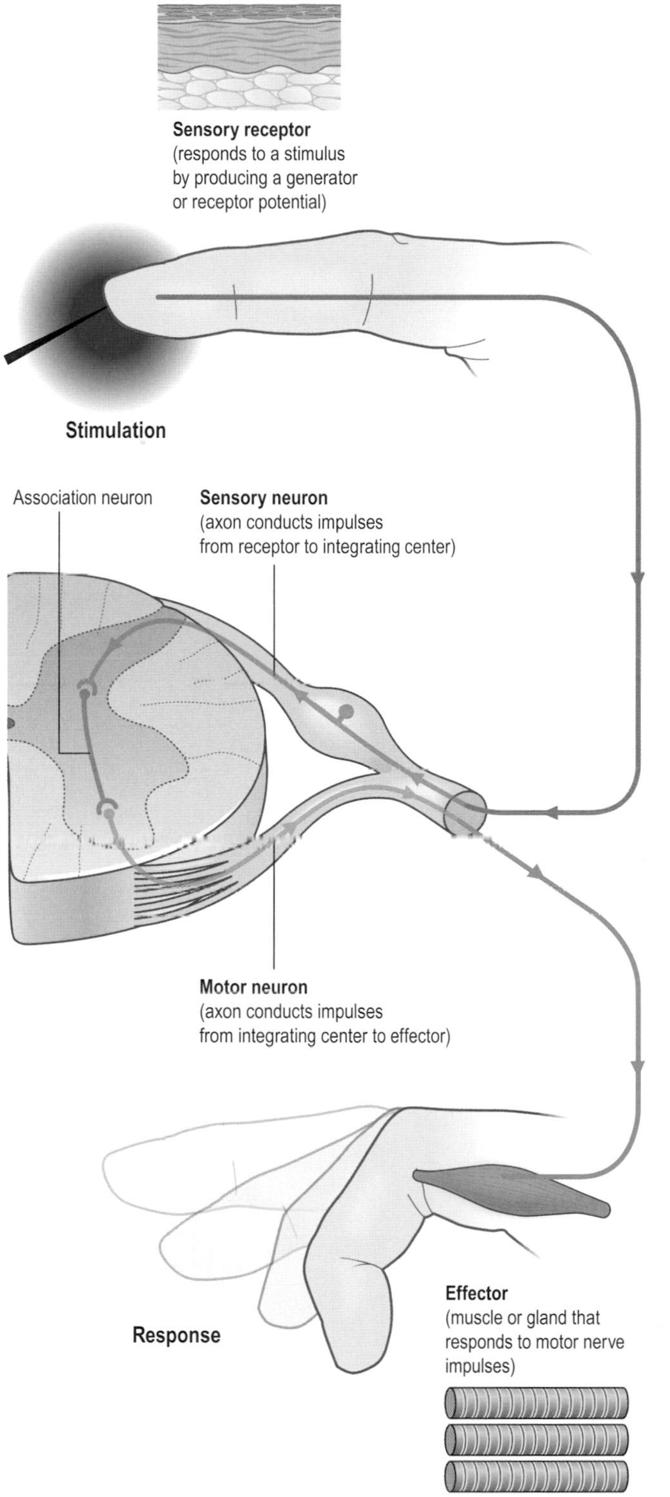

Sensory receptor
(responds to a stimulus by producing a generator or receptor potential)

Stimulation

Association neuron

Sensory neuron
(axon conducts impulses from receptor to integrating center)

Motor neuron
(axon conducts impulses from integrating center to effector)

Effector
(muscle or gland that responds to motor nerve impulses)

Response

FIGURE 2.9
Reflex reaction.

body functions rely upon reflexes, most of which we are not even aware of. Common reflexes include:

1. the gag reflex

2. blushing, dilation of facial blood vessels with psychological stress

3. blinking when something touches the eyeball

4. pulling the hand back after touching something hot

5. knee-jerk reflex, a sudden kicking movement (quadriceps twitch) when the kneecap is tapped lightly

6. dilation of skin capillaries when the skin is exposed to hot water or a hot object

7. sneezing when in contact with dust or allergens.

How does this information relate to hydrotherapy? Because the skin and the internal organs underneath both receive their sensory innervation from the same segment of the spinal cord, applications of heat or cold to skin areas reflexly related to the viscera can influence their function. Internal organs are usually reflexly related to the skin directly over them, but every part of the skin surface is also reflexly related to some internal organ or vascular area (Figure 2.10). An application of heat or cold to the skin will affect the tissue directly under it to a much greater extent than it affects the reflexly related organ – for example, an ice bag applied over the stomach may cause a brief change in the size of the blood vessels of the brain, but the greatest effect will be on the abdominal muscle directly under the ice. While massage therapists do not apply heat or cold for extended periods of time and only treat problems in body systems other than the musculoskeletal, it is still helpful for us to understand how the body works as a whole, and how to take advantage of the body's reflex relationships when performing hydrotherapy treatments.

PHYSIOLOGICAL EFFECTS OF HEAT AND COLD

When the air temperature is 82°F (28°C), a naked person who is not moving generates exactly as much heat through metabolic processes as he or she loses through radiation, and no additional effort is needed to maintain a 98.6°F (37°C) core temperature. Although 98.6°F is the ideal temperature for vital organs deep in the body, tissues nearer the body surface are cooler: normally 94°F (34.4°C) for muscle tissues, 92°F (33.3°C) for subcutaneous tissues, and 90°F (32.2°C) for the skin. The body

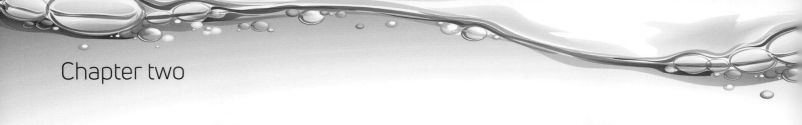

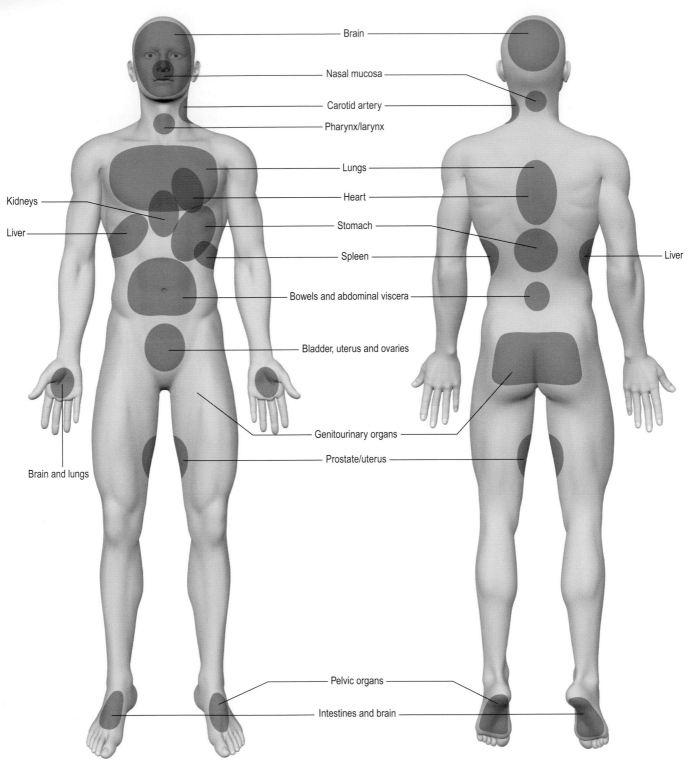

FIGURE 2.10
Skin areas reflexly connected to specific organs and parts of the body.

constantly makes adjustments to maintain the right temperature in each part of the body. (Most hydrotherapy treatments are thermal: that is, they use temperatures above or below normal body temperature. Hot and cold treatments can cause dramatic changes in the blood vessels, chiefly **vasodilation**, widening of the blood vessels, or **vasoconstriction,** narrowing of the blood vessels – (see Figure 2.11.)

Because the circulatory system is a closed system and the amount of fluid in it does not change, changes in the sizes of blood vessels in one area of the body can affect the entire system. Any time that one or more "pipes" becomes larger through vasodilation or smaller through vasoconstriction, fluid has to be redistributed within the system. For example, when the blood vessels in the feet are widely dilated by a hot footbath, more blood flows that direction. Then, as there are only five quarts (five liters) of blood in the person's circulatory system, and a large portion of that amount just shifted into the vessels in the feet, other regions of the body will experience a reduced blood flow. Immersion in a hot bath causes widespread dilation of skin vessels, and as more blood flows to the skin there is less blood available to flow to the brain. This is why a bather may become lightheaded. Putting an ice pack on the back of the head causes vasoconstriction, and may relieve migraine pain by shifting blood flow away from swollen cranial vessels. Old-time hydrotherapists used this closed-system principle in many of their treatments, and termed these actions **derivation** (increasing blood flow in another area of the body) or **depletion** (decreasing blood flow in another area of the body).

Whole-body heat

Whole-body heat treatments have a number of distinct effects on the body which are often linked together in a chain of reactions. For instance, when a person is immersed in a hot bath, the skin temperature quickly begins to rise, which stimulates the heat receptors in the skin, which begin to relay that information to the brain. Sympathetic nervous system activity causes blood vessels under the skin to contract, so there is a small rise in blood pressure. As the heat penetrates further, more tissue heats up, sympathetic activity decreases, blood vessels near the body's surface dilate, and deeper arteries contract while warm blood radiates excess heat from the skin. At this point, as much as two

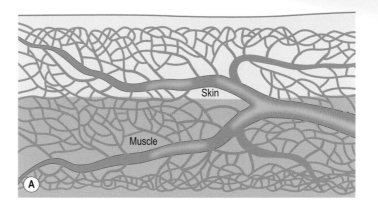

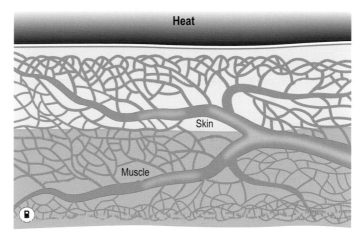

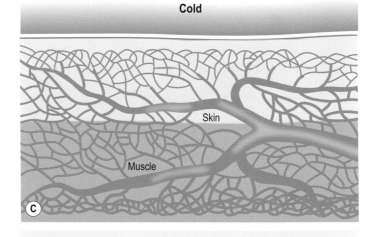

FIGURE 2.11

The effects of hot and cold applications on the blood vessels of the skin and underlying muscles. **(A)** Before application. **(B)** After hot application. **(C)** After cold application.

thirds of the body's total blood supply is in the skin's blood vessels so the skin becomes pinker. When a person is in a neutral-temperature environment, the heart pumps approximately 1 quart (1 liter) of blood to the skin every minute, but when that same person becomes overheated, the amount can increase to 6 quarts (6 liters) per minute! When the body responds by dilating so many blood vessels, it is like a tank that has suddenly become larger. The circulatory system can now hold more blood, and that blood is therefore under less pressure. After a 10-minute immersion in a 104°F (40°C) hot bath, blood pressure falls an average of 28 points systolic and 25 points diastolic (Shin, 2003). At the same time, the heart beats faster in order to maintain blood supply to body tissues, as well as to send more warm blood to the skin for heat loss.

If the core temperature still continues to rise, so does the heart's efforts to pump blood to the skin more quickly: for every 1 degree that the core temperature increases, the pulse goes up about 10 beats per minute. In a hot environment such as a hot bath, total cardiac output can increase by 60–70% compared to that of a neutral environment (see Case histories 2.2 and 2.3). During fever treatments, which involve periods of prolonged immersion in very hot water (104–108°F; 40–42.2°C), a person's heart rate may double. As the heart pumps faster and faster, there is not time for it to completely refill after each beat, and so it pumps less blood each time. Although sweating can normally cool the body a great deal, it is less effective in this case because the skin is surrounded by hot water and no heat can be lost through evaporation of sweat. Breathing also adapts, speeding up as the body works to eliminate heat through the lungs: for every degree the core temperature rises, the bather will take 5–6 more breaths

---

THE HOT BATH HOMEWORK ASSIGNMENT   CASE HISTORY 2.2

BACKGROUND

Sixteen students in a hydrotherapy class were given a homework assignment: to study the effects of a hot bath on their physical and emotional states. Each student recorded his or her pulse, respiratory rate and oral temperature three times: first, before getting into a hot bath, second, after 20 minutes in the hot bath, and finally after getting out of the bath, then having a cold shower and 30-minute rest period.

FINDINGS

When the class assembled again, each student shared his or her experience, and the teacher wrote the change in their vital signs on the board. Almost all reported that at the end of the 20 minutes in the hot bath, their heart rates had increased significantly, their oral temperature rose by at least 1 degree Fahrenheit, and their respirations were faster. Human skin blood flow can range from almost zero in extreme cold to 60% of the total cardiac output in very hot conditions. The only exceptions were students who were taking baths that were much cooler than their normal bath, students who were very cold when they got into the bath, or students who could not keep their bathwater warm. For those students, their heart rates, respirations and core temperatures did not rise, because their bodies never became sufficiently warmed by the bath water.

In addition to the information on vital signs, all students except two reported that they felt much more relaxed mentally afterwards, and many fell asleep. The two who did not feel relaxed were the ones who could not keep their bathwater warm and were chilled and tense when they left the bath.

Along with these similarities were some surprising differences. Preferred bath temperature varied widely among the students: one reported his comfortable bath temperature was 98°F (36.7°C), while another's was 108°F (42.2°C). One student felt so hot when he got out of the tub that he almost fainted, and the cold shower felt wonderful to him; while another student forgot to take the cold shower, cooled off rapidly in the cold air, and soon began to feel quite cold. The two who never became sufficiently warm in the bath found the cold shower extremely unpleasant.

DISCUSSION QUESTIONS

1. Why did the student who forgot to take the cold shower cool off rapidly?

2. What does the case history tell us about the best way to help a client take a safe and effective hot bath?

| A CLIENT WITH STRESS AND HIGH BLOOD PRESSURE | CASE HISTORY 2.3 |

BACKGROUND

45-year-old Sangheeta has a very stressful job as a high-level administrator at a large university. She receives Swedish massage on a regular basis to help her relax and relieve chronic back pain from an old injury. She is currently taking her blood pressure numerous times a day, and has found that it goes up when she is stressed and goes down (and her "stress headache" disappears) each time she takes a long hot bath. When she arrives for a session at the end of one particularly stressful day, her blood pressure reading is 150/89. After her whole-body Swedish massage, her reading drops to 119/85. Other sessions follow a similar pattern, with her readings changing from 134/80 to 118/80 one day, and from 141/89 to 117/65 on another. However, if

Sangheeta's session is on a Sunday afternoon after she has had a relaxing weekend, her blood pressure is lower at the start of the session, and her blood pressure is not significantly different afterwards (125/75 followed by 124/71).

DISCUSSION QUESTIONS

1. How does stress cause Sangheeta's blood pressure to rise?

2. How would a hot bath relieve a high blood pressure headache?

3. Explain the effect of massage on Sangheeta's blood pressure, and why it is not as pronounced after a relaxing weekend.

TABLE 2.1 The effects of whole-body heat treatments versus short whole-body heat treatments		
	Long whole-body heat treatment	**Short whole-body heat treatment**
Duration	Longer than 5 minutes	5 minutes or less
Vasodilation	Complete	Not complete
Redness of skin	Present	Present
Heart rate	Increased	Decreases initially
Stroke volume	Decreased	No significant increase
Systolic blood pressure	Normal or decreased	No significant increase
Respiratory rate	Increased	Decreased
Muscle tone	Decreased	Increased
Blood flow	Up to 400% faster	No significant increase
Sweating	Profuse	None
Migration of white blood cells	Increased	No significant increase
Core temperature	Elevated	No change
Primary effect	Thermal, actual warming of the tissues	Stimulation of nervous system (tissue not significantly heated yet)
Physiological effect	Depressant and excitant	Depressant

per minute. Should he or she begin to hyperventilate, the oxygen saturation in the blood will rise as well. The number of white blood cells in the general circulation rises significantly, and remains that way for at least a few hours. This is the reason that whole-body heating treatments have been used for some immune system disorders (see Appendix C).

Connective tissue softens and muscles relax as they warm, so musculoskeletal pain is often greatly reduced. A very short hot bath or shower will not raise the core temperature very much, however, and thus will produce very different effects than a longer one. A summary of the physiological effects of both long and short whole-body heat treatments is presented in Table 2.1.

Local heat

Using moist heat on small areas can soften muscles and other soft tissues before they are massaged or manipulated while relieving muscle and joint pain. Because hot packs, water bottles, local baths, compresses, moist towels and moist heating pads are applied directly on the skin, it absorbs most of the heat, but deeper tissues gradually warm as well. If the application is hot enough, it takes about 15 minutes to fully penetrate muscles, depending upon how dense the tissue is. Heat can also penetrate joints that are not covered with much soft tissue, like those in the hands and feet. The client's initial skin temperature also makes a difference: for example, if a hot fomentation is put over an area that has just been iced, it takes longer to heat the tissues underneath than if the area was warm to begin with. The hotter the area becomes, the greater the reaction: every time a limb becomes 4 degrees warmer, its blood supply doubles. Blood flows from other parts of the body to supply the warm area and radiate more heat off its surface (Petrofsky, 2003). These reactions are caused by the local effects of temperature directly on the blood vessels and sweat glands, as well as by spinal cord reflexes conducted from the skin receptors to the spinal cord and back (Figure 2.12).

Below are some of the body's protective reactions to local heat:

1. Sensory nerves are stimulated and cause local vasodilation. Not only is blood flow to the area under the heat increased, but the blood itself grows warmer; when it is carried off to other areas of the body, this also prevents overheating. If the application is too hot, of course, even vasodilation will not prevent tissue damage.

2. Local sweating.

3. As heat sinks in, dilation of deeper blood vessels in muscle tissue. Local muscle blood flow can triple.

4. Reduced muscle tension, tone, spasm and pain. For this reason, hot packs applied to trigger points can reduce pain when they are pressed on.

5. Increased local metabolic rate.

6. Increased oxygen delivery to tissues.

7. Heat applied to one limb causes vasodilation to the other limb as well. This is known as the **contralateral reflex effect.** The effect will not be as strong in that limb, however.

8. Increase in core temperature if the application is very large or very hot.

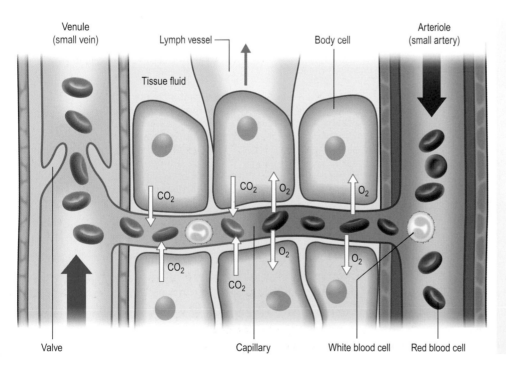

FIGURE 2.12
Supplying the cells with nutrients. Red blood cells pass from the arteriole to the venule, dropping off oxygen and other nutrients, and picking up carbon dioxide for elimination.

9. Reflex effects of prolonged heat on deeper organs include dilation of the blood vessels where the application is actually placed, as well as in related viscera. Deep internal organs are more influenced by reflex effects than by actual changes in the temperature of the tissues. For example:

    • Prolonged heat to the abdominal wall causes decreased intestinal blood flow, decreased intestinal movement, and decreased production of stomach acid.

    • Prolonged heat over the lower abdominal wall causes an increased production of urine.

    • Prolonged heat to the chest makes breathing and expectoration easier.

    • Prolonged heat over the kidneys increases production of urine.

    • Prolonged heat over the pelvis relaxes the muscles of the bladder, rectum and uterus, dilates their blood vessels, and can increase menstrual flow.

    • Prolonged heat over the **precordium** increases the heart rate and decreases its force.

Whole-body cold

The body has twenty times as many receptors for cold as for heat, showing that the body is more vigilant about the core temperature going down than going up. Cold receptors are stimulated the most when the surface of the skin is below 77°F (25°C), but stop working when the skin temperature is below 41°F (5°C). Because the body also reacts to cold temperatures more vigorously than to hot temperatures, cold treatments are more stimulating than hot ones. For example, a warm bath is far more relaxing than an icy-cold shower, but the longest-lasting feeling of warmth comes when the bath is followed by a cold shower.

When you first get into a cold bath or shower and the skin over the entire body comes into contact with cold water, the cold receptors in the skin fire, and the nervous and circulatory systems quickly respond. Reflexes immediately increase the temperature of the body by shivering, inhibiting sweating and constricting skin blood vessels. As the blood vessels in the skin constrict (reflex action), the sympathetic nervous system kicks in: blood pressure rises, muscle tone increases, and the heart begins to pump out more blood with each stroke.

If you get out of the water after only one minute, you feel invigorated. The generalized vasoconstriction floods your internal organs with nutrient-carrying blood, and your entire metabolism is stimulated. Then, a reactive vasodilation of the blood vessels in the skin gives you a prolonged sensation of warmth. These changes will last for a few hours. Your body rose to the challenge of maintaining a healthy core temperature by increasing many body functions, and the amount of time you were in the water was not long enough to cause any actual chilling. So, with a brief exposure, cold immersion has been stimulating, not depressing.

If you stay in the water longer, however, an entirely different reaction will take place. Vasoconstriction of blood vessels at the periphery of the body (skin and muscles of the arms and legs) keeps blood near to the body core, but the little that is coming back from the periphery is cold, and gradually that will reduce the core temperature. If the cold is too extreme, the core temperature decreases and the entire metabolism slows down: breathing and heart rate slow, the muscles become clumsier and harder to move, the receptors in the skin do not work as well, and thinking becomes muddied. Clients who are in cold showers or baths too long may begin to experience this chilling and will be highly uncomfortable: shivering and pale, they are likely to be tense, cross, and difficult to warm.

If they continue in cold water, the body can become colder and colder, and an even more extreme reaction can happen. When the muscles in the blood vessels run out of oxygen and other nutrients, they dilate because they are unable to constrict anymore, the cold blood on the surface of the body returns to the body core, and real hypothermia sets in. Cold has become a depressant rather than a stimulant. Interestingly, induced hypothermia has actually been used by Russian doctors as a way of depressing body functions to allow open-heart surgery without a heart–lung machine, as is done in the West (Figure 2.13). A summary of the physiological effects of long and short whole-body cold treatments is presented in Table 2.2.

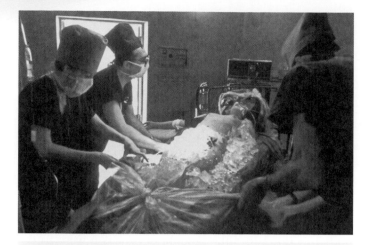

FIGURE 2.13
A 12-year-old girl being packed in ice before open-heart surgery, Novosibersk, Russia, 1994. Photo by Heidi Bradner, reprinted with permission from Panos Pictures, London, England. As the ice cools this girl's body, her core temperature and heart rate will slowly drop, her metabolism will slow down greatly, and eventually her heart will stop beating altogether. When her core temperature has reached 84°F (29°C), her heart can be safely operated on without a heart–lung machine, because her cells' demands for oxygen and other nutrients has been reduced to almost zero, and therefore her brain and other vital organs can survive for an extended period of time without her heart supplying them with blood.

Effects of local cold treatments

Applications of local cold to small portions of the body are powerful tools to help reduce edema, numb painful areas, and prepare muscles, joints and other soft tissues to be massaged or manipulated. These reactions are caused by spinal cord reflexes and by the direct effect of cold touching blood vessels and sweat glands.

Because local cold applications are applied on the surface of the skin, their greatest cooling effect takes place there, on the subcutaneous tissues underneath the skin to a lesser degree, and finally, if the application is cold enough, on the muscles underneath. Ligaments that are not covered with dense tissue may also become very cold, affecting how well a sprained joint will heal.

These responses may vary to some extent, depending on how cold the skin is at the beginning, how cold

the application is, and how long it is left on. For example, if you want to cool an area with an ice pack, it will take longer if the area is already very warm. Local cold penetrates far more deeply than local heat, as once the small blood vessels are constricted, less warm blood can flow from the heart into the area. Table 2.3 compares the effects of local cold and hot treatments. When tissues are cooled for a long time, vasodilation will occur intermittently. For example, when fingers are immersed in an ice-water bath, their skin temperature will decrease for 15 minutes. Then, however, when the tissue becomes cold enough that it might become damaged – about 59°F (15°C) – arterioles react to preserve the tissue by dilating for long enough to raise the tissue temperature and supply the tissue with some nutrients. This is known as the reactive vasodilation or the "hunting reaction." No treatments in this book will use extremely long, cold applications that could lead to this reaction. Below are some of the body's reactions to local cold:

1. Sympathetic nervous system stimulation occurs as a result of the cold input to the cold receptors in the skin, resulting in increased levels of norepinephrine, vasopressin, angiotensin and other hormones.

2. Constriction occurs in many skin blood vessels. This shuts off much of the blood flow to the chilled areas, just as shutting off a faucet cuts off water flowing into a hose. The skin becomes pale and white due to the reduced blood flow. A hand immersed in a 41°F (5°C) cold water bath for 30 minutes will have a 78% decrease in blood flow (Kamler, 2002). Meanwhile internal blood vessels nearer to the heart are filled with more blood, and so dilate. This is an example of **depletion.**

3. Constriction of blood vessels in muscle tissues as the cold penetrates deeper. In the case of an immersed hand, reflex vasoconstriction will occur in the other hand as well. One study found that after ten minutes of ice packs, blood flow in the knee joints of dogs had halved (Michlovitz, 1996).

4. In a limb, cold applied to that limb will cause vasodilation to the other limb as well. This is known as the **contralateral reflex** effect.

5. When local cold treatments are given on a regular basis, such as a hand being regularly immersed

TABLE 2.2 Comparing and contrasting the effects of long whole-body cold treatments versus short cold whole-body treatments

	Longer than one minute whole-body cold treatment (cold-water bath or plunge; cold shower)	One minute or less whole-body cold treatment (cold-water bath or plunge; cold shower)
Vasoconstriction	Initially vasoconstriction is present, but when the body is completely chilled, muscles of blood vessels are without oxygen and cannot contract	Peripheral vasoconstriction followed by vasodilation
Circulation	Slower	Increased
Heart rate	Decreased	Decreased
Speed of nerve conduction	Decreased	Increased
Skin sensitivity	Decreased	Increased
Muscle effects	Sluggish and clumsy	Toned
Sensation	Cold	Warm
Blood pressure	Decreased	Increased
Shivering	Begins once the body is chilled, continues until too cold to continue	No shivering
Metabolism	Decreased	Increased
Migration of leukocytes through capillary wall	Decreased	No change
Physiological effect	Depressant	Stimulant
Core temperature	Decreased	Slightly increased or no change

TABLE 2.3 Comparison of effects of prolonged local applications of hot and cold

Effects	Long local heat treatment	Long local cold treatment
Local blood flow	Increased	Decreased
Muscle spasm/guarding	Decreased	Decreased
Local inflammatory response in acute injuries	Increased	Decreased
Joint stiffness in arthritis	Decreased	Decreased
Edema production	Increased	Decreased
Pain	Reduced	Reduced
Metabolic rate	Increased	Decreased
Nerve conduction velocity	Slowed	Slowed
Muscle strength	Reduced	Reduced
Tissue elasticity	Increased	Decreased
Joint stiffness	Decreased	Increased for a very short time, then decreased
Local sweating	Present	Absent

in cold water, the blood vessels contract faster and harder.

6. Reflex effects of cold applications occur directly under the cold and in reflexively related organs as well, and may be used for therapeutic effect. A short cold application to a reflex area causes active dilation of the blood vessels in the related viscera, with tonic and stimulating effects. A long, continuous application of cold affects both the skin and the underlying organs: the blood vessels constrict

during the application and afterwards, nerve conduction is slowed and muscles are firmly contracted. Table 2.4 shows the reflex effects of both short and long applications of local cold on various parts of the body.

In addition to the body's protective mechanisms discussed above, here are some other effects that stem from chilling of tissue and the lack of blood flow:

1. *Lowered temperatures.* Skin temperature will decrease within a minute, followed by cooling of subcutaneous tissue and finally deeper muscle tissue. It can require as long as 30 minutes for ice packs to cool muscle tissue to a depth of 1.6 inches (4cm).

2. *Decreased oxygen to tissues.*

3. *Decreased muscle spasm* due to slowing of motor nerve activity.

4. *Decreased blood flow* to joints and surrounding soft tissues.

5. *Less sensitivity of receptors* for touch, pressure and stretch.

6. *Stiffer, less supple connective tissue.*

7. *Decreased core temperature* if the application is very large or very prolonged.

Contrast treatments

Contrast treatments involve alternating heat with cold in a single treatment. Whole-body contrast applications consist of rapid alternations of whole-body hot and whole-body cold, such as a hot bath followed by a cold plunge, usually repeated three or more times. By combining the advantages of short hot and short cold exposures, they create a dramatic increase in circulation, reflex stimulation of related tissues and organs, decreased musculoskeletal pain, and a strong feeling of invigoration.

Local contrast treatments consist of local heat (fomentation, paraffin dip, hot compress, heat lamp, hot local

TABLE 2.4 Reflex effects of long versus short local cold treatments		
Site of local cold application	**Reflex effects of long cold treatments**	**Reflex effects of short cold treatments**
Face, forehead, scalp, and back of the neck	Contraction of blood vessels of the brain	
Abdominal wall	Increases intestinal blood flow, intestinal movement, and production of stomach acid	
Nose, back of neck, and hands	Contraction of blood vessels of nasal mucosa	
Main trunk of artery	Contraction of the artery and its branches	
Pelvic area	Stimulates muscles of pelvic organs	
Precordium (anterior chest)	Slows heart rate, increases stroke volume	
Acutely inflamed joints or bursae	Contraction of blood vessels and provides pain relief	
Acute injuries such as bruises and sprains	Vasoconstriction and decrease of hemorrhage and edema	
Face and head		Stimulates mental activity
Chest		First increases respiratory rate, then decreases and deepens it
Sacrum or feet		Dilation of the uterine blood vessels
Abdomen, hands, or feet		Constriction of muscles of the bladder, bowel and uterus
Over the liver		Increased liver activity
Stomach		Increased gastric secretion
Over the precordia		Increases rate and force of heartbeat

bath, etc.) followed by local cold (ice packs, ice massage, cold compresses, cold baths or cold mitten frictions), always repeated three or more times. The circulatory effects of short hot applications (vasodilation) are combined with the effects of short cold, and will at least double the resting amount of local blood flow.

When arterioles are dilated by heat, blood flow has a tendency to slow down and congest tissues, but when a cold application causes the arteriole muscles to contract, this has the effect of pushing the increased blood flow through the capillaries and into venules and lymphatic ducts; this temporarily empties the arterioles and creates a suction effect, pulling more fresh blood into the arteries. Contrast baths, therefore, increase local circulation more than hot baths. A contrast footbath increases local circulation more than a hot footbath, and so does a contrast full-body shower compared to a hot one. These changes in circulation can not only be measured with a variety of instruments but can also be seen with the naked eye: the skin turns a much brighter red after a contrast treatment than after a warm application alone. This increase in blood flow is especially marked on the first change from hot to cold, suggesting that the muscles of the arterial walls can become fatigued (Fiscus, 2005).

Contrast applications combine the advantages of heat and cold without their disadvantages: for example, while hot applications increase circulation, they can also promote congestion and edema; and while cold applications decrease edema, they also decrease local blood flow and deprive tissues of oxygen and other nutrients. However, when hot applications are combined with cold applications in a contrast treatment, local circulation is greatly increased without increasing edema.

While some of these circulatory changes may seem so transitory that they could not have any long-term effect, they can actually be significant for someone with a circulatory problem if performed on a regular basis. For example, patients with varicose veins who received alternating hot and cold showers to the legs for a period of 25 days experienced significant improvements in the circulation to their legs, and this effect lasted one month or more (Saradeth, 1991).

Almost everyone who receives a local contrast treatment reports a strong feeling of invigoration and relaxation in the area, and often considerable pain relief as well. Contrast treatments complement bodywork, since both enhance circulation, relieve tension and musculoskeletal pain, and provide sensory stimulation (see Case history 2.4).

Neutral treatments

Neutral treatments are neither hot nor cold: in a neutral bath, the water is 94–98°F (35–37°C). Neutral baths, showers and body wraps have traditionally been used for sedative purposes because they are very soothing and non-stimulating. With nothing to stimulate thermal receptors and little or no mechanical stimulation or noise, a tense person may be able to truly relax. Unlike a hot or a cold treatment, the person's temperature and vital signs remain stable.

PHYSIOLOGICAL EFFECTS OF MECHANICAL AND CHEMICAL TREATMENTS

Like hot and cold treatments, mechanical and chemical treatments provide an extra tool for the massage therapist to achieve his or her therapeutic goals, and are often much enjoyed by clients.

Mechanical treatments

There are two types of **mechanical treatments**:, those that use friction on the skin, and those that use water to apply pressure on the skin. Early hydrotherapists often prescribed friction treatments to stimulate both nerve reaction and blood and lymphatic circulation, thus increasing the effects of heat and cold. For example, an overheated patient who was put in a cold bath might be rubbed vigorously with a cold wet cloth to bring blood nearer to the surface, where heat could be lost through the skin. Bedridden patients might be given a cold mitten friction or a salt glow to stimulate the circulation of blood and lymph one would normally get from physical exercise. Salt glows, brushings and cold mitten frictions have a stimulating effect that is similar to tapotement and vibration strokes.

Percussion treatments include showers, tubs with jets, and sprays. When something strikes the skin, the body reacts defensively: muscle tone and nerve reaction

Chapter two

THE FLUID-SHIFTING EFFECT OF A CONTRAST TREATMENT TO THE LEG CASE HISTORY 2.4

BACKGROUND

Janet was a healthy, athletic, 57-year old biologist. She usually received massage once a month for chronic neck and shoulder tension and general wellness. One day she came to her massage therapist with a specific problem: she was experiencing pain and edema in her left lower leg. There was a reddish blotch about the size of a quarter on her left lower leg, just medial to the tibia. Her doctor had already evaluated her thoroughly, ruled out bone disease, injury, and phlebitis, and approved massage and hydrotherapy: he suspected Janet had a ruptured varicose vein that was leaking blood.

TREATMENT

The massage therapist noticed that the affected left lower leg was noticeably larger than the right. Gentle pressure with an index finger along the left tibia produced dents that remained for some time, a condition known as pitting edema, and Janet's hamstring muscles were also swollen to the touch. Janet lay in the prone position, and the massage therapist performed 5 minutes of effleurage and petrissage on her left hamstring muscles. They checked her leg at this point, and noted a slight reduction of lower leg edema and a distinct lightening of the color in the discolored area. Janet's hamstring muscles also felt less swollen to her. Another 5 minutes of massage was performed on Janet's gluteal muscles while she was still in the prone position, followed by massage of her quadriceps muscles while she was supine. Another reduction of edema and lightening of coloring in the blotch was noted by both therapist and

client. Clearly the massage had dilated the blood and lymphatic vessels in Janet's upper leg.

The massage therapist then began a mild contrast treatment of the lower leg. She had already heated a gel pack in hot water and she now placed it on the entire medial surface of the left tibia. It was covered with a dry towel to keep it from cooling off and left for 2 minutes. Then the therapist removed the hot pack and performed ice massage over the area for 1 minute. This round of hot-followed-by-cold was repeated four times. When the therapist was not placing the gel packs or performing ice massage, she massaged Janet's head and neck.

Each time the hot or cold was changed, Janet's leg was evaluated again. The discolored area became slightly lighter-colored after each application, and the entire area gradually became pinker. After the last hot and cold round, the area was a healthy pink, the ankle was back to its normal size, and the discolored area could no longer be seen. Janet felt no pain in the area. Note that no hands-on massage was performed over the lower leg.

DISCUSSION QUESTIONS

1. Explain the change in appearance of Janet's lower leg.
2. What does the case history tell us about the fluid-shifting effect of contrast treatments?
3. Why was a contrast treatment of the lower leg a better way to affect circulation than using massage techniques?

increase, and the area's blood vessels dilate. John Harvey Kellogg described the mechanical effect of a strong stream of water on the skin in these words: "… At the exact point upon which the column of water falls, the skin becomes instantly blanched, the color re-appearing as soon as the stream is allowed to fall on any other part … The blood-vessels are not only made to contract by the thermic impression of the water, but the weight of the stream of water, the force of the impact, compresses the tissues and forces the blood out of the vessels, leaving them free to dilate again as soon as the pressure is

removed. Thus the tissues are alternately compressed and released … the thermic effect of the douche is thus materially aided by the mechanical or percussion effects of the moving water … A powerful reflex effect is produced by the stimulation of the various sets of nerves which recognize temperature, pressure, pain, and tactile impressions" (Kellogg, 1923).

The effects of mechanical treatments are difficult to measure, and perhaps have to be felt to be truly appreciated. They are most often performed to increase the thermal, fluid-shifting, and nervous system effects of other hydrotherapy treatments. If one treatment employs hot or cold water, mechanical stimulation may also help warm or cool the tissue faster. For example, a cold mitten friction keeps the cold water in contact with the skin even better than simply laying a cold towel over the skin. Whirlpool jets keep hot water in contact with the skin far more than still water. These treatments also provide a great deal of sensory stimulation and many massage clients enjoy them. They are less appropriate for clients who are highly sensitive or tactile-defensive. Examples of whole-body treatments that rely on mechanical stimulation:

- exfoliating treatments such as salt glows, cold mitten frictions and dry brushing

- sprays, showers and whirlpool jets (Europe)

- massage balls, rollers and percussion vibrators.

Chemical treatments

Chemical-containing substances can be dissolved in water and then applied to the skin using compresses, poultices, packs, ice massage, steam inhalation, local baths, or whole-body baths. Each chemical has a separate and distinct effect upon the skin or deeper tissues, and effects vary widely. Below are a few of the most common substances used in hydrotherapy treatments, along with their effects:

- Oatmeal contains essential fatty acids and other chemicals that have a soothing and re-moisturizing effect upon the skin itself. It is used in full-body baths and body wraps.

- Essential oil of eucalyptus contains terpene alcohols and other chemicals that give it anti-inflammatory, expectorant and anti-viral actions. Eucalyptus and other essential oils can be applied through local baths, steam inhalations, compresses, ice massage, and full-body baths.

- Dried or fresh herbs contain a wide variety of chemicals and are used in steam inhalations, compresses, ice massage, and various kinds of baths.

- Mustard seed powder, used in baths and plasters, contains allylglucosinolates that cause dilation of the blood vessels of the skin and thus relieve muscular and skeletal pain. Capsaicin, used in compresses, baths and massage lotions, is the pungent ingredient in cayenne pepper. It binds to vanilloid receptors on nerve endings and causes both vasodilation and a sensation of heat. It is used in compresses, fomentations and baths. For more information about the use of herbal preparations in massage practice, see Box 12.4 (page 306).

CHAPTER SUMMARY

In this chapter, you have reviewed the anatomy and physiology of several body systems that are key to hydrotherapy. You have also learned how the body's natural defenses can be used to our clients' advantage. You have learned, too, how the body responds to hot and cold, and to mechanical and chemical treatments. Making use of the body's own talents, hydrotherapy treatments help provide our clients with such benefits as overall relaxation, increased pliability of tissue, increased local circulation, pain relief, reduction of muscle spasm and plain old enjoyment. In the next chapter, we move on to learning how to get ready to perform a wide variety of these treatments.

REVIEW QUESTIONS

Short answer

1. Name six different sensations for which there are separate receptors in the skin.

2. Give an example of a reflex and explain how it keeps the body out of danger.

3. Explain the physiological effects of whole-body and local exposure to heat.

4. Explain the physiological effects of whole-body and local exposure to cold.

Fill in the blanks

5. Prolonged applications of heat can cause _____ of blood vessels in the area where it is actually placed, as well as in _____.

6. The brain has to constantly receive a high proportion of the body's entire blood supply because it has high _____ needs and an inability to store _____.

7. A neutral bath is relaxing due to its lack of _____.

Multiple choice

8. The circulatory system protects the body's:

   A. Core temperature

   B. Skin temperature

   C. Blood supply to the brain

   D. All of the above

9. The body's immediate response to a drop in skin temperature is:

   A. Vasodilation of skin blood vessels

   B. Increased blood flow to the brain

   C. Vasoconstriction of skin blood vessels

   D. Sweating

10. Reflexes are useful because they increase the speed at which the body reacts to external threats such as:

    A. High heat

    B. Blood loss

    C. Object in the eye

    D. All of the above

11. An application of ice can relieve pain and muscle spasm. Which of these does it *not* affect?

    A. The skin

    B. The spinal cord and brain

    C. The digestive system

    D. The muscles

Matching

12.

1.	Artery	A.	Carries blood towards the heart
2.	Valve	B.	Most plentiful vessel in body
3.	Lymph	C.	Contains oxygenated blood
4.	Vein	D.	Found in blood vessels going against gravity
5.	Capillary	E.	Tissue fluid

REVIEW QUESTIONS *continued*

13.

1. Brain
2. Reflex arc
3. Parasympathetic
4. Peripheral
5. Hypothalamus

A. Autonomic nervous system
B. Temperature center
C. Central
D. Far away from center of body
E. Shortcut

14.

1. Mechanical
2. Thermal
3. Fluid-shifting
4. Chemical

A. Absorption into or through skin
B. Stimulation of skin and nerves
C. Redistribution of blood or lymph
D. Warming or cooling of tissue

Chapter two

References

Allen MT, Patterson SM. Hemoconcentration and stress: a review of physiological mechanisms and relevance for cardiovascular disease risk. Biol Psychol 1995; 41(1):1–27

Andreone B et al. Neuronal and vascular interaction. Ann Rev Neurosci 2015; 38: 25–46

Benson H. Body temperature changes during the practice of g-Tummo yoga. Nature 1982; 295: 234–6

Brown F et al. The role of skin absorption as a route of absorption for volatile organic compounds (VOCs) in Drinking Water. Am J Public Health 1984; 74(5)

Cobos B, Haskard K, Howard K. White coat hypertension: improving the patient–healthcare practitioner relationship. Psychol Res Behav Manag 2015; 8: 133–41

Cox, L. Swimming to Antarctica. New York: Knopf, 2004

Fiscus KA. Changes in lower-leg blood flow during warm, cold, and contrast-water therapy. Arch Phys Med Rehabil 2005; 86(7): 1404–10

Fitzsimmons M. Gynaecomastia in industrial workers. British Journal of Industrial Medicine, 1 October 1944

Guyton AC, Hall JE. Textbook of Medical Physiology, 11th edition. Philadelphia, PA: Elsevier, 2010

Hao J, Ghosh P, Li SK et al. Heat effects on drug delivery across human skin. Expert Opin Drug Deliv 2016; 13(5): 755–68

Kamler K. Surviving the Extremes: A Doctor's Journey to the Limits of Human Endurance. New York: St. Martin's Press, 2002

Kellogg JH. Rational Hydrotherapy. Battle Creek, MI: Modern Medicine Publishing Company, 1923, p. 439

Lynch J. The Language of the Heart. NY: Basic Books, 1985

Michlovitz S. Thermal Agents in Rehabilitation. Philadelphia, PA: FA Davis, 1996

Mobius-Winkler et al. Coronary Collateral Growth Induced by Physical Exercise. Circulation 2016; 133: 1438–48

Muldoon MF, Herbert TB, Patterson SM, et al. Effects of acute psychological stress on serum lipid levels, hemoconcentration, and blood viscosity. Arch Intern Med 1995; 155(6): 615–20

Nyboer JH, Keatinge WR. Arctic cold swim from Alaska to Soviet Union. Proceedings of the First Alaska Regional Chapter of the American College of Sports Medicine, 1989

Ozturk ET. Human cerebrovascular function in health and disease: insights from integrative approaches. Journal of Physiological Anthropology 2018; 37: 4

Pastore MN et al. Transdermal patches: history, development and pharmacology. Br J Pharmacol 2015; 172(9): 2179–209

Patterson SM, Krantz DS, Gottdiener JS et al. Prothrombotic effects of environmental stress: changes in platelet function, hematocrit, and total plasma protein. Psychosomatic Medicine 1995; 57(6): 592–9

Petrofsky J et al. The use of hydrotherapy to increase blood flow and muscle relaxation in the rehabilitation of neurological and orthopedic patients. Journal of Neurologic and Orthopedic Medicine and Surgery 2003; 21(3): 188

Roe C. A Poultice for A Healer. Penguin: New York, 2003

Saradeth B et al. A single blind, randomized, controlled trial of hydrotherapy for varicose veins. Vasa 1991; 20(2): 147–52

Scheindlin S. Transdermal drug delivery: past present future. Molecular Interventions 2004; 4(6): 308–12

Shin T, Wilson M, Wilson T. Are hot tubs safe for people with treated hypertension? CMAJ 2003; 169(12): 1265–8

Taub E. Feedback-aided self-regulation of skin temperature with a single feedback locus. Biofeedback Self Regul 1976; 1(2): 147–68.

Taub E. Feedback treatment of vasospastic syndromes. Biofeedback and Self-Regulation 1978; 3(4)

Thrash A, Thrash C. Home Remedies: Hydrotherapy, Massage, Charcoal and Other Simple Treatments. Seale, AL: Thrash Publications, 1981

Vogel S. Vital Circuits: On Pumps, Pipes, and the Workings of Circulatory Systems. New York/Oxford: Oxford University Press, 1992

Recommended resources

Buchman D. The Complete Book of Water Healing. New York: Instant Improvement Incorporated, 1994, p. 206

Caring Medical. Rest Ice Compression Elevation; Rice Therapy and Price Therapy. https://www.caringmedical.com/prolotherapy-news/rest-ice-compression-elevation-rice-therapy/ [Accessed: March 2020]

Charkoudian N. Skin blood flow in adult human thermoregulation: how it works, when it does not, and why. Mayo Clin Proc 2003; 78: 603–12

Guyton AC, Hall JE. Textbook of Medical Physiology, 11th edn. Philadelphia, PA: Elsevier, 2011

Hayes B. Five Quarts: A Personal and Natural History of Blood. New York: Ballantine Books, 2005

Kee K et.al. Influence of nicotine on cold induced vasodilation in humans. Experimental Biology 2004 [Abstract]

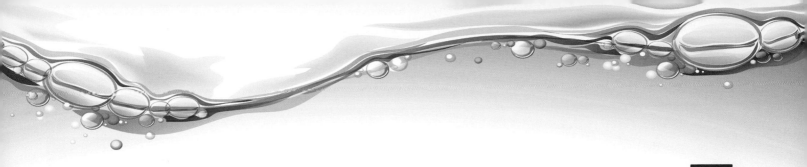

Preparing to give hydrotherapy treatments 3

In the scientific use of water in the treatment of disease, elaborate apparatus is not essential for effectiveness. It is possible to secure the most valuable of the therapeutic advantages of water by the aid of sheets, towels, blankets, a pail, a bathtub and a thermometer, if coupled with the consummate skill that comes from long experience.

John Harvey Kellogg, *Rational Hydrotherapy*

CHAPTER OBJECTIVES

After completing this chapter, the student will be able to:

1. Describe several properties of water and how these make it useful in hydrotherapy treatments
2. Explain that water can be used in each of its three forms: liquid, solid, and vapor
3. Explain conduction, convection, condensation, evaporation, and radiation, and give an example of each
4. List the equipment needed for basic and more elaborate hydrotherapy treatments
5. Describe several considerations when selecting hydrotherapy equipment
6. Explain guidelines for sanitization of hydrotherapy equipment
7. Describe general cautions when giving hydrotherapy treatments to clients with specific conditions
8. Explain several contraindications to hydrotherapy treatments
9. Describe safety precautions to be used when giving hydrotherapy treatments
10. Explain factors that influence the body's response to hot and cold treatments
11. Describe additional questions that need to be added to the standard massage therapist's health intake form before giving clients hydrotherapy treatments
12. Explain the basic guidelines for hydrotherapy
13. Describe the decision-making process for choosing which hydrotherapy treatments are best suited to individual clients
14. Explain how hydrotherapy can be used in a variety of different environments.

In a single day, as you move from treating a chronically ill person at home or in a nursing facility, giving massages at a sporting event or treating clients in your private office, hydrotherapy treatments can enhance each and every session (see Figure 3.1). Preparing to perform these treatments means selecting and maintaining the appropriate equipment as well as knowing how to choose a treatment that is fine-tuned to the unique needs of each of your clients (see Case history 3.1). After reading this chapter, you will be able to select the hydrotherapy equipment that works for your individual practice, whether you are an independent practitioner in a one-person office or an employee of a facility such as a massage franchise, chiropractic clinic, hospice, health club, or spa. By taking a thorough medical history and taking note of cautions and contraindications, you will also be able to determine which treatments are safe for which clients. You will also understand basic guidelines and how to perform treatments in different settings.

Many hydrotherapy treatments use water in its liquid form, which occurs at temperatures between 32°F (0°C) and 212°F (100°C) (see Table 3.1).

EQUIPMENT

A massage therapist who intends to make hydrotherapy an integral part of their practice can choose from a wide variety of hydrotherapy modalities. Depending upon where you practice, the access you have to running water, and the types of clients you see, there are many different ways to incorporate hydrotherapy treatments. This section will help guide you as you make decisions about what hydrotherapy equipment to purchase. We present three different levels of investment in equipment, and discuss factors to consider when shopping for equipment. Directions for sanitizing and maintaining your hydrotherapy equipment are included as well.

Water and its unique characteristics

What are the unique properties of water as a healing agent? First of all, water can readily change form: it can be a liquid (water), a vapor (such as steam), or a solid (ice). In a process called the **water cycle**, the overall amount of water on earth remains constant, but the water frequently changes form. Heat from the sun causes surface

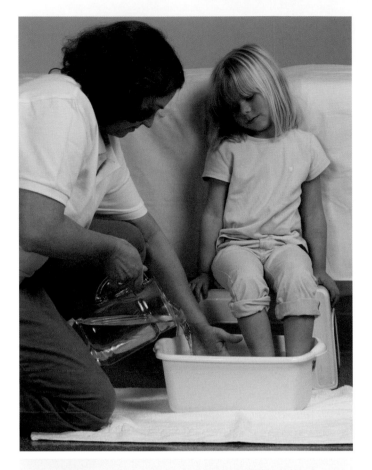

FIGURE 3.1
Massage therapist providing a footbath for client.

water – water in lakes, rivers, and oceans – to evaporate. Warm air holds more water vapor than cold air, so as air rises and cools, the water vapor condenses. Fine droplets may appear as clouds or mist; larger droplets fall as rain

TABLE 3.1 Forms of water			
Form of water	Solid	Liquid	Gas
Name	Ice	Water	Steam
Temperature range	Less than 32°F (0°C)	Between 32°F and 212°F (0°C and 100°C)	Greater than 212°F (100°C)
The effect of temperature changes	Molecules move farther apart, making it less dense than liquid water; volume increases by 11% over liquid water (100 spoonfuls of liquid water make 111 spoonfuls of ice)	Expands slightly when heated and contracts slightly when cooled	As they get hotter, molecules move faster and then separate, forming a vapor
Action when applied to the body	Absorbs body heat	Below 98°F (36.7°C) water absorbs body heat; at neutral temperature it neither absorbs body heat nor transfers heat to the body; above 98°F (36.7°C) it transfers heat to the body	Transfers heat to the body

| MANY CONDITIONS CAN BE HELPED WITH MORE THAN ONE HYDROTHERAPY TREATMENT | CASE HISTORY 3.1 |

BACKGROUND

Susan, a 45-year-old physical therapist, had widespread cancer, which had begun with breast cancer and then metastasized into her liver and the bones of her spine. She was experiencing not only tremendous emotional stress but a great deal of pain in her spine, but she enjoyed her hospice massages very much, and they reduced her nervous tension and relieved her back pain for a time. Normally local heat is contraindicated for persons with cancer, but the hospice's supervising physician had approved warm fomentations to Susan's spine before massage as a last-stage comfort measure. Susan has a hot tub in her back yard, normally kept at 104°F (40°C).

TREATMENT

Before each massage, the massage therapist placed a fomentation on Susan's back, then massaged her feet for a few minutes while the heat seeped into her spine. The therapist then removed the fomentation and gently massaged Susan's back. After her massage, Susan was helped into her hot tub for 15–20 minutes. She sometimes soaked in the hot tub before her massage: because of her bone cancer, just being freed from the pull of gravity for a while relieved some of her back pain and was wonderfully soothing. This helped her to begin her massage in a more relaxed state. Since the water also raised her core temperature slightly, it was also easier to keep her warm during her massage sessions. At other times, Susan floated in her hot tub after a massage, which helped her feel even more relaxed than with the massage alone.

DISCUSSION QUESTIONS

1. What steps would you need to take to ensure that hydrotherapy treatments are safe for a patient such as Susan?

2. What other hydrotherapy treatments might help relieve her pain?

or – if the air is cold enough – as ice crystals clumped together as snow.

Here are some of the amazing characteristics of water.

Water is abundant

Running water is available in virtually every office or home in the United States and Europe, and virtually every household has a bathtub or shower which can be used for basic low-cost hydrotherapy treatments such as warm baths or contrast showers. (That said, this precious natural resource should never be wasted.)

Water is affordable

A warm bath is an inexpensive treatment compared to other products which can help a client relax, such as prescription medications, nutritional supplements, or products containing herbs or essential oils. For someone with inflamed muscles, the numbing and anti-inflammatory effects of ice massage are cheaper than the gels, creams, herbal products or medications often used to get the same effects.

Water has weight

As anyone who has had to carry water for a long distance can testify, water is heavy, weighing 1 kilogram per liter or 8 pounds per gallon. When you are in a pool, the pressure of water on your tissues is called **hydrostatic pressure**.

Water is versatile

Water can be used therapeutically in everything from cooling wet compresses to sponges full of holes, and from steamy hot packs stored in a metal tank to a hose that can apply water at high pressure.

Water is easy to use

Water is easy to work with and even to transport in its different forms, from ice massage cups in a cooler to warm water in a foot tub.

Water stimulates the skin

Cold, warm or hot water stimulates the temperature receptors in the skin: the classical hydrotherapists called this stimulation the "thermic impression" and made great use of it. For example, a very short cold shower or bath did not chill the person, but was often used to give a brief impression of chilliness, which stimulated a strong vasoconstriction. Pressure receptors can be stimulated by treatments which friction, spray or strike the skin, and proprioceptors in muscles and joints are stimulated by the weightlessness we feel when floating in water. Many hydrotherapy treatments such as a hot shower or a cold mitten friction combine thermal and mechanical effects.

Water provides buoyancy

Floating in water is deeply soothing and can relieve discomfort in conditions such as osteoarthritis, obesity and pregnancy.

Water affects both mind and body

(see Chapter 1, Box 1.1)

Water can absorb, retain, or give off heat and cold

Water can absorb and give off heat more easily than any other substance. (To understand ways that water can work its magic in treatments, see Box 3.1.) This means that when water is heated to a hot but safe temperature, it is capable of heating a body part or the entire body very efficiently. Cold water also has a great capacity to absorb heat: for example, if an overheated athlete is treated for heatstroke by immersion in an ice water bath, his or her temperature can fall as much as 8°F (-13°C) in 15 minutes. While a lot of heat is needed to raise the temperature of liquid water, it holds heat better than most substances: for example, hot water holds twice as much heat as liquid paraffin, and when water does cool down it gives off a lot of heat. Therefore a hot moist treatment such as a hot gel pack or **fomentation** gives off a lot of heat as it cools. To change one gram of liquid water to one gram of water vapor (steam) at the same temperature of 212°F (100°C), requires approximately 540 calories, which is stored in the water vapor.

When one gram of liquid water cools to 33.8°F (1°C), one calorie of heat is given off. Then should that one gram of water reach 32°F (0°C), approximately another 80 calories of heat must still be lost in order to change the water to its solid form, ice. These extra calories are known as "latent heat." Therefore freezing water gives off large quantities of latent heat and melting ice absorbs large quantities of latent heat. One gram of melting ice absorbs 80 times more heat than one gram of water being raised from 32°F (0°C) to 33.8°F (1°C). This makes ice a very powerful treatment.

Water is a powerful solvent

Because more substances can be dissolved in water than in any other liquid, it is known as the "universal solvent." (Unfortunately, for this reason water can also become polluted with an almost unlimited number of noxious substances.) For millennia, healers have used water to move chemicals through the skin into the body. A wide variety of medicinal substances – salts, minerals, vinegar, seaweed, clays, baking soda, oatmeal, essential oils and a huge variety of herbs – have been added to whole-body baths or mixed with smaller amounts of water for compresses, body wraps, plasters, and poultices.

What type of equipment is right for your practice?

With advance planning and your equipment carefully laid out, you can add water treatments to each and every session without sacrificing hands-on massage time. Begin with simple equipment and try it in your practice before you go on to more expensive or complicated equipment. (Figure 3.2 shows a variety of simple hydrotherapy items.) Then, if you plan on incorporating hydrotherapy treatments into a significant portion of your massage sessions, or perform more advanced treatments, you can invest in more elaborate equipment. Some massage therapists happily use only minimal hydrotherapy equipment, but in a variety of ways—for example, with nothing more than hot and cold running water, Epsom salts, a dish tub, a water thermometer, and a few towels, you can make compresses that are hot, cold, or contrasting, for use over different parts of the body; you can make cold mitten frictions and salt glows; and you can perform hot, cold, or contrasting baths for the hands or feet.

BOX 3.1	POINT OF INTEREST

HOW HEAT AND COLD ARE TRANSFERRED TO AND FROM THE BODY

Water is able not only to absorb and retain heat, but to transfer it to a person or thing in one of the following ways:

- The transfer of heat by direct contact of one heated or cooled substance with another is called **conduction**. This is the primary way that temperature exchange is done in hydrotherapy. For example, when an ice pack is applied to one part of the body, heat is conducted away from the skin into the ice pack.

  When a hot pack is applied to one part, heat is conducted from the hot pack onto the skin. Water can conduct heat onto the body many times better than air, so moist heat penetrates more deeply than dry heat: hot, moist applications such as moist heating pads heat body tissues much more than even the very hottest dry cloth.

- The transfer of heat onto or off a body by moving air or gas is called **convection**. "Wind chill" is one example of how body heat can be lost by convection – to determine how cold it is outside, we must calculate not only the air temperature but also how hard the wind is blowing, since wind will strip warm air directly off a person's body. When we get out of a hot sauna and stand in a breeze, we become much cold much faster than if there is no breeze at all.

- **Condensation** is the process which changes water vapor (a gas) into liquid water. Examples of condensation include your eye glasses fogging up when you enter a warm building from outside on a cold winter day and the cold glass comes into contact with warm air. Another is when you walk outside on a cold day and see your breath as you exhale: the air leaving your lungs is much warmer than the outside air temperature, causing the water vapor to condense into a small mist. Similarly, when you take a hot shower the bathroom mirror will often steam up as moist air comes into contact with the cool mirror and condensation occurs.

- **Radiation** is the transfer of heat through space, without two objects touching. If you warm yourself by a fireplace without touching the fire (always a smart strategy), the heat is reaching you through radiation. When a person who is overheated steps out of a warm bath, heat is transferred into the air through radiation. (If a wind comes along, heat will be lost even faster through convection, as discussed above.) Radiation is one of the main ways that humans lose body heat.

- **Evaporation**, the reverse of condensation, is the process of changing liquid water into water vapor. Sweating in hot weather cools the body through evaporation; and the hotter the air, the more you sweat and the more evaporation and cooling take place.

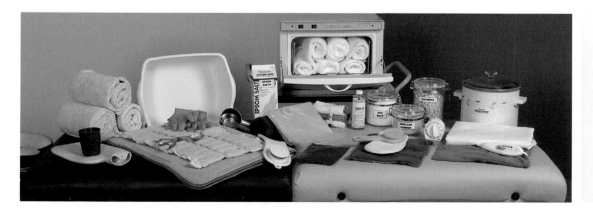

FIGURE 3.2
Various kinds of hydrotherapy equipment suitable for local treatments.

Chapter three

SPA-LEVEL EQUIPMENT

Many spa treatments use very expensive equipment: specialty showers, special hoses for percussion, sophisticated hydrotherapy tubs and tiled "wet rooms" are not usually found outside of spas. However, it is important that you know about these treatments because they have been practiced for centuries or more in both the United States and Europe, and are still used in many modern spas. For more about these treatments, see *Spa Bodywork* by Anne Williams.

Here is a list of spa-level equipment, in order of increasing cost:

1. A **Swiss shower** with 16 heads: about $5,000 for the equipment itself, plus a minimum of $2,000 for tiling a shower enclosure.
2. A **Vichy shower**: about $4,000 and also requires a wet room (see Chapter 8).
3. A **Scotch hose or percussion douche**: about $4,000, and it requires a wet room.
4. **Mud baths**: about $5,000 to construct each bath, and a lot of upkeep.
5. **Jetted hydrotherapy tub**: $15,000 dollars. The tub must be cleaned, sanitized and dried between clients; in addition, the jets must be flushed out (see Figure 6.16).
6. **Watsu** pool: $10,000 to $30,000, depending upon whether the pool is part of an existing building or if a new building must be created for it (see Figure 6.18).

Other therapists, though, may be excited about having more elaborate pieces of equipment such as a sauna or hot tub. To help you determine what is ideal for your practice, lists for three different levels of hydrotherapy equipment follow. To see how spas utilize their more sophisticated equipment, see Box 3.2.

Basic level equipment

Having running water in the therapy room is not absolutely necessary, but you will need to have a sink close at hand.

- Water thermometer, essential for safety. Figure 3.3 shows both Fahrenheit and Celsius temperature scales.
- Extra linens, including about 20 washcloths, four small hand towels, and four large bath towels.
- Counter space or a cart for hydrotherapy equipment.
- A large tray to carry materials to and from the therapy room, such as hot water bottles, pitchers of water, bowls, and used linens or other items which need to be cleaned. Brand-new baking sheets which are both sturdy and completely washable work well for this purpose.

- At least three one-quart-size metal bowls. They may be used for water, ice cubes, salt for local salt glows, etc.
- Pitchers, a 4-cup size and an 8-cup size.
- Plastic tubs that can go underneath the table to hold used towels, and can double as containers for local water baths.
- One form of local heat: choose between a slow cooker or turkey roaster for hot water (useful for salt glows, hot compresses, silica gel packs, and hot water for hot water bottles and hand and footbaths), a microwave oven (useful for heating fomentations and some types of hot gel packs), a hot towel cabinet (holds many hot moist washcloths), or a moist heating pad.
- Local cold options: choose between very cold water (useful for cold mitten frictions, cold water bottles, cold compresses and cold local baths), iced compresses, ice packs and ice cups. Some kind of refrigeration is needed for all these forms of local cold. A miniature refrigerator can hold all of these items, or a small ice chest may also be used to hold ice packs and ice cups during a session (see Figure 5.2).

- Zipper closure bags of various sizes are useful for making ice packs and iced compresses, as well as heating fomentations in a microwave.

- Local friction treatment options: choose Epsom salts and two washcloths for salt glows, cold water and two washcloths for cold mitten frictions, a loofah glove or mitt and two washcloths for loofah scrubs, or a soft natural bristle brush and two washcloths for dry brushing.

- Plastic sheets may be used to protect the massage table if desired: just place them under your fabric sheets. Towels are also effective unless a large amount of water is spilled on the table.

- Floor covering: anytime that liquid water is being used for treatments, linoleum is a better floor covering than carpet because it is easier to clean. Many people do not care for the colder feel of linoleum, however. In that case, washable rugs can be put over the linoleum so that they can be easily removed and cleaned, but they should have a non-skid backing.

- Grab bars near showers, hot tubs or bathtubs – the more the better.

Basic-plus equipment

Simply add items for several additional local treatments. By choosing just one more local heat treatment, you have many more options for adding hydrotherapy to your sessions. For example, one type of local heat treatment – such as a Fomentek flat hot water bottle – may be appropriate for warming a cold person or increasing circulation to a person's entire back before massage, but it is too large for a hot or contrast treatment in a small body area, and will not wrap around an area as liquid water will do. A paraffin bath is excellent for deep heating of the hands, feet and face, general body warming, and even contrast treatments of the hands, feet and face, but it is not practical to use for someone with a stiff neck. Whole-body heating treatments such as hot blanket packs can be performed without having to purchase more expensive equipment such as steam cabinets or showers. One additional source of cold, an ice machine, makes it far easier to perform contrast treatments, but it is possible to place a bag of ice in a

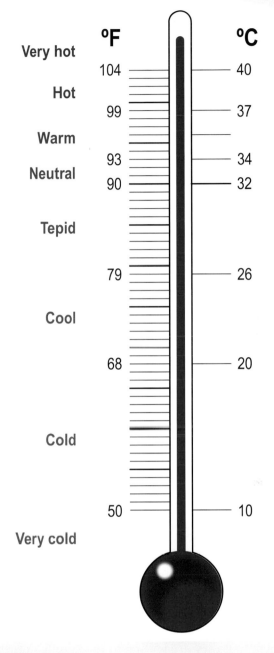

FIGURE 3.3
General sensations associated with cold, neutral, and hot water.

small ice chest instead. Except for the hand-held shower attachment, having running water in the therapy room is still not absolutely necessary, but you will need to have a sink close at hand. Contrast applications with a shower attachment can be performed easily by your clients in their homes.

Below is a list of additional equipment which is still relatively inexpensive:

- *Equipment for one additional local heat treatment,* such as a Fomentek flat hot water bottle, a paraffin bath, a hot towel cabinet, or a hydrocollator tank which holds four hot packs or a hand-held shower attachment. (This requires a room with a bathtub or shower stall.)

- *Equipment for one additional local cold treatment,* such as an ice machine or a cold therapy gel pack and an ice chest to keep it cold.

Advanced-level equipment

Simply add one of the many types of whole-body heating treatments listed below. This can be as simple as a standard shower (which can be used for local or whole-body heating, cooling or contrast treatments), or as elaborate as a soaking tub, flotation tank, **Watsu** pool, sauna or hot tub. Other facilities for whole-body treatments include individual steam canopies and cabinets. A large shower with a steam bath attachment is perhaps the most versatile of all, because it can be used for steam baths, hot showers, cold showers, contrast showers, and whole-body salt glows.

When purchasing any of the whole-body hydrotherapy items, there are many things to be considered. They are more expensive and require more office space, water, energy, and linens; and time to clean and sanitize everything after the session. Since the cost can be divided up among more than one practitioner these added expenses may be more practical in a health club or a clinic with multiple practitioners. However, some practitioners may feel so strongly about the value of a particular treatment that they are willing to invest in it. A therapist who spends $5000 to install a tiled sauna and shower, or $20,000 for a Watsu pool will have to practice for some time in order to make back the original investment, but may be more than willing to do so.

Below is a list of different equipment for a variety of whole-body treatments, in order of increasing cost. Equipment may have several cost components: at the outset, the cost of purchase and the cost of installation, perhaps; and in use, the running costs of energy, water, and maintenance. (For spa-level equipment, see Box 3.2.)

1. Japanese soaking tub: this type of tub uses less space than a standard bathtub, but more water. Heating the water with gas or electricity is an ongoing cost. Since the surface of the water–where heat radiates from–is smaller, it may lose less heat than a standard bathtub.

2. Standard bathtub: these use about 30 gallons (115 liters) of water. Heating the bath water with gas or electricity is an ongoing cost.

3. Steam canopy, which can be laid over the client as he or she lies on the massage table. This item is highly energy-efficient, using a maximum of 5 cups of water and the same amount of energy as a small kitchen appliance.

4. Standard tiled shower: showers in general use less water than baths. Heating the shower water with gas or electricity is an ongoing cost.

5. Multi-head shower panel: this can be added on to a basic shower to make a multi-spray shower. Because multi-head showers use a great deal of water, larger pipes must be installed and heating the water with gas or electricity is more expensive than for a standard shower.

6. Individual steam cabinets: these use little water, but quite a lot of energy.

7. Individual stainless-steel whirlpool tubs: extremity whirlpools use approximately 50 gallons (190 liters) of water and whole-body whirlpools use twice that amount. Energy to heat water and run pumps is an jets is an additional cost.

8. Steam shower with steam generator.

9. Hot tub or spa: upfront costs include installation and energy to heat water. (A shower must also be provided for the client's use.)

10. Dry sauna: a sauna – basically a small room with a heater – is a major investment, and uses a lot of electricity. (A shower must also be provided for the client's use.)

Factors to think about when selecting hydrotherapy equipment

Selecting equipment is an important decision. Below are some key factors to consider as you make this decision.

Goals of therapy

This answer will be different depending upon the type of clients that you treat. For example, a therapist who specializes in sports massage can use ice treatments to help athletes with injuries, while a therapist who specializes in working with the elderly can use warming treatments to help them tolerate being partially or completely disrobed. The sports therapist does not need to help his athletic clients, who likely have excellent circulation, to stay warm, and the therapist for elders is not likely to be treating his clients for athletic injuries.

Cost

To calculate this, figure the total cost of purchasing and installing equipment. For example, to do heating treatments using steam rooms, or hot tubs or multi-head showers, a large hot water tank with large pipes is needed. Also figure upkeep and laundry expenses. You might even have to raise your rates to pay for expensive equipment.

Maintenance time and expense

Any time that your clients use a shower, either before or after a massage session, it must be cleaned and dried before the next use. The shower may also need some type of periodic maintenance, such as replacing grout or cleaning drains. Local whirlpools must be sterilized after each use. A steam cabinet must be cleaned and dried after each use, and a steam canopy wiped off with cleanser and air-dried between clients. Parts may wear out and need to be replaced. These are just a few examples of maintenance issues that need to be considered. Especially for large specialty equipment such as Vichy showers or saunas, be sure to ask the manufacturers how they will help you if something functions poorly or needs to be replaced. Consider how much time you, as a therapist, are willing to spend doing maintenance. Perhaps you would prefer to stay with a few simple local treatments that require little or no maintenance, rather than cleaning large pieces of equipment or being responsible for them should they break.

How much water will you use?

This factor is important not only to keep your expenses low, but also to conserve natural resources. By reducing your consumption you save water and the energy that

would otherwise be used to treat, heat, and distribute to your home or office. (Waste water also has to be treated after it goes down the drain.)

The amount of water used for various treatments varies widely. A standard 10-minute shower uses about 25 gallons (95 liters) of water, while a shower with 15 jets uses over ten times that much. Perhaps the most water-wasteful of all hydrotherapy treatments are top-of-the-line showers complete with multiple jets and "waterfall" features, which use up to 80 gallons (303 liters) of water per minute.

Letting tap water run down the drain while it warms up is wasteful: collect it in a pitcher or bucket until it warms, then use that clean water to drink or to water your garden.

Energy consumption

The single biggest use of electricity in the average Western home is heating water, mostly for showers. Heating water with an electric steam boiler to do one Russian steam bath takes 68 kilowatts of energy. Making ice also uses a lot of energy, but not as much as using electricity to generate heat.

Sanitation protocols

Just as with any other equipment used during a massage session, hydrotherapy equipment should be sanitized after each use. This protects your client's health and your own. Below are some specific directions on sanitizing your hydrotherapy equipment after a session:

1. Any surface that comes into contact with the client's skin should be sanitized, including floors. All steam cabinets, showers, tubs or other whole-body heating equipment must be cleaned with a bacteriocidal agent and then dried before use. Follow the manufacturers' specific instructions on how to clean them.

2. All bowls, lotion bottles, and other containers should be washed in hot soapy water and wiped with alcohol. Any leftover substance that is in an open bowl, such as salt that was used for a salt glow, should be thrown away if your hands touched it during a session. If you handled the substance without touching it with your hands—for example, if you

Chapter three

TABLE 3.2 Thermal sensations			
Terms	**Temperature range**		**Comments**
	Fahrenheit	Celsius	
Freezing	32	0	
Very cold	32–55	0–13	Painfully cold
Cold	55–65	13–18	Tolerable but uncomfortable. Prolonged immersion in water less than 60°F (15.5°C) may lead to hypothermia
Cool	65–80	18–27	Produces goose flesh
Tepid	80–92	27–33	Slightly below skin temperature (92°F; 33°C)
Warm or neutral	93–97	34–36	Comfortable
Hot	98–105	37–41	Tolerable, but parts turn red
Very hot	105–110	41–43	Tolerable for short periods
Painfully hot	110–120	43–46	Intolerable – this is likely to cause injury to diabetic feet
Dangerously hot	125 or above	52 or above	Likely to burn skin
Boiling	212	100	

used a scoop to remove Epsom salts from a container–then the rest of it can still be used. The reason for this rule is that if you touched the salt with your hands, touched your client as you applied the salt, and then touched the salt again, that salt is now contaminated. It should not be used on anyone else.

3. All cloth items, such as robes, sheets, towels, washcloths and shower mats, must be washed in hot water with an appropriate detergent and then dried using heat. Keep them on shelves or in cabinets that are at least 4 inches (10 cm) off the floor and used only for storage. Throw away items such as disposable shower caps or slippers after your client has used them.

GENERAL CAUTIONS AND CONTRAINDICATIONS

Hydrotherapy is generally very safe, and you can use it with almost all of your clients. Since clients are all different, before you give someone a hydrotherapy treatment for the first time, be sure to ask if he or she has had that treatment before, and what the response was (for an example of factors to consider, see Case history 3.2). When clients are receiving a whole-body heating treatment such as a sauna for the first time, limit their time to 15 minutes. During the treatment, ask clients for feedback frequently, and be ready to terminate any treatment that does not seem to be working. Signs of a poor reaction

include nausea, headache, dizziness or lightheadedness, and clients feeling too warm or too cold. Table 3.2 shows whether a water temperature will be perceived as hot, warm, neutral or cold.

Below we discuss both cautions and contraindications to hydrotherapy.

Cautions

Hydrotherapy treatments are not necessarily ruled out, but the special needs of the client must be carefully considered. An initial treatment may need to be milder: for example, using warm water rather than hot water, or cool water rather than ice water. No treatment should ever be painful or unpleasant.

Attention deficit disorder

Many medications for this condition promote vasodilation, so heating treatments should be avoided. All other treatments are fine.

Aversion to cold

Clients who have a strong negative reaction to the idea of cold treatments can generally be accommodated by modifying the treatment. For example, for a cold application, begin with water that is a bit warmer than you

CHOOSING THE RIGHT TREATMENT FOR A CLIENT WITH NERVOUS TENSION AND SCIATIC PAIN	CASE HISTORY 3.2

BACKGROUND

Gene was a 70-year-old woman who sought massage because she was under a great deal of stress and because she hoped massage could reduce the chronic pain in her low back, buttock and upper thigh she calls "sciatica." She had similar discomfort once years ago, but had gone many years without experiencing it until she had hip joint replacement surgery 6 months before: although she healed very well from the surgery, the "sciatica" began afterward and had not gone away since then. She also told the therapist that she was often colder than the people around her.

DISCUSSION QUESTIONS

1. What additional questions should the therapist ask Gene when interviewing her?

2. Some traditional hydrotherapy treatments for sciatica include ice massage. Is it safe to perform any of these hydrotherapy treatments with her? What steps should the therapist take to determine this?

3. If approved, which of the hydrotherapy treatments would be appropriate and effective for her?

---

want it to be. If the client's reaction is good, wait a bit and then add a few ice cubes to the water. For a contrast treatment, use warmer water, and increase the length of the treatment. For example, a contrast treatment of 2 minutes of heat followed by 30 seconds of cold could be changed to 2 minutes of heat followed by 1 minute of cool water. When treatments are going to be done in a series or if the patient is going to do them daily at home, their aversion to cold will probably be decreased as they enjoy the good feelings afterwards.

Children

Children not as able to regulate their body temperature than adults: since they have thinner skin and more surface area relative to their body mass, they can become chilled more easily in cold temperatures. However, young children also heat up more easily than adults when exposed to heat (Tsuzuki-Hayakawa, 1995). Monitor children carefully while they are receiving hydrotherapy treatments. In general, make local hot and cold applications less extreme, check their skin frequently, and ask them for more feedback than you would with an adult. Local salt glows are a good choice for children and warm baths are very soothing and relaxing and fun. Saunas and steam baths should last no longer than 10 minutes and should be supervised by a parent (Jokinen, 1991). Also, note that children tend to dislike cold applications, although individual responses can vary. For more information on

hydrotherapy and children, see *Pediatric Massage Therapy* (Sinclair, 2004). Massage therapists should not perform hydrotherapy treatments with infants unless they have special training in this area.

Small body size

When smaller adults are exposed to cold, they get cold more easily than larger adults. The United States Army's research in environmental medicine has found that rates of peripheral cold injury in female soldiers are twice that of men: since women have a greater surface area relative to their body mass than men, they lose proportionately more heat from their skin. This means body temperature falls faster in extreme cold conditions, and this often leads to more peripheral cold injuries.

Elders

Some of the physical changes associated with aging may make it more difficult for older people to adjust to extremes of hot and cold. Loss of subcutaneous fat means it is easier for them to be burned by hot applications or chilled by cold applications. The muscles of the blood vessels may not function as well, and so vasodilation and vasoconstriction are less efficient in controlling body temperature (Proctor, 2003; Inoue, 2004). However, this does not mean that gentle hydrotherapy treatments are not appropriate. In a small study at Kagoshima

Chapter three

University in Japan, researchers studied the effects on elderly people of 10-minute hot baths at 106°F (41°C). They found that elders, with or without heart disease, felt less fatigue and leg pain and improved their exercise endurance. Researchers concluded that the hot water had stimulated greater vasodilation, which caused more blood flow to skeletal muscles, which made them better able to contract (Norton, 2002). In general, be more vigilant with elderly people. Keep treatments shorter – no more than 15 minutes in a sauna, hot tub, or steam bath – and temperatures more moderate. Be sure to check the elder's skin frequently, and ask for more feedback than you would with a younger person.

HIV/AIDS

Because people with HIV/AIDS generally have a variety of body systems that are affected by the virus, hot baths or other whole-body heating treatments should be undertaken only with their doctor's approval. Hyperthermia (whole-body heating) is currently being studied for treatment of this condition. Researchers at John Bastyr College of Naturopathic Medicine found that a regimen of very hot baths that raised patients' temperatures to 102°F (39°C) and kept it there for 40 minutes caused a significant inactivation of the HIV virus (Standish, 2002).

Cancer

Massage is used by cancer patients for relaxation and to ease anxiety, discomfort and pain, so it is a situation in which the massage therapist may be tempted to give hydrotherapy treatments for the same benefits. Both whole-body and local treatments may be used for some people with cancer. Whole-body heating treatments have been given to strengthen the immune system, and local heat, ice massage and warm baths are sometimes used for pain. It is likely that the client's doctor will approve hydrotherapy treatments, but she or he should be consulted first. For more information, see Chapter 13.

Pregnancy

Except for hot applications over the abdomen, local treatments which do not raise the core temperature are safe for pregnant women. Neutral baths and hand- and foot-baths with added Epsom salts are a traditional treatment for local edema in the last stage of pregnancy. There is concern that increased core temperature in the early months of pregnancy could harm a fetus, so prolonged hot baths, hot tubs, steam baths or saunas are contraindicated. One study investigated this risk and found that exposure to heat in the form of hot tub, sauna or fever in the first trimester of pregnancy was associated with an increased risk of neural tube defects, with the hot tub having the strongest effect of any single heat exposure (Milunsky, 1992).

Overweight clients

Because overweight people have more fat covering their muscles than thin people have, it often takes longer for a local heat application to penetrate into their tissues, and once that area is warmed, it takes longer for the heat to dissipate. The same is true of cold applications. For the same reason, overweight people may heat up faster during whole-body heat treatments such as saunas and hot tubs and may not tolerate them as well. Check their medical histories carefully to rule out other contraindications, avoid extremes of temperature, and monitor them closely.

Clients with limited mobility

In conditions such as muscular dystrophy, cerebral palsy, post-polio syndrome, spinal cord injuries, Parkinson's disease, advanced arthritis and even obesity, our clients' ability to move easily is reduced. Hydrotherapy treatments can be enjoyable and treatments such as salt glows and contrast treatments can be wonderful forms of skin stimulation. However, someone who has trouble moving might not be able to get out of a hot bath quickly or easily remove a local application that is too hot. Be especially attentive to such clients and assist them as needed.

Contraindications

Contraindications are special symptoms or conditions that make a procedure or other remedy risky. Below we discuss some specific conditions that rule out certain hydrotherapy treatments. Specific contraindications will also be given with the instructions for each hydrotherapy treatments. Avoid treating clients who are intoxicated from drugs or alcohol, are acutely ill, or have eaten a large meal recently. (No massage or hydrotherapy treatments should be given until at least one hour after eating a full meal.)

Acute local inflammation

Heat applications are contraindicated in cases of acute local inflammation as they can encourage edema.

Artificial devices

Do not apply heat over implants, pacemakers, defibrillators, medication pumps or other artificial devices. Heat and cold may be safely applied over artificial hip and knee joints.

Asthma

Many people with asthma find moist heat (such as a warm fomentation over the chest) or whole-body heating very comforting. These treatments are safe to use – however, inhaling cold dry air can sometimes trigger asthma attacks, and even stepping from a warm sauna or steam bath into cold air may not be helpful. Do not let a person with asthma become chilled for even a moment during or after a hydrotherapy treatment.

Circulatory system conditions

The high temperatures experienced in a sauna, steam bath or hot bath can create extra demands on the circulatory system. This includes significant changes in how fast and how forcefully the heart beats, how much blood the heart pumps with each beat, the size of different blood vessels, and where blood is distributed in the body. Typically a larger amount of the person's blood supply than usual is shifted to the blood vessels of the skin for cooling. Even a large or very warm local application such as a silica gel hot pack causes a response throughout the circulatory system (Smith, 1993).

Therefore, for persons with the following heart or blood vessel problems, some hydrotherapy treatments are contraindicated unless approved by the client's doctor.

1. Whole-body heating treatments are contraindicated for:

    • *High blood pressure*. At the very beginning of a whole-body heating treatment, the blood pressure rises for a very short time, and this could be dangerous for some people. In addition, clients may be taking medications that change how the blood vessels react to heat and cold, such as beta blockers and calcium channel blockers.

    • *Low blood pressure*. Many medications can contribute to this problem, including those for depression and hypertension, and so can alcohol. Long hot baths or other treatments that raise the core temperature significantly may cause fainting, and are not recommended.

    • *Heart disease* such as coronary artery disease or congestive heart failure. The client's heart may not be strong enough to meet the demands of whole-body heating. In addition, clients with these conditions may be taking medications that alter heart function.

    • *Phlebitis*. Local treatments are contraindicated.

    • *Varicose veins*. Local treatments may be used with caution–avoid extremes of hot and cold.

2. Local heat to the feet is contraindicated for:

    • **Arteriosclerosis of the feet and legs** Do not apply local heat to the feet in the form of hot footbaths, hot water bottles, heating pads or paraffin dips.

    • **Buerger's disease** is a rare disorder in which medium-sized arteries become inflamed and swollen, and this can result in clots, occlusions and gangrene. Do not apply heat to the feet.

3. Local cold is contraindicated for **Raynaud's syndrome,** a simple vasoconstriction disorder of the extremities which affects 5–10% of the general population. Spasm of the smallest arteries that supply the hands or feet can be triggered in situations which would not affect someone without Raynaud's syndrome. For example, as discussed in Chapter 2, constriction of blood vessels in the hands can accompany emotional stress in many people; however, in a person with Raynaud's syndrome, it can also trigger an episode of vasospasm. Exposing the hands or feet to even mild cold can have the same effect; the muscles of the arteriole walls spasm,

drastically reducing blood flow, and the area turns blue and is numb and/or has a tingling, burning sensation. The arteriole spasm does not go away readily, and may last for an hour or longer. Soaking the hands or feet in warm water to rewarm them may stop an episode of vasospam, but the area often throbs painfully when it is rewarmed. The bottom line: exposure to a local cold treatment, such as a cold hand bath or an ice pack over the ankle, could trigger an episode of vasospasm in a person with Raynaud's syndrome.

Diabetes

Diabetes can lead to cardiovascular disease, so even without an official diagnosis, it is better to assume that the client has it and not to give hot baths. However, warm and neutral-temperature baths are a good choice for diabetics, as are whole-body salt glows (for more on this, see Chapter 13). With diabetes, the small blood vessels just under the skin narrow, and do not dilate as well as usual. Here's what could happen with higher temperatures: a local heat treatment such as a hot footbath leads to increased tissue metabolism, which increases the need for oxygen and other nutrients, but the blood vessels in the feet cannot dilate well. This situation could lead to tissue death and is to be avoided at all costs. Also, diabetics often have less ability to sense heat, cold and pressure in their feet and might not be able to tell when hot applications are dangerously hot. Therefore, hot footbaths, heating pads, hot water bottles, paraffin dips and hot moist packs on the feet are contraindicated, along with steam cabinets where the client sits upright and steam enters through the floor of the cabinet. However, warm footbaths of 102°F (39°C) or less are safe for diabetics. Several medical clinics in the US and Europe use alternating footbaths to treat diabetic ulcers of the feet: alternating warm (102°F; 39°C) and cold (55°F; 13°C) footbaths promote circulation without dangerously high temperatures. However, this treatment should only be performed with a doctor's permission.

Inability to sense heat or cold

Several conditions can cause the loss of normal sensation, including spinal cord injury, multiple sclerosis, arteriosclerosis, nerve injury, exposure to toxic substances and diabetes. The potential danger in dealing with clients who cannot feel heat or cold very well is that they won't be able to tell you if a hot application is burning their skin or a cold application is freezing their skin. Therefore, temperature extremes are contraindicated. Mild heat (no more than 102°F; 39°C), cool (but not ice cold) water, and neutral applications such as salt glows and neutral baths are safe.

Lymphedema

Lymphedema is an accumulation of lymph in subcutaneous tissues, most commonly seen after cancer surgery that removed lymph nodes. Doctors advise patients with this condition to avoid exposure to heat. For example, patients with lymphedema of the arm are advised to wear a long, insulated glove when removing something hot from the oven. Local heat to a limb leads to vasodilation and increased blood flow, followed by an increase in fluid leaking out of the capillaries and into tissue spaces. This is a normal process and ordinarily the lymphatic system returns this fluid to the heart: however, when lymphatic vessels or nodes are destroyed, fluid does not flow out so easily, and the surrounding tissues swell, causing discomfort and possible tissue damage. Therefore, such treatments as hot fomentations, hydrocollator packs, hot water bottles, hot footbaths and paraffin dips are contraindicated. All whole-body heating treatments result in dilation of skin blood vessels, including the vessels of the affected limb. However, local treatments such as a warm footbath or a warm whole-body bath to 102°F (39°C) are safe, and aquatic therapy in a 92°F (33°C) pool can be an effective treatment to help move blood and lymph through an affected limb (Rymal, 2002). Prolonged applications of ice should also be avoided because a freezing temperature could damage the small blood vessels under the skin. For more information, see the section on lymphedema in Chapter 13.

Multiple sclerosis

Any application of heat that is very large or is on the person's skin for a long time can raise the core temperature, and can cause extreme fatigue in those with multiple sclerosis, and thus is contraindicated. Neutral or cold treatments, including neutral temperature whirlpools, cold compresses, and exercise in cold water, are indicated. (For more information, see *Multiple sclerosis* on page 343.)

Nerve or crush injuries to the extremities

Sometimes clients with these injuries are permanently hypersensitive to cold. To promote circulation, contrast treatments may be effective because a brief cold immersion will not actually chill the client's tissues. The water temperature should be tailored to the person, so begin with cool, not cold water, and if the client tolerates it, the water temperature may be lowered gradually. Salt glows at a mild temperature may be even more effective. Paraffin dips are commonly used in physical therapy of the hands and feet.

Prescription medications

Clients who are taking certain medications should not receive hydrotherapy.

Cold treatments that promote vasoconstriction should not be combined with medications that promote it, such as migraine headache medications that include caffeine. Heat treatments that promote vasodilation should not be combined with medications that promote that, such as decongestants and some migraine headache medications. Clients with high blood pressure should not be treated in any case, but especially if they are taking medications which lower blood pressure.

Seizure disorders

Seizures can be caused by a variety of factors, including head trauma, infections, alcohol poisoning and brain tumors, but for one third of clients with seizures there is no known cause. Whole-body treatments should not be very hot or very cold because they might trigger a seizure. Mild sedative treatments such as salt glows, warm baths, neutral baths, and wet sheet packs taken to a neutral stage are indicated, however someone must be present at all times in case of the unlikely event of a seizure.

Skin conditions

1. *Infections or rashes.* Do not apply any hydrotherapy treatment over skin that is infected or has a rash, except with a doctor's permission.

2. *Recent injection sites.* For the first 24 hours, do not apply hot or cold over injection sites or less than 4 inches away from them. This includes injections that are subcutaneous, intramuscular (botox, vaccines), or into joints (cortisone) (Salvo, 2013).

Thyroid disorders

Whole-body heating treatments are contraindicated for patients who- already have low thyroid activity or hypothyroidism. Although a one-time heating treatment will have little effect on a thyroid condition, regular saunas, steam baths, hot baths or other heating treatments can depress thyroid activity. However, people with underactive thyroid glands often feel cold all the time, making it more challenging to keep them warm during a session. Whole-body cooling treatments stimulate thyroid activity and are contraindicated for anyone with overly high thyroid activity (hyperthyroidism). A one-time cold treatment will have little or no effect on a thyroid condition, but regular cold baths may (DeLorenzo, 1999).

Topical applications

Do not apply heat over any kind of topical application, and stay at least 4 inches away from transdermal patches (Salvo, 2013).

Safety precautions

A few simple safety precautions should be observed when performing hydrotherapy treatments:

1. Since many hydrotherapy treatments use liquid water, there is a chance some might be spilled on the floor. Mop up any spills immediately so that there is no chance of anyone slipping.

2. Use metal tongs or gloves so your hands are not burned, and always exercise caution when handling hot packs (Figure 3.4).

3. When clients receive a massage before going into a hot tub, steam room, or sauna, they should be sure to wash off the massage oil or lotion thoroughly before going in. This prevents bath water from being contaminated, and there will be no slippery film left

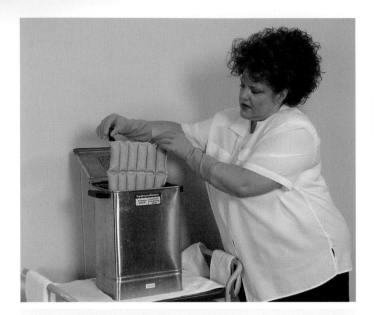

FIGURE 3.4
Using gloves to protect the hands while handling hot packs.

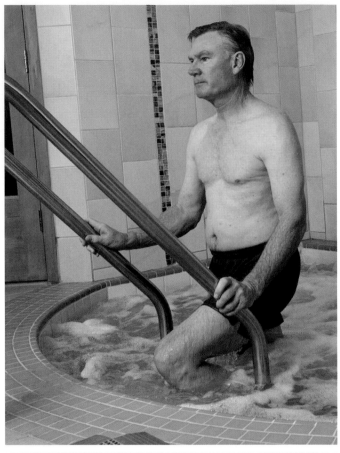

FIGURE 3.5
Client using grab bars.

on floors or benches. In most cases, if the client is going to have a whole-body heating treatment it is better to have it before bodywork begins, because then the client begins the session already relaxed and warm, with more pliable soft tissue and greater joint range of motion.

4. Clients should not be barefoot, especially if they have just had a massage. Oily feet should not be on the floor of your facility, and if a client is going to walk to a sauna or hot tub or shower, he or she could slip. Clients should be wearing socks at the end of the massage, and then wear shoes with non-slip bottoms.

5. As seen in Figure 3.5, grab bars in bathrooms, showers, hot tubs and bathtubs may help stabilize someone who is obese, unsteady on his or her feet, or lightheaded and dizzy from overexposure to heat, or who has poor balance.

6. Clients are more likely to complain of chilling after showers or baths in the winter, so make sure they have a towel or dry clothing to put on as soon as they get out.

7. To prevent burns, saunas should always have a railing or fence around the heater.

FACTORS AFFECTING THE BODY'S RESPONSE TO HEAT AND COLD

When you give a hydrotherapy treatment, you hope for a vigorous reaction.

While we cannot always predict how an individual will respond to our treatments, here are some factors to keep in mind.

Client's hydration status

Water makes up at least two thirds of our total body weight. Our blood, cerebrospinal fluid, tears, sweat, saliva and other secretions are largely water, most body parts are more than half water, and the cells that make up every one of our vital organs need water to carry out basic chemical reactions. An average adult needs to take about 8 cups (almost 2 liters) of water every day, although this amount can vary depending upon the person's body size, lifestyle, and whether the weather is hot or cold. Clients should never become dehydrated in your sessions: the client's response may be weaker, and he or she may not feel as well. For example, someone with low blood pressure will be more likely to be dizzy when they stand up if they are dehydrated. Provide the client with water before, during and after sessions.

Body composition and genetics

Just as individuals vary widely in their response to tactile stimulation, their tolerance of different temperatures can also be quite individual. One client may feel comfortable receiving a massage in a cool room with open windows and minimal draping, while another client in the same room, at the same time of year, feels comfortable only when the room is warmed, the windows are closed, warming devices (such as hot water bottles or hot fomentations) are placed on her body, and she is covered with extra blankets. The same is true of water temperatures. Over many years, students in hydrotherapy classes have reported a range of "ideal" bath temperatures, from 98°F to 110°F (37°C to 43°C). See Case history 2.2.

These individual differences are a combination of many factors. A very thin person will feel usually cold much more acutely than someone with a high percentage of body fat. Some people actually have thinner skin than others, with thermal receptors that are closer to the skin surface, so their experiences of heat and cold will be different from those of people with thicker skin.

Differences in the body's response to temperature have been found in groups such as Asians, Inuit peoples, African-Americans and Caucasians. These differences reflect the different climates where their ancestors originated (Charles, 2003; Kelsey, 2001; Marino, 2004; Nguyen, 2003). Our ability to generate body heat and to cool ourselves by sweating, and the extent to which our blood vessels react to cold, are all genetically influenced. (However, as therapists our first responsibility is to rely on our client's feedback as we work with them, not on assumptions or stereotypes.) Every client is an individual and we cannot always predict how anyone will respond. Asking about your client's past experience with heat and

cold, and paying close attention to their response, is the best guide to the appropriateness of the treatment.

Seasonal considerations

Clients who are regularly exposed to very hot or cold temperatures tend to respond to them better. For example, we start to sweat more when we begin to spend more time outside in the spring and summer and then we can tolerate heat better, while people who work in severe cold develop an increased ability to tolerate it. Over time, repeated cold hand baths cause the blood vessels of the hand to react faster and harder, so your clients may react to a treatment better if they have recently been exposed to hot or cold temperatures, compared to someone who has not (DeLorenzo, 1999; Geurts, 2005; LeBlanc, 1975).

For this reason, you may need to think about the season when applying some hydro treatments. The client who comes in on a warm day – already overheated – is not likely to enjoy that hot fomentation which usually feels wonderful in the dead of winter, and a client who enters your office on a cold winter's day – already chilled – is not likely to be receptive to ice massage unless his or her body has been thoroughly warmed first. One of the most effective ways you can use hydrotherapy treatments in your office is to maintain your clients' body temperatures so they are neither chilled nor overheated. For example, a client who is already warm but needs a heating treatment as part of his or her massage session can receive a cooling treatment at the same time On a hot day, hot moist packs will aid in stretching the large dense muscles of a football player, and using a cold footbath at the same time can prevent him from becoming overheated. For more on this topic, see Boxes 3.3 and 3.4.

Client's physical condition

Healthy people are stronger and react to hydrotherapy faster. Clients who are frail, inactive, very old or very young, or who have major health problems, are likely to have a weaker response. For example, a young vigorous person may be able to tolerate a cold plunge after a hot bath, and then enjoy the prolonged feeling of warmth that the cold plunge usually gives: a weaker person, however, may become chilled during the plunge and take a long time to warm up again.

Chapter three

USING HYDROTHERAPY TO COOL THE CLIENT DURING A SESSION

1. When clients enter your office on a hot day, a simple way to help them cool down before massage is a brief cold foot soak. Even 5 minutes of soaking can reduce body temperature and feel soothing. This can be performed with clients seated or lying supine on the massage table with knees bent.

2. A cool shower before or after the massage session will reduce body temperature.

3. A Fomentek filled with cold water may be placed on the therapy table, then covered by the sheet the client will lie on. A hot water bottle filled with ice water may be used on any part of the body.

4. Washcloths or round cotton pads that are dipped in ice water can be used to cool the eyes and upper face. Miniature ice packs with a thin layer of cloth underneath, or cooled gel masks made specifically for the eyes, are also effective.

5. Ice packs can be used for almost any part of the body, if they are the right size: small ones can go over the eyes, long narrow ones can go behind or around the neck or on any other part of the body, and larger ones may be used on areas such as the upper thigh or back. Always protect the skin with a thin layer of cloth directly on the skin and the ice pack on top of that.

6. Chilled gloves (made of loofah, very thin wool or cotton) for the hands or chilled cotton socks for the feet provide cooling that may be more acceptable for some clients than cold nearer the center of the body. Both the gloves and the socks can be soaked in water, wrung out, and kept in the freezer until they are needed. Thaw them slightly until they are limp but still cold, and put them on the client's hands or feet. When they warm up, they can be re-dipped in ice water or iced herbal teas and applied again.

7. A large towel dipped in ice water and well wrung out is effective for cooling the back. Compressions, pressure points and other massage techniques may be used through the cold towel. To cool the chest and abdomen, use a slightly smaller towel dipped in ice water and wrung out. Massage may be done through the cold towel.

8. Spray ice water from a mister bottle over the client's body at the same time. This is especially effective if you have a fan blowing cool air over the client's body. Some therapists add a few drops of cooling essential oils such as peppermint. Do not spray the face.

9. Wash each portion of the body off with a washcloth dipped in ice water as you finish massage—especially effective if you have a fan blowing cool air.

10. Salt glows can be performed with ice water, on individual areas of the body or the entire body. Ice water is used to moisten the salt, and to wash the client off before and after the salt application.

11. Ice massage can be used on individual areas.

12. Use an iced sheet wrap, using a sheet which has been wrung out in cold water, then put in the freezer for 10 minutes or in an ice chest half-full of ice cubes for 10 minutes or in the refrigerator for 20 minutes. A sheet can also be soaked in a large container of very cold water (made with plenty of ice cubes) and used right away. The iced sheet is placed on the massage table, and the client lays on the iced sheet, is wrapped, and then receives massage on face, hands and feet before the sheet is removed.

13. Cold plunges are extremely cooling. If taken after a massage session, clients should shower first to remove massage oil or lotion.

Client's skin and core temperature before a treatment

If the client's skin is very cold or very hot at the beginning of a treatment, he or she will probably have a slower or weaker reaction. If the skin is very hot, it will take longer for a cold application to chill it, and if the skin is very cold, it will take longer for a hot application to cool it.

The client's core temperature is also important: if it is low before a cold immersion, he or she is likely to react weakly (Belanger, 2002). Clients should be thoroughly warm but not overheated before a treatment begins. Keep the treatment room at about 70°F (21°C).

BOX 3.4	POINT OF INTEREST

USING HYDROTHERAPY TO WARM THE CLIENT DURING A SESSION

1. Hot foot soak prior to massage. This can be done with the client sitting in a chair or supine on the massage table.

2. A hot bath, shower, sauna or steam bath prior to massage. Don't let clients become chilled on the way out.

3. A Fomentek filled with warm water may be placed on the therapy table, then covered by the sheet the client will lie on.

4. Warmed gel eye masks, moist, round cotton pads or washcloths dipped in hot water, or small gel packs with layers of cloth underneath, can warm the eyes and upper face.

5. Moist local heat applications include hydrocollator packs and hot fomentations, moistened hot towels which have been kept in a cooler, and washcloths that are either heated up in a crockpot that has a small amount of water in the bottom, or dipped in hot water and then wrung out before being applied to the client's skin.

6. Paraffin treatments of the hands or feet are effective at warming the whole body, especially if prolonged.

7. Hot water bottles of various sizes, filled with warm water.

8. Large towels dipped in hot water and wrung out may be used to warm the entire back or front of the body. They will cool off rapidly, however, and should be replaced when cold by another warm towel. As soon as the last towel is removed, the client should be dried thoroughly, and covered immediately with a drape.

9. Wash off each area after you massage it, using a washcloth dipped in hot water. Dry the skin immediately and cover the client to keep the area warm.

10. A full-body warming wrap, with massage of the feet or head while the client rests in the wrap.

Part of the body treated

Different areas of the body have different amounts of warm and cold receptors, so some parts are more sensitive to temperatures. For example, an ice pack laid upon the chest is likely to chill the client far more than the same ice pack laid upon the foot.

Treatment temperature

The hotter or colder the water, the faster and stronger the client's reaction. For example, a neutral temperature shower (98°F or 37°C), tends to create much less of a reaction than a very hot or very cold shower.

How fast the water temperature is switched

The more sudden the application of a hot or cold treatment, the greater the client's reaction. For example, if a person is standing in a warm shower and the water temperature is gradually changed to cold, his reaction will not be as strong as if the water temperature were quickly changed from warm to cold. The more abrupt the change, the more stimulating the treatment will be.

Length of treatment

In general, the shorter the application lasts, the more stimulating it is to the circulation. For example, a short hot bath is more stimulating than a long hot bath, and a short cold shower is more stimulating than a long cold shower. A short hot application, such as a hydrocollator pack laid on an area for 2 minutes, is more stimulating to the circulation than a longer hot application; and ice massage, where the cold continually moves to new areas, is more stimulating to the circulation than an ice pack which remains in one place for many minutes.

Proportion of the body that is treated

All other factors being the same, the larger the application, the greater the reaction. For example, a client who lies on a bed of three fomentations that warm him from his knees to his neck will have a much stronger reaction than a client who has a small warm compress over the eyes.

Use of friction or percussion

Adding friction or percussion to a hot or cold treatment is much more stimulating to the nerves, and the blood vessels in the skin then react more strongly and this increases the warming or cooling of the skin. A cloth wrung out in ice water and rubbed briskly over the lower back will cause a stronger reaction then if you simply lay the cloth on the area and leave it alone.

Body temperature after a whole-body treatment

Being uncomfortably hot after a sauna or freezing cold after a long ice application would make anyone uncomfortable and tense, undermining even the best bodywork. Check in with the client and make sure he or she is comfortable.

Dislike of heat or cold

Some people have an aversion to heat or cold, sometimes stemming from a bad experience with hot or cold applications in the past. This might make them unwilling to try a hydrotherapy treatment. For example, in *Pediatric Massage Therapy,* Sinclair quotes a woman who was physically abused as a child, and every hot bath had made her welts and bruises sting. Due to these painful memories, when she grew up she avoided hot baths altogether (Sinclair, 2004). Similarly, as a very young child, Suzanne Pike was admitted to Warm Springs Rehabilitation Institute for treatment of her clubfeet. Pike regularly received painfully hot paraffin footbaths followed by painful massage and manipulation. At age 73, she disclosed that this experience had caused a lifelong fear of medical treatments and doctors, and the thought of heat being applied to her extremities was unpleasant (Pike, 2005). If your client has such an aversion to a particular treatment, it may be better to use a different one that will achieve the same end. For example, if your client has an aversion to a local heat treatment such as a fomentation, local circulation can be enhanced by a salt glow performed with neutral temperature water instead. Perhaps if you explain the purpose of a treatment the client may be willing to give it a try, but never try to coerce anyone.

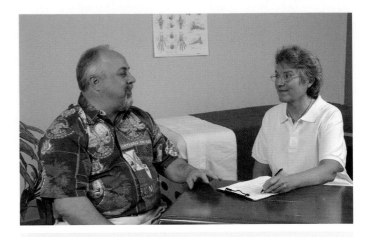

FIGURE 3.6
Interviewing the client.

CLIENT HEALTH HISTORY

Taking a careful health history will alert you to any conditions that might contraindicate hydrotherapy treatments (an interview with a client is seen in Figure 3.6). Additionally, at the end of the form, several questions are included that can help you explore how the client may feel about certain treatments (Figure 3.7 gives a sample health history form). Take a few minutes to discuss the history form with your client and address any particular health concerns. Should there be any question about a treatment that the client would like to have but that you suspect is unsafe, take time to explain your concerns to the client. For example, a client with **lymphedema** or a history of stroke may not know that she should not go in the sauna at your facility, even if she and her friends were planning on going in together after their massage sessions. (You may wish to read her the information from this book or another source to make your concerns completely clear.)

BASIC GUIDELINES FOR HYDROTHERAPY

Following these basic guidelines will ensure that you give your client a safe and effective treatment:

1. While you are giving the hydrotherapy treatment, explain what you are doing and why. This may be as simple as saying, "Now I'm going to put an ice pack over your bruise. It will feel cold at first, but it will help relieve the swelling and discomfort."

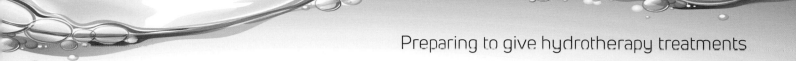

Health history

Name

Address

Date

Telephone number(s)

How is your health in general?

Do you have any conditions that are being monitored by a healthcare practitioner? (Please list)

Please check if you have any of the following conditions:

☐ Arteriosclerosis
☐ Arthritis
☐ Artificial devices (joint prosthetics, implants, pacemaker or other)
☐ Asthma
☐ Bursitis
☐ Cancer
☐ Diabetes
☐ Heart disease (history of heart attack, congestive heart failure, coronary artery disease)
☐ Hepatitis
☐ High blood pressure
☐ HIV/AIDS
☐ Joint pain or swelling
☐ Loss of feeling in any part of the body
☐ Lymphedema
☐ Migraine headaches

☐ Multiple sclerosis
☐ Nerve or crush injury to an extremity
☐ Phlebitis
☐ Pregnancy
☐ Raynaud's syndrome
☐ Seizure disorders
☐ Skin disease
☐ Stroke
☐ Tendonitis
☐ Tension headaches
☐ Tension or soreness in a specific area
☐ Thyroid conditions
☐ Whiplash injuries
☐ Other conditions
☐ Other pain

Comments

Surgical procedures undergone

Traumatic injuries such as bruises, sprains, broken bones, dislocations and concussions

FIGURE 3.7
Client health history.

Or "I'm going to put this hot pack over your lower back. It will help relax those muscles before I massage them."

2. Always check the temperature of hot or cold applications against your own skin before applying them to clients. When you use liquid water in a treatment, always use a thermometer to check its temperature.

3. When using a hot application, tell your clients, "Let me know if this starts to feel too hot." Do this even if you have given that person the same hot application many times before.

4. During treatments, carefully observe the client. Check occasionally under a hot application to see what the skin looks like, especially during the first 5 minutes when a pack is at its hottest. Also ask the client how it feels. For example, with either a hot pack or a cold pack you could ask, "How does this feel on your skin now?" Make sure your clients are comfortable during any hydrotherapy treatment. For example, if they are not entirely comfortable with ice, reassure them that you will keep the rest of their body extra warm. Drape carefully around areas where you are doing ice massage to keep trickles of ice water from dripping into sensitive areas.

5. Never start or end treatment with a chilled client: no one will be able to relax during a massage if he or she is cold. A client should never leave your office with wet hair or damp clothing.

6. Observe all contraindications.

7. Remind clients to follow safety rules. For example, in a facility such as a health club, clients should take seriously a warning on a sauna door saying that people with hypertension or cardiac problems should not go in.

SESSION DESIGN

Choosing which treatments to give your client during a massage session is not difficult. Taking a good history at the first session (including the client's past experience with hydrotherapy), listening carefully to your client's concerns, and getting feedback on the treatments makes it easy to pick the right one. Hydrotherapy applications should always complement massage technique and work towards the same goals. First, try to determine whether the client is more interested in relief from stress, help with a musculoskeletal issue, or simply needs to be touched. If relief from stress is the help he or she needs, ice massage is probably not called for: a more soothing treatment would be a warm bath, hot shower, or body wrap followed by massage. If the client has a musculoskeletal injury, ice massage or a contrast bath may be the best initial treatment to increase circulation and relieve discomfort in the injured area: afterwards massage techniques may also be applied around the injured area. If the client is seeking massage to receive nurturing touch, perhaps a local salt glow, which provides additional stimulation to the skin, would complement your touch.

Some specific examples:

1. A client arrives for an appointment that was scheduled a month ago, only to tell you that she was in a car accident yesterday. She was evaluated at a hospital emergency room and found to be free of serious musculoskeletal injuries; however, except for her hands and feet, the rest of her body still hurts too much to be touched. In addition, she is very stressed and upset by the accident. Any vigorous massage techniques are obviously contraindicated. A simple, deeply comforting session could begin by placing three small bath towels in warm Epsom salts water, placing them gently on her trunk, abdomen and legs, and covering each with a warm fomentation or a thin sheet of plastic and a heating pad. Then the client could receive massage on her hands and feet or energy work. This hydrotherapy treatment would help with her pain and allow her to have a relaxing session.

2. A client with a painful shoulder arrives straight from her doctor's office. Her doctor has ruled out a sprained shoulder, bursitis, or rotator cuff syndrome, and diagnosed her with a muscle strain: she is a nurse and lifted a heavy patient that morning. A session that meets her needs could combine a contrast treatment on her shoulder, using a moist hot pack followed by ice massage, with gentle massage around her neck, shoulder and upper arm. This will desensitize the area somewhat, improve circulation and help relieve pain.

3. A client arrives with a lower back spasm so severe that he is practically carried in by a friend. He has come directly from his chiropractor, who found the client's muscles too tense for an adjustment

and recommended massage. A salt glow of the lower back followed by ice massage would help increase circulation, relieve pain and decrease muscle spasm, thereby making your massage much more effective. Another possibility, in a facility that has steam cabinets or full bathtubs, would be for the client to take a steam bath or a hot Epsom salts bath first, followed by ice massage over the back muscles and then hands-on techniques. Still another possibility would be to place a towel soaked in Epsom-salts-saturated water on his back, then cover the towel with a thin piece of plastic and a hydrocollator pack, fomentation or hot water bottle on top of that. After a 15–20 minute application, his back muscles would be far more relaxed and ready for massage. At the same time, while the heat relaxes the spasmed areas, massage could be performed on related muscle groups, such as gluteals, piriformis, and spinal erectors. A study of 117 people who were hospitalized for lower back pain found that patients with chronic back pain had shorter hospital stays when treated with ice massage, and patients with acute back pain had shorter hospital stays when treated with moist hot packs (Lander, 1967).

When determining the best hydrotherapy treatment to meet a client's needs, it is helpful to follow a three-step reasoning process. Step 1: review the client's medical history; Step 2: interview the client; and Step 3: select the appropriate treatment. Below are two examples of how you might use this process, one for a relaxation massage and the other for a therapeutic massage.

Choosing hydrotherapy treatments for a relaxation massage session
Step 1: review the client's medical history

- Does the client have any contraindications to hydrotherapy treatments?

- Has the client had hydrotherapy treatments before, and if so, how has he or she reacted to them?

Step 2: interview the client

- In what part of the body does the client tend to store stress?

- Which of the client's muscles are particularly tight?

- What type of massage does the client prefer: light touch techniques such as energy work or gentle Swedish massage, or deep pressure techniques such as myofascial release or deep Swedish massage? A highly sensitive person who prefers light touch techniques would be more likely to prefer a hydrotherapy technique which is not highly stimulating, such as a warm compress. A not-so-highly sensitive person who prefers deeper techniques may enjoy, and tolerate well, such highly stimulating techniques as contrast applications and sprays and showers.

Step 3: select the appropriate treatment

- Decide which hydrotherapy treatments are options for this relaxation massage session. Of course, the treatments you can give are also determined by the hydrotherapy equipment that you have in your office. Review contraindications.

- Choose a treatment that is safe and appropriate.

- Obtain client permission.

Case history 3.3 shows the thinking process used by a therapist in an unusual situation.

Choosing hydrotherapy treatments for a therapeutic massage session
Step 1: review the client's medical history

- What soft tissue condition(s) is the client experiencing?

- Is this condition acute or chronic?

- Does the client have any contraindications to hydrotherapy treatments?

- Has the client had hydrotherapy treatments before, and if so, how has he or she reacted to them?

Step 2: interview the client

- In what part(s) of the body is the client experiencing pain or discomfort?

- Is there anything that increases or decreases the pain or discomfort?

Chapter three

BACKGROUND

Sarah is an active 54-year-old schoolteacher who is also hypermobile and prone to musculoskeletal pain for that reason. Sam has treated her many times for muscle spasms, injuries, and stress. Nine years previously, Sarah lifted a very heavy box and strained her right shoulder: she has had pain, muscle tightness and a "catching" sensation in the joint ever since. Diligent physical therapy did not relieve these symptoms, and she finally had surgery one week ago for a torn glenoid ligament. Her orthopedic surgeon found that the ligament was torn anterior-to-posterior, her supraspinatus tendon was somewhat frayed, and the cartilage lining her right distal clavicle had eroded over time. He operated to repair the glenoid tear and also removed about 8 mm of her distal clavicle. Sarah went back to her doctor one week later because she was concerned about increasing pain and swelling of her right upper extremity. Her doctor examined her, decided that her swelling was not abnormal and suggested she begin physical therapy in four weeks' time, in order to manage her pain and muscle spasm. He did state that as long as the shoulder joint was not disturbed massage was safe that very day. Since she was still just as uncomfortable, Sarah has requested that Sam give her a treatment at her home. When he arrives, Sarah is unhappy: she has stopped taking her prescribed medication because it was causing constipation, and her pain is now 7/10. She is also very constipated, cannot seem to get warm (her house is cold), has not slept well for a week, and cannot even lie down to rest. (She is wearing a sling, and is not supposed to lie flat.)

TREATMENT

Sam considers how to proceed. Massage of the shoulder is out, since it has only been a week since surgery. Ice massage of the shoulder area is out, because Sarah is quite cold. He must adjust his usual massage procedure because she cannot lie down. Sam decides to offer Sarah a hot foot soak along with hands-on treatment. Sarah's husband assists with a plastic tub and 104°F (40°C) water. As soon as Sarah's feet are placed in the hot water, she begins to feel warmer and less irritable. Sam proceeds to perform gentle lymphatic massage on her upper body for about 30 minutes, all the while avoiding the operated areas and working far enough away to avoid pulling on internal stitches. Her husband adds more water to the footbath to keep it at 104°F (40°C). Before Sam is finished with the session, Sarah exclaims how warm and relaxed she feels, how much less swollen her shoulder is, and how much her shoulder pain has decreased. Gentle lymphatic massage paired with the soothing, warming and fluid-shifting effect of the hot footbath was an unbeatable combination.

DISCUSSION QUESTIONS

1. What other type of massage or hydrotherapy treatment might have been suitable for Sarah's situation?

2. Could the therapist have addressed Sarah's constipation during this session? How?

Step 3: select the appropriate treatment

- Determine which part(s) of the body to treat.

- Decide which hydrotherapy treatments are options for this therapeutic massage session. Of course, the treatments you can choose from are also determined by the hydrotherapy equipment that you have in your office.

- Review contraindications.

- Choose a treatment that is safe and appropriate.

- Obtain client permission.

ADAPTING HYDROTHERAPY TREATMENTS TO DIFFERENT SETTINGS

Most of this discussion of hydrotherapy has been directed to a massage therapist working in an individual practice or sharing an office with others. However, individual hydrotherapy treatments can be performed in many other environments where a massage therapist might practice. Remember that treatments, in any setting, offer positive sensory stimulation along with their physiological benefits. Below are some examples of different settings and how hydrotherapy treatments could be adapted for use there. Careful sanitizing is very important, so always be sure to use hand sanitizer and/or sanitizing sprays according to safety protocols.

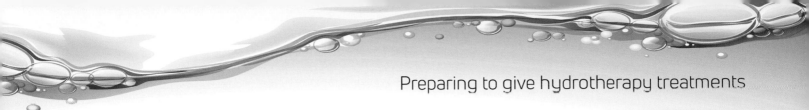

Outdoor sports events

A massage practitioner working outdoors at a sports massage event can take bags of ice and bottled water in an ice chest, along with extra towels and washcloths, Epsom salts and plastic dishtubs for footbaths. A nearby hose or other running water source is helpful. With these few simple tools items, you can perform:

- Ice massage to relieve sore and aching muscles.

- Local salt glows of the back, legs and feet to increase circulation and relax those areas.

- Ice-cold foot soaks for aching and burning feet, and to cool overheated athletes on a hot day.

- Epsom salt foot soaks for tired and aching feet. Water does not need to be hot for these foot soaks – even tepid water will be effective. Perhaps athletes who are waiting for a massage would like to soak their feet while they wait.

Hospitals

An individual massage practitioner practicing in a hospital setting may see patients who have access to a whirlpool.

For example, some hospitals that offer jacuzzis for women during labor may have them available after the birth to help with perineal and low back discomfort. Massage therapy for new mothers after a warm soak is a wonderful complement to this service. With the permission of the nursing staff, warm moist towels may also be used with any hospitalized patient to provide mild local heat, and to wash off massage lotion at the end of the massage. These treatments are very comforting for patients, and practical even if the patients are in bed. See Box 3.5 for an example of a hospital that incorporates hydrotherapy and massage extensively in the care of their patients.

Chiropractic or physical therapy clinics

An individual massage practitioner practicing in a chiropractic office or physical therapy clinic will often have access to a hydrocollator unit with hot packs, and possibly ice cups or ice packs as well. The hot packs are great for relieving muscle tension and increasing local circulation, and are easy to place on one part of the body while massage is being performed on another part. Ice massage is also very useful in this setting, where many clients are experiencing severe musculoskeletal pain.

BOX 3.5	POINT OF INTEREST

HYDROTHERAPY AND MASSAGE IN A HOSPITAL SETTING

Founded in 1942, Wildwood Hospital is an acute care hospital, outpatient clinic and health education center operated as a ministry of the Seventh-Day Adventist Church. Because Wildwood's guiding philosophy is to use natural treatments to promote health and provide an alternative to the use of prescription medication, hydrotherapy and massage are integral parts of treatment.

Each patient's case is reviewed by staff physicians (MDs), who prescribe natural remedies: there are specific hydrotherapy treatments for patients with common conditions such as liver cirrhosis, cancer, high blood pressure, asthma, diabetic ulcers, varicose ulcers, musculoskeletal complaints and diseases of

the immune system. After surgery, once a doctor has determined that the danger of bleeding is past– generally after 36 hours–many patients receive contrast treatments over their incisions to reduce pain and speed healing. Generally the incisions are covered with a sheet of plastic to keep them dry, then warm fomentations are alternated with cold or iced cloths, for a total of three changes.

Whole-body treatments are performed using large whirlpools, multi-jet showers and Russian steam baths. Local treatments are performed using small whirlpools, sitz baths, hot fomentations and ice. Many of the patients receive a contrast shower at the end of their other treatments. Patients who are strong enough to walk or be taken by wheelchair have their treatments in the hydrotherapy department of the hospital. However, if they are too weak or have too many intravenous

BOX 3.5 *continued*

lines, monitors, or other equipment to be moved, they receive treatments in their rooms. In that case, nurses or specially trained therapists generally use heat and ice to perform treatments.

Fomentations are heated in the hydrotherapy department, placed in a large cooler, and taken in a rolling cart to the patient's room, along with a supply of ice cubes. The hydrotherapy department, which is managed by a physical therapist, is a heavily used area of the hospital. It has separate men's and women's sides, each containing a multi-jet shower, a Russian steam bath, and five massage rooms. These rooms contain treatment tables where patients may receive bodywork after their water treatments. A common area used by both men and women contains porcelain sitz baths and large and small steel whirlpools. The entire hydrotherapy department is tiled from floor to ceiling, and its walls contain built-in niches with shelves for gloves, massage oils, and other small items.

Those who are staying at Wildwood while they attend health education programs also receive hydrotherapy treatments, either in the hydrotherapy department or in a nearby bathhouse equipped with showers, a jacuzzi, and a sauna.

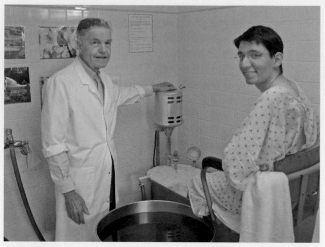

FIGURE 1
Physical therapist Earl Qualls, director of the hydrotherapy department, gives a cold friction to a patient. Mr. Qualls graduated from physical therapy school in 1951 and was still performing hydrotherapy treatments more than 50 years later. Photo courtesy of Earl Qualls, PT and Wildwood Hospital, Wildwood, Georgia.

Assisted living facilities

Clients in assisted living facilities may receive massage in their rooms, which usually contain a small kitchenette, and so here you have access to running water and ice. You may need to bring containers for water, or you may find them already in the kitchenette.

A simple, effective, and much-loved treatment in this setting is a warm footbath that incorporates a salt glow of the feet and lower legs. Place a large towel on the floor, place a chair on top of it and then have the client sit in the chair. Sitting on the ground in front of the client, treat each lower leg and foot in turn. One foot may be taken out of the footbath and an Epsom salts glow performed with the foot resting on the edge of the tub or bucket: then put that foot back and repeat with the other foot and lower leg. Rinse off with clean water, cooler water if possible, dry the feet, and finish with hands-on massage techniques.

Nursing homes

Clients are generally given massages in their rooms, which are smaller and have no kitchenette, however there is always a bathroom close by. With the hot and cold water coming out of the tap, simple treatments such as the local salt glow described above are feasible, and washing off massage lotion is simple. A hot cloth on the forehead on a cold winter day or a cold cloth on a hot summer day is easy and very comforting. You may wish

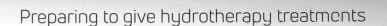

to bring a container for water, or obtain one from the nursing staff.

Health clubs or spas

Most health clubs or spas that offer massage have at least one hot tub, shower, steam room, or sauna. First review the client's health history. If there are no contra-indications, you can suggest that he or she use those facilities before or after massage sessions. Many clubs and wellness centers have signs on sauna doors that list contraindications, such as:

- *Do not use the hot tub or sauna under the influence of alcohol or drugs.*
- *Do not use the hot tub or sauna if you have an infectious disease, high or low blood pressure, or very low blood sugar, as this can decrease your tolerance to heat.*
- *Understand your own heat tolerance and do not exceed 15 minutes in the heat without a cooldown.*

Clients may also be asked to sign a consent form. Spas that offer foot treatments before foot massage, including warm soaks, salt glows, paraffin dips and mud applications should also notify clients of any safety issues. For example, the notice from the Barefoot Sage Spa, in Portland, Oregon, says this:

Any person with diabetes, nervous system or cardiovascular disorders, skin conditions, or cancer (including chemotherapy and radiation therapy) that may affect the sensation, circulation, or health in the feet may need a physician's release before some therapies can be provided. If you neglect to inform us of such conditions you do so at your own risk.

The point to remember here is that any spa or health club that offers hydrotherapy treatments asks clients to waive liability.

Clients' homes

With a little preparation, a massage practitioner who does house calls can perform many basic treatments. (Figure 3.8 shows the contents of a portable hydrotherapy kit.) Here are some items that can be kept together as a kit for home visits:

1. Container of hand sanitizer and water thermometer.
2. Ice chest, to transport ice to your client or to hold pre-heated moist towels, hydrocollator packs or fomentations.
3. Heat-resistant gloves.
4. Resealable plastic bags, one quart and one-gallon sizes, to make ice packs from ice cubes and to microwave fomentations.
5. Moist hot packs (fomentations or hydrocollator packs), with towels to wrap them in.
6. Washcloths, small towels, and bath towels, if linens are not available at the client's home.
7. Epsom salts.
8. Spray bottle of sanitizer and plastic bag for used linens.

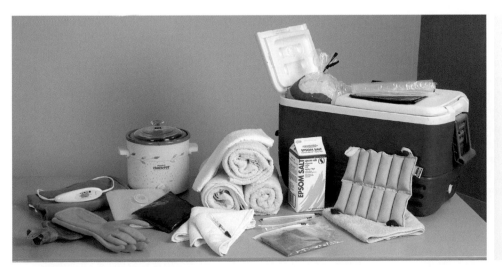

FIGURE 3.8
Portable hydrotherapy kit.

9. If running water is not available, take a plastic gallon jug with fresh water and a bag of ice. If you only have cold water available, you can make hot water by mixing boiling water with cold water as follows. Boil water on a stovetop. Mix in the proportions listed below to reach the desired temperature, and check the water with a thermometer before using it (see Case history 3.4 for an example of how this method was adapted to help bathe and soothe a cranky baby):

- One quart of boiling water plus four quarts of cold tap water = five quarts of water at 85°F (29°C).

- One quart of boiling water plus three quarts of cold tap water = one gallon of water at 92°F (33°C).

- One quart of boiling water plus two quarts of cold tap water = three quarts of water at 106°F (41°C).

Even though the water will gradually cool off, you can keep it at the same temperature: for example, if you are giving a footbath, take the client's limb out of the water, scoop out 1 cup of the cooled water, replace it with 2 cups of boiling water and check the temperature again before putting the limb back in the water.

10. Hot water bottles. In a pinch, any clean plastic bottle may be used for a hot or cold water bottle.

11. Optional: portable steam canopy in carrying container. It weighs 20 pounds, can be set up on any comfortable towel-covered surface, and requires only electricity and a little water.

12. Optional: slow cooker or turkey roaster to heat water, in a box for easier carrying.

13. Optional: plastic garbage bag, cardboard box and sturdy tape to construct a local bath such as an arm bath or sitz bath.

| CREATING A HYDROTHERAPY TREATMENT IN A CAMPGROUND | CASE HISTORY 3.4 |

BACKGROUND

David is a healthy 8-month old boy, who is on a 3-day car camping trip with his mom and dad and a group of their friends. David is usually happy and easy-going, but for some unknown reason is very unhappy tonight. He has been crying loudly and inconsolably for over an hour. His parents are at their wits end trying to soothe him, and are concerned about the disturbance to the other campers.

TREATMENT

David's mother suddenly has an idea: she remembers that the ice in their 4-gallon capacity cooler has all melted (it now holds 1.25 gallons (5.68 liters) of cold water) and she decides to heat water on a campfire to make David a bath. Everyone rushes to take all the food out of the cooler and fill it to three-quarters capacity (3 gallons; 13.6 liters) with cold water from a faucet. About 1 gallon of water is heated on the campfire to boiling (212°F; 100°C) as David continues to scream. The boiling water is poured into the ice chest, which is now almost full, and the water temperature is checked with David's baby thermometer. The water is 92°F (33°C). David has now been crying for an hour and a quarter and shows no sign of letting up. His mother undresses him and gently places him in the cooler. He gives a couple of astonished squawks, sighs, stops crying and gives every sign that the water feels good. He is supervised for 15 minutes while he splashes delightedly and his back is rubbed. He is then taken out of his "bath," dried, and put into pajamas. He falls right to sleep and sleeps well all night.

DISCUSSION QUESTIONS

1. What steps were taken to ensure that this hydrotherapy treatment was safe?

2. What other hydrotherapy treatments might have helped David stop crying?

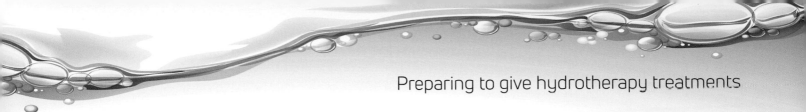

CHAPTER SUMMARY

In this chapter, you have learned about important qualities of water that make it effective for bodyworkers, and then how to select and maintain hydrotherapy equipment. You know how to recognize cautions and contraindications for hydrotherapy treatments, and how to obtain a thorough client health history. You have also learned some basic treatment guidelines, how to design a session to meet your client's unique needs, and how to adapt hydrotherapy treatments to various situations. Equipped with this knowledge, you can begin to use your own creativity to help your clients in ways that are fine-tuned for their individual needs. In the chapters to come, we will explore many hydrotherapy treatments in far more detail, and deepen your understanding of their potential.

REVIEW QUESTIONS

Short answer

1. Describe several characteristics of water and how these characteristics of water make it useful in hydrotherapy treatments.

2. Explain how water can turn from liquid to vapor or liquid to solid and back again.

3. Explain conduction, convection, condensation, evaporation, and radiation.

4. Name six factors that affect a person's response to a hydrotherapy treatment.

5. Describe the additional questions you will need to add to a standard health intake form if you are going to give a hydrotherapy treatment.

Multiple choice

6. Water treatment is partly a chemical application. in all but one: Which of these is the exception?

A. Epsom salt bath

B. Mud bath

C. Whirlpool bath

D. Aromatherapy compress

7. Buoyancy relieves discomfort in three of these conditions. Which condition does it *not* help?

A. Obesity

B. Arthritis

C. Measles

D. Pregnancy

8. Some hydrotherapy treatments are contra-indicated for certain conditions. Which is the exception?

A. Chilled person

B. Multiple sclerosis

C. Lymphedema

D. Inactive person

E. Raynaud's syndrome

9. All but one of these factors could cause a poor response to some hydrotherapy treatments. Which is the exception?

A. Sedentary lifestyle

B. Cold skin at the beginning of the treatment

C. Chronic illness

D. Dehydration

E. Emotional stress

F. Highly athletic person

10. All but one of the people below might be easily chilled. Which would not? Someone who ...

A. Has a hypothyroid condition

B. Is from a family where everyone gets cold easily

C. Is small and thin

D. Is obese

E. Is not accustomed to cold

11. All but one of these are effective ways to conserve water when you perform hydrotherapy treatments. Which is the exception?

A. Collecting water as it runs until it has reached the desired temperature

B. Using appliances that do not waste water

C. Flushing trash down the toilet

D. Choosing hydrotherapy treatments that use less water

E. Warming the client, not the air

12. Which heat treatment is the most expensive?

A. Paraffin bath

B. Steam room

REVIEW QUESTIONS *continued*

C. Hot footbath

D. Steam canopy

E. Homemade fomentation

Matching

13.

1.	Solvent	A.	Treats heatstroke
2.	"Hypnotic"	B.	Warms body parts
3.	Absorbs heat	C.	Dissolves other substances
4.	Heat conducting	D.	Whole-body warm bath

14.

1.	Convection	A.	The process which changes water vapor (a gas) into water (a liquid)
2.	Conduction	B.	The transfer of heat through space, without two objects touching, through the emission of heat
3.	Radiation	C.	The transfer of heat by direct contact of one heated or cooled substance with another
4.	Condensation	D.	The giving off of heat by the actual movement of heated liquid or gas

15.

1.	Crushing injuries	A.	No heat to abdomen
2.	Asthmatics	B.	Thicker insulation
3.	Limited mobility	C.	Thinner skin
4.	Obesity	D.	No cold dry air
5.	Pregnancy	E.	Difficult movement
6.	Children	F.	No local cold treatments

16.

1.	Scalding	A.	92°F (33°C)
2.	Very cold	B.	60°C (15.6°C)
3.	Neutral	C.	110°F (43°C)
4.	Very hot	D.	97°F (36°C)
5.	Cold	E.	125°F (51.6°C)
6.	Tepid	F.	212°F (100°C)
7.	Boiling	G.	32°F (0°C)

17.

1.	Mop	A.	Prevents falling onto heater
2.	Gloves	B.	Prevents chilling
3.	Grab bars	C.	Prevents slipping in a puddle
4.	Towel or dry clothing	D.	Prevent falling
5.	Guard rail around heater	E.	Prevent burning the hands

18.

1.	Local heat	A.	Steam bath
2.	Whole-body cold	B.	Ice massage
3.	Hot air bath	C.	Sauna
4.	Local cold	D.	Paraffin
5.	Whole-body moist heat	E.	Wet sheet pack

Discussion questions

19. Describe the physical changes that might cause a client to become light-headed or nauseous during a whole-body heating treatment.

20. Discuss the factors you need to take into account to select a hydrotherapy treatment for a client.

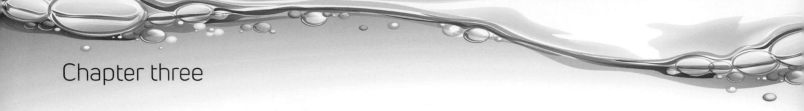

REVIEW QUESTIONS *continued*

True/False

21. Local cold is contraindicated in Raynaud's syndrome.

22. Local heat to the feet is safe for people with diabetes.

23. Salt glows can be used to improve skin circulation and provide sensory stimulation for bedridden people.

24. The most important hydrotherapy tool is one basic heat treatment.

25. After a massage session, all cloth items should be washed in hot water and hung up to dry.

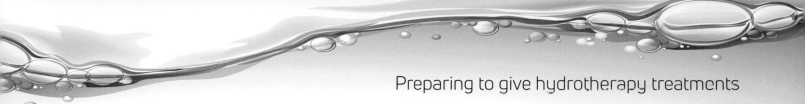

References

Belanger A. Evidence-based guide to therapeutic physical agents. Baltimore: Lippincott, Williams and Wilkins, 2002, p. 269

Charles K. Fanger's Thermal Comfort and Draught Models. Ottawa: Canada: Institute for Research in Construction, National Research Council of Canada, 2003

DeLorenzo F et al. Haemodynamic responses and changes of haemostatic risk factors in cold-adapted humans. Q J Med 1999; 92: 509–13

Geurts C. Local cold acclimation of the hand impairs thermal responses of the fingers without improving hand neuromuscular function. Acta Physiol Scand 2005; 183: 117–29.

Inoue Y, Kuwahara T, Araki T. Maturation and aging-related changes in heat loss effector function. J Physiol Anthropol Appl Human Sci 2004; 6: 289–94

Jokinen E. Children in sauna: hormonal adjustments to intensive short thermal stress. Acta Physiol Scand 1991; 142(3): 437–42

Kellogg J. Rational Hydrotherapy: A Manual of the Physiological and Therapeutic Effects of Hydriatic Procedures. Battle Creek, MI: Modern Medicine Publishing Company, 1923

Kelsey R, Alpert B, Patterson S, Barnard M. Racial differences in hemodynamic responses to environmental thermal stress among adolescents. Circulation 2001; 101: 2284

Lander BR. Heat or ice for relief of low back pain? Physical Therapy Review 1967; 47(112): 1126–8

LeBlanc J et al. Autonomic nervous system and adaptation to cold in man. J Applied Physiology 1975; 39(2): 181–6

Marino FE, Lambert MI, Noakes TD. Superior performances of African runners in warm humid but not in cool environmental conditions. J Appl Physiol 2004; 96(1): 124–30

Milunsky A et al. Maternal heat exposure and neural tube defects, JAMA 1992; 268(7): 882–5

Nguyen MH, Tokura H. Sweating and tympanic temperature during warm water immersion compared between Vietnamese and Japanese living in Hanoi. J Human Ergol (Tokyo) 2003; 32(1): 9–16

Norton A. A nice warm bath may be good for the heart. Reuters Health Information, 3 November 2002

Pike S. Personal communication/interview with author. Warm Springs, GA, 23 Feb 2005

Proctor D et al. Impaired leg vasodilation during dymanic exercise in healthy older women. J of Applied Physiology 2003; 95

Rymal C. Can patients at risk for lymphedema use hot tubs? Clin J Oncol Nurs 2002; 6(6): 369

Salvo S. Mosby's Pathology for Massage Therapists. Edinburgh: Elsevier, 2013

Sinclair M. Pediatric Massage Therapy. Baltimore: Lippincott, Williams and Wilkins, 2004, p. 157

Smith E. The cold pressor test: vascular and myocardial response patterns and their stability. Psychophysiology 1993; 30(4): 366–73

Standish L. AIDS and Complementary Medicine. Edinburgh: Churchill Livingstone, 2002

Tsuzuki-Hayakawa K et al. Thermoregulation during heat exposure of young children compared to their mothers. Eur J Apply Occup Physiol 1995; 72(1–2): 12–15

www.usareim.army.mil: Prevention and Treatment of Cold-Weather Injuries [No author given. Accessed July 2018]

Recommended resources

Kandel R. Water from Heaven: The Story of Water from the Big Bang to the Rise of Civilization and Beyond. New York: Columbia University Press, 2003

Michlovitz S. Thermal Agents in Rehabilitation. Philadelphia, PA: FA Davis, 1996

Pielou EC. Fresh Water. Chicago: University of Chicago Press, 1998

Qualls E. Hydrotherapy. Wildwood, GA: College of Health Evangelism, 1985

Thrash A, Thrash C. Home Remedies: Hydrotherapy, Charcoal, and Other Simple Treatments. Seale, AL Alabama: Thrash Publications, 1981

Williams A. Spa Bodywork. Baltimore: Lippincott, Williams and Wilkins, 2006

www.awwa.org Website of the American Water Works Association, contains information on a variety of topics related to water

www.epa.gov/watrhome/you/chap3

www.unwater.org United Nations website on water issues

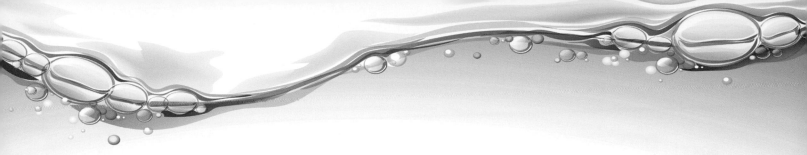

Fomentations, hot packs, compresses, and other local heat treatments 4

Castor oil packs should be considered the treatment of choice, the first line of defense, for all local pain and inflammation … I like to think of castor oil as imparting nourishment to organs that have been starved due to over-activity of the sympathetic nervous system, and gentle detoxification to organs that have been smothered due to over-activity of the parasympathetic nervous system.

Thomas Cowan, *The Fourfold Path to Healing*

CHAPTER OBJECTIVES

After completing this chapter, the student will be able to:

1. Describe why heat is used in modern medicine
2. Describe the effects of local heat treatments
3. Explain the contraindications for local heat treatments
4. Name and describe local heat treatments, mustard plasters, castor oil packs and charcoal packs
5. Perform all local treatments using the procedures described in this chapter.

This chapter covers various treatments that apply heat to a single part of the body. They are relatively simple and inexpensive, so they are more accessible than whole-body treatments that require more elaborate and expensive equipment. They are also versatile and can be used to treat your clients in many different ways (Figure 4.1).

How can local heat improve a massage session? Here are some examples: heat makes tissues far more pliable and stretchable; it relaxes muscles, including smooth muscle; it makes myofascial trigger points less painful to pressure while they are treated and less sore afterwards; it improves local circulation; it relieves the joint stiffness and discomfort of osteoarthritis; and, finally, it reduces nervous tension. Even short but consistent application

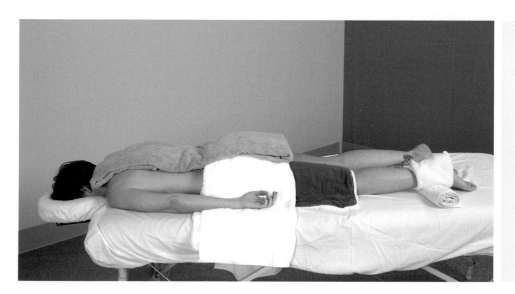

FIGURE 4.1
Client with a silica gel pack on the posterior thigh, fomentation on the entire back, and a hot compress on the ankle.

BOX 4.1	POINT OF INTEREST

THE PRIMARY EFFECTS OF LOCAL HEAT APPLICATIONS

Heat has a wide range of uses in modern medicine due to its five main effects.

1. Moist heat hydrates tissues. ENT doctors recommend steam inhalation for sinus problems and dry, irritated throats, while pediatricians recommend breathing steam for runny noses and other symptoms of the common cold and croup. Aestheticians use steam to hydrate the skin for cleansing and removing dead skin cells.

2. Heat warms tissues. Opthalmologists can treat dry eyes with heat to melt the secretions of the oil-producing glands at the rim of the eyelids. Frostbitten tissues are gradually warmed with footbaths, which although tepid are actually very warm compared to the temperature of the frozen tissue. During operations, many patients become chilled by uncovered skin, cold intravenous fluids and medications: to reduce surgical site infections and other problems, many patients are now warmed with electric blankets, forced air or warmed intravenous fluids. Warmed muscles are more elastic and easier to stretch, and require less force applied to the joint to do so, so local heat is favored before exercise and hands-on treatment by chiropractors, physical and massage therapists. Athletic trainers recommend steam baths for post-workout muscle soreness when the muscles are too sore to be touched.

3. Heat dilates blood vessels, especially moist heat: one study found that when skin stayed dry, blood flow under a heat lamp almost tripled, but when the skin was wet, it quadrupled (Petrofsky, 2009). By increasing absorption of inflammatory chemicals, warm moist compresses are used to soothe the discomfort of conjunctivitis (pink eye), and to speed healing of skin abscesses, particularly after they have been drained. Warm compresses over clogged milk ducts are recommended by lactation consultants to treat painful and engorged breasts, discomfort and clogged milk ducts: by increasing circulation, heat eases swelling, unclogs ducts and helps milk to flow. Compresses are also recommended by dentists and oral surgeons after oral surgery such as tooth extractions: ice is used for the first 36 hours, then warm moist compresses are used to improve bloodflow. Phlebotomists use warm packs to draw blood to the surface and make veins stand out from the skin. Warm sitz baths and heat lamps reduce perineal discomfort after labor and delivery. Hot moist applications to the ear during airplane flights dilate vessels around the ear—this helps pressure stabilize and eases ear pain during takeoff and landing. Moist warm skin absorbs more chemicals from herbal concoctions, essential oils and medication patches (Hao, 2016; Scheindlin, 2004). Using a warm moist pack relieves soreness after trigger point treatment (Simons, 1999).

4. Heat decreases muscle tension. It is used by osteopaths, physical therapists and chiropractors to relax muscles before adjustments and by midwives during labor and delivery. Daily use of hot packs can gradually quiet active trigger points (Simons, 1999) Kidneystone pain is caused by a spasm of the smooth muscle which lines the ureter, and can be relieved by heat in the form of hot fomentations, hot sitz baths and electric blankets (Kober, 2003).

5. Heat applications can increase the core temperature, and heating body wraps are especially effective for hypothermic patients. There is currently great interest in treating cancer with hyperthermia (HeetalJha, 2016). See Appendix C, for more on this topic.

can help many aches and pains. For example, English researchers found that patients with chronic mechanical neck pain who used heating pads 20 minutes a day for 14 days had significant pain relief compared to a non-heating-pad group (Cramer, 2012). Rheumatologists sometimes recommend three hot baths a day for flare-ups of arthritis and pain from old injuries. Furthermore, hot applications can be combined with cold ones to form contrast treatments which stimulate circulation and relieve pain more than either hot or cold alone.

Because heat applications are so helpful, they are used in almost every kind of medical setting (for more on this, see Box 4.1), and also in spas, which offer creative and enjoyable ways to integrate them into massage sessions.

Of course there are local heat treatments that can be performed without water (hot stones, heated bricks, rice-filled microwaveable bags, dry heating pads) but those that use water transmit heat better. For example, heated dry cloths do not warm the body nearly as much as heated moist ones.

The advantages of any type of hot application must always be weighed against two potential problems—applications that are too hot can burn, and prolonged application of heat to the body surface raises the core temperature. For more on overuse of heat, see Box 4.2.

Indications

The indications are similar to those for all heat applications:

1. Nervous tension. Perhaps the fastest and most effective way to help a client settle and relax during a session is to apply local heat: a warm pack over the eyes, hot compresses over the back, a heating pad over the abdomen or a warm footbath, etc., warm and soothe in a way that powerfully complements bodywork. As discussed in Box 1.2, page 6, warm applications also create positive emotions.
2. Muscle spasm.
3. Poor local circulation.
4. Musculoskeletal pain (muscle soreness, chronic pain, stiff, sore or arthritic joints).
5. Muscle tightness.
6. Tissue that needs to become more pliable and stretchable before massage, such as thick, sensitive scar tissue or the dense muscles of an athlete.
7. Post-treatment soreness after deep massage.
8. Menstrual cramps.
9. Active trigger points.
10. When a derivative or fluid-shifting effect is desired, to encourage more blood to flow away from congested areas. Useful for migraine headaches.
11. A chilled area, such as cold feet or hands.
12. A chilled client.

Contraindications

1. Lack of feeling (numbness) in a specific area. Never put a hot application on a numb area: this can easily lead to a burn. Diabetics with numbness in their feet have been burnt simply by walking barefoot on hot sand, and paraplegics burnt on their buttocks by using heated car seats.
2. Rashes or other skin conditions that could be worsened by heat.
3. Inflammation.
4. Swelling.
5. Broken skin, i.e. burns, wounds, sores, cracked skin from eczema or severe chapping.
6. Cancerous tumor, unless approved by the client's doctor.
7. Implanted devices such as cardiac pacemakers, stomach bands and infusion pumps.
8. Peripheral vascular disease, including **Buerger's disease**, and arteriosclerosis of the lower extremities.
9. Diabetics should not receive hot applications to the legs or feet.
10. Sensitivity to heat, especially in those with thinner skin who could burn more easily. This includes many elderly people and small children.

Cautions

1. Elderly (over 60 years old).
2. Children.

Special safety note

Use extreme caution with electrical appliances such as kettles, hot pack heaters, towel steamers and slow cookers! Never immerse cords in water; do not let cords hang over the edges of tables or counters; unplug appliances from wall outlets when they are not in use; and keep them out of reach of children.

BOX 4.2	POINT OF INTEREST

WHEN HEAT IS TOO MUCH OF A GOOD THING

Like anything, local heat can be overused. Remember to observe the guidelines given here and you will never risk burning a client. Here are a few examples of overuse of heat.

Burns

Thermal burns can occur when too-hot liquids, steam or objects come in contact with the skin. The amount of tissue damage depends upon how hot the water or the heated object is, and how long our skin is in contact with it. A footbath at 156°F (69°C) can cause a significant burn in a single second, while at 120°F (48.8°C) a footbath takes 5 minutes to do the same damage. Touching hot objects can cause burns at temperatures as low as 109°F (43°C) over a long time, but if we touch an object that is 140°F (60°C), we will burn in 5 seconds. Hot objects should never be left directly on bare skin, and hot stones should never be used when they are hotter than 105–110°F (40.5–43.3°C: Defrin, 2006; Yarmolenko, 2011).

Reduced sperm production

Laptops and cellphones placed over the groin area, daily hot baths or saunas, overuse of electric blankets, and even standing by open fires for long periods of time can all reduce sperm production. If the heat exposure stops, sperm production will rebound in about 2 weeks (Hefi, 2007; Thrash and Thrash, 1981).

Damage to blood vessels

Toasted skin syndrome is a condition in which red, permanently raised patches on the skin are created when skin is exposed for many hours a day to heat not quite hot enough to burn for many hours a day (usually less than 119°F or 48°C) – see Figures 1 and 2. This chronic exposure damages superficial blood vessels and collagen and encourages pooling of blood. In the past, this condition developed when older people spent hours sitting close to coal stoves or tradespeople worked near open fires, but today it happens most often from space heaters, heated car seats, heating pads, hot water bottles, heated blankets and portable electric devices. One patient developed toasted skin syndrome on her chest after carrying her cell phone in her bra; another on his thighs from his laptop computer. Although this condition is not painful, it is usually permanent (Riahi, 2013; Rudolph,1998).

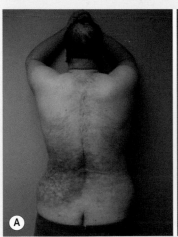 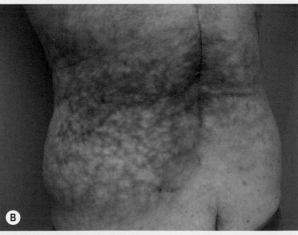

FIGURE 1
Toasted skin syndrome. The 32-year-old patient had severe back pain associated with a rare nervous system tumor at L1 level, and had been using a heating pad eight hours each night for one year. Photos courtesy of The Dermatologist, East Windsor, New Jersey.

SILICA GEL HOT PACKS

Marketed under brand names such as *Hydrocollator* and *Thermollator*, hot packs filled with silica gel are one of the most popular ways for hands-on therapists to apply heat to the body. Because they are easy to heat up and apply to clients, they provide a simple way to relax them while reducing muscle tightness prior to treatment. In offices with multiple practitioners, it is common to see a hot pack heater left on throughout the day while the packs are being used, returned to the heater to rewarm, and used again. Different sizes and shapes are available so packs can be adapted to treat almost any part of the body, and the packs can be combined with cold applications to create contrast treatments.

Underneath the packs, the client's tissue generally increases in temperature by as much as 20°F (11.1°C) at the skin, 15°F (8.3°C) in the tissue just under the skin, and 6°F (3.3°C) in the muscle tissue underneath that. As with all local heat treatments, muscles become more relaxed, joints become warmer and less stiff, and collagen fibers become easier to stretch. Studies have found that by combining silica gel pack applications with gentle prolonged stretching, there is greater long-term improvement in flexibility than by stretching alone. Silica gel packs, however, may not always be the best choice when applying moist heat, because they don't conform to body curves as well as fomentations or hot compresses, they are too heavy to be applied to very sensitive areas, and they cannot be used underneath the client. Clients should not lie on them for three reasons: (1) the packs are bumpy and uncomfortable; (2) the client's body weight could squeeze water out of the pack and possibly cause a burn; and (3) the skin cannot be monitored without constantly rolling the client to one side to examine the back.

The packs are made of canvas material and filled with silica granules which absorb hot water, then form a gel-like substance which holds heat very well. They are placed on wire racks in special metal tanks with electrical heating elements. Once the metal container is filled with water and turned on, it is heated to 160–166°F (71.1–74.4°C) in 1–2 hours. The packs can then be removed from the hot water, wrapped in towels, and applied to clients right away, while they are still hot. They can also be wrapped in towels and kept hot in an ice chest for up to 20 minutes before using. If the metal container is left turned on overnight, the packs will be hot and ready to use the next morning. If you are not seeing many clients in a row and need only one silica gel pack at a time, it saves money and energy to buy individual silica gel packs and heat them in hot water on a hot plate or stovetop. Silica gel pack heaters require a fair amount of energy (the heaters in the smallest containers use as much energy as ten 100-watt light bulbs). If you use your hot silica gel packs for just a few hours every day, save both energy and money by filling the heater with hot rather than cold water each time you use it. You can also buy an insulating foam wrapper to reduce heat loss from the tank (NAIMCO, 425-648-7730). For larger tanks that hold more than four packs, it requires more energy to turn them off at night and try to reheat cold water in the morning than to leave them on overnight so that the water in the tank stays hot.

The procedure below shows you a step-by-step procedure for using a silica gel pack on the upper back.

SNAPSHOT

Temperature Silica gel packs are hot when you take them out of the water and stay hot for about 30 minutes, but they cool at different rates depending upon how hot they are when they come out of the water and how thick the towels are. It is always safer to assume they could burn you or your clients, so handle them carefully and monitor your client frequently.

Time needed 15–20 minutes for a relaxing, sedative effect.

Equipment needed Metal hot pack container; hot pack; tongs or gloves to remove hot pack from the container; enough towels to make 4–6 layers of towel between the pack and the client's skin, or terrycloth covers may be purchased from the manufacturers.

Effect Primarily thermal.

Cleanup Return the silica gel pack to the metal container; launder used towels. The water in the tank should be changed periodically, depending upon how frequently you use it, as eventually it will become contaminated with small silica particles.

Procedure

1. Check with the client to make sure there are no contraindications for the use of local heat.

2. Explain the use of local heat to the client and get his or her consent.

3. Check the water temperature on the heater's digital display or use a water thermometer.

4. Carefully remove the silica gel pack from the hot water with tongs, or put on gloves and pick the pack up by the loops on the edges (Figure 4.2A).

5. Wrap the pack in folded towels. You may fold a large bath towel in half and wrap the hot pack in it or use several smaller towels. The layers of towel will protect the client's skin from burning, and also prevent the pack from cooling off too fast. Silica gel packs generally require about 6 layers of towels, but keep extra towels on hand to use if needed. For example, more towels may be needed for an elderly person or a child (Figure 4.2B).

6. Check to make sure the hot pack is not too hot by feeling it with your own hand or wrist (Figure 4.2C).

7. Warn the client the hot pack is going on, and tell him or her, "Be sure to tell me right away if this feels too hot."

8. Check the area visually before applying towel-wrapped pack (Figure 4.2D). This allows you to see what the client's skin normally looks like.

9. Place the hot pack on the client's lower back (Figure 4.2E).

10. At first, check the skin every 2–3 minutes: lift up the pack and check the client's skin. It will be pinker due to increased blood flow, which is normal, but be alert for any signs of blistering or burning. Also ask the client how it feels. Add more towels to protect the skin if needed. Although the hot pack will begin to cool off right away, it will stay warm for 20–30 minutes (Figure 4.2F).

11. As the hot pack cools off, you may remove some of the towels to keep the treated area warm, but continue to monitor the client's skin.

12. Remove the hot pack if there are any signs of damage to the skin, or if the client tells you the area is too hot.

13. Dry the skin, apply oil or lotion, and begin massage. You will find the client's tissues warm, relaxed and pliable.

FOMENTATIONS

A fomentation is a large pad made of many layers of thick laundry flannel, toweling, or other heavy absorbent material. Fomentations have been used in various forms by many ancient medical traditions. They were used extensively in "water-cure" institutions, for rehabilitation of wounded soldiers during the First and Second World Wars, and during 20th century polio epidemics (see Box 4.3).

"Fomies" absorb hot water from steam and hold heat effectively (see Case history 4.1). Like other moist heat applications, hot fomentations raise local tissue temperature, improve local circulation, relax and soften muscles and fascia, and relieve many kinds of musculoskeletal pain. See Box 4.4 for directions on how to make your own fomentations.

Some practitioners prefer silica gel packs to fomentations, and each has its advantages: for example, silica gel packs need to be wrapped in towels, whereas fomentations need a layer of wool and a layer of towels; fomentations can cover larger areas and drape to fit body curves, while silica gel packs are smaller and more rigid; however, it takes more time to prepare fomentations and they cool off faster.

When they are ready for use, fomentations are very hot, so they are wrapped in a layer of heat-retaining wool felt and then in additional layers of towels. Once applied, fomentations won't cool off if you cover them with a waterproof material (such as a sheet of heavy plastic) and then a heating pad over that. At this stage, they can also be put in a cooler for 10–20 minutes before you use them.

To prepare fomentations, first soak them in water so they are wet all the way through; second, wring them out so that they are thoroughly wet but not dripping (Figure 4.3), and third, heat them.

Below are four options for heating a fomentation:

- Wet the fomentation, then place it inside a gallon-size resealable plastic bag. Heat this in a microwave oven for approximately 5 minutes.

- Wet the fomentation, roll it up in heavy-grade aluminum foil, and heat in a 425°F (220°C) oven for 25 minutes.

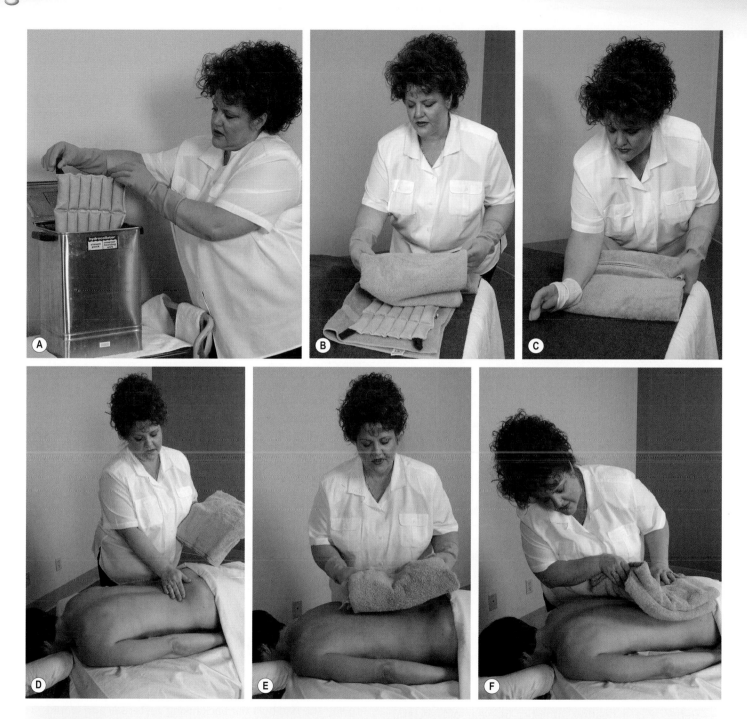

FIGURE 4.2
Silica gel hot pack. (**A**) Remove the silica gel pack from the hot water with tongs, or put on gloves and pick the pack up by the loops on the edges. (**B**) Wrap it in one or more towels. (**C**) Check to make sure the hot pack is not too hot by feeling it with your own hand or wrist. (**D**) Check the area visually before applying the towel-wrapped pack. (**E**) Place the hot pack on the client's lower back. (**F**) Check the skin every 2–3 minutes at first: lift up the pack and check the tissue.

BOX 4.3	POINT OF INTEREST

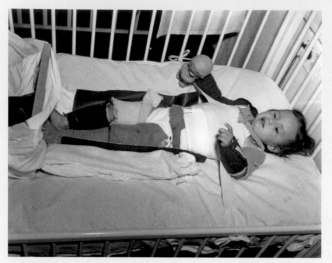

FIGURE 1
Fomentation and stretching treatment for polio, San Angelo, Texas, 1949. Photograph courtesy of March of Dimes Birth Defects Foundation.

FOMENTATION AND STRETCHING TREATMENT FOR POLIO

In the 1930s an Australian army nurse named Elizabeth Kenny developed a treatment for polio victims that involved wrapping the limbs of acutely ill polio sufferers with hot fomentations to reduce muscle spasms and the pain they caused. "Foments" were made of wool blankets, individually cut to fit each patient. Wool was used because it retained heat well. The wool pieces were heated in very hot water, removed with tongs, run through a wringer twice, and then placed on the patient. During the acute phase, hot packs were reapplied once an hour, around the clock. In the 1949 March of Dimes picture above, the young girl in the acute phase of polio is shown receiving this treatment in a hospital in San Angelo, Texas. Even though the fomentations gave relief to tight, painful muscles, they were meant to be very hot and unfortunately burns sometimes occurred. As soon as the initial fever receded, nurses and physical therapists began to work with patients by applying fomentations and moving limbs passively to maintain range of motion. Later, the fomentations were used again to relax tight spasmodic muscles before stretching, active exercise and massage, which were used to restore muscles to their full function.

Sister Kenny's regimen was quite different than the standard medical treatment for polio sufferers, which consisted of prolonged bed rest and immobilization of the limbs with splints and casts. The standard treatment actually did more harm than good, as it caused atrophy and contractures in limbs which were already weak. The medical profession grudgingly accepted Sister Kenny's techniques and they became standard treatment for polio victims by the mid-1940s. Sister Kenny became a world-famous healer (Wilson, 2005).

A HOT FOMENTATION FOR A PAINFUL MUSCLE SPASM	CASE HISTORY 4.1

BACKGROUND

Rebecca is a healthy, athletic, 64-year-old secretary. After a long winter spent indoors, and even though her muscles were completely unconditioned, she walked 20 miles (32 km) yesterday. She had received bodywork from the massage therapist only once before, but called to say she had hurt her back hiking yesterday and would like a massage for that reason. She arrived in severe pain, half-carried by her husband. Every movement was excruciating and getting up on the massage table

continued

A HOT FOMENTATION FOR A PAINFUL MUSCLE SPASM

or even undressing was unthinkable. Her mid-back, where the pain was located, was also very sensitive to the touch. Her chiropractor would later diagnose a torn sacral ligament and muscles which were spasming to splint the area.

TREATMENT

Rebecca was able to sit straddling a chair, and so the massage therapist draped a hot fomentation around her mid-back and secured it in place with an elastic bandage while listening to her history. Although her mid-back was still very painful and getting on the massage table was impossible, the fomentation reduced Rebecca's pain slightly after just a few minutes. She remained seated on the chair and her husband helped her to remove her shirt so that the therapist could

massage her back above and below the fomentation. Rebecca's pain gradually began to decrease. After 15 minutes of heat, and massage above and below the painful area, the therapist removed the fomentation: with her husband's assistance Rebecca was able to get on the massage table so that the therapist could give more specific massage to the painful muscles. Her mid-back muscles were pink and pliable, and ready for treatment.

DISCUSSION QUESTIONS

1. How did the fomentation relieve Rebecca's pain?
2. What other local heat or cold applications could have been used in this situation?

- Wet the fomentation, roll it up, and place it upright in a steamer basket over a 1 gallon (4 liter) pot of simmering water for about 20 minutes.

- For a large homemade fomentation, you will need protective gloves and a large bath towel. Put on the gloves, then carefully twist the towel, dip it in very hot water, and twist it again to squeeze out excess water. Herbal preparations such as ginger tea or water with essential oils or salts can also be added to the soaking water. If you use common sense, a hot, wet towel can go directly against the client's skin, rather than being wrapped in wool and dry towels. First check the hot, wet towel against your own skin to make sure it is not too hot, and then monitor the client's skin carefully for burning. Hot towels lose heat faster than ready-made fomentations, but they can also be kept warm longer by covering them with a waterproof material and then a heating pad.

The procedure below shows you how to use a hot fomentation on the anterior thigh, but fomentations can be adapted to treat almost any area of the body. They can

be especially useful if you wish to apply heat to the front and back of the body at the same time. They can also be combined with cold applications to create contrast treatments.

SNAPSHOT

Temperature Once fomentations have been properly heated, they are very hot.

Fomentations cool off at different rates, depending upon how hot they are to begin with and how thickly they are wrapped, so it is best to assume they have the potential to burn and monitor your clients at all times. When checking the client's skin, slide your hand under the wrapped fomentation and feel the client's skin, as well as checking it for signs of blistering or burning.

Time needed 15–20 minutes for a relaxing, sedative effect.

Equipment needed Protective gloves; fomentation; wool felt to wrap it in; one or two towels. As discussed above, you will need a safe way to heat the fomentation.

BOX 4.4	POINT OF INTEREST

HOW TO MAKE FOMENTATIONS

Fomentations are relatively easy to make, and a miniature fomentation made be made on the spot from a few simple ingredients. Directions are included for making both a miniature and a full-size fomentation.

Miniature fomentation

Equipment needed Boiling water; protective gloves; kitchen sponge; hand towel; microwave oven.

Effect Thermal.

Cleanup Wash the hand towel.

Procedure

1. Lay the sponge on the hand towel.
2. Using gloves, wet the sponge with a small amount of boiling water.
3. Now fold the towel around the sponge to make a small pack, and pick it up by the dry ends of the towel.
4. Microwave it for 30 seconds.
5. Remove it from the microwave by holding the dry ends of the towel.

6. Check the temperature of the mini-fomentation against your own skin before applying it to your client's skin, and – as with all hot applications – monitor the skin carefully.

Standard-size fomentation with cover

Equipment needed 1 (1 metre) of heavy cotton laundry flannel, terrycloth material or a thick towel for the fomentation; and 1 (1 metre) of wool or polar fleece for the cover.

Procedure

1. Cut the fabric into a piece measuring 25 × 40 inches (63 × 100cm).
2. Fold it in half and then in half again, so the finished size is 10 × 25 inches (25 × 63cm).
3. Sew the pack together around the edges (a serger is good for this) or make about six quilting stitches through all the layers to hold them together.
4. Cut the wool or polar fleece material so it measures 30 × 32 inches (76 × 80cm), which is large enough to overlap the fomentation on all sides.
5. Once you have made the fomentation, follow the directions in this chapter for preparing and applying it.

Effect Primarily thermal.

Cleanup Hang the fomentation and the felt cover up to dry: because they never touch the client's skin, they only need to be laundered occasionally. Used towels need to be laundered.

Procedure

1. Check with the client to make sure there are no contraindications for the use of local heat.
2. Explain the use of local heat to the client and get his or her consent.
3. Soak the fomentation and wring it out (Figure 4.3A).
4. Place it in a zipper closure bag and heat it in a microwave (Figure 4.3B), or roll it up and stand it in a steam basket over boiling water.

5. Using gloves, carefully remove the fomentation from its heat source (microwave oven, steamer, or oven – see Figure 4.3C).
6. Wrap the fomentation in a layer of wool felt or polar fleece (Figure 4.3D), and then in towels (Figure 4.3E). You may double a large bath towel and wrap the fomentation in it. The towels will protect the client's skin from burning and prevent the fomentation from cooling off too fast. Fomentations generally require about four layers of towels, but keep extra towels on hand to use if needed. Work quickly to prevent the fomentations from losing too much heat.
7. Check to make sure the fomentation with its covers is not too hot by feeling it with your own hand or wrist (Figure 4.3F).

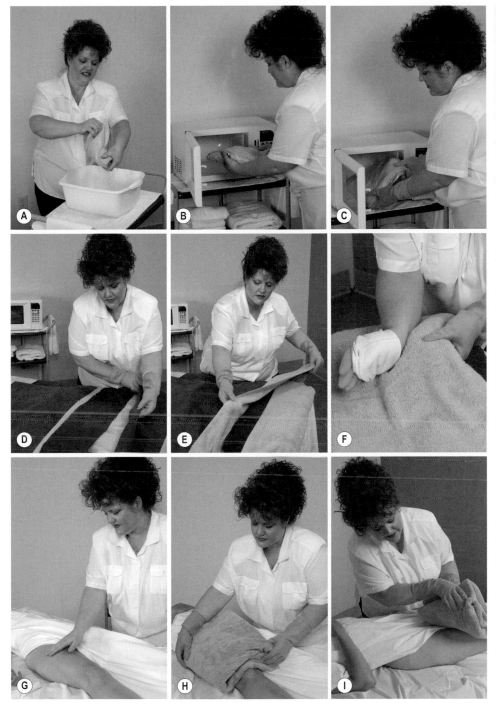

FIGURE 4.3
Fomentation. (**A**) Soak the fomentation and wring it out. (**B**) Place it in a zipper closure bag and heat it in a microwave oven (shown), or roll it up and stand it in a steam basket over boiling water (not shown), or roll it up in aluminum foil and heat it in an oven (not shown). (**C**) Remove the fomentation from its heat source (microwave oven, steamer, or oven) using gloves. (**D**) Wrap the hot fomentation in a layer of wool felt, or polar fleece. (**E**) Wrap the hot fomentation in towels. (**F**) Check to make sure the fomentation with its covers is not too hot by feeling it with your own hand or wrist. (**G**) Check the area visually before applying the towel-wrapped fomentation. This allows you to see what the client's skin normally looks like. (**H**) Place the fomentation on the client's thigh. (**I**) Check the skin every 2–3 minutes at first: lift up the pack and check the tissue.

8. Warn the client the fomentation is going on, and say, "Be sure to let me know if this ever feels like it is too hot."

9. Check the area visually before applying the towel-wrapped fomentation (Figure 4.3G). This allows

you to see what the client's skin normally looks like.

10. Place the fomentation on the client's thigh (Figure 4.3H).

11. Check the skin every 2–3 minutes at first: lift up the pack and check the tissue (Figure 4.3I). It will

be bright pink due to increased blood flow and this is normal, but check for any signs of blistering or burning. Also ask the client if it feels as though it is too hot.

12. The fomentation will stay warm for about 20 minutes. It will begin to cool off right away, so the danger of burning decreases as time goes on. As the fomentation cools off, you may remove a layer of towels to keep the area warm, but you will need to keep checking the client's skin.

13. Remove the fomentation if there are any signs of overheating, if the client tells you the area feels too hot, or if he or she feels overheated.

14. Dry the skin, apply oil or lotion, and begin massage. You will find the client's tissue warm, relaxed and pliable.

HOT COMPRESSES AND HOT TOWELS

Hot compresses

A hot **compress** – a folded cloth dipped in water – is a milder version of the intense moist heat of the silica gel pack or the hot fomentation. You may prefer hot compresses over silica gel packs or fomentations because compresses may be easily made and applied with even less trouble. To make a hot compress, all the massage therapist needs is towels, hot water, and gloves to protect the hands when wringing out the cloths. However, one disadvantage to hot compresses is that they cool off faster than silica gel packs or fomentations. They have been used since ancient times to apply various substances to the skin by simply soaking the cloths in water mixed with herbs, essential oils, minerals, salts and other materials. Compresses have also been combined with various cold applications to create contrast treatments.

You can easily make compresses to suit individual clients. For example, a tiny hot compress to cover the eyes may be made by soaking a washcloth in hot water and then wringing it out. Small or medium-size hot compresses may be made with a few layers of cloth or small towels. Hot compresses that can cover the entire back can be made with a large bath towel. There are many ways to prepare hot compresses: water can be heated using a stovetop, electric teakettle, microwave oven, or slow cooker on a low setting; or you can even use very hot tap water. You can soak towels in a bowl of hot water and then wring them out, or you can roll them up dry and place them in an ice chest or slow cooker and pour boiling water over them. Dampened towels can also be heated in a resealable plastic bag or in a Pyrex dish in a microwave oven. Commercial heating cabinets marketed under such names as Hot Towel Cabi not only heat small and medium-size cloths that you have wrung out in water, they also keep them warm until needed. Commercial hot towel steamers used by barbers are another option.

To make sure clients are not burned, always check the compress against your own hand or wrist before applying, monitor the client's skin, and let the client determine if the hot compress is uncomfortably hot: this is the reason it should never be applied to an area of poor sensation.

Wring-as-you-go method

Below is an overview of treatment details and a sample procedure, using the abdomen.

SNAPSHOT

Temperature Hot (110–120°F; 43.3–48.9°C).

Time needed 10–20 minutes, depending upon the size of the compress, and if more than one is to be used. Small compresses will cool off faster.

Equipment needed Water thermometer; hot water; 6–10 towels of appropriate sizes; gloves to protect your hands. Thin towels do not hold heat: be sure to purchase towels that are thick enough to retain heat for 1–2 minutes.

Effect Primarily thermal.

Cleanup Clean and sanitize the water containe; dispose of used towels.

Procedure

1. Check with the client to make sure there are no contraindications for the use of local heat.

2. Explain the use of local heat to the client and obtain their consent.

3. Check the water temperature and adjust if it is not within 110–120°F (43.3–48.9°C).

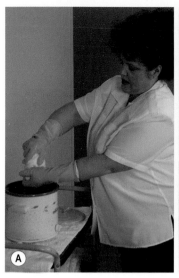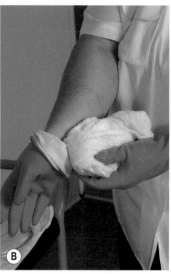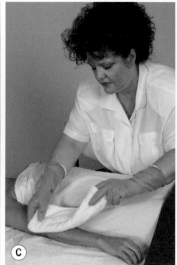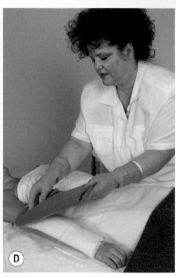

FIGURE 4.4

Hot compress. (**A**) Check the water temperature; then, wearing gloves, wring out the cloth in hot water. (**B**) Check to make sure the hot cloth is not too hot by feeling it with your own hand or wrist. (**C**) Place the hot cloth on the client's skin. (**D**) Place a warm gel pack pad over the piece of plastic (optional).

4. Wearing gloves, wring out the cloth in hot water (Figure 4.4A). Rotating your wrists as you wring out the cloth provides your joints with an excellent range-of-motion exercise.

5. Check to make sure the cloth is not too hot by feeling it with your own hand or wrist (Figure 4.4B). If it is, let it cool to a safe temperature.

6. Warn the client the compress is going on, and tell them to let you know if it ever feels too hot.

7. Check the area visually before putting on the hot application. This allows you to see what the client's skin normally looks like. Warn the client before applying the hot cloth, and tell them to let you know if it ever feels too hot.

8. Place the hot cloth on the client's skin (Figure 4.4C). Covering it with a small sheet of plastic or polar fleece, which retains heat and does not absorb water, slows heat loss.

9. Monitor the client's skin, and ask for feedback occasionally.

10. Replace with a new hot cloth every 1–2 minutes if a heating pad is not used. If a heat lamp or heating pad is placed over the sheet of plastic

(Figure 4.4D), the compress does not need to be replaced and can stay on 10–20 minutes.

11. When you remove the compress for the last time, gently dry the area with another dry cloth. You will find the client's tissue warm, relaxed, and pliable.

Variation 1: Using a slow cooker as a towel steamer

Step 1: Towels are tightly rolled and placed in a slow cooker.

Step 2: One quart (1 liter) of very hot water is poured on top.

Step 3: The slow cooker is turned onto a high setting for 15 minutes, then switched to a warm setting; towels will stay hot until ready to use (Figure 4.5).

Variation 2: Making compresses with additives

1. Ginger compress – add 1 teaspoon of powdered ginger to 1 quart (1 liter) of hot water. Ginger has been found to be anti-inflammatory and

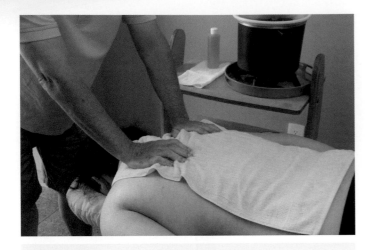

FIGURE 4.5
Hot towels are easily placed in the slow cooker ahead of time, and used when needed during a session.

helpful for arthritis (Altman, 2001; Therkleson, 2014).

2. Epsom salts compress – Use 1 cup of Epsom salts mixed with 2 quarts (2 liters) of hot water. Helpful for bruises and inflammation.

HOT TOWELS
Hot towel rolls

A hot towel roll is a useful massage tool; as you gently massage an area with the roll you also warm it deeply. Each of five hand towels are rolled tightly, cinnamon-roll fashion, around another towel to make a large roll, then hot water is poured into the center of the roll. The towels will now be warm all the way through, and the outermost towel will be warm but not overly hot. As each outer towel cools, it is unrolled onto the area being massaged, then removed so the next innermost towel can be used. The roll is used to perform gentle massaging movements such as compressions, gliding strokes and stretches (Figure 4.6). This is an excellent technique for lifting injuries that feature strained back muscles – especially if you end the treatment with a cold application over the spine and surrounding muscles.

SNAPSHOT
Temperature Hot (110–120°F; 43.3–48.9°C).
Time About 15 minutes.

Equipment needed Water thermometer; electric tea kettle; six towels of appropriate size; gloves to protect your hands. Thin towels do not hold heat: be sure to purchase towels that are thick enough to retain heat.

Effect Primarily thermal.

Cleanup Dispose of used towels.

Procedure

1. Check with the client to make sure there are no contraindications for the use of local heat.

2. Explain the use of local heat to the client and get her consent.

3. Prepare the hot towel roll by laying out six over-lapping towels. Begin rolling the first one very tightly and continue one by one until you have a tight long cylinder (not shown).

4. Using an electric tea kettle, pour about 1 quart (1 liter) of boiling water into the center of the towel roll. Use care not to splash water (Figure 4.6A). For clarity, gloves are not shown in the photo; however, you should always wear them for this step.

5. Check to make sure the roll is not too hot by feeling it with your own hand or wrist. The innermost towels will be very hot, but the outer towel will be warm.

6. Check the area visually before applying the towel roll (Figure 4.6B). This allows you to see what the client's skin normally looks like.

7. Warn the client the roll is going on their back, and tell them to let you know if it ever feels too hot.

8. Place the hot roll on the client's lower back (Figure 4.6C). Perform gentle massaging movements.

9. Monitor the skin every 2–3 minutes at first by lifting up the pack and checking the area. It will be pink due to increased blood flow, which is normal, but check for any signs of blistering or burning.

10. As the outer towel cools, unwind it and continue massaging; the next towel should still be warm. Always check the temperature before using the roll.

11. Continue until you are down to the last hot towel. Massage through it (Figure 4.6D), and then spread it over the treated area and leave it there until it has cooled off.

12. If possible, finish with an ice massage or a brisk rub of the area with a towel wrung out in very cold water.

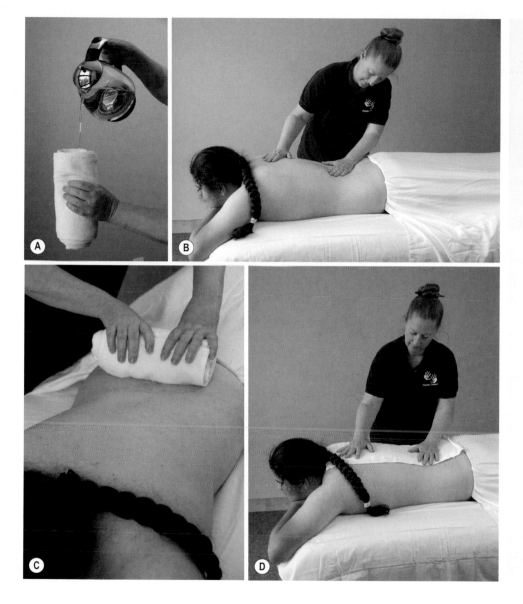

FIGURE 4.6
Hot towel roll. Prepare the hot towel roll by laying 6 towels out. Begin rolling the first one very tightly and continue one by one until you have a tight long cylinder (not shown). (**A**) Pour boiling water into the center of the towel roll. Do not splash the water. (**B**) Checking the area visually before applying towel roll. (**C**) Performing gentle massaging movements with the hot towel roll. (**D**) Spreading the last hot towel over the treated area.

Individual hot towels

Hot towels are an even milder form of heat than hot compresses, which are meant to stay on for 15–20 minutes. The massage therapist can create deep relaxation and mild vasodilation at the skin by draping the towel on the client and massaging through it using compressions, kneading, pressure points, skin rolling or a variety of massage tools. (These techniques cannot be done over a heating pad, fomentation, or therapy gel pack) (Figure 4.7). As the towels cool off in 1–2 minutes, replace with as many hot towels as you desire. Creative massage therapists have designed all sorts of other helpful procedures to enhance bodywork with hot towels, such as sliding rolled hot towels under the neck and lumbar areas to support and warm them, wrapping the face in warmth before a facial massage, tractioning the neck, or cleansing the feet of massage oil or lotion as a last relaxing touch at the end of a session. Clients love them all! Many of these techniques will be discussed in later chapters.

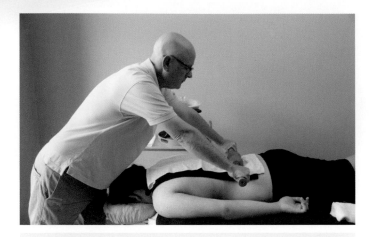

FIGURE 4.7
Massage over a hot towel.

MOIST HEATING PADS

Electric heating pads are another way to apply heat to a single area. They are portable, get hot with the flip of a switch, and are flexible enough to drape around many parts of the body. Because they are not wrapped in layers of towels they are less bulky and easier to work around than silica gel packs or hot fomentations. However, heating pads lack the penetrating intense heat of silica gel packs or fomentations and cannot be used in a setting without electricity, and the therapist must be careful not to trip or pull on the cord while working. Like all local heat treatments, heating pads can also be combined with various cold applications to create contrast treatments, although the client's reaction will be milder because the heat is less intense.

There are two different kinds of electric heating pads: moist and dry ones. Moist heating pads have outer covers that draw humidity from the air and then retain it. When the pad is turned on, the moisture goes out of the cover and onto the area being treated. Any dry electric heating pad can be made into a moist one by laying a wet cloth over the area to be treated, covering that with a thin sheet of plastic, and then putting the dry heating pad on top of that. Moist heat penetrates farther into tissues than dry heat (Petrofsky, 2009). To prevent burns, many heating pads now come equipped with digital temperature readouts and an automatic shutoff, so after a

period of minutes or hours they simply turn off. A client who will be using one at home should always check if this feature is available, and should never fall asleep while using a heating pad. Persons with reduced sensation, such as those with neuropathy or nerve injuries, should not use heating pads.

Below is an overview of treatment details and a sample procedure, in this case treating the abdomen. For reasons of hygiene, a thin layer of cloth or a sheet of plastic is placed between the client's skin and the heating pad for hygienic reasons.

SNAPSHOT

Temperature Settings vary from (78°F; 25.5°C) to high (125°F; 51.7°C).

Time needed 15 minutes or longer, depending upon the condition.

Equipment needed Heating pad in a cloth cover; small sheet of plastic or cloth.

Effect Primarily thermal.

Cleanup Anything that has touched the the client's skin should be sanitized. If a layer of cloth was put between the heating pad and the skin, it should be laundered; if a sheet of plastic was used, either wash it with hot water and soap or throw it away.

Procedure

1. Check with the client to make sure there are no contraindications for the use of local heat.

2. Explain the use of local heat to the client and get his or her consent.

3. Inspect the heating pad (Figure 4.8A).

4. Plug in the heating pad and turn it on to the desired setting (Figure 4.8B).

5. Warn the client before applying the heating pad, and tell him to let you know if it ever feels too hot.

6. Check the area visually before putting on the heating pad (Figure 4.8C). This allows you to see what the client's skin normally looks like.

7. Place the heating pad on the abdomen (Figure 4.8D).

8. Check the skin every 5 minutes: lift up the pad and check the client's tissue (Figure 4.8E).

HOT WATER BOTTLES

Often a drug will be taken which risks injury of the health for all future time, when a hot water bottle would have been even more effective, more economical, and entirely safe.

Agatha and Calvin Thrash, *Home Remedies: Hydrotherapy, Massage, Charcoal and Other Simple Treatments*

Hot water bottles are another tried and true, hydrotherapy treatment. Before there were plastic or rubber ones, hot water bottles were most often made of earthenware, with a cork for a stopper. They were used to warm beds and to soothe all manner of aches and pains. Extremities could be kept warm with them, too – some ceramic water bottles were even made with footprint-shaped indentations – and miniature water bottles were put in muffs to keep the hands warm.

Today's hot water bottles are made of rubber or plastic and are a simple, cheap, and versatile way to use local heat in your massage sessions. They can be used to heat a massage table, to warm a cold client, to put on an aching part of the body while another area is being massaged, or be laid on top of compresses or packs to keep them warm. They are readily available; they are lightweight and portable; they come in a variety of sizes; and in a pinch they can be made from any leak-proof plastic bottle. They cool off in 30–60 minutes, so if someone falls asleep on them, there is far less potential for burns than with a heating pad. Clients who avoid electric devices on their skin, such as heating pads, love hot water bottles.

Rubber hot water bottles

A rubber hot water bottle can be put over or under any part of the body. When air is expelled from it and the right amount of water is put in, it becomes flexible and can conform to different parts of the client's body. For example, a small hot water bottle can be placed under the chin, atop a small area of the arm or on the abdomen in the supine position, or on the back of the neck or behind a knee in the prone position. A larger one may be placed on the client's chest, abdomen or legs in the supine position, or on the back or legs in the prone position. During a massage, a hot water bottle placed over the chest or

---

A MOIST HEATING PAD FOR "PINCHED NERVE" PAIN	CASE HISTORY 4.2

BACKGROUND

Mario, a 25-year-old computer consultant, had had severe pain in his midback for days. One week previously his doctor diagnosed him with a pinched nerve and prescribed muscle relaxant and pain medications. However, Mario's pain continued to be so severe that he had not gone to work for the last five days and he now had referred pain in his right hip and torso. He visited Susan, a new massage therapist who had never seen anyone in such severe pain before.

TREATMENT

Susan decided to begin with Mario in a prone position. She placed a moist heating pad on his mid-back area, and because his pain was so severe that she was actually afraid to touch his back, she then performed gentle joint mobilization on his legs for 30 minutes. Near the end of the session, with his pain essentially unchanged, Susan asked him to roll over into the supine position. Mario took a very deep breath and began to turn, rotating his spine in the process. As he did, they both heard his back make a series of extremely loud popping sounds, after which he sat up and said in a shocked voice that his pain was completely gone. He got off the massage table carefully, dressed, thanked Susan and left her office. On a follow-up call a week later, Mario told Susan his back was still pain-free. The intense heat on Mario's severely cramped muscles had greatly relaxed them, freed his severely fixated vertebrae, and relieved his pain, all without any direct hands-on treatment.

DISCUSSION QUESTION

1. Name two other treatments that Susan could have tried for Mario's problem.

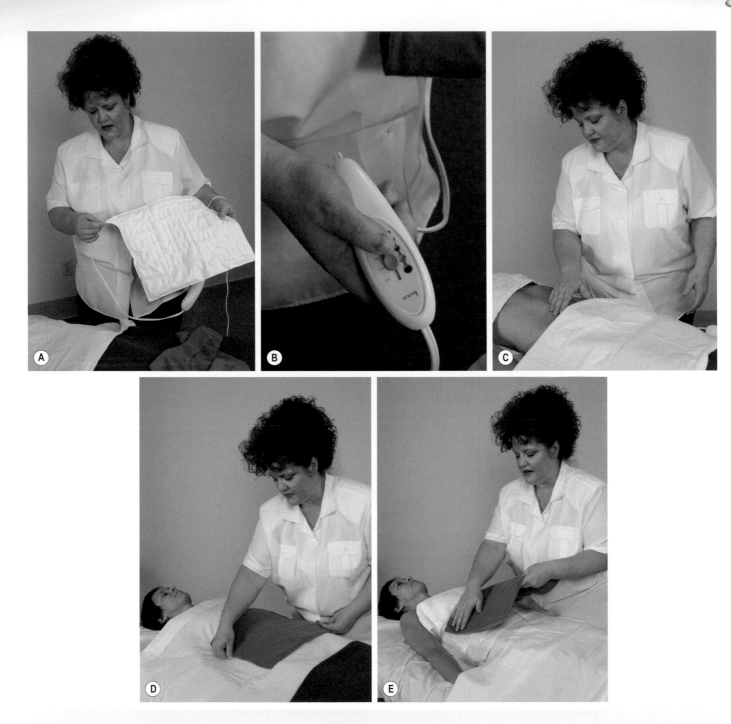

FIGURE 4.8
Moist heating pad. (**A**) Inspect the heating pad. (**B**) Plug in the heating pad and turn it on to the desired setting. (**C**) Check the area visually before applying the heating pad. (**D**) Place the heating pad on the client's abdomen. (**E**) Check the skin every 5 minutes at first: lift up the pad and check the tissue.

abdomen gives the client a convenient, comforting place to place the hands while the bottle warms the body core at the same time.

Do not put weight or pressure on a rubber hot water bottle and never put it in any type of oven. To extend its life, never fill it with boiling water, check it before using to make sure there are no splits in it, and do not fold it. If a bottle bursts it could scald the client!

Below is an overview of treatment details and a sample procedure, using an application to the lower back.

SNAPSHOT

Temperature Hot (110–120°F; 43.3–48.9°C).

Time needed 10–30 minutes.

Equipment needed Water thermometer; hot water bottle; a thin cloth to wrap it in.

Effect Primarily thermal.

Cleanup-Launder the cloth. Empty the water bottle and hang it upside down for storage. Keep it in a cool dry location.

Procedure

1. Check with the client to make sure there are no contraindications for the use of local heat.

2. Explain the use of local heat to the client and get his or her consent.

3. Fill the bottle about one half to two thirds full with hot water from the tap (Figure 4.9A). Use the thermometer to ensure the water is 110–120°F (43.3–48.9°C). Expel all the air and check to make sure the top is properly seated and firmly closed so the bottle does not leak (Figure 4.9B).

4. Wrap the hot water bottle in a thin cloth or pillowcase (Figure 4.9C).

5. Warn the client the hot water bottle is being placed, and tell him or her to let you know if it ever feels too hot.

6. Check the area visually before placing the bottle on the client. This allows you to see what the client's skin normally looks like.

7. Place hot water bottle on the lower back (Figure 4.9D).

8. Even though burns are uncommon with rubber hot water bottles, be sure to monitor the client's skin.

Flat plastic hot water bottles (come in two sizes)

When filled with hot water at the appropriate temperature, this simple device is safe to lie on. When laid flat on a massage table before a session begins, it warms the table; during the session, it can warm the client's

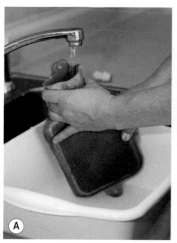
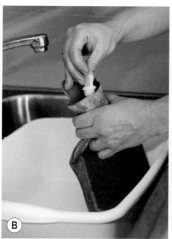
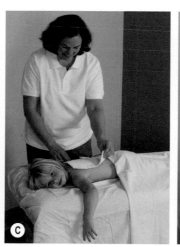
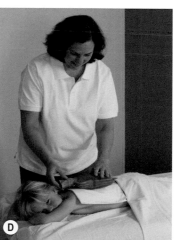

FIGURE 4.9
Rubber hot water bottle. (**A**) Check the temperature of the hot water at the tap, then fill the bottle about one half to two thirds full with it. (**B**) Expel all the air and check to make sure the top is properly seated and firmly closed, so it does not leak. (**C**) Wrap it in a thin cloth or pillowcase. (**D**) Place the hot water bottle on the lower back.

entire body; and it warms and softens local areas before they are massaged. It will stay warm for up to 2 hours, and can also be laid on the anterior surface of the body.

A smaller size can be draped around a joint or over the abdomen prior to massage, or under the neck or lumbar region or wrists as a cozy support. An advantage of this particular treatment is that it is inexpensive and fairly low-tech: all the therapist needs is the bottle and hot water. This hot water bottle may even be used with two clients, if it is put in a cooler to retain its heat after the first session (never put it in a microwave). It can also be combined with various cold applications, including another bottle filled with chilled water, to create contrast treatments. A larger hot water bottle may heat a larger proportion of the client's body, and so it has even more potential for raising the core temperature.

SNAPSHOT

Temperature Very hot (water at 108–113°F; 42.2–44°C).

Time needed 10–30 minutes. The client's tissue will begin to warm after about 5 minutes.

Equipment needed Water thermometer; a hot water bottle; a thin cloth to cover or wrap the hot water bottle in (a pillowcase is ideal).

Effect Primarily thermal.

Cleanup Launder the cloth. Empty the water bottle and lay it flat with the lid off, so the last drops of water will evaporate. Then it can be folded for storage.

Procedure

1. Check with the client to make sure there are no contraindications for the use of local heat.

2. Explain the use of local heat to the client and get his or her consent.

3. Fill bottle about one third full with hot water from the tap (Figure 4.10A). About 6 cups of water will be needed for a large 18 × 24 size bottle. Use a thermometer to ensure the water is 108–113°F (42.2–44°C).

4. Carry the open bottle carefully to the massage table, lay it flat on the table, use your hand to expel all the air bubbles, and check to make sure the top is snapped on securely so the bottle does not leak (Figure 4.10B).

5. Cover it with a cloth or pillowcase, or place it inside a pillowcase (Figure 4.10C).

6. As the client lies on the cloth that is covering the hot water bottle, tell her to let you know if it ever feels like it's too hot (Figure 4.10D).

7. Even though burns are highly unlikely if the correct water temperature is used, be sure to monitor the client's skin and ask for feedback. The area will warm up more slowly than if a silica gel pack or fomentation is used.

Cleanup Launder the towel; clean the outside of the bottle if necessary, following the manufacturer's directions.

HEAT LAMPS

Heat lamps were invented in the late 1800s and soon became popular physical therapy devices because they are so easy to use (see Figure 4.11). Like other local heat treatments, they can enhance bodywork by easing musculoskeletal discomfort, warming cold areas, and making tissues easier to stretch and massage. Make the application a moist one to increase blood flow: in one study, subjects' forearms were covered with either moist or dry towels and kept under a lamp for 15 minutes, resulting in a skin temperature of 104°F (40°C). Skin blood flow was then compared, and when a moist rather than a dry towel was used, blood flow increased by 25% (Petrofsky, 2009). Below is an overview of treatment details and a sample procedure using the knee joint.

SNAPSHOT

Indications Same as with other local heat treatments, especially a cold client, dense muscle tissue, very sensitive scar tissue, joint pain, and stiffness.

Contraindications

1. Do not use with babies or small children.

2. Do not use on the abdomen of a pregnant woman.

3. Do not use over a drug patch, because this increases drug absorption (Hao, 2016).

4. Do not use over skin cancers or rosacea.

5. Do not use over medical devices such as pacemakers or medication ports.

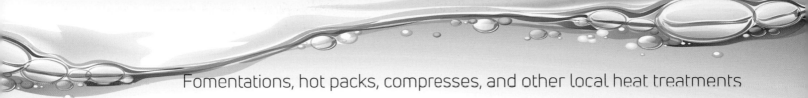

Cautions

1. Always use a heat lamp that has a guard over the bulb, so neither you nor your client ever touch it with bare skin when it is hot.

2. Treat the lamp gently and don't screw the bulbs in too tightly.

3. Place the lamp at least 25–30 cm away from the area. The suggested time is 15–20 minutes.

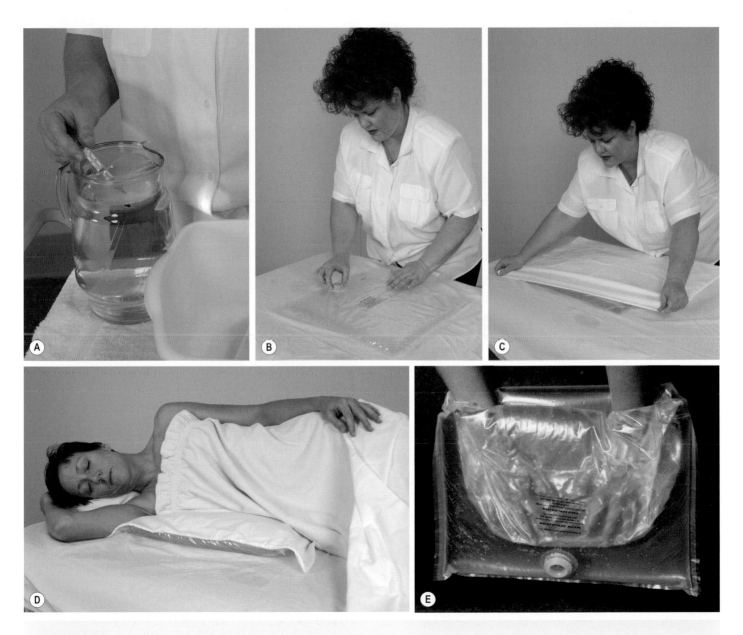

FIGURE 4.10

Flat plastic hot water bottle. (**A**) Check the temperature of the hot water at the tap, then fill the bottle about one half to two thirds full with it. (**B**) Expel all the air, snap the lid on, and check to make sure the lid is firmly closed and water does not leak out. (**C**) Cover the hot water bottle with a pillowcase. (**D**) Client lying on the hot water bottle. (**E**) When the client's hands are pushed up into the folds of the bottle, warmth surrounds them on all sides. This is easily done during a session if the client is supine and the bottle rests upon the abdomen. Photo courtesy of permission from Fomentek Company.

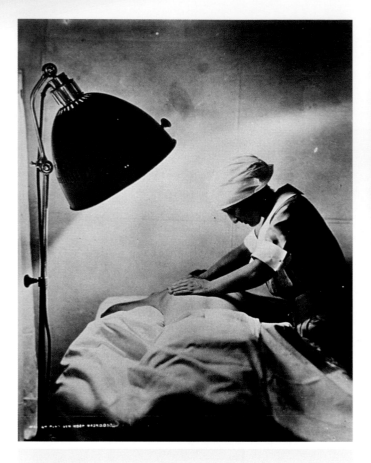

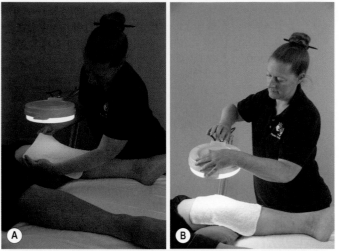

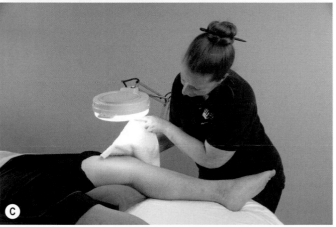

FIGURE 4.11
Rehabilitation aide treating a soldier, Walter Reed Army Hospital, 1922. Image from History of Medicine, National Library of Medicine. Sourced from ihm.nlm.nih.gov/images 101449253.

FIGURE 4.12
Figure 4.12 Heat lamp. (**A**) Positioning the heat lamp over the knee and placing a moist cloth. (**B**) Setting the heat lamp timer. (**C**) Checking the knee area.

4. Do not use the lamp on the head, and do not shine it in the client's eyes.

5. Monitor the client's skin, and do not keep the lamp on one spot if the client feels a burning sensation.

Temperature Hot.

Time needed 15–20 minutes.

Equipment needed Heat lamp; a thin moist cloth.

Effect Primarily thermal.

Cleanup Launder the cloth.

Procedure

1. Check with the client to make sure there are no contraindications for the use of local heat, and check the area visually.

2. Explain the use of local heat to the client and get his or her consent.

3. Place a moist towel over the knee, then position the lamp so heat will be directed toward it, keeping at a distance of 12–16 inches (25–30 cm) (Figure 4.12A).

4. Turn on the heat lamp and set the timer for 20 minutes (Figure 4.12B).

5. Tell the client to let you know if the lamp ever feels too hot.

6. Check the area (Figure 4.12C), then check the skin every 5 minutes.

7. When the timer sounds, turn off the heat lamp and move it away from the treatment table.

8. Remove the moist cloth and begin the massage.

MUSTARD PLASTERS

When the sheet-bath failed to cure my cough, a lady friend recommended the application of a mustard plaster to my breast. I believe that would have cured me effectually, if it had not been for young Wilson. When I went to bed I put my mustard plaster – which was a very gorgeous one, eighteen inches square – where I could reach it when I was ready for it. But young Wilson got hungry in the night, and ate it up.

Mark Twain, *Curing a Cold*

A plaster is a paste-like herbal mixture that is spread on a protective cloth and then applied to the body. Plasters are an ancient remedy for local problems such as wounds, bruises, pneumonia and muscle aches. Hippocrates and famed Persian physician Avicenna (980–1037 AD) used plasters not only for local problems but also to get herbal medicines into a patient who could not swallow them. (Many herbs are so well absorbed via plasters that they can later be detected in the patient's urine). A German pharmacopeia of 1872 listed 28 different plasters, including ones made with capsicum, mustard, opium, belladonna, and oil of peppermint (Schcindlin, 2004).

When combined with water, chemicals and enzymes in ground mustard seeds encourage blood flow to the surface of the skin. Ground mustard seed was once listed in the US Pharmacopeia (list of approved medications) as the main additive in many baths, liniments, plasters and massage oils, and was also used by US Army doctors.

When applied to the skin, mustard plasters not only encourage blood flow, they also function as a **counter-irritant**, stimulating superficial nerves and distracting the central nervous system from deeper-seated pain. Originally mustard plasters were thought to draw out "bad humors." Practically speaking, however, they were used to provide soothing heat, increase local circulation, and relieve arthritis pain. In pre-antibiotic days they were used to treat respiratory ailments such as pneumonia, chest colds and bronchitis by deeply warming the chest (Duke, 2002). Today's massage therapist can use a mustard plaster before massage to ease a painful muscle or joint and to bring heat to deeper layers of muscle. You can buy ready-made mustard plasters or make your own, as shown here. They are indeed very hot and can even cause blistering, so you must monitor the skin underneath the plaster carefully and not keep it on for longer than the recommended time. Be especially careful with children, monitoring their skin frequently.

Below is an overview of treatment details and a sample procedure, using the anterior shoulder area.

SNAPSHOT

Indications

1. Poor local circulation.
2. Painful muscles that will be massaged after the plaster is removed.
3. Frozen shoulder.
4. Gout.
5. Acute lower back pain of muscular origin, chronic back pain, arthritis pain.
6. Raynaud's syndrome.

Contraindications

1. Sensitive skin.
2. Allergy to mustard seed.
3. Open skin (wounds, rashes, eczema, etc.).
4. Any area where heat is contraindicated, such as in diabetic neuropathy or spinal cord injury.

Temperature Hot (110°F; 43.3°C).

Time needed 14–30 minutes.

Equipment needed 1 tablespoon of mustard powder, 4 tablespoons of wheat flour, and enough tepid water to make a paste; spoons for measuring and stirring the paste; thin cotton cloth, approximately 10 × 12 inches (4 × 5cm); a piece of plastic that is slightly larger; small towel; fomentation, hot water bottle, or heating pad to keep the plaster warm (optional); small tray.

Effect Primarily chemical from the ground mustard, but also thermal due to the application of heat over the plaster.

Cleanup Dispose of the plaster and plastic sheet; launder the thin cloth and towel.

Procedure

1. Check with the client to make sure there are no contraindications for the use of local heat.

2. Explain the use of local heat to the client and get his or her consent.

3. Mix mustard powder, flour, and water to make a paste that can be spread on the cloth but is not so thin that it will run. A disposable bed pad or incontinence pad cut to the same size may also be used (Figure 4.13A).

4. Place the cloth on a tray (Figure 4.13B).

5. Spoon the mustard mixture onto the cloth, and spread it out, leaving enough dry cloth to fold over well on all four sides. Only one thin layer of cloth will be between the skin and the plaster (Figure 4.13C).

6. Warn the client before applying the plaster, and tell him to let you know if it ever feels too hot.

7. Check the area visually before applying the plaster (Figure 4.13D). This allows you to see what the client's skin normally looks like.

8. Place the plaster on the client's anterior shoulder (Figure 4.13E).

9. Cover it with the piece of plastic (Figure 4.13F), and cover the plastic with a small towel.

10. Place a source of heat on top of the plaster, plastic and small towel (Figure 4.13G).

11. Check the skin after 10 minutes and leave the plaster on for a total of 20 minutes.

12. Monitor the client's skin carefully—if the skin becomes very red before the 20 minutes is up, the reaction is finished and the plaster may be taken off. If the client feels any stinging or burning, remove the plaster immediately.

13. To clean the skin, apply a tissue or small cloth dipped in vegetable oil, and wipe off all the mustard (Figure 4.13H).

CASTOR OIL PACKS

Castor oil is a thick clear oil extracted from crushed castor beans. The oil is easy to obtain because the castor-oil plant grows well in many parts of the world. It has been used medicinally for centuries in both Ayurvedic and European folk medicine, and is commonly found in drugstores. It has a high concentration of fatty acids, especially ricinoleic acid. Castor oil packs have long been

---

A MUSTARD PLASTER FOR RIB MUSCLE PAIN   **CASE HISTORY 4.3**

BACKGROUND

Oscar is a healthy 25-year-old deliveryman for a vending machine company. One day a broken service elevator caused him to drag a heavily loaded hand truck up two flights of stairs by hand. By the time he reached the top stair, he was in such excruciating pain on the right side of his chest and torso that he was taken by ambulance to a hospital emergency department. Oscar was diagnosed with torn pectoral muscles and strained rib cartilage. He was given a prescription for narcotic medication and a referral for physical therapy to begin in ten days. Almost every movement was very painful, especially breathing and rolling over. Although Oscar had begun taking the narcotics, he had once struggled with drug addiction and now avoided strong painkillers, so he reduced his dosage and then found sleeping almost impossible.

TREATMENT

Fortunately for Oscar, his brother was a massage therapist and treated him each night, beginning by applying a mustard plaster over the right upper chest and ribcage for about 20 minutes. Oscar's discomfort eased during that time and his brother was then able to perform gentle but thorough massage on the intercostals, serratus anterior, pectorals and other nearby muscles. This allowed Oscar to sleep without medication, and the pain gradually began to recede, making life tolerable while he waited to begin physical therapy.

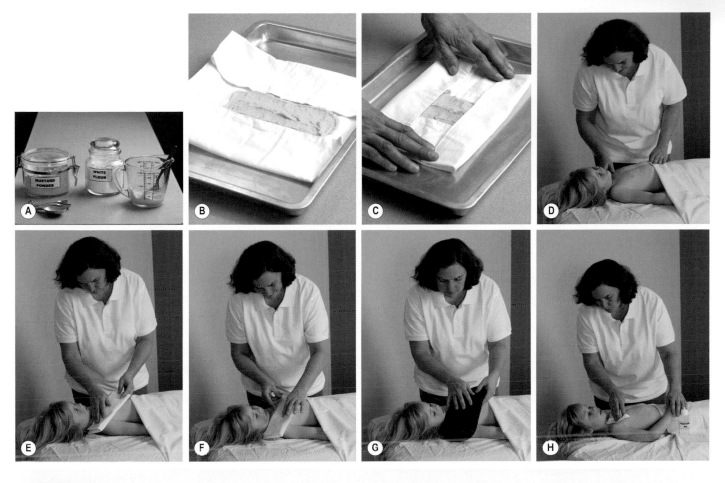

FIGURE 4.13
Mustard plaster. (**A**) Mix mustard powder, flour, and water to make a paste that can be spread on the cloth but is not so thin that it will run. (**B**) Place the cloth on a tray. (**C**) Spoon the mustard mixture onto the cloth, and spread it out, leaving enough dry cloth to fold over well on all four sides. Only one thin layer of cloth should be between the skin and the plaster. (**D**) Check the area visually before applying the plaster. (**E**) Place the plaster on the client's anterior shoulder. (**F**) Cover it with the piece of plastic and a small towel. (**G**) Place a source of heat on top of the plaster, plastic and small towel. (**H**) At the end of the treatment time, remove the pack, apply a tissue or small cloth dipped in vegetable oil, and wipe off all the mustard.

used for increasing local circulation of blood and lymph, relaxing smooth muscle, softening scar tissue, relieving muscle and joint pain, and helping to relax specific areas. Hot applications laid over the packs increase absorption of chemicals in the oil, as well as creating all the effects of local heat.

Some practitioners of natural medicine prescribe months-long regimens of daily castor oil packs, because these packs are believed to have strong detoxifying properties; however, no research has been done to investigate this claim. Others feel castor oil is beneficial for the immune system because it stimulates the body's production of lymphocytes: for example, the Balance Spa in Boca Raton, Florida, offers an "ImmunoMassage" treatment which combines massage with castor oil packs and essential oils specifically for the immune system. An important consideration for the massage therapist is the use of castor oil packs to soften fibrotic nodules and adhesions: packs are applied at the beginning of a massage session to prepare these tissues for treatment, and then taken off after 30 minutes or more.

Rather than using castor oil packs in massage sessions, a simpler method is to thickly cover the area to be treated with castor oil and cover it with plastic wrap. Now use a hot water bottle, heating pad, heat lamp or other local heat application to apply heat on top. Remove after 30 minutes, cleanse the area, and begin massage. Below is an overview of treatment details and a sample castor oil pack procedure using the calf, showing you how to incorporate it into a massage session.

SNAPSHOT

Indications

1. Muscle pain, including menstrual cramps.
2. Tight, fibrous tissue which is going to be treated with massage, including fibrotic knots, scar tissue, tight iliotibial bands and adhesions. Clients may follow up treatment at home by massaging the tissue with castor oil for a few minutes each day.
3. Arthritis, especially painful arthritic hands and knees.
4. Neck and back injuries, including sprains and strains, after 24 hours (ice would be used for the first 24 hours).

Contraindications

1. Any area where heat is contraindicated, such as in acute injury, diabetic neuropathy or where there is local inflammation.
2. Broken skin.
3. Tumors (unless approved by the client's doctor).
4. Ulcers.
5. The lower abdomen in pregnant women.

Temperature Warm (from a heating pad).

Time needed 45 minutes to 1 hour.

Equipment needed Flannel cloth (wool is preferred, but cotton may be used); bottle of castor oil; metal pan or tray large enough to hold the flannel; a piece of plastic wrap, or a thin sheet of plastic cut from a garbage bag, that is slightly larger than the flannel; local heat source to keep the pack warm, such as a fomentation, hot water bottle or heating pad; washcloth; soap or half a teaspoon of baking soda, which

can be added to one cup of water to cleanse the skin after the pack has been removed.

Effect Primarily chemical, due to the action of the castor oil itself, but also thermal, due to the application of heat over the entire pack.

Cleanup Dispose of the plastic sheet and the bed pad if used; wash the metal pan with soap and water; launder the washcloth. If flannel was used, it can be taken home in a plastic bag and reused by the client up to 10 times, provided it is kept in a plastic container in the refrigerator between uses; otherwise, it should be thrown away. No one else should use the flannel.

Procedure

1. Check with the client to make sure there are no contraindications for the use of local heat.
2. Explain the purpose of the castor oil pack to the client and get his or her consent.
3. Cut or fold the flannel to the appropriate size so there will be three layers of cloth. A disposable bed pad or incontinence pad may be used instead. Cosmetic pads may be used for very small areas. Place the pad on a metal pan or tray.
4. Pour castor oil over the flannel and leave it until it is well saturated: the cloth should be wet but not dripping (Figure 4.14A). The oil may be warmed first by putting it in a bowl of warm water or in the microwave for a few seconds.
5. Warn the client before applying the flannel, and tell them to let you know if it ever feels too hot.
6. Check the area visually before applying the flannel. This allows you to see what the client's skin normally looks like.
7. Apply the flannel to the calf (Figure 4.14B).
8. Cover it with the piece of plastic (Figure 4.14C).
9. Apply heat on top of the plastic-covered flannel. Use a heating pad on the highest safe setting: a high setting is preferable but a medium setting is allowed. A heat lamp, hot water bottle, warm gel pack or other source of heat may be used instead (Figure 4.14D). If a heat lamp is used, simply cover the area with the castor oil, put the lamp 8–12 (20–30 cm) inches from the oiled area, and switch it on.
10. Proceed with massage on other areas of the body.
11. Remove the pack after 30–90 minutes (Figure 4.14E). If using a disposable bed pad or incontinence pad, simply throw it away.

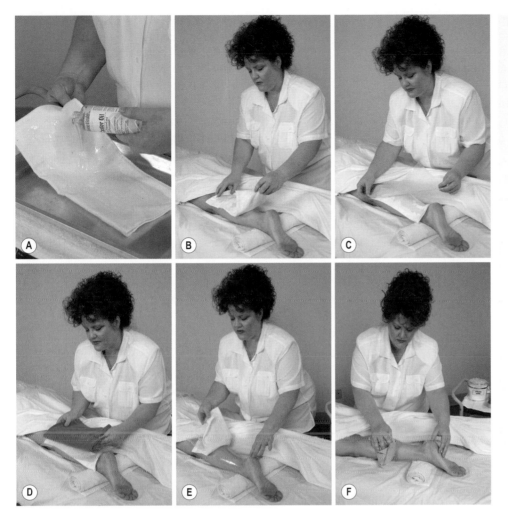

FIGURE 4.14
Castor oil. (**A**) Soak the flannel in castor oil. (**B**) Apply it to the skin. (**C**) Cover the flannel with plastic. (**D**) Cover the plastic with a heating pad or water bottle. (**E**) Remove the treatment. (**F**) Clean the skin with one cup of cool water mixed with one half teaspoon of baking soda.

12. Clean the skin with one cup of cool water which has had half a teaspoon of baking soda added to it (Figure 4.14F) or simply massage the castor oil in.

13. Proceed with local massage.

CHARCOAL PACKS

Charcoal is without a rival as an agent for cleansing and assisting the healing of the body.

Agatha Thrash, *Encyclopedia of Natural Remedies*

Activated charcoal is cheap, is easy to obtain, and has been used for centuries in many different cultures. Charcoal has an impressive ability to absorb body wastes, chemicals, and drugs of various kinds. It is used in medicine to absorb poisons and to remove toxins in various metabolic problems such as kidney and liver diseases. Charcoal is used in gas masks to filter poisons in the air,

and in water filters for the same purpose. As bodyworkers, we can use charcoal poultices to absorb inflammation and reduce pain when fluid and toxins may be impairing the healing process (Howell, 2013; Thrash and Thrash, 1981). We can make charcoal packs ourselves, or buy pre-made packs of different sizes and shapes.

SNAPSHOT

Indications Charcoal is helpful for arthritis, sprains, strains, bruises, and any type of musculoskeletal pain, especially when heat is not recommended.

Contraindications Charcoal is contraindicated for open skin wounds, rashes or eczema.

Temperature Room temperature.

Time needed 20 minutes to 1 hour.

Equipment needed Stain-proof surface to mix charcoal on; 4 tablespoons charcoal powder; one quarter cup of water; zip-closure bag; measuring spoon and cup; one paper towel; one disposable bed pad (incontinence pad) cut to 5 × 8 inches (13 × 20cm); a piece of plastic that is slightly larger than the charcoal pack, used to protect linens (optional).

Effect Primarily chemical, as charcoal absorbs inflammation and toxins.

Cleanup Throw the pad away.

Procedure

1. Charcoal can be messy and should be handled with that in mind. Using a stain-proof surface such as a metal tray or ceramic plate, slowly measure charcoal and water in a zipper-closure plastic bag (Figure 4.15A). Put the charcoal powder in first, gently add water to the bag, close it, and knead the mixture until it is the consistency of peanut butter.

2. Spread the charcoal paste on the incontinence pad and cover that with a single layer of paper towel.

3. Place it charcoal-side down on the client's skin (Figure 4.15B), and cover the linens underneath the client with a piece of plastic so they are protected against drips.

FIGURE 4.15
Charcoal pack. (**A**) Measuring and adding charcoal and water into a zipper-closure plastic bag. (**B**) The finished charcoal pack has been applied to the client's wrist.

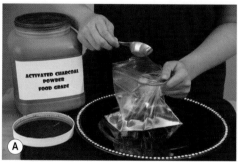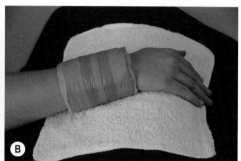

A CHARCOAL PACK FOR INFLAMMATION AND PAIN

CASE HISTORY 4.4

BACKGROUND

Ken is a 73-year-old retired farmer who has Type 2 diabetes, early-stage Parkinson's disease, and congestive heart failure. He normally uses a walker, but yesterday he tripped on an uneven ramp and fell very hard onto his knees. Not only were his knees too sore to touch (he rates his pain 8/10) but they were so stiff that, as he sat in a chair, he could not bend his knee and put one foot on top of the other thigh. His therapist gently examined the front of his legs and they were indeed very sore to the touch, while the back of his legs were not.

TREATMENT

While Ken finished undressing and got on the massage table, the therapist made two long charcoal packs. Using powdered charcoal mixed with water, he spread the mixture on two bed pads made from one pad cut in two. He covered the top with a single layer of paper towel, and put a piece of plastic under each pack. With Ken in the prone position, he slid the packs, with the charcoal on top, underneath each leg, covering the area from mid-thigh to mid-calf. (The plastic sheet prevented the charcoal packs from staining the linens.) The therapist then gave Ken a Swedish massage of his back and the back of his legs. When Ken rolled over into the supine position, the therapist held the charcoal packs in place, and they were left over Ken's knees for the remainder of the massage session. The therapist then gave Ken a Swedish massage of his upper body. At the end of the session, he removed the charcoal packs, which had now been in place for 60 minutes, and gently washed and dried Ken's legs. Once dressed, he stated that not only was his pain reduced (he rated it 3/10), but his legs were also much less stiff, so that he could now place each foot on top of the other thigh to put on his socks and shoes.

DISCUSSION QUESTIONS

1. What other treatments could the therapist have safely selected?

2. Why did the therapist decide not to give Ken a hot footbath for this problem?

CHAPTER SUMMARY

In this chapter you have learned about a variety of treatments that can heat a single part of the body without immersing it in liquid water, and the effects and benefits of each. Therapeutic heat can help relieve musculoskeletal pain and promote mental relaxation and increased local circulation. It also helps to warm and soften stiff muscles before exercise and stretching. Your therapy "toolbox" has just begun to expand; however, in each of the chapters ahead we will learn more new treatments, and learn even more about how to fine-tune them for you personally and for your clients. Soon you will even be able to combine treatments, if desired, for particular clients.

REVIEW QUESTIONS

Short answer

1. What is the number one hazard of heat applications?

2. Name five different conditions for which local heat is contraindicated.

3. Name three conditions for which local heat may be indicated.

4. Discuss the difference between the heat provided by hot stones or a dry hot water bottle, and that of a silica gel pack or fomentation.

5. Describe the effect of local heat on myofascial trigger points.

6. Discuss one treatment in this chapter that does not use heat.

Multiple choice

7. Local application of heat:

    A. Relaxes connective tissue

    B. Improves healing

    C. Causes local vasodilation

    D. Relieves pain

    E. All of the above

8. Which of these treatments has a heating effect?

    A. Local salt glow

    B. Cold footbath

    C. Charcoal pack

    D. Hot compress

    E. Castor oil pack

9. Local application of heat is indicated for all but one of these conditions. Which is the exception?

    A. Chronic arthritis

    B. Increased circulation

    C. Acute sprain

    D. Prior to exercise

10. The desired effects of a mustard plaster include all of these but one. Which is the exception?

    A. Provide soothing heat

    B. Prepare muscles for massage

    C. Increase local circulation

    D. Cause a blister

    E. Relieve arthritis or muscular pain

11. For which of these would a charcoal pack *not* be used? for all but one:

    A. Decrease pain

    B. Detoxification

    C. Treat kidney failure

    D. Reduce inflammation

True/False

12. True/False   Moist heat has the same effect as dry heat.

13. True/False   A cold pack application prior to massage aids in muscle relaxation.

14. True/False   Mustard plasters must be carefully monitored because they can burn the skin.

15. True/False   Castor oil packs are used to soften adhesions.

16. True/False   Local heat treatments decrease core temperature.

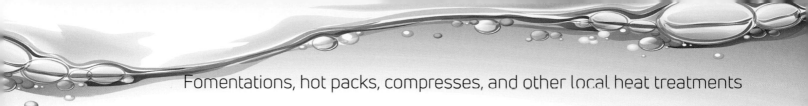

References

Altman RD, Marcussen KC. Effects of a ginger extract on knee pain in patients with osteoarthritis. Arthritis Rhem 2001; 44(11): 2531–8

Cowan T. The Fourfold Path to Healing. Brandywine, MD; New Trends Publishing, 2004

Cramer H et al. Thermotherapy self-treatment for neck pain relief–a randomized controlled trial. European J of Int Med 2012; 4(4): 371–3

Defrin R, Shachal-Shiffer M, Hadgadg M, Peretz C. Quantitative somatosensory testing of warm and heat-pain thresholds: the effect of body region and testing method. Clin J Pain 2006; 22: 130–6

Duke JA. Handbook of Medicinal Herbs, 2nd edn. Boca Raton, Florida FL: CRC Press, 2002

Hao J, Ghosh P, Li SK et al. Heat effects on drug delivery across human skin. Expert Opin Drug Deliv 2016; 13(5): 755–68

Hefi S, Tarapore PE, Walsh TJ et al. Wet heat exposure: a potentially reversible cause of low semen quality in infertile men. Int Braz J Urol 2007; 33(1): 50–6; discussion 56–7

Howell CA et al. Nanoporous activated carbon beads and monolithic columns as effective hemoadsorbents for inflammatory cytokines. Int J Artif Organs 2013; 36(9): 624–32

Jha S, Sharma P, Malviya R. Hyperthermia: role and risk factor for cancer treatment. Achievements in the Life Sciences 2016; 10(2): 161–7

Kober A et al. Local active warming: an effective treatment for pain, anxiety and nausea caused by renal colic. Journal of Urology 2003; 170(3): 741–4

Petrofsky JS. The effect of the moisture content of a local heat source on the blood flow response of the skin. Arch Dermatolog Res 2009; 301(8): 581–5

Riahi R, Cohen J. What caused this hyperpigmented reticulated rash on this man's back? The Dermatologist 2013

Rudolph C et al. Hot water bottle rash not only a sign of chronic pancreatitis. The Lancet 1998; 351 (9103)

Scheindlin S. Transdermal drug delivery past, present, future. Molecular Interventions 2004; 4(6): 308–12

Simons DG, Travell JG, Simons LS. Travell and Simons' Myofascial Pain and Dysfunction: the Trigger Point Manual, Vol 1: Upper Half of Body, 2nd edn. Baltimore, MD: Lippincott, Williams and Wilkins, 1999, pp. 133, 170

Therkleson T. Topical ginger treatment with a compress or patch for osteoarthritis symptoms. J Holist Nurs 2014; 32(3): 173–82

Thrash A. Encyclopedia of Natural Remedies. Fort Ogelthorpe, GA: TEACH Services Publishing, 2015

Thrash A, Thrash C. Home Remedies: Hydrotherapy, Massage, Charcoal, and Other Simple Treatments. Seale, AL: Thrash, 1981, p. 75

Twain M. Curing a Cold. The Golden Era (weekly literary journal). San Francisco, 20 September 1863

Wilson D. Living with Polio: The Epidemic and its Survivors. Chicago, IL: University of Chicago Press, 2005

Yarmolenko P et al. Thresholds for thermal damage to normal tissues: an update. Int J Hyperthermia 2011; 27(4): 320–4

Recommended resources

Belanger A. Evidence-Based Guide to Therapeutic Physical Agents, Baltimore: Lippincott, Williams and Wilkins, 2002

Boyle W, Saine A. Lectures in Naturopathic Hydrotherapy. Sandy, Oregon: Eclectic Medical Publications, 1988

Doub L. Hydrotherapy. Self-published manuscript. Fresno: California, 1971

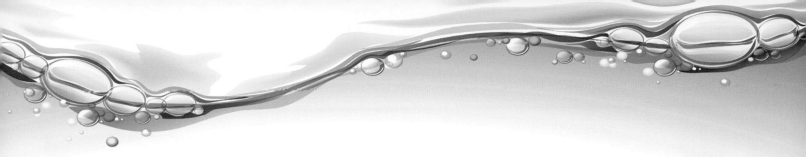

Cold packs, compresses, and ice massage: 5
local cold applications

What actually happens when you apply cold to an area? Not to oversimplify, but what happens is the cold constricts the local blood vessels which results in a decrease of bleeding of an injury and swelling. This holds true for both internal bleeding such as bruises and open wounds. Cold immediately decreases the painful spasm of an injured muscle. It provides a numbing effect on nerves just below the skin thereby reducing the pain. Taking into consideration all of the aspects of cold therapy as stated above; you are now helping to provide an environment where the body helps to rebuild and repair damaged tissue.

Harold Packman, *Ice Therapy: Understanding Its Application*

CHAPTER OBJECTIVES

After completing this chapter, the student will be able to:

1. Describe the effects of local cold applications
2. Describe how local cold is used in modern medicine
3. Name and describe local cold applications
4. Explain why cold might be contraindicated for some local cold applications
5. Name and describe local cold applications
6. Explain the four stages of ice massage
7. Describe four different procedures for ice massage, and when you would use one rather than another
8. Perform local cold treatments using the procedure included with each treatment.

In this chapter, you will be introduced to some common local cold applications whose benefits have been recognized since ancient times (see Figure 5.1). Like the local heat applications covered in Chapter 4, these are effective, inexpensive, and in most cases quite portable. They require little preparation and can be easily incorporated into your massage sessions. Cold applications affect the body differently than local heat treatments. Because of these effects, modern medicine uses cold, especially ice, for numerous conditions (see Box 5.1).

How can applying local cold treatments improve a massage session? Here are some examples:

- Before working with a muscle that is in spasm, cold gel packs, ice packs, ice bags, ice massage, or iced compresses (frozen wet cloths) can relieve the spasm.

- Stroking the length of a muscle with ice can temporarily de-activate trigger points so you can stretch taut muscles to their full length.

- Ice massage can be used to prepare tissue for deep massage and prevent possible soreness in a muscle after it has been treated with deep transverse friction.

- Cold applications may relieve arthritis pain even better than heat (numbness begins when the skin temperature drops to 36°F (2.22°C)).

- Before you massage near a sprained ankle, cold applications can help reduce tissue swelling and pain.

- A flat plastic water bottle filled with chilled water or an ice water compress can cool an overheated client.

- Under a hot application, blood vessels are dilated and cooler blood can flow in readily. But under a cold application, blood vessels are constricted, and this actually reduces the amount of fresh warm blood that can flow in to feed cells. This means that the area will rewarm slowly even after the cold has been removed. It also means that cold applications can penetrate more deeply into tissues than warm applications. Thus, after an ice pack has been on

Chapter five

FIGURE 5.1
Client with cold gel pack on upper back, ice pack on hamstring muscles, and ice massage being performed on the gastrocnemius.

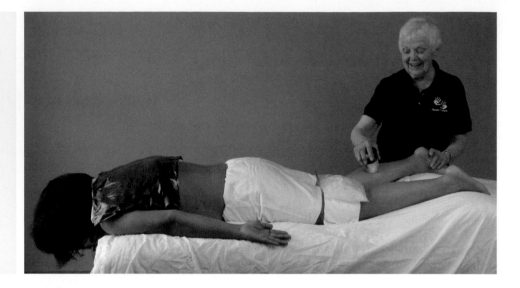

BOX 5.1	POINT OF INTEREST

THE FIVE PRIMARY EFFECTS OF COLD APPLICATIONS

Cold applications have a wide range of uses in modern medicine due to these effects:

Cold reduces sensation

Cold reduces sensation by cooling nerves, which slows their messages to the brain (Herrera, 2010). The numbing effect of ice is widely used in medicine to reduce the discomfort of:

1. Musculoskeletal injuries such as bruises, muscle strains, hematomas, and fractures, and soreness after vigorous physical therapy (Anava-Erroba, 2010).
2. Post-orthopedic surgery pain.
3. Mouth pain after root canal surgery, using 36°F (2°C) water to rinse the surgery site (Keskin, 2016).
4. Phantom limb pain (Tolis, 2018).
5. Shingles pain.
6. Labor pain, when used over the perineum.
7. Nipple soreness after breastfeeding or expressing milk.
8. Injections and blood draws: a small device called a Buzzy combines a small flat ice pack and a small vibrator placed on top; it reduces pain as much as anaesthetic creams, in both children and

adults (McGinnis, 2016; Sahiner, 2015). Ice packs are used on needle puncture sites after bone marrow biopsies.
9. The unpleasant taste of certain bad-tasting medications.
10. Stinging sensations after laser treatments or chemical peels.

Ice reduces inflammation

This anti-inflammatory effect is widely used in medicine to reduce swelling or itching due to:

1. Musculoskeletal injuries such as bruises, sprains, strains, and torn muscles.
2. Orthopedic surgery.
3. Joint inflammation: six studies have shown that ice packs and ice-water hand baths reduced joint pain significantly when repeated over a period of days (Guillot, 2014).
4. Some cancer medications and some types of cancer that cause itching.
5. Wounds that are healing.
6. Mild poison ivy, hives, eczema and psoriasis.
7. Dry eye syndrome, considered an inflammatory disorder.

Ice reduces local bloodflow

This effect occurs because of reflex vasoconstriction. For example, in one study the effect of an

BOX 5.1 *continued*

ice wrap applied to one knee was compared to a room-temperature wrap on the other knee. Researchers found that the ice wrap caused a 38% decrease in arterial blood flow, a 25% decrease in soft tissue blood flow, and a 19% reduction in blood flow to the bone itself (Ho, 1994). Icing a knee can decrease blood flow to both soft tissue and bone in the knee in as little as 5 minutes (Ho, 1990). The reason ice applications are generally limited to 15–20 minutes is because the tissues under the ice may become damaged from lack of blood: frostbite and nerve damage have resulted from longer applications. Even packages of frozen vegetables left on too long have caused frostbite (Graham, 2000). This effect of ice is currently used in medicine to decrease blood flow into tissues such as:

1. Areas which may still be bleeding after musculoskeletal trauma or surgeries which cause bruising, such as facelifts.

2. The arteries which supply blood to the brain. Decreasing the flow helps control migraine headaches. Researchers have used both ice and liquid coolant pumped up the nostrils to decrease blood flow, while the classic bodywork approach is to use ice packs, cold gel packs, or cold stones to the back of the neck and to the face.

3. The joints of hemophiliacs during a bleeding episode.

4. The nose during a nosebleed.

5. Injection sites, in order to slow the absorption of medications just injected.

6. The scalp, as ice applied to the skull with "cooling caps" during chemotherapy lessens absorption of chemotherapy medications and reduces hair loss. A "cooling helmet," using either icepacks or liquid coolant pumped through tubes, is a recent invention used to cool the brain after a traumatic brain injury in order to decrease edema and bleeding (Kurland, 2012; Urbana, 2012).

7. The hands and feet. Since chemotherapy drugs can cause peripheral neuropathy and nail damage, icy-cold gloves and socks are worn during infusions to reduce absorption into the hands and feet. When the frozen glove or sock is applied to only one hand or foot, the other side will have more peripheral neuropathy (Hanai, 2018).

8. Erupting herpes blisters. Ice applications arrest their development and shorten healing time.

Ice reduces muscle spasm

This effect is used in medicine to: deactivate trigger points and release muscle tension long enough for individual muscles to be gently but thoroughly stretched; to increase range of motion before stretching; and to ease muscle spasticity before physical therapy for cerebral palsy. Massage therapist Harold Packman combined ice massage over the facial nerve and manual massage to successfully treat a woman with longstanding spasmodic contraction in her eye and face (Packman, 2007). Conversely, ice is sometimes used to stimulate muscle tone. (For more on this, see page 348.)

Ice reduces body temperature

This effect is used in medicine to reduce the core temperature in high fevers, heatstroke and heat exhaustion. Local scrotal cooling is helpful to improve sperm production in men with low counts. Special cooling vests containing ice packs or gel packs are used in operating rooms to keep surgeons and nurses from becoming overheated by hot operating lights and layers of clothing such as gowns, protective suits and lead aprons. Patients with multiple sclerosis often experience fatigue when they become very warm: cooling gloves and vests reduce this problem so they can leave their air-conditioned homes in the summer and participate in outside activities again (Robinson, 2017). Finally, to prevent their deterioration before surgery, severed fingers and toes which are going to be reattached, and organs which are going to be transplanted, are cooled in bags that are kept in iced water.

it for only 20 minutes, a muscle may take an hour or more to reach normal temperature again. The more superficial areas will begin to warm up as soon as an ice pack is removed, but muscle tissue that is 1.2 inches (3cm) deep will not begin to warm up even 30 minutes after the ice pack has been removed (Myrer, 2001).

Cold applications can often be creatively combined with hot ones to fine-tune a session for a specific client's needs. For example, when a hot application is needed for clients who are likely to become overheated, adding an application of cold somewhere else on the body will help keep them comfortable. Hot and cold applications can also be combined to form contrast treatments which stimulate local circulation and relieve pain. After you learn how to use local cold treatments, you can not only design an in-office massage session using them, but also give your clients simple instructions for doing them at home.

INDICATIONS, CONTRAINDICATIONS AND CAUTIONS FOR LOCAL COLD APPLICATIONS

Below are the primary indications, contraindications, and cautions for local cold treatments. The advantages of any type of cold application must always be weighed against three major disadvantages:

- most cold applications reduce nearby blood flow
- prolonged application of cold to the body surface can drop the core temperature
- many clients dislike cold and shy away from it altogether.

For more on overuse of cold, see Box 5.2.

Indications

1. Pain and edema in musculoskeletal injuries including muscle strains, joint sprains and contusions, used for the first 4 hours only.
2. Numbing of areas before light therapeutic exercise (**cryokinetics**). Temporary relief of pain may allow helpful range of motion exercises in injured joints and conditions such as arthritis, while exercises dilate blood vessels and rewarm tissues, avoiding vasoconstriction in deep tissues.
3. Preventing muscle soreness after heavy exercise.
4. Acute low back pain.
5. Chronic low back pain, including sciatica.
6. Rheumatoid arthritis, if beneficial for the client (heat may work better for some).
7. Osteoarthritis, if beneficial for the client (heat may work better for some).

8. Bursitis, if beneficial for the client (heat may work better for some).
9. Chronically stiff or spastic muscles, due to damage to the brain or spinal cord.
10. Stimulation of low muscle tone from stroke, spinal cord injury, muscular dystrophy, cerebral palsy, birth defects and other conditions.
11. When stimulation of local circulation is called for, using cold as part of a contrast treatment.
12. When a derivative (fluid-shifting) effect is desired to reduce blood flow in congested areas. For example, when cold is applied on the back of the neck it causes local vasoconstriction and may be helpful in treating a migraine headache.
13. Overheated client.

Contraindications

1. Cold client – warm every chilly client before applying cold, otherwise expect a weaker reaction and a distinct dislike of your treatment. Your treatment room must be warm at all times. Any local heat treatment, from a heat lamp to a hot water bottle, will prevent chilling of the client who has a cold application.
2. Aversion to cold.
3. Sensitivity to cold, common in clients with fibromyalgia.
4. Headache upon contact with cold.
5. Numbness in the treated area. This can be caused by spinal cord injury, diabetic neuropathy or other medical conditions. Some medications could also cause the person to be unable to feel the pain of a too-cold application. Never put a cold application on a numb area.
6. Poor circulation. Because cold decreases blood flow, do not use it over areas where the circulation is already poor. For this reason, cold is contraindicated with any peripheral vascular disease, including diabetes, Buerger's disease, and arteriosclerosis of the lower extremities.
7. Raynaud's syndrome.
8. Previously frostbitten areas.

Continued

BOX 5.2   POINT OF INTEREST

WHEN COLD IS TOO MUCH OF A GOOD THING

Like anything, local cold can be overused. Remember to observe the guidelines given here and you will never risk injuring a client. Here are a few examples of overuse of cold.

Slower healing of injuries

RICE – Rest, Ice, Compression and Elevation – has been recommended since 1978 by sports doctors: using ice immediately after a sprain or strain was thought to delay swelling and reduce pain. The latest research, however, shows that icing injured tissue leads to restriction of blood flow by contraction of blood vessels. Gabe Mirkin, MD, the physician who originally coined the term RICE, now recommends that the injured person skip ice unless pain is very severe, and then use ice packs only two or three times, for 15–20 minutes each. Short-term, Dr. Mirkin recommends over-the-counter non-steroidal anti-inflammatory medications, but only for the first 24–48 hours, since they too slow down recovery by suppressing inflammation. Compression and elevation are still recommended, while gentle exercise is preferred over complete rest (Consumer Reports, 2015). Physiatrist and prolotherapy expert Ross Hauser, MD, has also maintained for many years that ligamentous injuries heal poorly when iced over time – he recommends ice for only the first 4 hours after injury, then compression and elevation, gentle movement, and helpful treatments such as hot-and-cold contrast treatments and acupuncture (Hauser, 2017).

Tissue damage

Cold therapy machines are frequently used after surgeries, including rotator cuff repairs, joint replacements and even amputations. These machines feature a reservoir with an ice-and-water slush: this is connected to a tube that continually circulates chilled water to selected areas just under a cloth pad. The typical patient uses the machine 3–4 hours a day for 4 weeks. Skin temperature may go as low as 68°F (20°C). Khoshnevis et al. found that cold machines lead to deep vasoconstriction, which can persist long after cooling is stopped (Khoshnevis, 2015). Cold is used to reduce blood loss to decrease the need for pain medication after surgery or acute injuries (including amputations) and to decrease muscle soreness after strenuous workouts or vigorous physical therapy (Chen, 2014). Unfortunately, cold machines are often overused, resulting in frostbite and damage to skin, nerves and other tissues. Skin temperatures below 20°F (−6.7°C) can cause frost bite (Dundon, 2013; Brown, 2009; McGuire, 2006). Machines typically carry warnings such as: "Warning: this device can be cold enough to cause serious injury, including full skin necrosis … Inspect the skin under the cold therapy pad every 1–2 hours. Do not let any part of the pad touch the skin … stop using if you experience any adverse reactions such as: increased pain, burning, increased swelling, itching, blisters, increased redness, discoloration, welts or other changes in skin appearance."

However, because of existing nerve damage or desensitization from prior surgery or injury, patients may not always feel how cold the pad is on their skin, so unfortunately nerve and skin damage occurs before the pad is removed. Patients without sufficient guidance sometimes suppose that the colder the pad is the better; or the longer it is on, the better. Some patients have required reconstructive surgeries, and numerous lawsuits have been pursued against the manufacturers (Schmidt, 2018). In addition, tissues with less blood supply than muscles, including tendons, ligaments, cartilage and other connective tissues, will likely suffer from prolonged vasoconstriction, and may heal more poorly. Dr. Ross Hauser maintains there is no proof that tissues will be healthier in the future by using cold machines (Hauser, 2018).

9. Where an analgesic cream has been applied to the skin.

10. Wounds that are not healed.

11. Malignancy in the area to be treated.

12. Heart disease – applying cold over the heart can cause a reflex constriction of the coronary arteries.

13. Implanted devices such as cardiac pacemakers, stomach bands and infusion pumps. Artificial joints are fine.

14. Marked hypertension – ice applications anywhere on the body usually cause a brief rise in blood pressure.

Cautions

1. Children have difficulty describing their bodily sensations and so may not tell you if cold is causing pain.

2. Elders (those over 60 years old) may have less ability to keep their body warm when cold is applied, so make sure that they do not become chilled.

3. Use caution when applying cold over superficial nerves: do not exceed recommended times and do not tie cold applications over them.

4. Clients may have decreased muscle strength and slower reflexes for 30 minutes after ice treatment, and can be prone to injury if they exercise right away.

5. Always check tissues periodically for cold damage: if an area has been cooled too much, blotchiness, redness or welts can occur.

Just how cold is cold?

A 2005 study compared the effect of three different forms of cold on skin temperature. Ice packs, gel packs kept in the freezer, and packages of frozen peas were each wrapped in towels wetted with room-temperature water and laid on subjects' skin. Skin temperature was measured at the beginning and again after 20 minutes. All cold devices cooled the skin, but ice packs caused the largest drop in skin temperature, from 90°F to 50°F (32°C to 10°C). Next coldest were the packages of frozen peas, which caused the subjects' skin temperature to drop from 90°F to 56°F (32°C to 13.3°C). The least

cooling were the gel packs, which reduced the skin temperature to only 57°F (13.9°C). Numbness began after 9 minutes (Kanlayanaphotporn, 2005). When applied for 20 minutes, a cold whirlpool (50°F; 10°C) also does not chill muscle tissue as much as an icepack (Meyrer, 1998). Because numbness does not begin until the skin temperature is lowered to 56°F (13.6°C), this study showed that all three cold applications could numb or begin to numb an area. To slow the metabolism down, which truly combats swelling, skin temperature should be maintained at 50°F (10°C) (Meyrer, 1998). Meyrer found that after 20 minutes of ice pack, the calf muscle temperature 0.4 inch (1cm) underneath the skin was 56°F (14.4°C) colder, and the deeper muscle (1.2 inch (3cm) under the skin) was only 43°F (6°C) colder. However, after a 30-minute rest period, the muscle 0.4 inch (1cm) under the skin had warmed up almost back to normal, but the deeper muscle tissue was actually colder than when the ice pack was taken off, reflecting deep vasoconstriction (Meyrer, 2001).

SILICA GEL COLD PACKS

Typically these packs have washable plastic or vinyl covers, and are filled with a gel which remains flexible even when frozen. Aside from those for musculoskeletal

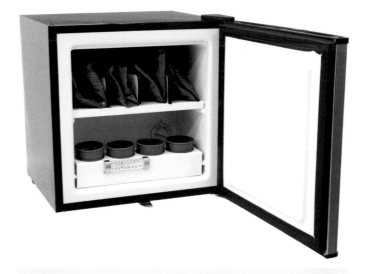

FIGURE 5.2
Small freezer for storing cold gel packs and ice cups.
Photo courtesy of Whitehall Mfg Company.

problems, gel packs are made for many other specific areas, such as whole-face masks to use after facial or dental surgery, specially shaped ones to drape around painful jaws, round ones for nipple soreness in breast-feeding mothers, and small ones to go over the eyes or sinuses. They are popular because they mold to body curves, are an effective source of cold, and require almost no preparation: all that is necessary is to place them in a freezer for 2 hours before you use them. Small freezers are inexpensive and take up little space in an office (Figure 5.2). When they are ready for use, gel packs remain cold for 15–20 minutes. While it is helpful to have such an efficient source of cold, they can also cause tissue damage and must be monitored.

Gel packs are most efficient at cooling large flat surfaces such as the thigh or the back (see Figure 5.3). Never let clients lie on a cold gel pack. Never tie a cold gel pack on any part of the body: this can compress the cooling tissues underneath and further reduce blood flow. A whole-face gel pack may be used in a face cradle to ease sinus congestion or to eliminate "cradle face" – puffiness as a result of laying supine during a session.

The procedure below shows you a step-by-step procedure for using a cold gel pack on the upper back. However, gel packs can be adapted to treat almost any area of the body. They can also be combined with hot applications to create contrast treatments.

SNAPSHOT

Temperature 25–32°F (−3.9–0°C).

Time needed 10–20 minutes. To prevent cold damage, do not exceed this time.

Equipment needed Cold gel pack (see also Case history 5.1); a thin cloth or towel to put between the gel pack and the client's skin. A cold wet cloth conducts cold better than a dry one.

Effect Primarily thermal.

Cleanup Launder the cloth covering; clean the surface of the gel pack with soap and water if it has come in contact with the client's skin.

Procedure

1. Dampen a thin cloth.
2. With the client in the prone position, place the cloth on the upper back (A).
3. Place the cold gel pack on top of the cloth (B).
4. Remove the pack every few minutes to inspect the skin (C).
5. Remove it after a maximum of 20 minutes.

ICE PACKS AND ICE BAGS

Ice packs and ice bags are a popular method of treating many local musculoskeletal conditions and so they are widely used in doctors' offices, hospitals, athletic

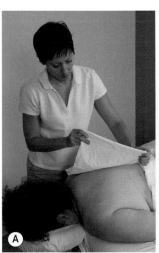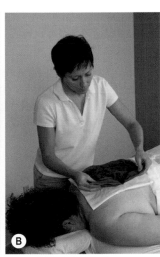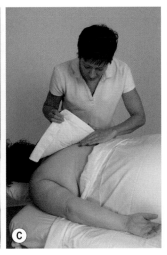

FIGURE 5.3
Large gel pack on the back.
(**A**) With the client in the prone position, place the cloth on the upper back. (**B**) Place the cold gel pack on top of the cloth.
(**C**) Remove the gel pack every few minutes to inspect the skin, then replace it.

Chapter five

BACKGROUND

Leila was a healthy 38-year-old woman with a history of constant, low-level lumbar pain. She was diagnosed with scoliosis at age 13, wore a brace for a few years, and at age 17 underwent surgery to fuse her spine at T4 to L3 level. Leila healed well from her surgery but although she experienced minimal pain prior to surgery, afterwards she was never pain-free. Her **physiatrist** – a doctor specializing in rehabilitation – recommended a program of regular aerobic exercise, periodic physical therapy and regular massage therapy. Leila managed her pain quite well on this program but experienced increasing pain during the latter part of each day, which sometimes kept her from falling asleep.

TREATMENT

After having a cold gel pack applied to her back during a massage session, Leila realized that its numbing quality could help reduce her pain at bedtime. She purchased a large gel pack, kept it in the freezer, and began to use it every night before bed. Sitting upright in a chair, Leila slid the pack behind her back, and when the painful area became quite numb, after about 15 minutes, she could then remove it and quickly fall asleep.

DISCUSSION QUESTIONS

1. Explain how the cold gel pack relieved Leila's pain.
2. What other local cold treatments could be added to Leila's massage sessions?

---

facilities, physical therapy clinics and massage therapy offices. Not only do they cool effectively, but they are also simple to prepare: ice packs can be easily made with only a towel and crushed or cube ice. When the packs are applied to the client's skin for 20 minutes, they can reduce the intra-muscular temperature by as much as 5–10°F (2.8–5.6°C). They also lead to deep vasoconstriction and should not be used repeatedly: experts used to recommend 20 minutes of ice followed by a 20-minute rest, repeated many times after an injury such as a sprained ankle. Researchers eventually found that this practice severely limits blood flow and tissue healing, so this is no longer recommended.

Either ice packs or bags can be applied to almost any area of the body, except over the eyes, and are especially suited for larger dense muscles that need real cold to chill them. Smaller areas without much insulation, such as the back of the hand, do not need to be iced for very long in order to become very cold.

Ice packs

Ice packs made with towels can be large or small, depending upon the size of the towel. You can even make a tiny ice pack by wetting a sponge, freezing it, putting it in a plastic bag, then wrapping it in a thin wet cloth. In Figure 5.4 we show a small ice pack which can be used on the back of the neck, the front of the knee joint, or other small areas. Never lie on an ice pack.

SNAPSHOT

Temperature Very cold (32°F; 0°C).

Time needed 10–20 minutes. To prevent cold damage, do not exceed this time.

Equipment needed One damp towel; one dry towel; crushed ice or ice cubes. Larger towels can be used to make larger packs.

Effect Primarily thermal.

Cleanup Launder the towel.

Procedure

1. Dampen a small face towel, then lay it on a flat surface. Place about 4 cups worth of ice cubes on one end of the towel (Figure 5.4A). Fold it over to make an ice pack which will fit easily over a small area (Figure 5.4B).
2. Place the ice pack on the client's skin (Figure 5.4C).
3. Cover the ice pack with a dry towel of the same size (Figure 5.4D).
4. Remove the pack every few minutes to check for cold damage, then replace.
5. Remove after a maximum of 20 minutes. For an injury such as a sprain, muscle strain or contusion, use only once or twice during the first 4 hours, then do not use during healing.

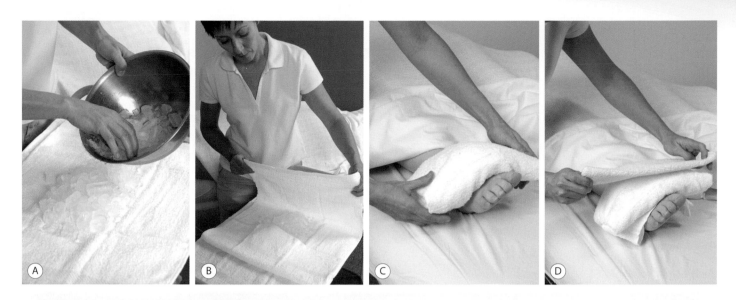

FIGURE 5.4
Home made ice packs. (**A**) Placing ice cubes on a towel. (**B**) Folding the ice inside the towel to form an ice pack. (**C**) Placing the ice pack on the client's skin. (**D**) Placing a dry towel on top of the ice pack.

Ice bags

Ice bags are simple, easy-to-find items, and they come in various sizes.

SNAPSHOT

Temperature Very cold (32°F; 0°C).

Time needed 10–20 minutes. To prevent cold damage, do not exceed this time.

Equipment needed Pre-made ice bag or plastic re-sealable bag; crushed ice cubes to fill the bag; a thin cloth to be placed between the ice bag and the client's skin (optional). Figure 5.5 shows various types of ice bags.

Effect Primarily thermal.

Cleanup Launder the cloth coverings and any other linens used; clean the surface of the ice bag with soap and water if it has come in contact with the client's skin; dispose of the resealable plastic bag, if used.

Procedure

1. Fill the pre-made ice bag or the resealable plastic bag with crushed ice or ice cubes. Remove as much air as possible from the bag before you seal it.

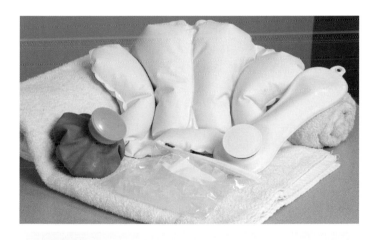

FIGURE 5.5
Pre-made ice bags come in various sizes.

2. Place a thin wet cloth on the client's skin (Figure 5.6A).
3. Place the ice bag on the cloth (Figure 5.6B).
4. Remove the bag every few minutes to check for cold damage. Remove after a maximum of 20 minutes. As with ice packs, use only during the first 4 hours after injury.

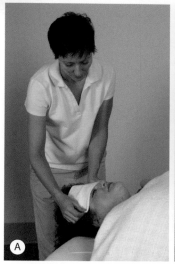
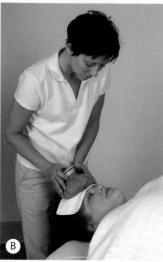

FIGURE 5.6
Applying an ice bag. (**A**) Placing a cloth on the client's skin. (**B**) Placing the bag on the cloth.

FLAT PLASTIC WATER BOTTLES

In Chapter 4 (page 106) you learned how to use a flat plastic water bottle filled with hot water, but it can also be used to apply cold. When laid flat on a massage table, the bottle can cool the client's entire torso or back. It will stay cool for approximately 30 minutes.

An advantage of this particular hydrotherapy treatment is that it is inexpensive and low-tech: all the therapist needs is the bottle and cold water.

Some therapists keep a filled bottle in the refrigerator, ready to use, or place it in a cooler with a bag of ice, where it will stay cold and ready for use for hours.

To create contrast treatments, bottles can be filled with cold water and then combined with various heat applications, including another bottle filled with hot water.

The following sequence shows an effective way to use a cold water bottle: simply place it on the massage table under a sheet or in a pillowcase, where it can cool the client's entire back or the back of a leg. (This could be perfect for acutely strained back muscles or a torn hamstring.) Unlike gel cold packs or ice packs, the cold water bottle is safe to lie on because it begins to warm up as soon as the client lies on it.

SNAPSHOT

Temperature Cold (water is 42–55°F; 5–12.8°C).

Time needed 5–30 minutes. The client's tissue will begin to cool after about 5 minutes.

Equipment needed Water thermometer; water bottle; and a thin cloth to cover or wrap the filled water bottle (a pillowcase is ideal).

Effect Primarily thermal.

Cleanup Launder the cloth; empty the water bottle and lay it flat with the lid off, so the last drops of water will evaporate; then fold and store it.

Procedure

1. Check with the client to make sure there are no contraindications for the use of local cold.

2. Explain the use of local cold to the client and get his or her consent. Fill the bottle about one third full with cold water that has been chilled in a refrigerator, or use room-temperature water that has been mixed with crushed ice and then strained (Figure 5.7A). About 5 cups of water (1.25 liters) will be needed to fill an 18 x 24 inch (45 x 60cm) bottle. Use a thermometer to ensure the water is 42–55°F (5–12.8°C).

3. Carry the open bottle carefully to the massage table, lay it flat on the table, use your hand to expel all the air bubbles, and check to make sure the top is snapped on securely so the bottle does not leak (Figure 5.7B).

4. Cover it with a cloth or place it inside a pillowcase (Figure 5.7C).

5. As the client lies supine on the cloth-covered bottle, say, "Be sure to let me know if this ever feels like it is too cold."

6. Although the chance of cold injury is minimal, be sure to ask your client for feedback. The bottle will be intensely cold when it is first lain upon, but will begin to warm up almost immediately.

ICE MASSAGE PERFORMED FOUR DIFFERENT WAYS

Ice massage is a technique of cooling tissue with an ice cube or a chunk of ice applied to the skin. The ice is moved over and around the area to be cooled, using a gentle rotary motion but no downward pressure. Ice massage may be performed on any part of the body, from large dense muscles such as the quadriceps to small areas such as the back of the hand. After an injury such

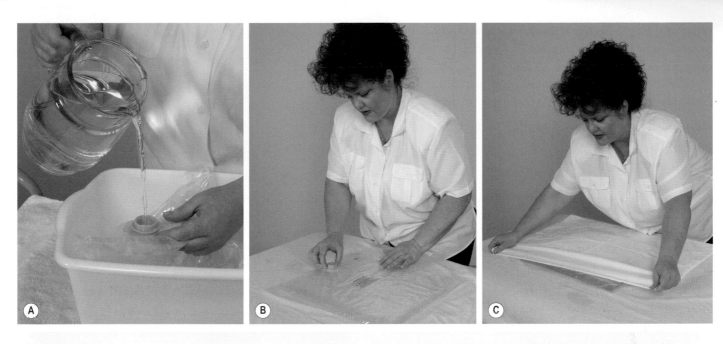

FIGURE 5.7
Flat plastic water bottle. (**A**) Fill the bottle about one third full with cold water. (**B**) Carry the open bottle carefully to the massage table, lay it flat on the table, use your hand to expel all the air bubbles, and check to make sure the top is snapped on securely so the bottle does not leak. (**C**) Cover the bottle with a cloth or pillowcase, or place it inside a pillowcase.

as a strained muscle, a torn muscle, a sprained joint or bruised soft tissue, ice massage reduces local swelling and inflammation and relieves spasm and pain. It can also help reduce post-treatment soreness after deep transverse friction has been performed. Ice massage is also an excellent home treatment you can teach to your clients. For example, a client who wakes up with an acutely stiff neck or other muscle spasm can easily perform ice massage on the area by himself.

Some practitioners prefer ice massage over ice packs or bags, and each has its advantages and disadvantages. Ice massage not only reduces tissue temperature as well as ice packs and ice bags do, but it does so much faster. One study comparing the cooling effect of ice massage to that of ice bags found that ice massage cooled the calf muscle as much as 10 minutes faster than an ice bag (Zemke, 1998). Therefore, using ice massage during a massage session means you will not have to wait as long for the area to cool. However, the advantage of rapid cooling must be weighed against the fact that ice massage is more intensely cold, and some clients will find the sensation too much. These clients may prefer a cold application that chills the area more slowly. In this case, you might

prefer to apply a cold gel pack in one area while performing massage on another part of the body until the area has cooled. You might also choose ice massage because herbs, essential oils or other chemical substances can be applied to the skin, if they are mixed with the water you use to make ice cups. As the ice melts, the dissolved chemical will come into direct contact with the skin. When choosing which cold application to use, remember that time will be taken away from manual massage while you are performing ice massage.

To begin, you will need to make a chunk of ice by freezing water in a paper cup, popsicle tray or a plastic cup that is designed especially for ice massage (see Figure 5.8A).

As you perform ice massage, keep in mind that the thicker the tissue you wish to cool, the more time it takes for cold to penetrate it. For example, tissues that are near the body surface and have little subcutaneous fat to insulate them, such as the front of the knee joint, will require less time; and tissues that are thick or covered by more subcutaneous fat, such as the gluteal muscles, will require more time. The tissues of a small, thin person who feels the cold readily will need to be treated differently than those of a larger person with well-developed muscles or a great deal of subcutaneous fat. Therefore, the *stages* of ice massage are a better guide to the right amount of time a client will need than a set number of minutes. However, never do more than 15 minutes of ice massage.

Generally, the client will gradually have four different sensations:

1. a sensation of cold
2. burning/pricking
3. aching
4. numbness – take the ice away as soon as this happens, then cover the area with a small dry towel until you begin massaging it.

It is important to explain the benefits of ice massage to clients before you begin, since they may want you to stop once the area begins burning or aching. When this stage is reached, tell them that this is beneficial because their tissue is just about to become numb. Once past the aching stage, clients will be happy with the relief that they receive.

Ice massage for muscle spasm, acute inflammation, and pain

Ice massage can also be performed on many other parts of the body, including the entire back, all four limbs, and the neck; but here we show a step-by-step procedure for the extensor muscles of the forearm (see also Case history 5.2).

SNAPSHOT

Temperature Very cold (32°F; 0°C).

Time needed 5–15 minutes, depending upon the thickness of the tissue and individual tolerance.

Equipment needed Ice in a paper cup or a specially designed plastic cup; medium- to large-sized towel.

Effect Primarily thermal.

Cleanup Dispose of ice, launder towel, sanitize plastic cup.

Procedure

1. Check with the client to make sure there are no contraindications for the use of local cold.
2. Explain the use of local cold to the client and get his or her consent.

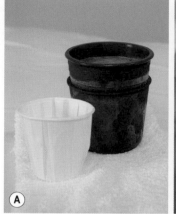
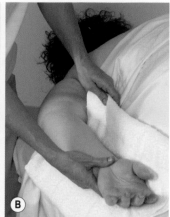
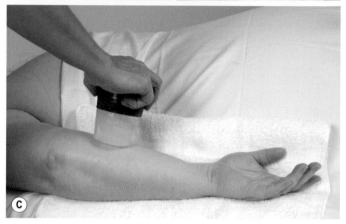

FIGURE 5.8
Ice massage. (**A**) Ice cups, made from paper cups or using commercial ice massage cups. (**B**) Drape towels around the area to be iced. (**C**) Hold the cup of ice in one hand and gently rub it in a circular motion. Here we show ice massage on the forearm.

3. Explain the four stages of ice massage to the client. It is important that he or she realizes that the ice massage must last to the point of numbness.
4. Drape towels around the area to be iced, so melting ice will not drip water onto other parts of the body (Figure 5.8B).
5. Hold the cup of ice in one hand and move it in a circular motion over the area you are treating and a few inches above and below the area as well (Figure 5.8C). Do not press down: you are using the ice to cool, not to manipulate the area.
6. Continue until the area is numb.
7. Remove the ice and dry the area.

BACKGROUND

Suzanne was a 28-year-old nurse who had received massage in the past for relaxation. Suzanne was generally very healthy, but had experienced mild whiplash from a sledding accident and was taking prescribed muscle relaxants and anti-inflammatory and pain medications. She was receiving physical therapy for neck and upper back pain and frontal headaches, but had never received massage therapy. She requested massage because she had a very uncomfortable feeling in her right mid-scapular region which felt as though the area "needed to be popped." Suzanne had never had this feeling (likely a muscle spasm stemming from her injury) until a few days ago, when she asked her father to "pop her back" in the mid-scapular region. He did so, but used tremendous force, and she immediately had a severe headache which lasted for 4 hours. She now knew that "popping" the area was not helpful, and she hoped that massage could help relieve her discomfort. Chiropractor David Bond has written about clients who constantly crack their own necks or other joints because of feelings of stiffness and muscular pain: he calls this habit "crack addiction." Unfortunately, constant cracking can create a vicious cycle in which the symptoms increase as ligaments and muscles become increasingly inflamed and uncomfortable. He recommends sufferers stop cracking their joints and use ice and manual massage to decrease discomfort instead (Bond, 2012).

TREATMENT

The massage therapist took Suzanne's history over the phone, then consulted with her physical therapist, who approved of ice massage as well as hands-on massage for Suzanne's entire back. The massage therapist began the session with 15 minutes of Swedish massage of the back, assessing Suzanne's muscles as she eased tension in the most superficial layers. Among other tight muscles, she identified active trigger points in the right rhomboid major and right lower trapezius muscles. At the end of the 15 minutes, Suzanne said her back felt more relaxed, but the uncomfortable sensation remained. The massage therapist then performed ice massage over the mid-thoracic region, concentrating on the right side. After 10 minutes of ice massage, Suzanne said the uncomfortable sensation was gone, and the massage therapist then proceeded to show her how to perform self-massage of the mid-scapular muscles by lying down and using a tennis ball. At the end of this time, Suzanne stood up and found that not only had the uncomfortable sensation still gone, but her back muscles felt comfortable and relaxed. The therapist gave her instructions on how to treat herself by using a cold gel pack or ice pack to cool her mid-thoracic muscles before using the tennis ball for self-massage.

DISCUSSION QUESTIONS

1. Why did ice massage relieve Suzanne's uncomfortable sensation?

2. What other hydrotherapy treatment that you have learned could be used in this situation?

Variation 1: Ice massage for chronic inflammation

This version of ice massage was refined by massage therapist and teacher Harold Packman over decades, as a way to take advantage of ice's virtues while avoiding deep vasoconstriction. Also, frail or elderly clients can tolerate this modified technique. Packman used a 5-minute on, 5-minute off method, with circular strokes which covered fairly large areas both proximal and distal to the area of concern: he then let the area warm for 5 minutes, and repeated this on-and-off procedure for a total of three times. He finished with Swedish massage to the area of concern. This method gave moderate cooling and stimulated the circulation, since the continually moving ice caused blood vessels to constrict and then, as the ice moved on, to dilate. Clients enjoyed the benefits of better circulation and reduced edema, as deeper tissues stayed cool while the skin went back to normal temperature (MacAuley, 2001). Clients got both relief of pain and tissue pressure, and Packman was successful in treating rheumatoid arthritis, advanced lymphedema, bursitis, passive swelling of the legs (common in some older clients) and other conditions (Packman, 2007).

Begin with the client warm and draped. Perform ice massage for 5 minutes only. For example, for chronic arthritis in the knee joint, use an ice cup or ice cube and move up and down the entire extremity for 5 minutes. Now let the area rest and rewarm for 5 minutes while you massage the opposite leg or another part of the body. Repeat 3 more times; then massage the arthritic knee and leg itself. Or for tennis elbow, the entire arm would be ice-massaged before Swedish massage of the entire extremity.

Variation 2: Ice massage with pressure before specific deep tissue massage

This technique makes deep tissue techniques more tolerable and less likely to cause soreness after the session. To use a cryocup or ice cube as a massage tool, first make sure the ice is very smooth, with no sharp edges. Make deeper, shorter strokes using fairly firm pressure on the area you wish to treat. (The dense paraspinal muscles are a common place to use this technique.) This technique is similar to thumb friction strokes. After 5 minutes, dry the area and proceed with manual massage.

Variation 3: Ice "massage" for the arch of the foot

To be used for plantar fasciitis, tightness of arch muscles, and arch muscle strain.

1. Fill a 20-ounce (590ml) plastic soft drink bottle with water and freeze it.
2. Have the client roll his or her foot over the bottle for 10–15 minutes. Rather than leaning the entire body weight onto the bottle, the pressure should be no more than will gently stretch the muscles, tendons and fascia.
3. Begin massage.

ICE STROKING (INTERMITTENT COLD WITH STRETCH)

Ice stroking is an additional technique which can temporarily release muscle tension and suppress pain. Normally, trying to stretch a tight muscle beyond its limited range of motion causes pain, an involuntary tightening of the muscle, and soreness afterwards: however, ice stroking can release or deactivate trigger points in individual muscles long enough for them to be gently, thoroughly, and painlessly stretched during a massage session. The ice is wrapped in plastic so the client's skin stays dry.

When ice is stroked over the muscle to be stretched, it causes a sudden drop in skin temperature, which is a strong tactile stimulation, and by keeping the ice moving, a continuous barrage of nerve impulses is sent to the spinal cord. This stimulus inhibits the normal reflex tightening of the muscle that would be present when you try to stretch it. Three sweeps with ice, each lasting 2–3 seconds, are made over the length of the muscle, and then it is gently stretched to its full length. Do not use ice stroking in acute injuries where tissue is inflamed, such as sprains or whiplash injuries. For more information on this technique, see *Travell and Simons' Myofascial Pain and Dysfunction* by (Simons, Travell, and Simons, 1999).

The procedure below shows you a step-by-step procedure for using ice stroking during trigger point treatment of the triceps muscle. This technique can be used for any muscles with active trigger points.

SNAPSHOT

Temperature 32°F (0°C).

Time needed 1 minute or less.

Equipment needed Ice cup or ice cube; a thin plastic bag to wrap ice in.

Effect Primarily thermal.

Cleanup Dispose of the ice and the plastic bag; sanitize the plastic cup if used.

Procedure

1. Treat trigger points with massage techniques.
2. Explain the use of ice to the client and obtain his or her consent.
3. Place the ice in a thin plastic bag (Figure 5.9A).
4. Gently stretch the muscle to the greatest extent possible without overstretching (Figure 5.9B).
5. Maintaining the muscle stretch, now stroke the entire length of the muscle three times with the ice, moving at about 4 inches (10cm) per second (Figure 5.9C).
6. Gently stretch the muscle to the greatest extent possible without overstretching (Figure 5.9D).
7. If the muscle is still not capable of fully lengthening without pain, try applying direct pressure to the trigger point, then gently stretching the muscle again, or have the client contract the antagonist muscle for 30 seconds and then relax completely as you gently stretch the muscle again.
8. Repeat steps 4, 5 and 6 until the muscle is pain-free when completely stretched.

9. Gently return the muscle to a comfortable position (Figure 5.9D) and massage the area further if desired.

10. Optional: to prevent post-treatment soreness, apply a heating pad or moist hot pack to the muscle for 5 minutes or more (Figure 5.9E).

COMPRESSES

Compresses are cloths that are soaked in water or other substances, wrung out, and then applied to various parts of the body. Compresses can be hot, warm, cold or iced, and are used to apply heat or cold over the skin or to apply a variety of chemical solutions to the skin. This section covers two cold compresses, one made with cold tap water only, and the other made with cold water and then frozen. (For information on a special type of cold compress which is more appropriate for a home treatment, see Box 5.3).

Cold compresses are milder than frozen gel packs and applications of ice. They may be more appropriate over delicate areas such as the eyes or for an especially cold-sensitive person. Because cloth molds to body curves well and has a slight weight, it may feel better to some clients. In the past, many different substances have been added to cold compresses for specific purposes, including herbs to reduce inflammation or to function as a counter-irritant, Epsom salts to counteract swelling of bruises and sprains, and essential oils to speed healing. Cold compresses have also been combined with various hot applications to create contrast treatments: for example, a client's foot can be treated with a paraffin dip followed by a cold compress, or a client's back can be treated with a hot silica gel pack followed by a cold compress.

You can easily make cold compresses to suit the individual client. For example, a tiny cold compress to cover the eyes may be made by soaking a washcloth in cold water and then wringing it out. Small or medium-size cold compresses may be made with a few layers of cloth or with small towels. Large cold compresses to cover the entire back can be made with a large bath towel.

Just as massage therapist Harold Packman developed a technique that takes advantage of cold's virtues without over-cooling an area, so physical therapist and lymphedema specialist Jean Yzer has developed an ingenious method of reducing swelling and pain before bodywork for lymphedema. Most people with this condition keep it in check with a combination of treatments that include exercises, stretching, lymphatic drainage massage, bandaging and compression wraps. Prolonged applications of ice are avoided, but mild cold is helpful in

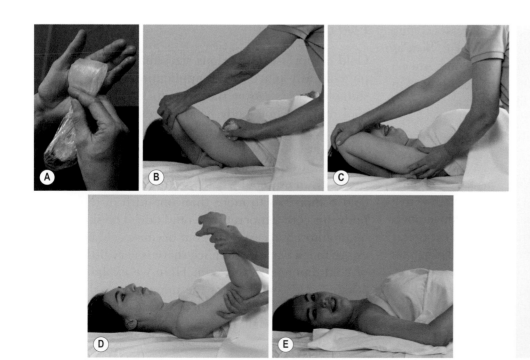

FIGURE 5.9
Ice stroking. (**A**) Place the ice in a thin plastic bag. (**B**) Gently stretch the muscle to the greatest extent possible without overstretching; then maintain that stretch while stroking the entire length of the muscle three times with the ice. (**C**) Gently, and without overstretching, stretch the muscle to the greatest extent possible. (**D**) Gently return the muscle to a comfortable position. (**E**) Apply a heating pad or moist hot pack to the muscle.

Chapter five

USING COLD TO CREATE HEAT: THE HEAT-TRAPPING OR DOUBLE COMPRESS

A heat-trapping compress is an ingenious application of cold which ultimately becomes a mild moist heat treatment. It was widely used in the days of the water-cure and is still an effective and safe home treatment. It begins by applying a cold compress – a cotton cloth dipped in cold water – to one part of the body, then covering that cold compress with dry cloth. The area underneath the two layers of cloth will be cooled initially by the cold cloth, but then the body will create a burst of heat in that area through reflex vasodilation and, because body heat cannot escape, the area will begin to warm up. The heat-trapping or double compress must be worn for at least several hours – overnight is ideal – so it is a good treatment for clients to use at home, but not practical for use during a massage session.

Heating compresses are used to warm and relax muscles and relieve musculoskeletal pain, and they also have a derivative effect since blood flow is increased once the compress becomes warm. They can be used on any part of the body and have no contraindications except skin rashes or other conditions that are irritated by moisture. Elke Fraser, LMT, who has been a massage therapist for 55 years, swears by the heating compress as a way to relieve hand and arm pain after a day of massage: she simply wraps her hands and forearms with cold cloths, covers them with dry cloths and sleeps with them on. In the morning, the heat trapped by the compress has completely dried the wet cloth, and her symptoms are greatly decreased (Fraser, 2015).

Heat-trapping compresses are effective for many musculoskeletal conditions, such as backache, arthritis, and joint injuries. They can be wrapped around the chest for sore or tight chest muscles, around the abdomen and lower back for backache, around joints such as the wrist, elbow, knee or ankle for stiffness and pain, and even around the throat to relieve muscle tension and strain. They help some patients with diabetic neuropathy. They also improve local circulation while they are on the skin, and so they can be used for cold feet and also for derivation. For example, using cold wet socks that are covered by dry socks is a classic treatment for sinus congestion. See illustrations on page 372.

---

reducing edema and pain. Yzer uses compresses wrung out in ice water and molded to the client's arm, then as each warms up, she switches to a fresh cold one. After 5 compresses over a period of about 15 minutes, the skin has cooled by about 45°F (7.2°C), fibrotic areas are easier to palpate, and myofascial lengthening and scar tissue release are easier, more comfortable and more effective (Mayrovitz, 2017; Yzer, 2017).

The first lymphedema patient Yzer was to use cooling on immediately welcomed the first cold washcloth with a sigh of relief. After three or four changes, her skin temperature was reduced, her pain had disappeared, her breast and upper arm tissue had become softer, and her pain level went from 10/10 to 1/10. Yzer was ecstatic, stating, "The physical agent of cold therapy for reducing swelling and pain trusted by rehabilitation specialists worldwide, had once again worked its magic!" (Yzer, 2017).

Cold compress

Cold compresses of various sizes may be used to apply cold any place where applications of ice are not suitable, such as over the eyes; to keep the forehead cool during whole-body heating treatments; to gently cool an overheated client; as part of a mild contrast treatment, along with hot compresses; to relieve itchy skin; and to treat clients who cannot tolerate applications of intense cold. (If for some reason you applied cold compresses to more than one-fifth of the client's body, his core temperature would fall.) The skin should be monitored occasionally, but because cold compresses are much warmer than ice there is very little danger of cold damage to the skin. Here we explain how to make a cold compress for the upper pectoral muscles, which are sometimes strained during heavy lifting or sports such as weight training, rowing or gymnastics.

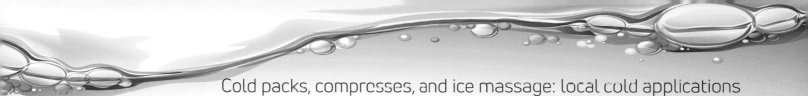

SNAPSHOT

Temperature Cold (40–50°F; 4–10°C).

Time needed 10–20 minutes, unless used as part of a contrast treatment. For a contrast treatment, leave on for 1 minute.

Equipment needed Water thermometer; container for water; a towel of suitable size to use for the compress; another towel which will be placed under the client to protect linens from drips.

Effect Primarily thermal.

Cleanup Launder used linens.

Procedure

1. Check with the client to make sure there are no contraindications for the use of local cold.

2. Explain the use of local cold to the client and get his or her consent.

3. Add crushed ice or ice cubes to a container of water until it is 40–50°F (4–10°C) (Figure 5.10A).

4. Soak a towel of the appropriate size in the water, then wring it out (Figure 5.10B).

5. Apply the towel to the client's upper pectoral area, and add a dry towel under the shoulder and rib-cage to catch drips (Figure 5.10C).

6. The towel will begin to warm up after a few minutes on the client's skin: reapply if desired, while you massage a related area.

7. Begin massage of the strained area.

Iced compresses

An iced compress is simply a wet towel which is placed in a resealable plastic bag and then frozen. When removed from the freezer and placed on the client's body, the compress remains cold for as long as 20 minutes. Although it is colder than the last compress we discussed, it is still not as cold as frozen gel packs or ice, and so it is useful for clients who cannot tolerate their intensity. Unlike cold gel packs or ice, cold compresses are safe for clients to lie on, since the compress will begin to warm up as soon as it comes into contact with the client's body. (Essential oils or herbal teas and tinctures may be mixed with the water when you make the compress.) If placed on an area at the beginning of a session, the compress can remain on that area for as long as 20 minutes while massage is performed elsewhere on the body. An iced compress for the hands can be made by wetting and freezing a pair of wool gloves; they can be taken from the freezer, wetted slightly to soften them, and worn on hands which are overworked, strained or arthritic. (Heat may work better for some arthritic clients.) A large compress can be made by dipping a medium-sized towel in cool water, wringing it out, folding it in half, then rolling it up using a sheet of waxed or parchment paper to keep the frozen layers from sticking together, and then freezing it for 2 hours. Begin by removing the paper, re-rolling the towel, laying it upon the client, and then slowly unrolling as it warms. Massage therapist Harold Packman made these from medium-sized terrycloth towels wrapped around the client's scalp and neck, and used them to treat migraines (Packman, 2007). Iced compresses are easy to make up ahead of time and you can simply take them from the freezer when needed. They are also an excellent home treatment for clients to use.

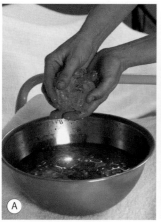
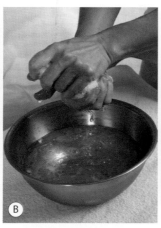
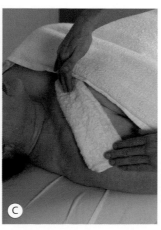

FIGURE 5.10
Cold compress. (**A**) Add crushed ice or ice cubes to a container of water until it is 40–50°F (4.4–10°C). (**B**) Soak a towel of the appropriate size in the water, then wring it out. (**C**) Apply the towel to the client.

To make a small iced compress, wring out a hand towel in cold water, fold it in quarters, and insert it into a resealable plastic bag. Lay it flat in the freezer. Chill for at least 2 hours. When it is ready to use, remove the iced compress from the bag and lay it directly on the body. It will be stiff at first but will soon warm up enough to conform to the part of the body. Here we demonstrate how to use one on the lateral aspect of the shoulder.

SNAPSHOT

Temperature Very cold (32 °F or 0 °C for a short period of time, then the compress will begin to warm up).

Time needed 20 minutes.

Equipment needed Hand towel; resealable plastic bag; freezer.

Effect Primarily thermal.

Cleanup Dispose of the plastic bag; launder the used towel.

Procedure

1. Soak a towel of the appropriate size in cold water, then wring it out (Figure 5.11A). It should be wet but not dripping.
2. Fold the towel in half lengthwise and in half again (Figure 5.11B).
3. Place it in a plastic bag, seal it, and then put it in the freezer (Figure 5.11C).
4. When ready to use the ice compress, first check with the client to make sure there are no contraindications for the use of local cold.
5. Explain the use of local cold to the client and get his or her consent.
6. Remove the iced compress from the bag and apply it to the client's shoulder (Figure 5.11D).
7. The towel will begin to warm up after a few minutes on the client's skin and become more flexible: wrap it more closely around the area as it softens.

Contrast compresses: another combination treatment

Here, a contrast treatment makes use of hot compresses alternated with cold ones. As noted in Chapter 3, contrast treatments can be used over many areas of the body to dramatically increase circulation. During a massage, contrast compresses are a simple way to prepare an area for massage by increasing blood flow, stimulating the skin and muscles underneath the compress, and relieving musculoskeletal pain. As with any hot and cold

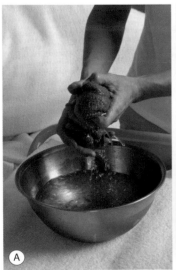
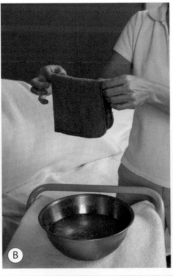
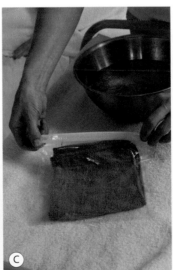
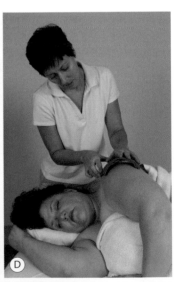

FIGURE 5.11
Iced compress. (**A**) Soak a towel of the appropriate size in cold water, then wring it out. (**B**) Fold towel in half lengthwise and in half again. (**C**) Place the folded towel in a plastic bag, seal it, and then put it in the freezer. (**D**) Remove the towel from the bag and apply the iced compress to the client's shoulder.

compress, chemical additives such as herbs, essential oils and salts can be easily applied with contrast compresses. For example, you could add different essential oils to each container of water.

A contrast treatment over the eyes is just one example of alternating hot and cold compresses (Figure 5.12). In this case, the goal is to dramatically increase blood flow around the eyes, helping to reduce discomfort from eye tension and strain. (This problem is very common in clients who look at computers, cell phones and other screens for long periods of time.) This also prepares the client's tissue for massage around the eyes. A similar treatment could be done to any part of the body for similar reasons. Here are two more examples: contrast compresses over the knee joint can be especially effective in stimulating healing after surgery, and contrast compresses over the lower back can increase blood flow to the lower back muscles and relieve pain. When would contrast compresses be preferred to contrast treatments using other types of heat and cold? When a slightly less intense treatment is preferred; when a small, irregularly shaped area needs treatment; or when the massage therapist has only hot and cold water and cloths available.

SNAPSHOT

Temperature Hot (102–110°F; 39–43°C) alternated with cold (32–55°F; 0–13°C).

Time needed 10 minutes.

Equipment needed Water thermometer; containers of hot and cold water; three washcloths; one towel to place under the head to prevent the sheets on the massage table from becoming damp. If you wish to perform massage seated at the client's head, place the containers of hot and cold water on a rolling cart that will be within easy reach. While the hot and cold treatment takes effect, you can easily treat the neck, shoulders, scalp and lower face.

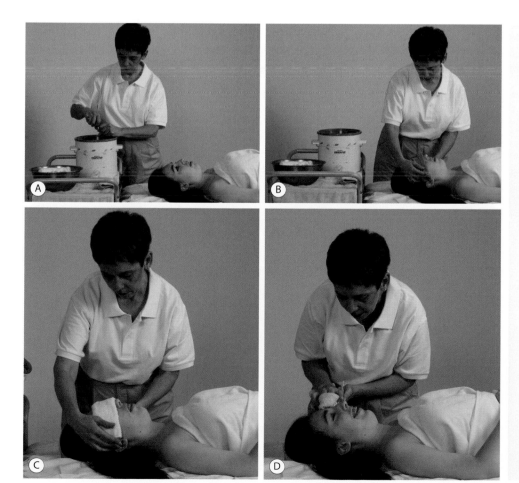

FIGURE 5.12
Contrast compresses. (**A**) Soak one washcloth in hot water and wring it out. (**B**) Fold the hot washcloth in half lengthwise and apply over the client's eyes. (**C**) Soak the other washcloth in cold water and wring it out, fold it in half lengthwise, and apply it over the client's eyes. (**D**) At the end of three rounds of hot followed by cold, gently dry off the area around the eyes.

Effect Primarily thermal.

Cleanup Clean and sanitize the containers; launder the washcloths and towel.

Procedure

1. Check with the client to make sure there are no contraindications for the use of local heat or cold.
2. Explain the use of local heat and cold to the client and get his or her consent.
3. With the client in the supine position, place a towel under the client's head.
4. Soak one washcloth in hot water and wring it out (Figure 5.12A).
5. Fold it in half lengthwise and apply it over the client's eyes (Figure 5.12B). Check with the client to make sure it is not too hot.
6. After 2 minutes, soak the other washcloth in cold water and wring it out, fold it in half lengthwise and apply it over the client's eyes (Figure 5.12C).
7. After the cold compress has been on for 30 seconds, remove it.
8. Repeat steps 2–5.
9. Repeat steps 2–5 again, for a total of three rounds.
10. Gently dry off the area around the eyes with the last washcloth (Figure 5.12D).

CHAPTER SUMMARY

In this chapter you have learned about a variety of treatments that cool just one part of the body, and about their effects and benefits. During massage sessions, therapeutic cold can help relieve acute inflammation, muscle spasm and musculoskeletal pain. It is also a great way to keep clients from becoming overheated, deactivating trigger points, and helping to increase local circulation when used in a contrast treatment. Your therapy "toolbox" has expanded with these cold treatments, and in each of the chapters ahead you will learn more treatments and ways to fine-tune these treatments for your massage practice.

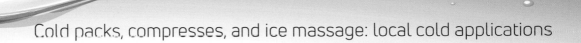

REVIEW QUESTIONS

Multiple choice

1. After application, cold gel packs retain their cold for how long?:
   A. 5 minutes
   B. 15–20 minutes
   C. 30–45 minutes
   D. 50 minutes

2. Local application of cold is most often used:
   A. To reduce swelling and pain for a few hours after an injury
   B. In chronic conditions
   C. To prevent hypothermia
   D. To torment your clients

3. Local application of cold is contraindicated for patients with:
   A. Inability to provide feedback about tissue temperature
   B. Chilled body
   C. Raynaud's syndrome
   D. Frostbite
   E. All of the above

4. In patients with acute muscle strains or contusions, cold is the best choice for:
   A. The first 4 hours
   B. The first few months
   C. The first 8 hours
   D. The first week

5. Which application is used to deactivate trigger points, allowing a muscle to be stretched to its full length?
   A. Cold flat water bottle
   B. Cold gel pack
   C. Contrast compress
   D. Ice stroking
   E. Iced compress

True/False

6. True/False — An iced compress can be used when pain is caused by acute swelling.

7. True/False — A flat water bottle filled with cold water cools tissues more than any other cold application.

8. True/False — The number one hazard of cold applications is cold-induced tissue damage.

9. True/False — Local cold applications can have effects on local tissue temperature, blood flow, edema, nerve function, muscle strength, and muscle tone.

10. True/False — Ice massage may be chosen over other cold treatments because it creates a mild relaxing sensation.

Chapter five

References

Anava-Erroba L et al. Effects of ice massage on pressure pain thresholds and electromyography activity postexercise: a randomized controlled crossover study. J Manipulative Physical Ther 2010; 33(3): 212–9

Bond W. Over Manipulation syndrome – can massage break the cycle? Massage and Bodywork Magazine. September/October 2012

Brown M, Hahn DB. Frostbite of the feet after cryotherapy: a report of two cases. J Foot Ankle Surg 2009; 48(5): 577–80

Caring Medical. Rest Ice Compression Elevation; Rice Therapy and Price Therapy. https://www.caringmedical.com/prolotherapy-news/rest-ice-compression-elevation-rice-therapy/ [Accessed: March 2020]

Consumer Reports. Is RICE still nice? On Health, December 2015; 8

Dundon JM, Rymer MC, Johnson RM. Total patellar skin loss from cryotherapy after total knee arthroplasty. J Arthroplasty 2013; 28(2): 376

Fraser E. Personal communication with the author, Corvallis, OR, 5 September 2015

Graham CA, Stevenson J. Frozen chips: an unusual cause of severe frostbite injury. British Journal of Sports Medicine 2000; 34: 382–3

Guillot X et al. Cryotherapy in inflammatory rheumatic diseases : a systematic review. Expert Rev Clin Immunol 2014; 10(2): 281–94

Hanai A et al. Effects of cryotherapy on objective and subjective symptoms of paclitaxel-induced neuropathy: prospective self-controlled trial. Journal of the National Cancer Institute 2018; 110(2)

Hauser R. Personal communication, November, 2018

Herrera F. et al. Motor and sensory nerve conduction are affected differently by ice pack, ice massage, and cold water immersion. Phys Ther 2010; 90(4): 581–91

Ho SS et al. Comparison of various icing times in decreasing bone metabolism in the knee. American J. of Sports Medicine 1990; 18: 375–8

Ho SS et al. The effects of ice on blood flow and bone metabolism in knees. American J. of Sports Medicine 1994; 22(4): 537–40

Kanlayanaphotporn R. Comparison of skin surface temperature during the application of various cryotherapy modalities. Arch Phys Med Rehabil 2005; 86: 1411–15

Keskin et al. Effect of intracanal cryotherapy on pain after single-visit root canal treatment. Australian Endodontic Journal, 4 October 2016

Khoshnevis S, Craik NK, Diller KR. Cold-induced vasoconstriction may persist long after cooling ends: an evaluation of multiple cryotherapy units. Knee Surg Sports Traumatol Arthrosc 2015; 23(9): 2475–83

Kurland et al. Hemmorhagic progression of a contusion after traumatic brain injury: a review. J Neurotrauma 2012; 29(1): 19–31

MacAuley DC. Ice therapy: how good is the evidence? Int J Sports Med 2001; 22: 379–84

Mayrovitz Hl, Yzer J. Local skin cooling as an aid to management of patients with breast cancer-related lymphedema. Lymphology 2017; (5)2: 55–666

McGinnis K, Murray E, Cherven B et al. Effect of vibration on pain response to heel lance: a pilot randomized control trial. Adv Neonatal Care 2016; 16(6): 439–48

McGuire DA, Hendricks SD. Incidences of frostbite in arthroscopic knee surgery postoperative cryotherapy rehabilitation. Arthroscopy 2006; 22(10): 1141

Meyrer et al. Temperature changes in the human leg during and after two methods of cryotherapy. J Athl Train 1998; 33(1): 25–29.

Myrer W et al. Muscle temperature is affected by overlying adipose when cryotherapy is administered. J Athl Train 2001; 36(1): 32–36

Packman H. Ice Massage-the Ultimate Cryotherapeutic Alternative. Bloomington, Indiana: Traford Publishing, 2007

Packman H. Ice Therapy: Understanding Its Application. Flushing, New York, self-published, 1987

Robinson D. Nursing student invents cooling vest to help surgeons beat heat stress. The Daily Case, 3 November 2017

Sahiner N, Inal S. The effect of combined stimulation of external cold and vibration during immunization on pain and anxiety levels in children. J Perianesth Nurs 2015 Jun; 30(3): 228–35

Simons DG, Travell JG, Simons LS. Travell and Simons' Myofascial Pain and Dysfunction: the Trigger Point Manual, Vol 1: Upper Half of Body, 2nd edn. Baltimore, MD: Lippincott, Williams and Wilkins, 1999

Tolis H. Personal communication with the author August 2018

Urbana LB. Therapeutic hypothermia for traumatic brain injury. Curr Neurol Neurosci Rep 2012; 12(5): 580–91

Schmidt and Clark. Cold therapy nerve damage. www.schmidtand-clark.com/cold-therapy-nerve-damage [Accessed 15 October 2018]

Yu S et al. Effect of cryotherapy after elbow arthrolysis: a prospective, single-blinded, randomized controlled study. Archives of Physical Medicine and Rehabilitation 2014; 96(1)

Yzer J. Cooling for Lymphedema. Charleston, SC Create Space Publications, 2017

Zemke J et al. Intramuscular temperature response in the human leg to two forms of cryotherapy: ice massage and ice bag. JOSPT 1998; 27(4): 301–7

Recommended resources

Belanger A. Evidence-Based Guide to Therapeutic Physical Agents. Baltimore: Lippincott, Williams and Wilkins, 2002

Michlovitz S. Thermal Agents in Rehabilitation. Philadelphia, PA: FA Davis, 1995

Taber C et al. Measurement of reactive vasodilation during cold gel pack application to nontraumatized ankles. Physical Therapy 1992; 72(4): 294–9

Thrash A, Thrash C. Home Remedies: Hydrotherapy, Massage, Charcoal, and Other Simple Treatments. Seale, AL: Thrash Publications, 1981

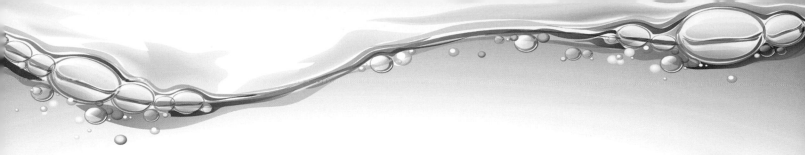

Immersion baths 6

Mollie McMillan [author of "Massage and Therapeutic Exercise" and founder of the American Physical Therapy Association] was arrested in Manila and put into a prison camp in 1942. Mollie made her bed on an inverted wooden filing cabinet to avoid sleeping on the ground, and she shared four toilets and three showers with 469 other women. But with her indomitable spirit, she still managed to set up a physical therapy clinic for the prisoners, performing miracles with her clever hands, hot water, a few pails and towels. As one admirer would later recall, 'Aching backs and arthritis from sleeping on cold cement, pulled muscles, painful feet, infected bedbugs bites and rashes—all manner of aches and pains were brought in. And every day people went away feeling better.

Wendy Murphy, *Healing the Generations: A History of Physical Therapy and the American Physical Therapy Association*

CHAPTER OBJECTIVES

After completing this chapter, the student will be able to:

1. Describe the effects of various local and whole-body baths
2. Explain the contraindications for various local and whole-body baths
3. Name and describe local baths of different temperatures including foot, hand, leg, arm and half-body baths
4. Describe a variety of applications for local baths
5. Describe the many conditions a hot footbath can be used for
6. Name and describe full body baths including a hot, warm, neutral, cold, and contrast baths
7. Name and describe various bath additives and their effects on the body
8. Describe a variety of applications for full-body baths
9. Demonstrate the procedure for each local and whole-body bath.

As noted in Chapter 1, baths are one of the most ancient and popular of all medical treatments, because they are convenient, effective for a variety of therapeutic purposes, and beloved by all. For the massage therapist, They complement hands-on techniques, since different baths can relax muscles and prepare them for massage, stimulate or depress blood flow, relieve muscular fatigue and soreness, relieve muscle pain, bring about a general relaxation response, and even stimulate muscle contractions. Dissolving therapeutic substances such as herbs, salts, essential oils, baking soda, oatmeal and charcoal in water is an easy method of incorporating them into your treatments. When liquid completely surrounds tissues (Figure 6.1) it is a better conductor of heat or cold than hydrotherapy applications that are merely placed on top of the area. (This is why immersion in cold water is the preferred method of cooling someone who is dangerously overheated.) We begin our discussion with the wide variety of partial-body baths, and then consider whole-body baths.

PARTIAL-BODY BATHS

For the massage therapist, baths which immerse only one part of the body are particularly convenient. They are inexpensive, require only basic equipment, and may be used for a variety of clients and situations. They are also safe, easy home treatments for your clients. Partial-body baths can be hot, warm, neutral, cold, or hot alternated with cold. They can be taken in all sorts of containers, from large bowls and plastic tubs to stainless steel whirlpools. The baths and the various types of additives given

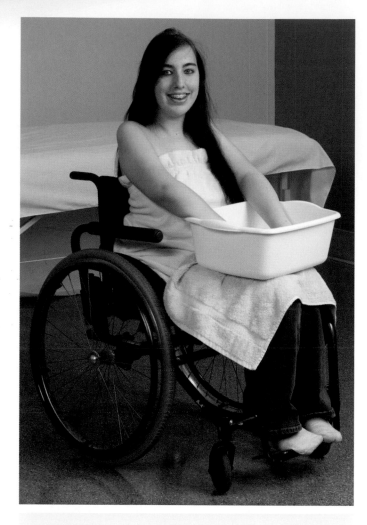

FIGURE 6.1
Hand bath.

2. When you do not have time to prepare a more elaborate treatment, such as a fomentation, partial-body baths are fast–simply get water at the correct temperature and you are ready to go.

3. When you do not have elaborate hydrotherapy equipment, a clean container, running water, a thermometer and a towel are all you need. Additives are easily added as well. When you wish to heat or cool an entire area, surrounding it with hot or cold liquid is the single most effective way to do that. In one study, the gastrocnemius muscle became much colder after a cold-water leg bath than an ice-pack application. Both were given for 20 minutes; then, while it took a full 3 hours for the bathed muscle to return to its normal temperature, the ice-packed muscle did the same thing in half that time (Zemke, 1998).

4. Massage and stretching can still be part of a local bath. Ischemic compression of trigger points will be more effective if the area is immersed in warm water, and tight muscles can be stretched while they are in a hot bath (Simons, 1999).

A note on sanitation

Tubs used for water baths, whether partial- or whole-body, must be cleaned, disinfected and dried between each use. This process is important to prevent transmission of pathogens such as athlete's foot fungus, coronaviruses and streptococcal bacteria. There are many different disinfectant solutions, from highly toxic ones which are intended for cleanup of blood or body fluids, to alcohol or citrus essential oils. You may need to consider what works best for your facility: for example, chlorine bleach is a common and effective disinfectant, but many find it too strong-smelling. If you buy a whole-body hydrotherapy tub, check with the manufacturer for recommended disinfectants.

Footbaths

For both hygienic and therapeutic reasons, baths for the feet have a long and rich history. Cold footbaths, called pediluvia, have met many a weary traveler on religious pilgrimages. In the home, foot-washing symbolized hospitality; and in the Christian religion it also

here are only a small sampling of the most common ones that have been used in the past. To learn more about some less commonly used baths, see Box 6.1.

When would you use one of these baths rather than another local hydrotherapy application? Here are some factors to consider when making your choice:

1. Water has a soothing feel on the skin that is enjoyed by most people, and hence is more enjoyable than many treatments that are laid on top of the skin, such as ice packs. In addition, tissue that is too sensitive to have any weight placed on it can be better treated with liquid water.

symbolizes humility and service to others. A footbath (Figure 6.2) is easy to integrate into a massage session, and can have a variety of effects depending upon the duration of the bath, the temperature of the water, and the use of additives such as Epsom salts, herbs, or essential oils.

BOX 6.1	POINT OF INTEREST

CLASSIC BUT LESS COMMONLY USED BATHS

The baths discussed below have been used not only for a thermal effect but also to apply a wide variety of chemicals, including herbal preparations, salts, essential plant oils, clays, seaweeds, and even muds.

Scalp baths

Scalp baths can be performed with the receiver supine, head hanging over the head of a massage table and resting in a bowl of water. This little-used bath can be used to warm or cool the scalp or to apply chemical preparations to it. For example, hot or warm scalp baths can be used to relieve some types of head pain and to encourage healing of injuries to the cranial bones or scalp; cold scalp baths can decrease circulation to the scalp to help relieve tension or migraine headaches; and contrast baths can increase circulation to the scalp. In Chinese medicine, stroke patients are sometimes given scalp baths with hot ginger tea to relieve head pain. Epsom salts scalp baths have been used to relieve swelling after head injury.

Eye baths

Eye baths, using bowls of water or glass eye cups, are used to warm or cool the eyes and the muscles around them, or to apply chemical preparations to them. Warm eye baths can be used to soothe muscle tension and eyestrain; cold eye baths relieve tired, itching eyes, and contrast baths stimulate circulation in the muscles around the eyes. Someone suffering from eye irritation from dust or allergies may find relief from bathing the eyes in cool water.

Sinus baths

Using bulb syringes, neti pots or special tips on Water Piks, sinus baths can be used to ease sinus congestion and improve local circulation, as well as to apply chemical preparations such as salt water or herb teas. Water may be hot, warm, or cool.

Throat baths

Throat "baths," performed by gargling, are used to warm or cool the throat or to apply chemical preparations such as salt water or herb teas. Warm throat baths can be used to relieve throat tension or irritation which occurs after overusing the voice or having a cold. Contrast baths can increase local circulation.

Sitz baths

Sitz baths immerse the pelvic region, covering about the same area as a pair of shorts. They are given in specially designed chair-shaped bathtubs (Figure 1, see over; Figure 1.9) and are used to warm or cool the muscles of the pelvic and lower back areas, as well as to apply chemical preparations such as salts, essential oils and herbal preparations to these areas. The pelvic area is large and more difficult to cover with other thermal applications such as moist heat packs or ice packs, and hence water baths to the pelvic area may sometimes be the most efficient solution. Hot sitz baths have been used to relieve coldness, sciatica, lower back pain, dysmenorrhea, spastic constipation, kidney stone pain, and poor local circulation, and also to create a fluid-shifting (derivative) effect. Warm sitz baths can also warm the entire body, soothe the perineum after labor and delivery, and speed healing of perineal stitches. Short cold sitz baths can be used to increase muscle tone in the smooth muscles of the uterus, bladder and colon, to relieve atonic constipation, and to stimulate circulation in the abdominal area. Long cold sitz baths can be used to treat pulled muscles in the groin area,

continued

Box 6.1 *continued*

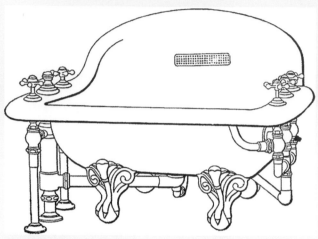

FIGURE 1
Porcelain sitz bath, manufactured in 1905 by Standard Sanitary Manufacturing Company of Pittsburg, Pennsylvania.

as well as to cool the entire body. Contrast sitz baths increase circulation to the muscles of the pelvis and lower back, to prevent menstrual cramps, and relieve chronic pelvic pain.

Arm and leg whirlpools

Stainless steel arm and leg whirlpools are most often used in physical therapy settings. They are used to relieve joint stiffness and muscle spasm in an arm or leg, to make therapeutic exercise easier, and to relieve pain. Warm local whirlpools may be used for post-traumatic pain, cleansing of wounds, swelling in the hands and feet, acute orthopedic trauma at the onset, acute edema, acute muscle spasm, scar tissue contractures from burns, wounds, or adhesions, and as a preparation for massage because tissues are left supple, warm, and relaxed.

Whirlpools have also proved very effective in the treatment of frostbite: tissue rewarming is achieved by submerging affected areas in a warm whirlpool at 100–106.5°F (38–41°C) for 15–30 minutes. If there is any dead tissue, a daily 104°F (40°C) whirlpool is used to remove it (Golant, 2008). Athletic trainers sometimes use whirlpools to treat athletic injuries, and may use hot, cold, or contrast temperatures. A typical whirlpool has at least six jets: some that use lower pressure to make the water swirl, and some

that have higher pressure for vigorous hydromassage. Unlike hot tubs, whirlpools are constructed of stainless steel and can therefore be sterilized after use.

Hubbard tank

The Hubbard tank (Figure 2) is a very large steel whirlpool with a turbine at one end, invented in the 1920s by American engineer Carl Hubbard. With a 425 gallon capacity, the tank is similar to a shallow swimming pool, and the entire body can be immersed. Because the person in a Hubbard tank is actively exercising, the water temperature is cooler than in a standard whole-body whirlpool, generally between 90 and 104°F (32 and 40°C), unless an artificial fever is being purposely created.

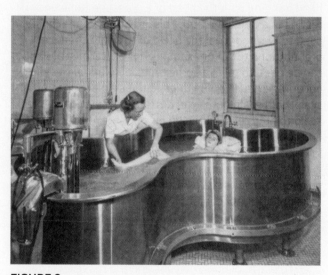

FIGURE 2
Physical therapist working with a polio patient in a Hubbard tank, 1949.

As can be seen in the 1949 photograph above, the unique figure-8 or butterfly shape of the tank allows a therapist to get close enough to work with the patient during the treatment but still stay dry. And because it is stainless steel, the tank can be sterilized after each use, making it suitable for people with open wounds and burns which could become infected if they were exercising in a swimming pool.

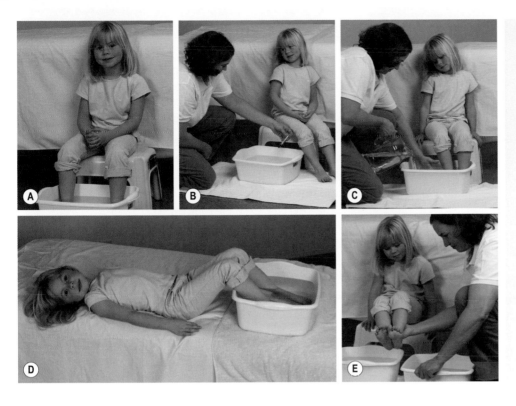

FIGURE 6.2
(**A**) Footbath. (**B**) Checking the water temperature. (**C**) Replacing the water to maintain the desired temperature. (**D**) Footbath with the client reclining on massage table. (**E**) The massage therapist moving the client's feet from one tub of water to another during a contrast treatment.

Hot footbaths

A hot footbath has many helpful bodywork applications. For more on this topic, see Box 6.2. A client with chronically cold feet will especially enjoy this treatment before a massage, and someone who is going to receive a cold treatment will be more receptive if a hot footbath is given first. When a client comes into your office who is feeling cold, a footbath can be performed with him or her sitting in a chair while filling out forms or talking to you, or it can be performed with the client lying down on the massage table. In a massage practice, a hot footbath before or after an evening massage would be an excellent way to help a client who struggles with insomnia. The author has successfully used hot footbaths combined with foot massage in places as diverse as first-world physical therapy clinics, children's camps, upscale spas, hospices, private massage practices, and homeless shelters, and even third-world settings with no running water—everyone loves this treatment. A large rectangular container such as a plastic dishpan provides space for both feet without crowding them, and has enough room for water to cover the feet up to the top of the ankles. Do not use footbaths with heating elements, as burns have occurred. Foot spas with jets are difficult and time-consuming to disinfect, and their use at some nail salons has led to bacterial infections. Therefore, do not use foot spas with jets.

SNAPSHOT

Temperature Hot (102–110°F; 39–43°C).

Time needed 20 minutes.

Equipment needed Water thermometer, container for water; 1½–2 gallons (5.5–7.5 liters) of water; large towel to go under the footbath; small towel for drying the feet; cold water and cloth for cold compress (optional). To make this a whole-body heating treatment, wrap the client in a blanket. If the client will be lying on the table, add anti-slip fabric (used to keep rugs from sliding) under the tub, and launder that as well.

Effect Primarily thermal.

Cleanup Clean, disinfect, and dry the tub; launder the towels.

Indications Chilled person, preparation for cold treatment, cold feet, foot and leg cramps, pain of gout or arthritis, menstrual cramps, migraine headache, insomnia (if given shortly before the client goes to bed), general relaxation. A hot footbath is an easy way to apply chemicals contained in herbs, salts, or essential oils.

BOX 6.2	POINT OF INTEREST

CLEVER USES OF A SIMPLE TREATMENT: HOT FOOTBATHS

Experienced hydrotherapists have long considered the hot footbath the most versatile of all water treatments. After many decades of experience, Agatha Thrash, MD, has stated: "If we had only one hydrotherapeutic measure available to us, we would have to select the hot footbath. It has so many uses, so few contraindications and is so readily available under all kinds of circumstances" (Thrash and Thrash, 1981). Traditionally used to warm cold clients, relieve pain, ward off colds, improve leg and foot circulation, and affect blood flow in areas above the feet (derivation), modern researchers have now confirmed its usefulness in other conditions. For example:

- Relieving symptoms of chemotherapy-caused neuropathy such as numbness, tingling, burning and prickling sensations (Oh, 2018).
- Decreasing anxiety (Mooventhan, 2014).
- Overcoming fatigue in women having chemotherapy for female cancers and patients undergoing dialysis (Shafeik, 2018).
- Improving lymphatic flow in the legs, even more than aerobic exercise (Olszewski, 1977).
- Relieving insomnia in a wide variety of people, including young adults, older adults, post-stroke patients at rehabilitation clinics, women having chemotherapy for female cancers, and adults with traumatic brain injuries. Researchers believe that the greater the dilation in the vessels of the feet, the less time it takes to fall asleep (Chiu, 2017; Karuchi, 1999; Rayman, 2005; Sung, 2000; Liao, 2013; Li, 2014; Ebben, 2006).

Contraindications Loss of sensation and /or peripheral vascular disease, which includes diabetes, Buerger's disease, and arteriosclerosis of the lower extremities.

Procedure

1. Check with the client to make sure there are no contraindications for the hot footbath.
2. Explain the use of the bath to the client and get their consent.
3. Have the client seated in a chair next to the massage table. Place a towel on the floor under the client's feet.
4. Put the container of hot water on the towel and rest the client's feet in the container (Figure 6.2A).
5. Monitor the water temperature from time to time (Figure 6.2B) and add more hot water if needed to maintain the desired temperature. Do not pour this water directly on the feet; have the client move their feet to the side of the container when you pour it in (Figure 6.2C).
6. If the client begins to sweat, add a cold compress to the forehead.
7. Massage of other parts of the body that can be done in a seated position may proceed at this time.
8. To finish, have the client lift their feet out of the water: move the container to one side, place the client's feet on the towel and cover with the towel.
9. Remove the container.
10. Dry the feet well.
11. Have the client move onto the massage table without stepping on the bare floor.

Variation 1: Footbath with client lying down

See Figure 6.2D: If a large towel is placed under the container of water to protect linens, a hot footbath can be easily given right on a massage table. The client simply reclines on the table and places his or her feet in the water. It is important that the container is heavy enough not to slide, and then clients can rest their feet in the water, without expending energy holding the legs up. A plastic milk crate can be used for this purpose: place the milk crate on the towel, place the footbath inside it, then have the client put his or her feet in the water. For hygienic purposes, any part of the milk crate that will touch the client's skin should be draped with a towel. Anti-slip fabric that goes under carpets can be used as well. To prevent the footbath from cooling off, a piece of wood may be pre-made to cover most of the top of the container, with a half-circle cut out for the legs. Then the person's feet go in the water and the wooden lid is put on top of the container.

Variation 2: Sweating footbath

When the footbath is used for this purpose, the client is seated in a chair, covered with a blanket, and given a cold compress to the head as soon as sweating begins. When the body is covered so that no heat escapes, the client's core temperature will soon begin to rise.

Variation 3: Vasodilating footbath

Mustard, ginger and cayenne are traditional vaso-dilating herbs. Ask if the client has sensitive skin, as burning and stinging sensations could result. If not, add two teaspoons (10ml) of mustard powder, one teaspoon (5ml) of powdered ginger, and one quar-ter teaspoon (1.25ml) of cayenne pepper to 2 gallons (7.5 liters) of water.

Warm footbaths

SNAPSHOT

Temperature Warm (98–102°F; 36–39°C).

Time needed 15–20 minutes.

Equipment needed Water thermometer; container; 1½–2 gallons (5.5–7.5 liters) of water; large towel to go under the footbath; small towel for drying the feet.

Effect Primarily thermal.

Cleanup Clean, disinfect, and dry the tub; launder the towels.

Indications Cold feet, mild warming of the body, or relaxation, when a hot footbath is contraindicated.

Contraindications None.

Procedure Same as for a hot footbath, simply adjust the water temperature to warm.

Variation 1: Epsom salts footbath

Use this for a client with soreness from poorly fitting shoes or vigorous exercise, plantar fasciitis (if part of a contrast footbath), arthritis, painful bruises, or for edema of pregnancy. Magnesium levels in the body rise after Epsom salts soaks (Waring, 2004).

Simply add 1 cup of Epsom salts per 1 gallon (4 liters) of warm water. For more information, see *Epsom salts baths* on page 169.

Variation 2: Charcoal footbath

A footbath with charcoal powder is helpful for bruises, swelling (such as for a sprained ankle), or gout, and is sometimes effective for the discomfort of peripheral neuropathy.

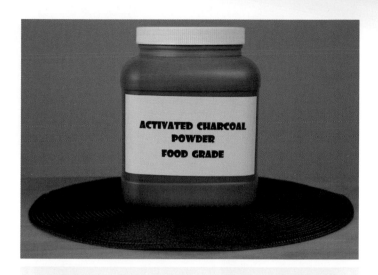

FIGURE 6.3
Bulk charcoal container. Courtesy of Charcoal House, Crawford, Nebraska.

Charcoal powder is messy, so follow the directions carefully:

1. Use dark-colored linens.
2. Using a scoop, remove 2 tablespoons (30 ml) of charcoal and add this to a small jar partially full of water. Close the lid tightly and shake so that the charcoal blends with the water, but does not escape the jar.
3. Let this sit while you prepare a warm footbath, then carefully add the charcoal water to it without splashing.

Variation 3: Sensory stimulation footbath

See Figure 6.4. This extended footbath is helpful for highly sensitive persons such as autistic children and frail elderly people who don't tolerate whole-body massage. It is also well suited for those who are new to massage, those who are uncomfortable disrobing, and those who have chronic pain. (Case history 6.1). A paraffin dip may be added at the end of the treatment. For other uses, see Chapter 14. The procedure and cleanup are the same as for a warm footbath, but lay out additional equipment on a tray covered with a clean towel: two extra washcloths, 1 cup (128g) of Epsom salts, a container of liquid soap, a soft brush or mesh bath sponge, textured massage tools or small handheld massagers, a pitcher of clean warm water, massage lotion or oil, and a pillow or chair for the therapist to sit on while facing the client

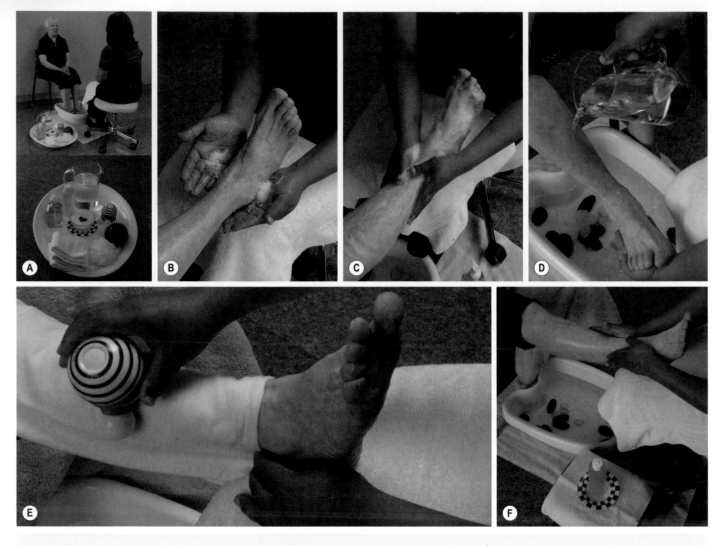

FIGURE 6.4
Sensory stimulation footbath. (**A**) Ingredients and seating position for the footbath. (**B**) Epsom salts glow. (**C**) Massaging with soap lather. (**D**) Rinsing off with clean water. (**E**) Covering the foot and leg so that the hand-held massager does not come into contact with the client's skin. (**F**) Using hands-on techniques.

(Figure 6.4A). Optional: river stones inside the container. The client may simply roll them around to stimulate the bottom of the feet, or you can oil them to massage the lower legs and feet. The stones will be just slightly warm from the footbath water. Do not use hot stones.

Put the container of warm water on the towel and rest the client's feet in the container. Begin by putting a little Epsom salts in your palm, moistening it slightly, and performing a salt glow of the lower legs and feet (Figure 6.4B). Let the feet rest back in the water and use the brush or bath poof and liquid soap to work up

a creamy lather, then massage the lower legs and feet through the lather (Figure 6.4C). Rinse off with half of the water from the pitcher (Figure 6.4D). Use washable massage tools or a hand-held massager to massage the lower legs and feet. Hand-held massagers can be used, but the client's foot and leg should be out of the water and covered with a thin towel (Figure 6.4E). Finally, use massage lotion to perform hands-on massage of the lower legs and feet (Figure 6.4F). Finally, rinse each limb off with clean water, towel dry briskly with a washcloth, put the client's socks on, and finish with tapotement. Repeat with the other limb.

BACKGROUND

Asha, 38, is a friendly cheerful woman with autism who lives in a group home. She is healthy but sometimes struggles with constipation due to medications, and has "meltdowns" – temper tantrums – that seem to others to come out of nowhere.

TREATMENT

At her first massage session, she gives many signs that she is is experiencing more stimulation than she can easily process – she thrashes about the massage table, squints against the light from a nearby window, repeatedly asks when she can go home, and does not appear to enjoy her massage at all. The therapist decides to try a gentler but still stimulating approach, so she prepares a sensory stimulating footbath for Asha's second session. She also closes the curtains, dims the overhead light, explains what she is going to do, then fills up the footbath with warm water. Asha sighs with happiness when the therapist places her feet in the water, and looks with interest at the other items that will be used. The therapist proceeds to give her a slow, gentle Epsom salts scrub, followed by the other parts

of the procedure. Asha loves her footbath and relaxes while the therapist massages her feet and legs. After a few more footbath sessions, a paraffin dip is added to her footbath, which she loves. Over time, she gradually becomes more comfortable with massage and happier to be there for her session; she tolerates more bodywork and relaxes better. In a few months she is able to relax during a whole-body massage that includes abdominal massage, which gradually reduces her constipation, plus a stimulating brushing of her hair. Staff at her home find that over time Asha begins to tolerate more stimulation. For example, in the past, abdominal discomfort from constipation would have led to meltdowns, but those gradually disappear, as do the ones that used to occur when a blowdryer was used on her hair. Her gradual tolerance of more stimulation would likely never have happened were it not for beginning with the footbaths.

DISCUSSION QUESTIONS

1. How did the footbath help Asha tolerate more stimulation?

2. What other bath treatment could have been used instead?

Cool footbaths

SNAPSHOT

Temperature Cool (66–98°F; 18.9–36.7°C).

Time needed 15–20 minutes.

Equipment needed Water thermometer; container for water; 1.5–2 gallons (5.5–7.5 liters) of water; large towel to go under the footbath; small towel for drying the feet. Smooth stones may be placed on the bottom of the footbath so that the client can stimulate and exercise the feet by rolling over the stones and picking them up with the toes.

Effect Primarily thermal.

Cleanup Clean, disinfect, and dry the tub (and the stones, if used); launder the towels.

Indications Uncomfortably hot feet, mild cooling of the body, general relaxation.

Contraindications None.

Procedure Same as for a hot footbath, but adjust the water temperature to cool.

Cold footbaths

Short cold footbaths stimulate local circulation and can also cause a reflex contraction of the blood vessels of brain, pelvic organs, bladder, liver and gastrointestinal tract: thus they were once used by hydrotherapists to treat uterine, bladder, or kidney bleeding. Any prolonged footbath with a water temperature of less than 98°F (36.7°C) will cool tissues, depress local blood flow, and lower the core temperature (see Case history 6.2). In one study, men with spinal cord injuries exercised until their core temperatures were elevated, then took cold footbaths which lowered their core temperatures by 4 degrees. Because of their injuries, their central nervous systems could not react to cold as usual, and so it was clear that the change in their core temperatures was

Chapter six

A COOLING FOOTBATH FOR HOT BURNING FEET	CASE HISTORY 6.2

BACKGROUND

A healthy, fit schoolteacher, 45-year-old Rachel received massage therapy regularly to help her deal with a highly stressful period in her life. One hot summer day she arrived for her regular appointment, and told the therapist that she had been on her feet for three hours that morning. She said her feet were swollen from the combination of prolonged standing on them and the summer heat, which always caused her to retain water, and she had had this problem for many years, and her family doctor had told her not to worry about it. However, as she lay down on the massage table, her discomfort was evident: she did not want anything covering her feet, complained that they were burning, and moved them restlessly.

TREATMENT

The therapist placed a plastic tub with 75°F (24°C) water – cool but not cold – on top of a towel at the foot of the table. Rachel placed her feet in the water, exclaimed that the water was cold for just a moment,

and then sighed with relief as her feet began to adjust to the temperature. The therapist began her massage routine at Rachel's head, while Rachel kept her knees bent and her feet in the footbath. After 2 minutes she said that her feet felt better, but were still somewhat hot. The therapist added 1 cup of ice cubes and 2 drops of oil of peppermint to the water, then continued the massage for another 5 minutes, when Rachel indicated that her feet felt "nice and cool" and that she was tired of holding up her legs. The tub was removed, and Rachel's wet feet were left to dry in the air. She quickly became more relaxed and commented on the wonderful sensation of a breeze blowing over her feet.

DISCUSSION QUESTIONS

1. Explain why the therapist chose the cool footbath for this situation.

2. Give examples of other hydrotherapy treatments you have learned that would also help Rachel's feet feel better.

from cooling of tissues only: cold blood in the feet was carried back to the heart and pumped from there out to the whole body (Livingstone, 1995).

SNAPSHOT

Temperature Cold (55–65°F; 13–18°C). Some clients may find this temperature hard to tolerate for very long. Crushed or cube ice may be used to cool the water.

Time needed 2–20 minutes (see above).

Equipment needed Water thermometer; container for water; a large towel to go under footbath; a small towel to dry the feet.

Effect Primarily thermal.

Cleanup Clean, disinfect, and dry the tub; launder the towels.

Indications When used for 2 minutes or less, stimulation of the entire body; when used for 2 minutes or more, cooling of the entire body; ankle sprains (the water must be over the top of the ankles); when one is learning to tolerate colder temperatures; as part of a contrast treatment; when stimulation of the toe, foot and ankle

extensor muscles is desired. (For more information, see the section on *Muscle weakness* on page 350.)

Contraindications Chilled client, Raynaud's syndrome, high blood pressure.

Procedure Same as for a hot footbath, but use cold water. Immerse the feet for 2 minutes or longer, depending upon the purpose of the footbath and the person's tolerance. Clients may tolerate cold water better if you cool it gradually by adding ice cubes or crushed ice after 1–2 minutes. Anytime the footbath water warms up too much, use a pitcher to remove some of the warmer water and replace it with colder water or ice.

Variation: Ice cold footbath to stimulate the tone of foot and ankle extensor muscles

This footbath can be used as part of a program to build muscle strength in clients with muscle weakness from stroke, muscular dystrophy, spinal cord injury, post-polio syndrome, or cerebral palsy. Muscle tone will be stimulated for about 20 minutes afterwards. (For more information, see the section on *Muscle weakness* on page 350.)

1. Explain the use of the ice-water bath to the client and get their consent. Because the cold is quite startling at first, it is very important to explain the purpose of this treatment.
2. Add equal parts of ice and water to a large container.
3. Place a towel under the ice-water bath and have the client sit in front of the bath.
4. Warn the client that the water will be very cold, then immerse the feet in the ice-water for 3 seconds.
5. Remove the feet from the cold water for 30 seconds, while the client exercises the extensor muscles of the feet and ankles.
6. Repeat steps 4 and 5 another five times, for a total of six ice-water "dips."
7. Dry the feet well.
8. The client's extensor muscles will be able to contract more strongly for about 20 minutes afterwards.

Contrast footbaths

A contrast footbath is simply a series of hot footbaths alternated with cold ones. As arteries dilate with heat and then constrict with cold, blood flow increases to roughly double that of someone who is not moving the feet. If this treatment is performed regularly, the muscles of the arterial walls will begin to contract more strongly. Since the baths are brief and deeper tissues are not directly in contact with the water, their temperature does not change very much: therefore, contrast footbaths do not produce edema as a hot treatment would. Because increased circulation is known to promote healing, foot ulcers, varicose ulcers and other poorly healing wounds have been treated with contrast foot and leg baths for generations. (Massage therapists should not treat these conditions unless directly under doctor's supervision.) The muscles of the arterial walls, which contract and relax with temperature changes, generally become fatigued after three or four rounds, and if the treatment needs to continue at that point, then the temperature contrasts will have to be greater–the hot water even hotter and the cold water even colder. To further increase the circulatory effect of a contrast footbath, have the client perform foot and ankle movements at the same time.

SNAPSHOT

Temperature Hot footbath at 110–115°F (43–46°C) and cold footbath 50°F (10°C).

Time needed About 10 minutes.

Equipment needed Water thermometer; two containers; enough water to cover the feet and ankles; two large towels to go under the containers; one small towel to dry the feet.

Effect Primarily thermal.

Cleanup Clean, disinfect, and dry the containers; launder the towels.

Indications Poor circulation in the feet; tendonitis in the feet or lower legs; tarsal tunnel syndrome; ankle sprains; derivation for migraine headache. For an acute ankle sprain, more rounds of hot and cold may be required to completely decrease swelling and pain, perhaps as many as ten rounds. In this case, pay extra attention to maintaining water temperature over time–otherwise the hot bath will begin to cool down and the cold bath will begin to warm up. (For more information, see *Sprains* on page 294.)

Contraindications Same as for hot and cold footbaths.

Procedure

1. Check with the client to make sure there are no contraindications for the contrast footbath.
2. Explain the use of the bath to the client and get their consent.
3. Set up everything just as you would for a hot footbath, but prepare one container of hot water and another of cold. To avoid drips, keep a towel under each container.
4. Begin with the hot footbath for 2 minutes.
5. Replace the hot footbath with the cold for 30 seconds.
6. Repeat steps 2 and 3.
7. Repeat steps 2 and 3 again, for a total of three rounds.
8. If any additives were used, rinse the client's feet with clean water, then dry the client's feet and put on socks.

Hand baths

Hand baths (Figure 6.5) are easy to integrate into a massage session. They have a variety of effects, depending upon the duration of the bath, the temperature of the water, and whether you put in any chemical additives.

FIGURE 6.5
(**A**) Hand bath. (**B**) Replacing water to maintain the desired temperature. (**C**) Adding ice cubes to maintain the cold hand bath temperature at 55–65°F (13–19°C).

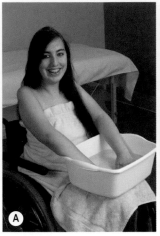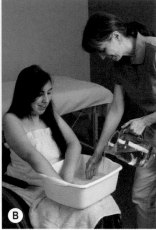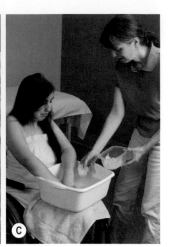

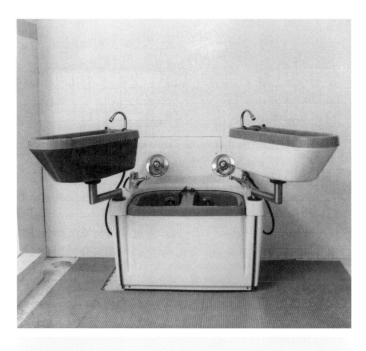

FIGURE 6.6
Combination arm and leg bath. Photo courtesy of HEAT Spa Kur Therapy Development, Inc., Bonita, California.

Figure 6.6 shows a combination arm and leg bath, which can be used to perform two partial baths at once. It might be used to treat someone with a migraine headache, by having both hands and feet in hot water at the same time.

Hot hand baths

A hot hand bath is another easy-to-perform treatment. It warms the hands, prepares them for massage, relieves hand pain, and, if prolonged, warms the entire body. A derivative effect is created when blood vessels in the hand dilate. One migraine sufferer discovered this effect by accident while she was washing dishes: "For years I have suffered from recurring migraine headaches …. [One day] I was struck by another migraine. I was determined to keep functioning – feeding my daughter, doing the laundry and washing the dirty dishes. I ran hot, hot water to rinse off my dishes, and, while rinsing, I felt my headache ebb. I could feel the blood draining out of my head like the tide washing away from the shore. It dawned on me that I was practicing my own biofeedback, by immersing my bare hands in the hot water. The blood vessels in my hands were dilating to allow blood to rush to the area and carry away the heat. That took the pressure out of my head. The dishes were clean and my headache was gone" (Bricklin, 1982).

SNAPSHOT

Temperature Hot (110°F; 43°C).

Time needed 15–20 minutes.

Equipment needed Water thermometer; container for water; 1 gallon (4 liters) of water; one large towel to go under the hand bath; one small.

Effect Primarily thermal.

Cleanup Clean, disinfect, and dry the tub; launder the towels.

Indications Cold hands; arthritis pain; cramps in the hand muscles; preparation for the stretching of muscles and fascia (the stretching of hand muscles can be performed in the hot water); as part of a contrast treatment; for a migraine headache (especially helpful at the beginning of a headache;

soak the full 20 minutes, then finish with a brief cold water pour).

Contraindications Loss of sensation in the hands.

Procedure

1. Check with the client to make sure there are no contraindications for the hot hand bath.

2. Explain the use of the hot bath to the client and get their consent.

3. Place the large towel on a table.

4. Fill a large bowl or plastic tub with hot water and place it on the large towel.

5. Have the client sit in a chair in front of the hand bath.

6. Have the client immerse their hands for 15-20 minutes. Massage may be performed on other parts of the body at this time. The container of water can be placed in the client's lap on a towel if desired (Figure 6.5A).

7. As the water cools, remove some and replace it with hotter water to maintain the temperature at 110°F (43°C). Do not pour hot water directly onto the hands (Figure 6.5B).

8. Remove the hands from water and dry them.

Variation: Epsom salts hand bath

This is helpful for sore or tired hands, painful bruises, or edema of pregnancy. Add 1 cup of Epsom salts per 1 gallon (4 liters) of warm water and finish by rinsing with clean water. (For more information, see *Epsom salts baths* on page 169.)

Cold hand baths

Short cold hand baths stimulate local circulation, and feel refreshing and invigorating, while long ones are very cooling but decrease local circulation. Both are easy to perform and especially welcome to clients who are overheated but would find a cold footbath intolerable. They can cause a reflex contraction of the blood vessels of the nasal mucosa, and thus were once used by hydrotherapists to treat nosebleeds. For clients who may not like colder water at first, try adding ice cubes or crushed ice after 1–2 minutes.

SNAPSHOT

Temperature Cold (55–65°F; 13–18°C). (The colder water may be hard for clients to tolerate.)

Time needed 15–20 minutes.

Equipment needed Water thermometer; container for water; approximately 1 gallon (4 liters) of water; one large towel to go under the hand bath; one small towel to dry the hands.

Effect Primarily thermal.

Cleanup Clean, disinfect, and dry the tub; launder the towels.

Indications Arthritis pain in finger joints (heat may work better for some); writer's cramp; poor circulation in the hands (use twice daily); strain of the hand muscles (use twice daily); cooling of the entire body if prolonged; as part of a contrast treatment.

Contraindications Chilled client, Raynaud's syndrome, high blood pressure.

Procedure

1. Check with the client to make sure there are no contraindications for the cold hand bath.

2. Explain the use of the bath to the client and get his or her consent.

3. Place the large towel on a table.

4. Fill a large bowl or plastic tub with cold water and ice. Place it on the large towel.

5. Have the client sit in a chair in front of the hand bath.

6. Have the client immerse their hands for 15–20 minutes. Massage may be performed on other parts of the body during this time. The container of water can be placed in the client's lap on a towel if desired.

7. As the water warms, remove some and replace it with ice cubes to maintain the temperature at 55–65°F (13–18°C) (see Figure 6.5C).

8. Remove hands from water and dry them.

Variation Cold hand bath and exercise, used to stimulate the fingers and improve wrist muscle tone

This hand bath and exercise routine can be used to help build muscle strength for clients with muscle weakness from stroke, muscular dystrophy, spinal cord injury, post-polio syndrome and some types of cerebral palsy. (For more information, see the section on *Muscle weakness* on page 350.)

1. Explain the use of the ice-water bath to the client and get his or her consent. The initial feeling of very cold water can be quite startling, so it is very important to explain the reason for this treatment.

2. Add equal parts of ice and water to the tub.
3. Place a towel under the ice-water bath.
4. Warn the client that the water will be very cold.
5. With the client seated, immerse the hands in the ice water for 3 seconds.
6. Remove the feet from the cold water for 30 seconds, while the client exercises the elbow, wrist and hand extensors.
7. Repeat steps 1 and 2 five more times, for a total of six cold water "dips."
8. Dry the body part briskly.
9. The client may now perform exercises for extensor muscles, as prescribed by his or her physical therapist. The extensor muscles will be stimulated and flexors inhibited for about 20 minutes.

Contrast hand baths

Figure 6.7 shows the contrast hand bath. This procedure is identical to that for the contrast footbath. A contrast treatment for the hands can be created from almost any heating treatment simply by dipping the hands in very cold water after using heat. For example, the hands could be dipped in paraffin or wrapped in hot fomentations instead of using hot water. Contrast hand baths can dramatically increase the circulation, and when performed regularly are a general tonic for the hands and wrists. They are effective for anyone performing heavy work with the hands. In fact, this treatment can be done immediately after a massage session if your hands feel tired or sore.

Making active movements of the hands and wrists while they are immersed increases blood flow even more.

SNAPSHOT

Temperature Hot (110°F; 43°C) followed by cold (55°F; 13°C).

Time needed 10 minutes.

Equipment needed Water thermometer; two containers; towel to dry hands.

Effect Primarily thermal.

Cleanup Clean, disinfect, and dry the tub; launder the towels.

Indications Muscular fatigue or pain from repetitive stress; arthritis pain; wrist sprain; poor circulation in the hands and wrists; healed hand or wrist fractures after the cast has been removed.

Contraindications Same as for hot and cold hand baths.

FIGURE 6.7
A contrast hand bath.
(**A**) Immersing the hands in hot water. (**B**) Changing from the tub of hot water to the cold.

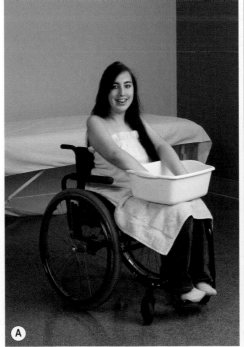
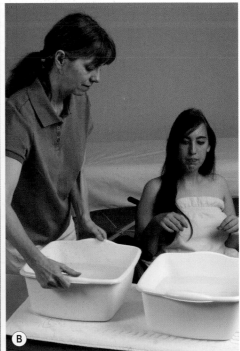

Procedure

1. Immerse the hands in hot water for 2 minutes (Figure 6.7A).
2. Immerse the hands in cold water for 1 minute (Figure 6.7B).
3. Repeat steps 1 and 2.
4. Repeat steps 1 and 2 another time, for a total of three rounds.
5. Dry the hands briskly.

Arm baths

An arm bath is also easy to integrate into a massage session, and can have a variety of effects depending upon the duration of the bath, the temperature of the water and if you use bath additives. You will need a somewhat larger container than for the hands alone, such as a rectangular plastic flowerbox (see Figure 6.8), an extra large plastic dishpan, a baby bathtub, or even a 5 gallon (20 liter) bucket.

Hot arm baths

A hot arm bath can warm the hands and arms, prepare them for massage, relieve hand pain, and, if prolonged, warm the entire body. After 20 minutes in a 111°F (44°C)

whirlpool, the temperature in the arm muscles can increase as much as 4°F (2.2°C) (Belanger, 2002). This is a significant finding, because anytime the temperature in a limb increases by 4 degrees, its blood supply will double. (This explains why a hot arm bath alone is not helpful for someone with lymphedema of the arm or a puffy, swollen wrist.)

SNAPSHOT

Temperature Hot (110°F; 43°C).

Time needed 15–20 minutes.

Effect Primarily thermal.

Equipment needed Water thermometer; container for water, such as a large bowl or plastic dishpan; 1–1½ gallons (5.5 liters) of water; large towel to go under the arm bath; small towel for drying the hands.

Cleanup Clean, disinfect, and dry the tub; launder the towels.

Indications Arthritis pain; muscle cramps after overuse of arm and hand muscles, such as in carpentry, massage or playing an instrument; preparation for stretching of arm muscles or fascia; derivation for migraine headache (use for 20 minutes at the beginning of a headache: finish with a brief cold water pour).

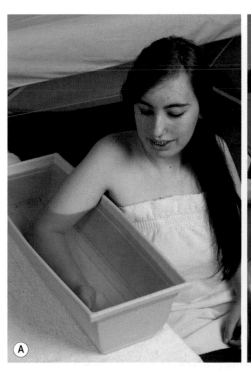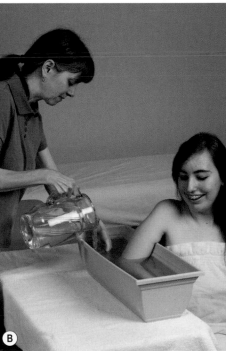

FIGURE 6.8
(**A**) Arm bath. (**B**) Replacing water to maintain the desired temperature.

Contraindications Lymphedema of the arm, loss of sensation.

Procedure

1. Check with the client to make sure there are no contraindications for the hot arm bath.
2. Explain the use of the bath to the client and get his or her consent.
3. Place the large towel on a table.
4. Fill a container with hot water and place it on the large towel.
5. Have the client sit on a chair in front of the arm bath.
6. Have the client immerse their arms as much as possible for 15–20 minutes. Massage may be performed on other parts of the body during this time.
7. As the water cools, take some out and replace it with hotter water to maintain the temperature at 110°F (43°C). Do not pour hot water directly onto the arms (Figure 6.8B).
8. Remove arm(s) from the bath and dry them briskly.

Cold arm baths

To perform a cold arm bath, first read the section on cold hand baths and follow the step-by-step directions given there. To treat the arms, simply use a larger water container and enough water to cover them; otherwise, all directions apply.

All indications and contraindications are the same. A cold arm bath will cool the entire body more than a hand bath alone.

Contrast arm baths

In a contrast arm bath, the hands and arms are immersed to the elbows first in hot water, then in cold water, for the purpose of increasing local circulation. Note that a contrast treatment for the arms can be created from almost any warming application, then following that with a cold-water immersion. For example, the arms could be coated with paraffin, soaked in hot water, or wrapped in hot fomentations, and after that plunged into cold water: all three methods would have a similar effect. To increase blood flow even more, have the client make active hand and arm movements.

SNAPSHOT

Temperature Hot (110°F; 43°C) alternated with cold (55°F; 13°C).

Time needed 10 minutes.

Equipment needed Water thermometer; two containers for water, each holding 1–1½ gallons (4–5.5 liters) of water; one large towel to go under each arm bath; one small towel for drying the arms and hands.

Effect Primarily thermal.

Cleanup Clean, disinfect, and dry the tub; launder the towels.

Indications Relieves muscular fatigue and pain in the arms, increases blood flow. Also indicated for wrist and elbow sprains, and for healed fractures after the cast has been removed.

Contraindications Same as for both the hot arm bath and the cold arm bath.

Procedure Same as for the contrast hand bath, but immerse the entire arm, or both arms, in the water.

Half baths

As shown in Figure 6.9, a hot half bath is one in which the client sits waist-deep in hot water. It is helpful when body warming is needed but the client cannot tolerate a full hot bath; when you wish to increase blood flow to the lower body, as when the client has a migraine headache; and to encourage skin absorption of substances such as herbs or essential oils. The tub is filled half-full using 104°F (40°C) water. In order to keep the top of the body warm, the client can either wear a shirt or use a small blanket or towel as a cover. Place a cold compress or ice bag on the head as soon as sweating begins. At the end of the bath, give the client a brief cold pour from just the waist down and finish with a rest of 20 minutes or more.

SNAPSHOT

Temperature Hot (104°F; 40°C).

Time needed 15 minutes.

Equipment needed Water thermometer; two large bath towels; a bowl of cold water and washcloth for a cold compress (optional); shorts or a bathing suit for the client; a shirt or small towel to cover the upper body if needed; one or more grab bars.

Effect Primarily thermal.

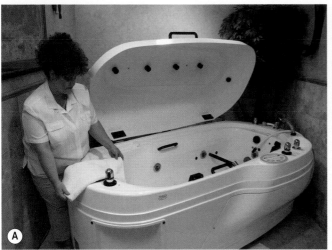
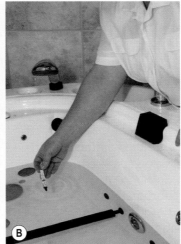
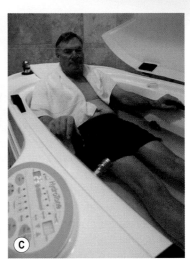

FIGURE 6.9
Half bath. (**A**) Placing towels. (**B**) filling the tub and checking the water temperature. (**C**) The client resting in a half bath.

Cleanup Clean, disinfect, and dry the tub; launder the towels.

Indications Arthritis of the lower extremities; acute or chronic low back pain; sciatica; chilled client; before a cold treatment; migraine headache. For an example of how to use the hot half bath for a migraine headache, see Case history 6.3.

Contraindications Diabetes, lymphedema in legs, loss of sensation, peripheral vascular disease (arteriosclerosis of the lower extremities or Buerger's disease).

Procedure

1. Check with the client to make sure there are no contraindications for the hot half bath.

2. Explain the use of the bath to the client and get his or her consent; then have client put on shorts or a bathing suit.

3. Place towels on the floor in front of the tub and behind where the client's head will be (Figure 6.9A).

4. Fill the tub to waist level, checking the temperature with a water thermometer (Figure 6.9B).

5. Have the client enter the tub, wearing a dry shirt or draped with a towel to keep the upper body warm if needed (Figure 6.9C).

6. After 15 minutes, have the client leave the tub, dry off vigorously, and lie down for a rest or massage.

Variation: Warm half bath

This bath is suitable for clients who would benefit from a half bath but suffer from diabetes or peripheral vascular disease. Simply follow the directions for the hot half bath, but use water that is 98–102°F (37–39°C).

Leg baths

Leg baths (not shown) are helpful for many aches and pains. They can warm or cool the legs, carry salts, herbs, essential oils or other substances, and affect the general circulation if they are significantly hot or cold. Leg baths are also an excellent home treatment for clients. Either a standard bathtub or a stainless steel whirlpool specifically designed for this purpose may be used. If only the lower legs are to be treated, use two deep buckets, one for each leg.

Hot leg baths

SNAPSHOT

Temperature Hot (102–110°F; 39–43°C).

Time needed 20 minutes.

Equipment needed Water thermometer; bath towel, shirt or small towel to cover the upper body if needed; grab bar if treatment is in a bathtub.

Chapter six

BACKGROUND

Christina was a healthy 53-year-old massage therapist who occasionally suffered a type of headache called an **occipital migraine**. Her optometrist had explained that a constriction of the basilar artery causes the sufferer to see vivid flashes of light or bright zigzag patterns, which slowly spread and move from the person's central vision to his or her peripheral vision. Sufferers may or may not have pain, and Christina felt fortunate that her head did not hurt when she had these migraines. She had not been able to connect them to any particular event in her life except eyestrain. One day, after typing at her computer for an hour, Christina again started to see flashing lights and bright moving zigzag patterns across her entire field of vision.

SELF-TREATMENT

Christina had read about using derivation to relieve migraine headaches and decided to try a hot half bath. After seeing the flashing lights for 10 minutes, she filled her bathtub partially full of 110°F (43°C) water. Leaving her shirt on, she got into a tub filled with about 6 inches (15cm) of hot water, which just covered her feet and legs. She took her watch into the tub with her, the better to observe the effects. She noticed the flashing lights starting to diminish after 4 minutes, and 2 minutes after that they were completely gone. Greatly relieved, Christina stayed in the water for another 5 minutes – a total of 11 minutes in the bath – and then got out tentatively, afraid that the migraine would recur at any moment. However, she dressed and continued her day with no further problem: the flashing lights did not recur and she felt entirely normal.

DISCUSSION QUESTIONS

1. Explain how hot water to the legs and feet affected this migraine headache.

2. What other hydrotherapy treatment could be used for the same purpose as the hot half bath?

Effect Primarily thermal.

Cleanup Clean, disinfect, and dry the tub; launder the towels.

Indications Stiffness and poor circulation after the removal of a leg or ankle cast, muscle soreness after vigorous exercise, arthritis pain in legs or feet, pain (including phantom pain) in an amputation stump, tight muscles or thick contracted scar tissues which are going to be treated with massage. Warming of the entire body if the leg bath is prolonged.

Contraindications Diabetes, lymphedema in legs, loss of sensation, peripheral vascular disease (arterio-sclerosis of the lower extremities or Buerger's disease).

Procedure

1. Check with the client to make sure there are no contraindications for the hot leg bath.

2. Explain the use of the bath to the client and get his or her consent

3. Place towels on the floor in front of the tub and behind where the client's head will rest.

4. Fill the tub to a level that covers the legs, checking temperature with a water thermometer.

5. Have the client enter the tub, wearing a dry shirt or towel to keep the upper body warm if desired.

6. After 20 minutes, help the client to leave the tub and dry off vigorously, and then he or she can lay down for a rest or massage.

Variation 1: Warm leg bath (98–102°F; 36–39°C)

This bath is safe for clients who would benefit from a leg bath but suffer from diabetes or lymphedema of the legs.

Variation 2: Epsom salts leg bath

A leg bath with Epsom salts can be used for soreness after vigorous exercise or painful bruises. Add 2 cups (256g) of Epsom salts to a warm, not hot, leg bath. (For more information on Epsom salts and their effects, see *Epsom salts baths* on page 169.)

Variation 3: Lower leg bath

Use two buckets and immerse the lower legs up to the knee.

Cold leg baths

Cold leg baths are not for everyone, as many people find exposure of such a large portion of the body to cold temperatures hard to take; however, they help prevent muscle soreness after vigorous exercise and are popular with athletes (see Figure 6.18). A classic study of their effects found that leg muscles were much stronger right afterwards. Subjects were given 54°F (12°C) leg baths for 30 minutes. Each subject was tested for leg strength many times during the bath, and for 3 hours afterwards as they relaxed. It turned out their leg muscles were stronger during the cold bath and afterwards for as long as 6 hours. The researchers concluded that the increased strength was due to increased blood flow to deeper leg muscles, as when superficial capillaries constricted, blood was shunted to deeper vessels (Fiscus, 2005).

SNAPSHOT

Temperature Cold, 50–60°F (10–15.5°C) for a strong reaction; up to 70°F (21°C) if the client cannot tolerate a very cold bath.

Time needed 5–20 minutes.

Equipment needed Water thermometer; bath towel, shirt or small towel to cover the upper body if needed.

Effect Primarily thermal.

Cleanup Clean, disinfect, and dry the tub; launder the towels.

Indications To prevent muscle soreness after vigorous leg exercise (15–20 minutes); to stimulate circulation in legs (2–5 minutes); overheated client (5–15 minutes).

Contraindications Marked hypertension, Raynaud's syndrome.

Procedure Follow the procedure for the hot leg bath, but use cold water.

Variation Lower leg bath

Use two buckets; immerse the legs up to the knee.

Contrast leg baths

Contrast leg baths can have a powerful influence on the circulation in the legs. For example, one study conducted in 2005 examined arterial blood flow in the lower legs during hot, cold, and contrast treatments. The contrast treatment consisted of 4 minutes of hot water (104°F; 40°C) alternated with 1 minute of cold (55°F; 13°C). There were significant fluctuations in arterial blood flow throughout the 20-minute treatment: it increased during the first hot water bath, then decreased when the water was changed to cold, and this occurred with each round. The increase was greatest on the first change back from a cold bath to a hot one, and then the increase was less with each successive hot bath, suggesting that the muscles of the artery walls began to tire. Contrast baths caused a greater increase in local circulation than a simple hot bath, and at the end of the bath, it was twice that of subjects who took no baths and were simply sitting quietly (Fiscus, 2005). Making active movements during the bath increases blood flow even more.

In the following directions for the contrast leg bath, we assume that the therapist has two tubs, one for hot and one for cold, but this can also be done using a bathtub for the hot water followed by a cold leg shower.

SNAPSHOT

Temperature Hot (102–110°F; 39–43°C) alternated with cold (55–70°F; 13–21C).

Time needed 10 minutes.

Equipment needed Two bathtubs; water thermometer; bath towel, shirt or small towel to cover the upper body if needed.

Effect Primarily thermal.

Cleanup Clean, disinfect, and dry the tub; launder the towels.

Indications Plantar fasciitis; muscular fatigue in legs; poor circulation in legs; joint sprains; passive swelling in legs; stiffness and poor circulation in the leg muscles after a cast has been removed; when prescribed by a doctor, to promote healing of infections.

Contraindications Same as for hot and cold leg baths.

Procedure

1. Follow the procedure for a hot leg bath, then, while the client is in the hot leg bath, fill the other container with cold water

2. Help the client to leave the tub of hot water after 2 minutes, and move into the tub of cold water.

3. After 30 seconds, help the client to switch back to hot.

4. Repeat steps 3 and 4.

5. Repeat steps 3 and 4, for a total of three rounds.

6. Dry the lower body briskly and have the client lie down for a rest or massage.

Chapter six

Variation Contrast lower leg bath

Use two deep buckets and immerse the lower legs up to the knee. Some clinics use two leg whirlpools side-by-side, with a platform built above them, and the client simply sits on the platform and slides from one to the other.

Paraffin baths

A paraffin bath is a special tank (see Figure 6.10) which keeps melted paraffin at a therapeutic temperature (125°F; 52°C). We use paraffin which also contains mineral oil, which makes the wax easy to remove and leaves the skin soft. Dipping a body part into paraffin repeatedly creates a coat of wax that not only warms the tissue underneath, but prevents heat from radiating off the skin; instead, heat goes deep into joints. It raises the temperature of the skin and the muscles and joint capsules underneath (see Box 6.3).

When might a massage therapist use this treatment with a client? The deep heating of a painful or stiff body part makes paraffin an excellent treatment for relieving joint stiffness in conditions such as arthritis, poorly healed sprains, non-acute bursitis, and fractures after casts have been removed. It is an ideal treatment for uneven areas such as the feet, where a hot pack or heating pad cannot contact all surfaces. When paraffin is combined with mobilization techniques to treat post-traumatic joint stiffness, results are better than with mobilization alone (Rashid, 2013). The deep heat of the bath also makes tissues softer and more pliable, which is especially helpful when you treat scar tissue. A combination of paraffin baths and stretching helps patients with burn scars gain significant increases in their joint range of motion (Belanger, 2002). Another time you might choose paraffin is for a client who does not have pain but is stressed and would like to try something that feels soothing or pampering. Cold hands will love this treatment. Clients with osteo- or rheumatoid arthritis would benefit from having a paraffin bath at home and using it daily. Children love and are fascinated by paraffin, but be sure to obtain parents' permission first, and let the child immerse one finger and remove it to see if they want to try it. Some children's hospitals recommend paraffin for children, while others never do. The author has used paraffin with hundreds of children older than six years old without a single problem, but this is a grey area. If there is any doubt or discomfort, one dip will not burn. Just stop the treatment right away. Paraffin can also be painted on an area that is difficult to immerse, such as a knee, then covered with plastic wrap and a heating pad. Some spas even offer paraffin facials!

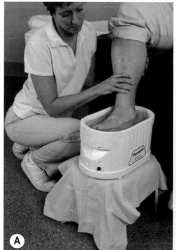 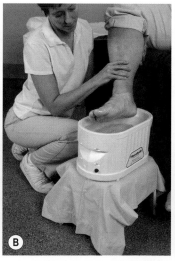 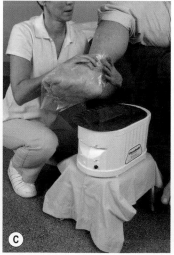 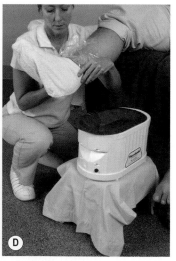

FIGURE 6.10
Paraffin footbath. (**A**) Dipping the client's foot in a paraffin bath. (**B**) The paraffin-coated foot drying. (**C**) Wrapping the foot in a plastic bag. (**D**) Placing a bootie on the client's foot.

BOX 6.3   POINT OF INTEREST

HISTORY OF THE PARAFFIN BATH

According to English physical therapist Olive Millard, who practiced in Europe from 1913 to 1940, the melted paraffin bath was first introduced into the practice of physical medicine in 1916. Mr W.L. Ingle, of an English firm that tanned and finished leather, noticed that a number of workers at his plant were immersing their hands and feet in a vat of wax that was used for preparing animal skins (probably for relief of arthritic pain). Mr Ingle then presented one to the Commanding Medical Officer of the 2nd Northern General to treat wounded soldiers (Millard, 1952).

Paraffin baths were enthusiastically adopted for physical therapy, and became very common. They were used throughout Europe and North America, by physical therapists, athletic trainers and massage therapists. At Warm Springs Rehabilitation Institute, a state-of-the-art facility founded in 1926, paraffin was one of the treatments used for musculoskeletal problems. For example, a patient with clubfeet might be treated with serial casting, which is used to gradually straighten out twisted limbs. To begin, the feet were each bent as much as possible towards a normal position and then put in a cast for a week or two. Then each foot would be taken out of its cast and dipped in hot paraffin to make the tissue more pliable, and then massaged, stretched and bent even more towards a normal position, and then put into another cast. Melted paraffin was also used to treat arthritis pain and soften scar tissue prior to stretching.

However, paraffin does have some disadvantages too. For example, melted paraffin is easy to spill, difficult to clean off surfaces, and more expensive than water; a paraffin bath must be plugged in for three hours before the wax will have completely melted; only the hands and the feet can be easily immersed in a paraffin bath.

The procedure below describes a paraffin bath for the feet, but this treatment is also very effective for the hands.

SNAPSHOT

Temperature Hot (123–126°F; 50.5–52°C).

Time needed 15 minutes.

Equipment needed Footbath supplies, as you will use a warm footbath to warm and clean the feet first; paraffin bath, containing three pounds of paraffin; two small plastic bags and two booties or oversized socks to slip on the feet. New paraffin baths often include all these supplies when they are purchased. Warmed electric booties are available from therapy suppliers.

Effect Primarily thermal.

Cleanup Throw away the plastic bags and used paraffin; launder the towel and booties or socks.

Indications Cold hands or feet; poorly healed sprains; non-acute bursitis; fractures after cast removal; thick, tight scar tissue; muscle strains and spasm; gout pain; joint stiffness; arthritis.

Contraindications Peripheral vascular disease, including diabetes, Buerger's disease, and arteriosclerosis of the lower extremities; skin with cuts or sores; loss of sensation (lack of feeling); sensitivity to heat, especially in those with thinner skin, such as the elderly and small children. Do not use with children under six years old.

Procedure

1. Check with the client to make sure there are no contraindications for the paraffin bath.

2. Explain the use of the bath to the client and get their consent.

3. Have the client seated in a chair next to the massage table. Place a towel on the floor under the client's feet.

4. Put the container of warm water on the towel, rest the client's feet in the container, and soak them for a few minutes. If running water is not available, spray the feet with a sanitizer. This step begins heating the feet, feels good to the client, and keeps the paraffin bath clean.

5. Dry one foot, then quickly dip it in paraffin and remove it (Figure 6.10A).

6. Wait about 3 seconds for the wax to harden slightly (the wax will just start to lose its shine). Check in with the client that it is OK to continue. If so, then dip the foot again (Figure 6.10B). Do 6–10

dips in all: with fewer dips, the wax coating will be too thin to retain heat

7. Encase the foot in a plastic bag or cellophane wrap, then in an oversized sock, cloth bootie, or electric bootie (Figure 6.10C).

8. Repeat steps 5–7 with the other foot.

9. Leave the paraffin on for about 10 minutes, then remove the outer cover, bag or cellophane, and paraffin from one foot.

10. Massage that foot and slip a sock over it.

11. Repeat steps 9 and 10 on the other foot.

Variation 1: Paraffin dip on massage table

The client may disrobe, wrap in a sheet, and sit up on the side of the table while you bring the paraffin bath to her. Carry it very carefully and do not let the cord trail on the floor: instead, place the bath and the cord on a tray and carry it that way. Paraffin spilled on a rug is very difficult to remove.

Variation 2: Contrast treatment

Paraffin foot dips can be used to create a contrast treatment by dipping the feet in cold water for 30 seconds after removing the paraffin. Perform three rounds of hot paraffin dips followed by cold water.

WHOLE-BODY BATHS

In this section, you will learn about a number of different bath treatments in which the entire body is immersed in water. The continuous bath, an ingenious use of the bathtub to treat a variety of problems, is not used today because it is extremely time-consuming, but it is a good example of how varied the effects of whole-body baths can be (see Box 6.4). Many different whole-body treatments work well in a standard bathtub, and all can complement massage treatments and deepen the effectiveness of bodywork. If you work in a facility that has a bathtub it is easy to add whole-body baths to your repertoire of hydrotherapy treatments. You may also give your clients instructions on how to take different types of baths at home.

Important note: every bathtub should have at least one grab bar that can be easily reached by the client.

Standard baths

An excellent example of how to use a standard bathtub to enhance bodywork is from the practice of a massage therapist in Oregon, USA. Next to her waiting room she had installed a small private garden-like alcove, which contained a green porcelain tub and many hanging plants. Clients came early, let themselves in, and soaked for 15 minutes before their session. They then put on a bathrobe and went back to the waiting room, already warm and relaxed before their session even began. Clients had signed a release form before they did this.

Hot baths

Almost everyone enjoys a full-body hot bath like the one pictured in Figure 6.11, especially clients who are cold or who have musculoskeletal pain. The combination of the warmth of the water, the soothing sensation of water on the skin, and the temporary release from the pull of gravity draws healthy and sick people alike. According to Patrick Horay, author of *Hot Water Therapy*, "There is something almost magical about hot water … slipping into a warm bath, a part of you remembers and allows itself to be supported and buoyed up, warmed and nurtured to the core. It reminds you to let go of physical and mental tension, to give up all the striving and activity, to be just held by the penetrating warmth" (Horay, 1991).

SNAPSHOT

Water temperature Hot (103–110°F; 39–43°C), depending upon the client's tolerance. Clients vary widely as to their ideal temperature, and what is an extremely hot bath to one person will be almost a cold bath to another. Also, if the water temperature is too hot, clients won't be able to stay in very long. For anyone who is not accustomed to taking a hot bath, begin with no more than 15 minutes to ensure they will react well.

Equipment needed Water thermometer; tub; two bath towels; bathmat; grab bar.

Effect Primarily thermal.

Cleanup Clean and sanitize the tub; launder the towels and bathmat.

Indications Before massage, use hot baths to soften connective tissue, relax muscles, enhance circulation and encourage mental relaxation. The whole-body heating effect also helps relieve many types of musculoskeletal pain, including pain from arthritis, gout, dysmenorrhea, back pain, sciatica,

BOX 6.4	POINT OF INTEREST

CONTINUOUS BATHS: INGENIOUS TREATMENTS FOR ANCIENT PROBLEMS

The continuous bath treatment was first developed by a Viennese doctor in 1861. Patients remained in a tub of neutral temperature water (98°F; 37°C) for extended periods of time, from a few hours to many days or weeks. They lay on a canvas stretcher that was suspended inside the tub by clamps or hooks, which formed a hammock-type sling. The stretcher was covered with a blanket, and rubber pillows were provided for the patient's head and feet. Once the patient was in the water, the top of the tub was covered with boards, which helped retain the heat and also provided a table for the patient (for an example, see Box 1.4, Figure 1). Warm water ran in continually as cooler water ran out, so that not only did the bath stay at a constant temperature, but water was constantly running gently over the skin. Normally a waterproofing ointment was applied to the patient's skin at the beginning of the bath, since he or she stayed in the water for many hours at a time. Sometimes patients would be removed periodically, but only long enough for the tub to be cleaned and more waterproofing ointment applied.

Continuous baths met some medical needs that today are treated by medications, but when they were developed, there were no effective medications for many of the problems they addressed. These included reflex spasms from spinal cord injuries, paralysis of the legs, and joint stiffness and pain from advanced arthritis. Because bacterial growth in infected areas was reduced while the person remained in the bath, before the advent of antibiotics the continuous bath was also a standard treatment for such conditions as non-healing pressure sores, gangrene, ulcers from radiation burns, fecal and urinary fistulas, and extensive burns (Baruch, 1920).

Floating in the bath also decreased pressure and pain on sores or wounds on the back part of the body, and reduced the number of painful dressing changes on badly infected wounds (Thrash and Thrash, 1981). The continuous bath has also been useful for relieving the pain and stiffness of rheumatoid arthritis and the pain, spasm, burning sensation, and tremors of Parkinson's disease (Jelinek, 1953). When hydrotherapy was popular in mental hospitals, continuous baths were used extensively to sedate agitated mental patients. Physical therapist Earl Qualls saw the continuous bath being used in California state mental hospitals as late as 1952, both for musculoskeletal pain and for a tranquilizing effect (Qualls, 2007).

Continuous baths have fallen out of use because of their time-consuming nature, but research is needed to find out whether they could be useful in cases where medication is not effective, such as pressure sores that do not heal even when treated with anti-biotics, or in cases where medication side-effects are very serious.

---

neuralgia, muscle soreness, sprains, strains, bruises and con-tusions, and it is known to help a person fall asleep faster and sleep more deeply (Rayman, 2005; Sung, 2000). Since this bath will cause clients to sweat, provide drinking water before, during and afterwards.

Contraindications Dehydrated client; systemic or chronic conditions, including cardiovascular problems, diabetes, hepatitis, lymphedema, multiple sclerosis, seizure disorders, and hypothyroid conditions; loss of sensation; great obesity; pregnancy; inability to tolerate heat; ingestion of alcohol or drugs; recent meal (wait at least an hour after a meal). The only exception is when the client's doctor has approved hot baths.

Procedure

1. Check with client to make sure there are no contraindications for the full hot bath.

2. Explain the purpose of the bath to the client and get his or her consent. If the bath might be too hot, in many cases a warm bath will work just as well and it is better to start with a milder temperature and see how the client does.

3. Place a bathmat on the floor in front of the tub and a towel behind where the client's head will rest (Figure 6.11A).

4. Begin filling the tub and check the water temperature with a thermometer (Figure 6.11B).

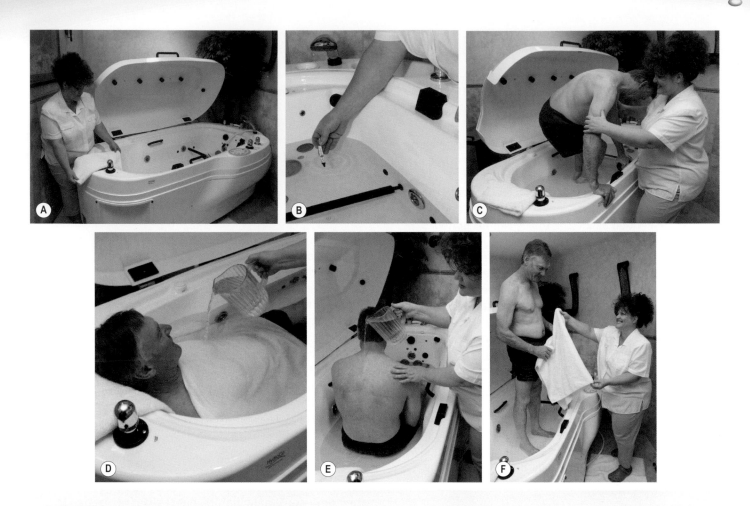

FIGURE 6.11
Hot bath. (**A**) Placing a bathmat and towel. (**B**) Filling the tub and checking the water temperature. (**C**) The client entering the tub.
(**D**) Covering the chest and shoulders with a towel. (**E**) Pouring cold water over the client. (**F**) Giving the client a towel to dry off with.

5. When the tub is half full, have the client get in the tub and sit down: assist as needed (Figure 6.11C).

6. Have the client adjust the temperature to a tolerable level as the bath finishes filling.

7. Have the client remain in the tub for 15 minutes or longer, depending upon tolerance.

8. If the bathtub is too small for someone to be entirely immersed, cover the chest and shoulders with a large towel and pour water over it frequently (Figure 6.11D).

9. A brief cold shower or cold-water pour will help re-invigorate someone who is feeling drained after a hot bath (Figure 6.11E). However, many clients find this step unpleasant, so it is optional.

10. If the client feels light-headed or dizzy, he should sit in the tub while the water drains, before getting out. This will bring down the core temperature slightly. The client should not try to get out of the tub until the light-headed or dizzy feelings pass, and then always should use a grab bar.

11. Provide a towel (Figure 6.11F).

12. Give the client water to drink.

Variation Cold water finish

A brief cold bath, a cold shower, or even just pouring cold water over the client. The cold water causes vasoconstriction of the blood vessels under the skin. This is difficult or unpleasant for many people, but results in a prolonged feeling of warmth and invigoration. The cold exposure should be about 30 seconds, and no longer than 2 minutes. Do not perform this treatment unless the client is quite warm.

Warm baths

Since maintaining the core temperature at 98.6F (36°C) is easier in a warm bath than in a hot one, a warm bath demands less of our adaptive powers. The client will still experience the bodily changes that come from adjusting to a higher-than-usual core temperature, such as vasodilation of the skin and sweating, but these changes will be less extreme. For this reason, warm baths are practical for many people for whom hot baths are contraindicated. However, musculoskeletal pain will be less dramatically affected by a warm bath. (Rayman, 2005; Sung, 2000). Provide water to all clients before the bath.

SNAPSHOT

Water temperature Warm (99–102°F; 37–39°C). Clients vary widely as to what is the most comfortable temperature for them. If the water temperature is beyond the client's tolerance, he or she won't be able to stay in very long. For someone who is not accustomed to taking a warm bath, begin with no more than 15 minutes.

Equipment needed Water thermometer; tub; two bath towels; bathmat; grab bar.

Effect Primarily thermal.

Cleanup Clean and sanitize the tub; launder the towels and bathmat.

Indications Before massage, to soften connective tissue, relax muscles, enhance circulation, and encourage mental relaxation; for musculoskeletal pain, including the pain of gout, dysmenorrhea, back pain, arthritis, neuralgia, sprains, strains, bruises and contusions. Relieves insomnia if taken before bed.

Contraindications Seizure disorders, due to the danger of a client having a seizure in the tub; loss of sensation; great obesity; inability to tolerate heat; ingestion of alcohol or drugs; recent meal (wait at least an hour after a meal).

Procedure Follow the procedure for hot baths, only using warm water.

Neutral baths

The neutral bath places the client in an environment with as little thermal or mechanical stimulation as possible. (For more on its use with mentally disturbed people, see Box 1.2.) Water surrounds the person's body evenly on all sides is unusually soothing and calming. Eliminating other sensory stimulation, such as noise, extraneous conversation or bright lights, is part of the treatment. The heart rate drops, while the skin blood flow, skin temperature and core temperature remain the same (Miwa, 1994). Blood pressure also normalizes. JG, a 65-year-old Jamaican patient who was being treated by MDs at Uchee Pines Health Center, originally arrived with high blood pressure (160/100), even though she was taking three hypertensive medications. After 3 weeks on a program of dietary changes, two neutral baths each day and a massage before bedtime, she was not taking any medications and her blood pressure averaged 145/80. One day, however, her blood pressure rose to 215/110 after an upsetting phone call. She was immediately given a neutral tub bath followed by a full body massage and a one-hour rest, and her blood pressure was then was measured at 150/75 (Thrash, 1998) Massage after a neutral bath is a wonderful complement to this relaxing treatment.

SNAPSHOT

Water temperature Neutral (95–100°F; 35–38°C) water will cool a bit during the bath, so start a bit warmer, adjust the temperature, and add more warm water as needed. Keep the bathroom warm and never allow the person to become chilled.

Time needed 20 minutes or more.

Equipment needed Water thermometer; tub; two bath towels; bathmat; grab bar.

Effect Primarily mechanical (lack of sensory stimulation).

Cleanup Clean and sanitize the tub; launder the towels and bathmat.

Indications Insomnia, nervousness, anxiety, and depression; and diseases of the heart and blood vessels where more extreme hot and cold temperatures cannot be used, such as arteriosclerosis or diabetes. When performed under a doctor's supervision, it is sometimes used to lower blood pressure in a hypertensive person.

Contraindications Severe cardiac weakness; eczema.

Procedure

1. Follow the procedure for a warm bath, and make sure the water is comfortably warm when the client first gets in. Next, adjust the temperature using a water thermometer and keep it the same throughout the bath.

2. Keep the environment calm and quiet.

3. Have the client dry off gently so as not to stimulate the skin, and then he or she may lie down to rest or to receive a massage.

Short cold baths

A short (30 seconds to 2 minutes) cold bath is a traditional way to stimulate the muscles of the superficial arteries to contract more strongly. A short cold bath has little or no cooling effect on the body, however, because the tissues are not chilled long enough to actually lower the core temperature. The body's defense mechanisms are stimulated, however, to such a degree that if a person takes a short cold bath and then immediately dries off and gets dressed, he or she will actually feel warmer than before. A feeling of invigoration is common, as the body's functions are stimulated, and for this reason a cold bath is a classic ending to a sauna. Longer cold baths have been used in the past to reduce fevers, because they actually cool the body and bring the core temperature down, but they are not recommended for massage therapy unless a client has become overheated in a hot bath, sauna, or steam bath.

SNAPSHOT

Water temperature Cold – generally below 65°F (18°C). Cold tap water is usually at 55–65°F (13–18°C).

Time needed 30 seconds to 2 minutes maximum.

Equipment needed Water thermometer; tub; two bath towels; bathmat; grab bar.

Effect Primarily thermal.

Cleanup Clean and sanitize the tub; launder the towels and bathmat.

Indications Stimulation of blood flow to the skin; invigoration; prevention of painful menstrual cramps (see page 342); prevention of delayed-onset muscle soreness.

Contraindications Chilled client; extreme fatigue; kidney disease; cardiovascular disease (the blood pressure will rise for a very short time, and may be too much of a demand for a person with heart disease or arteriosclerosis); hyperthyroid conditions (this is a disease in which the basal metabolic rate is too high, and a short cold bath will further increase the metabolism); client with an aversion to cold.

Procedure Follow the procedure for hot baths, only using cold water and keeping the bath short – just 30 seconds to 2 minutes in length.

Contrast baths

As with other contrast treatments, hot and cold are alternated, leading to dilation and constriction of the superficial blood vessels, stimulating the circulatory and other body systems and leaving the client both relaxed and invigorated. However, only the hardiest of clients can tolerate very hot alternated with very cold: someone who would like to try a contrast bath, but who is not accustomed to such a circulatory system challenge, would do better to try a warm bath alternated with a cool bath at first. If you do not have the two tubs that this treatment calls for, you can substitute a sauna or steam bath for the hot bath, and use a cold shower for the cold bath. In Scandinavia, rolling in the snow is a traditional method of cooling the body after heat exposure; however, as discussed in the introduction to this chapter, immersion baths are truly the most efficient way to warm and cool the body. Be sure to explain the benefits of the contrast bath to your client, because the first immersion into the cold bath is often quite a strong sensation! The muscles of the blood vessels generally become fatigued after three changes. To increase the circulatory effect of a contrast bath even further, have the client exercise gently at the same time.

SNAPSHOT

Water temperature Hot (104–110°F; 40–43°C) alternated with cold (65°F; 18°C or less).

Time needed About 15 minutes.

Equipment needed Water thermometer, two tubs (one filled with hot water, the other with cold water); two bath towels; bathmat; grab bar.

Effect Primarily thermal.

Cleanup Clean and sanitize the tub; launder the towels and bathmat.

Indications To decrease muscle soreness after strenuous exercise; when stimulation of blood flow to the skin or a feeling of invigoration is desired; when training the circulatory system to react better to cold, in order to stay warmer in the winter (see Chapter 11); as a general tonic.

Contraindications Because it combines the effects of hot and cold baths, the same as for both a hot bath and a short cold bath.

Procedure

1. Check with the client to make sure there are no contraindications for either hot or cold whole-body baths.

2. Explain the use of the contrast bath to the client and get his consent.

3. Place a bathmat in front of each tub and a towel for the client's head to rest on.

4. Fill both tubs, one with hot water and the other with cold, and check the water temperature in each.

5. Have the client enter the hot bath and remain for 5 minutes so that his body is thoroughly warm.

6. Have the client move to the cold bath for 30 seconds to 1 minute.

7. Have the client move back to the hot bath and remain for 2 minutes, for maximum skin vasodilation.

8. Have the client move to the cold bath for 30 seconds to 1 minute.

9. Repeat steps 7 and 8.

10. Hand the client a towel to dry off with, as they get out of the tub.

Baths with additives

To increase the therapeutic effects of a standard bath, consider adding one of the substances in this section. They are safe, easy to obtain, and inexpensive, and have beneficial effects on the skin, muscles, joints, or nervous system (see Figure 6.12 for examples of bath additives). Comfortably warm water is used for all the baths that follow, since the goal of the treatment is to bring the dissolved substance into contact with the client's skin, rather than create a treatment with primarily thermal effects. Warm water is helpful because it leads to dilation of the

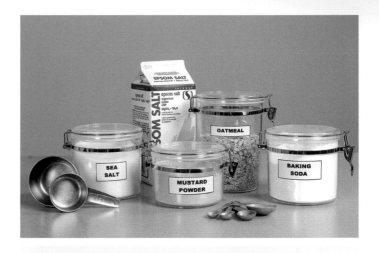

FIGURE 6.12
Containers with bath additives.

blood vessels under the skin, which increases absorption of the chemical. A warm bath also provides a relaxing environment for the client: not only does the water feel pleasant, but if it was very hot or cold, he or she might not remain in the bath long enough for absorption to occur.

Mineral water hot springs, mud baths and seawater baths have all been used to treat musculoskeletal ailments for thousands of years. Natural mineral springs contain various mixtures of chemicals such as potassium, magnesium, calcium and sulfate; mud baths are used to stimulate circulation and metabolism and to combat inflammation; and minerals found in seawater, including sodium chloride, are said to stimulate circulation of blood and lymph and speed elimination of toxins. Where these baths are available, massage therapy is almost always practiced as well.

Oatmeal baths

Because it contains essential fatty acids and other beneficial chemicals, oatmeal has an anti-inflammatory effect that makes it suitable for a variety of skin irritations (Vie, 2002). It soothes and re-moisturizes dry skin and relieves many types of itching for as much as several hours. Powdered oatmeal is an ingredient in many commercial bath products, but it is easily added to a bath using simple uncooked rolled oats (see Figure 6.13).

FIGURE 6.13
Oatmeal bath. (**A**) Adding a commercial oat product to bathwater. (**B**) Muslin bag containing oatmeal. (**C**) Patting the skin dry.

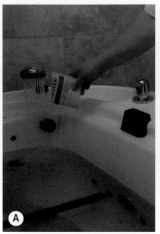
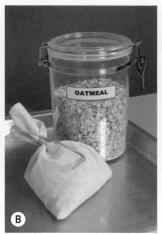
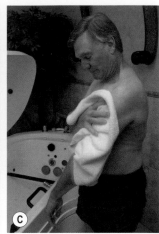

SNAPSHOT

Water temperature Warm (98–104 °F; 37–40 °C).

Time needed 15–20 minutes.

Equipment needed Water thermometer; bath towel; bathmat; grab bar; and one of the following:

1. One packet of commercial oatmeal preparation, which can be added to the bath as soon as it begins filling to make sure it dissolves fully.

2. One cup uncooked rolled oats ground fine in a blender and then mixed with three cups of cold water.

3. One cup of uncooked rolled oats in a muslin bag.

Effect Primarily chemical.

Cleanup Clean and sanitize the tub; launder the towels and bathmat.

Indications Skin irritations such as poison oak, poison ivy, chickenpox, shingles, psoriasis, rashes, eczema, diaper rash, icthyosis and sunburn.

Contraindications The same as for a full warm bath.

Procedure The same as for a full warm bath, except that now directions are included for adding oatmeal to the bath.

1. Check with client to make sure there are no contraindications for a warm whole-body bath.

2. Explain the use of the bath to the client and get his or her consent.

3. Place a bathmat on the floor in front of the tub and a towel behind where the client's head will be.

4. Begin filling the tub: check the water temperature with a thermometer and then add the oatmeal preparation (Figure 6.13A). If a muslin bag with oatmeal (Figure 6.13B) is used, it should put in the tub right away, so that it becomes thoroughly saturated with bathwater: during the bath, it should be squeezed occasionally to extract its beneficial properties.

5. Have the client enter the tub when it is half full: assist as needed.

6. Have the client adjust the temperature to tolerance as the bath finishes filling.

7. The client may remain in the tub for 15 minutes or longer.

8. Hand the client a towel to dry off with before he or she gets out of the tub. The skin should not be toweled off vigorously: instead the skin should be gently patted dry, so that some of the oat solution remains on the skin (Figure 6.13C). Do not let the client become chilled during this process.

Baking soda baths

As an anti-acid, sodium bicarbonate is widely used in medicine. For example, it is added to intravenous medication when a patient is in a state of acidosis, to many commercial preparations such as Alka-Seltzer to neutralize stomach acid, and to water which is used to decontaminate the skin after some chemical exposures. Because it can normalize the skin's acid/base balance and neutralize many toxins, and has mild anesthetic properties, baking soda is used to decrease many types of skin irritation. You can provide your clients with these benefits by adding it to a bath treatment, or you can suggest that clients take a baking soda bath at home. For example, a client who has previously scheduled a massage session but now believes his skin might be too irritated to be touched, could take a series of baking soda baths the day before his appointment, to see if this improves the condition of his skin and makes massage more comfortable.

SNAPSHOT

Water temperature Warm (98–104°F; 37–40°C).

Time needed 15–20 minutes.

Equipment needed Water thermometer; 1 cup of baking soda; bath towel; bathmat; grab bar.

Effect Primarily chemical.

Cleanup Clean and sanitize the tub; launder the towels and bathmat.

Indications Skin irritations such as sunburn, heat rash, eczema, itching, hives, poison oak, poison ivy, and reactions from chemotherapy or radiation treatments for cancer.

Contraindications The same as for a full warm bath.

Procedure Follow the procedure for the oatmeal bath, but add baking soda instead.

Epsom salts baths

"Epsom salts" is the common name for a mineral compound, magnesium sulfate heptahydrate, that was first prepared from the waters of a mineral spring in Epsom, England. That spring was discovered in the early 1600s, bubbling up through soil which contained the mineral Epsomite, and its waters were soon found to be both relaxing and purgative (Sakula, 1984; Childs, 1993).

Because they are a laxative when taken internally, they can be found in almost every grocery store and pharmacy and can be purchased without a prescription. Since the discovery of Epsom salts, hydrotherapists have used them in partial and whole-body baths, body wraps, compresses and constitutional treatments. As magnesium is a necessary element in some enzymes responsible for detoxification, they are often prescribed for that purpose. Because, like other salts, they can pull water from cells, Epsom salts are used as a fast-acting purgative in some types of poisoning, as a laxative to draw water into the intestines to soften feces, and as a substance that draws fluid. This action means it can improve conditions such as cerebral edema and bruised and injured tissues, and it can even draw out splinters. Magnesium reduces striated muscle contractions and thus is a muscle-relaxant, used to prevent convulsions in pregnant women with

pre-eclampsia, to treat overactive reflexes in spinal cord injury, and to ease some cases of **bronchospasm** (Childs, 1993; Azaria, 2004). Many parents of children with autism swear by its calming, sleep-inducing effects in baths. Flotation tanks use hundreds of pounds of Epsom salts per bath for buoyancy, and adding them to the bathwater is also an efficient way of raising blood levels of magnesium—one study found a hot 12-minute bath with one pound (454g) of the salts led to significant rises in the amount of magnesium and sulfate in the blood (Waring, 2004).

Dermatology professor E. Proksch found that when persons with dry, rough and red skin bathed their forearms in a concentrated Dead Sea salt bath, it moisturized their skin and reduced inflammation, and this effect lasted for as long as 6 weeks. Probably the high magnesium content of the Dead Sea salts is responsible for these effects (Proksch, 2005).

As massage therapists, we can use Epsom salts in baths for their relaxing effect, to reduce possible soreness after deep tissue massage and to reduce inflammation in cases of swelling, bruising and soreness after vigorous exercise. We can add herbal preparations and essential oils as well.

SNAPSHOT

Water temperature Warm (98–104°F; 37–40°C).

Time needed 15–20 minutes.

Equipment needed Water thermometer; bath towel; bathmat; one or more grab bars; 2 cups of Epsom salts for an adult or 1 cup of Epsom salts for a child. Use double that amount when the bath is taken specifically for detoxification.

Effect Primarily chemical.

Cleanup Clean and sanitize the tub; launder the towels and bathmat. Epsom salts are not corrosive to drain pipes.

Indications Bruises; sprains in the sub-acute stage; soreness after exercise; nervous tension; arthritis pain; general tonic; detoxification.

Contraindications Same as for a full warm bath.

Procedure Follow the procedure for the oatmeal bath, using Epsom salts instead of oatmeal. Afterwards, Epsom salts should be thoroughly rinsed off with a brief shower or by pouring clean water over the client. Then, apply a moisturizing lotion or oil to the skin: this is simple to do if the client is going to be receiving a massage.

Sea salt baths

Sea salt baths are a traditional hydrotherapy treatment given as a general tonic, and for calming and relaxing. One to three cups of salt are used in a tonic bath, which may be taken daily. The water holds the heat better because of the salt. Salt baths have been used in the past for patients with severe burns, as a way of providing them with electrolytes: in this case five pounds of water are added to 40 gallons (150 liters) of water, which is about the same concentration of salt as ocean water. However, below we give the amount for a tonic bath, which uses a smaller amount of salt. Herbal preparations or essential oils can be added as well.

SNAPSHOT

Time needed 15–20 minutes.

Water temperature Warm (98–104°F; 37–40°C).

Equipment needed Water thermometer; 1–3 cups (128–384g) of sea salt; bath towel; bathmat; grab bar.

Effect Primarily chemical.

Cleanup Clean and sanitize the tub; launder the towels and bathmat. Sea salt can be corrosive to drainpipes, so immediately after the bath the pipes should be thoroughly flushed with tap water so that no salt water remains.

Indications General tonic; chronic sciatica; fractures after removal of the cast; dislocations; gout; arthritis.

Contraindications Same as for a full warm bath.

Procedure Follow the procedure for the oatmeal bath, using sea salt instead of oatmeal. The salty water should be thoroughly rinsed off after the bath, with a brief shower or by pouring clean water over the client. Then apply a moisturizing lotion or oil to the skin: this is simple to do if the client is going to be receiving a massage.

Powdered mustard or ginger baths

Mustard paste is powerfully heating in a plaster (see *Mustard plasters*, page 109), but the smaller amount used in baths is mildly warming, encourages sweating, relieves muscle soreness and fatigue, and is an excellent home treatment for insomnia. You can make your own

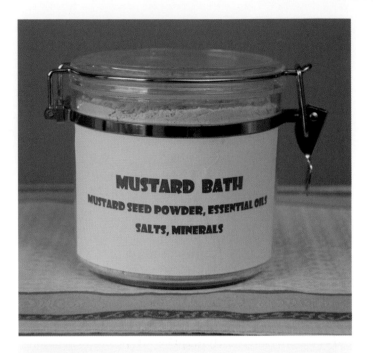

FIGURE 6.14
Mustard bath mixture.

mustard bath or purchase a ready-made preparation (Figure 6.14). Ginger is also mildly warming and is a traditional folk treatment for joint pain, as it has profound anti-inflammatory effects when taken internally; one study showed it reduced pain and stiffness in knee joints 40% better than a placebo: researchers concluded that ginger extract could one day be a substitute for nonsteroidal anti inflammatory medications (Altman, 2001).

SNAPSHOT

Water temperature Warm (98–104°F; 37–40°C).

Time needed 15–20 minutes.

Equipment needed Water thermometer; pre-made commercial mustard bath; 1/3 cup (76g) mustard powder or 1/6 cup (38g) ginger powder for an adult; bath towel; bathmat; grab bar. Fresh ginger tea may be used, but is time-consuming to prepare.

Effect Primarily chemical.

Cleanup Clean and sanitize the tub; launder the towels and bathmat.

Indications Muscle soreness or fatigue, insomnia.

Contraindications Same as for a full warm bath.

Procedure Follow the procedure for the oatmeal bath, using mustard or ginger powder instead of oats. Powder may be added directly to the water under the spigot or mixed in a bowl of water first to eliminate any lumps, then added to the bathwater. After the bath, mustard or ginger water should be thoroughly rinsed off with a brief shower or by pouring clean water over the client. Then apply a moisturizing lotion or oil to the skin: this is simple to do if the client is going to be receiving a massage.

Detoxification baths

Detoxification baths that combine salts and baking soda may be taken two or three times per week. This bath combines the detoxifying effects of three previous baths: baking soda neutralizes toxins; Epsom salts draw water and toxins, and provide magnesium and sulfate which are needed for detoxification; sea salts draw water and toxins; and the warm water promotes a moderate amount of sweating. Clients should replenish water and electrolytes afterwards. (For more information on detoxification, see *Detoxification treatments* on page 243.)

SNAPSHOT

Water temperature Warm (98–104°F; 37–40°C).

Time needed 15–20 minutes.

Equipment needed Water thermometer; 1 cup (128g) each of sea salt and Epsom salts and 1½ cups (192g) baking soda to put in the tub; bath towel; bathmat; grab bar.

Effect Primarily chemical.

Cleanup Clean and sanitize the tub; launder the towels and bathmat.

Indications As a general tonic, after recent exposure to toxins, or as part of a detoxification program.

Contraindications Same as for a full warm bath.

Procedure Follow the procedure for the oatmeal bath, using baking soda and both types of salt instead of oatmeal. Add them directly under the spigot as soon as the tub begins filling, to make sure all are dissolved. At the end of the bath, the bathwater should be thoroughly rinsed off with a brief shower or by pouring clean water over the client. Then apply a moisturizing lotion or oil to the skin: this is simple to do if the client is going to be receiving a massage.

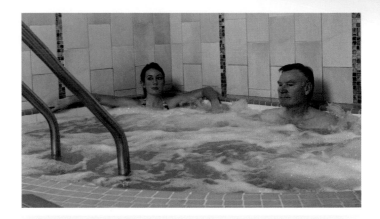

FIGURE 6.15
Hot tub.

Specialized baths

In addition to the standard bath treatments presented above, a massage therapist who is working in an athletic club or spa can perform other treatments that require special equipment. Here we cover baths that are taken in hot tubs, spa bathtubs, whole-body stainless steel whirlpools, and **Watsu** treatments that take place in pools.

Jetted tubs (hot tubs)

The terms used to describe tubs with jets are somewhat confusing: they may be called Jacuzzis (named after the first manufacturer of jetted tubs), hot tubs or spas. They are all small pools containing jets of water or air or both, and are big enough for more than one person to use at a time. Today, tubs with jets such as the one pictured in Figure 6.15 can be found in athletic clubs, health spas and some private homes. The bathwater is generally heated to about 104°F (40°C), which is comfortable for the majority of people, but it can easily be adjusted to lower or higher temperatures (see Case history 6.4). Some jetted tubs have tile walls and floors, while others are made of fiberglass or other synthetic materials. Unlike a standard bath tub, water is not drained out at the end of the bath, and instead the water is treated with disinfecting chemicals. Jetted tubs also contain equipment that heat and recirculate the bathwater. Using jetted tubs safely is important: water temperature must be carefully monitored, and covers put back on properly after use. Accidental drownings have occurred when tubs were left uncovered.

Chapter six

BACKGROUND

Susan was a 51-year-old woman with no previous history of health problems who had just been diagnosed with **multiple sclerosis.** She had many of its typical symptoms, including muscle weakness, spasticity, fatigue, and other problems. (For more on this condition, see the section in Chapter 13.)

TREATMENT

Even before she was diagnosed with multiple sclerosis, Susan had felt poorly for some time. She had been receiving hydrotherapy treatments and massage from Eva at a spa, and over time she and Eva tried a variety of treatment-and-massage combinations before finding the one which Susan felt was the most relaxing and helpful.

They began with a soak in a jetted tub of hot water, followed by a massage. However, people with multiple sclerosis are advised to avoid sunbathing, hot showers, hot tubs, hot swimming pools, saunas, and even electric blankets, because their symptoms worsen with elevations in body temperature of as little as 1°F (0.5°C). Even exercising on a warm day may raise body temperature enough to exacerbate symptoms: for example, Susan once had pain in her hands and feet, extreme fatigue, increased muscle spasms, and even tunnel vision after a short hike on a hot day. However, since she had not yet been diagnosed with MS, her first spa treatments were in warm water. She soon realized that these baths made her feel tired and weak, and then, trying different temperatures, she and Eva eventually found that soaking in a 97°F (36°C) whirlpool for 10 minutes was relaxing and did not make her symptoms worse.

Again, guided by how Susan responded, Eva and Susan found additional hydrotherapy treatment that helped meet Susan's needs. After Susan had taken the cooler soak, Eva gave her a salt glow using sea salt, oil of peppermint and grapeseed oil. Eva had this combination available at the spa and felt comfortable using it because peppermint is such a common, widely used, and safe essential oil. Menthol, which is the main chemical in peppermint oil, stimulates cold-sensitive receptors in the skin and gives a cooling effect.

After the cool soak, Susan's body would be scrubbed, rinsed, and then covered with plastic wrap, a sheet, and finally a blanket, and she would rest for 20 minutes. When uncovered, she was slightly warm and sweaty, but because of the peppermint oil she never felt hot, and she found the wrap very relaxing. Next she took a brief shower, and finally, received a Swedish massage from Eva. This combination of hydrotherapy and massage turned out to be relaxing and helpful for the emotional stress and spasticity that come with multiple sclerosis, but had unexpected benefits as well: if Susan was feeling a flare-up (temporary worsening of symptoms) coming on, the combination soak and wrap treatment resulted in her symptoms being milder and lasting a shorter time.

DISCUSSION QUESTIONS

1. How did Eva, as a massage therapist, determine which treatments were effective for Susan?

2. What information relevant to hydrotherapy should be part of the medical history of someone with multiple sclerosis?

SNAPSHOT

Water temperature Hot (104–110°F; 40–43°C).

Effect Thermal and mechanical.

Equipment needed Water thermometer; tub; two bath towels; bathmat; grab bar.

Cleanup Clean and sanitize the tub; launder the towels and bathmat. Periodic maintenance should be done according to the manufacturer's directions.

Indications Same as for a hot bath.

Contraindications Same as for a hot bath, but clients with rashes or skin infections should not be in bathwater that is agitated by jets, as this might spread the skin condition. Individual stainless steel whirlpools can be sterilized but jetted tubs cannot, so anyone with open skin (wounds, burns or pressure sores) should not use them. Clients who have been drinking alcohol should not use hot tubs!

Procedure Same as for a full hot bath.

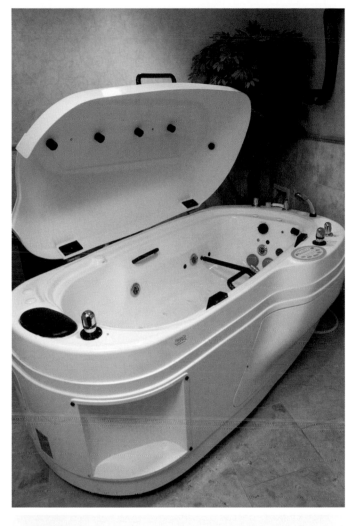

FIGURE 6.16
Spa bathtub.

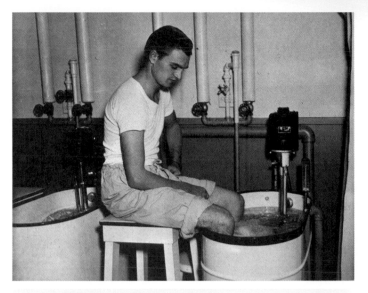

FIGURE 6.17
Contrast leg whirlpools, 1946: one pool is hot, the other cold. Image from the History of Medicine, National Library of Medicine. Sourced from ihm.nlm.nih.gov/images 101395644.

The tubs are the same size as a standard one-person bathtub, and can also be used for simple whole-body baths. See Figure 6.16 for a picture of one such tub. At the time of writing, they are very expensive, and suitable only for high-end spas. (For another type of spa bathtub, see Figure 8.2C.)

Spa bathtubs

Special European hydrotherapy tubs for one person may contain not only jets but specialized hoses so that a therapist can perform underwater massage. In this technique, the client lies in the warm water of the tub while a stream of pressurized water is applied to various tissues. In Europe this is also popular as an after-workout massage for athletes, and for injuries such as sub-acute fractures, dislocations, sciatica, low back pain, joint contractures, scoliosis and various types of paralysis. Underwater pressure massage may also be used for general relaxation and to promote lymphatic drainage.

Stainless steel whirlpools

A whirlpool is a stainless steel bathtub containing one or more turbines which mix air with the water in the tub, and jets of water which can be directed to specific areas (see Figure 6.17). Whirlpools are most often used in medical settings because they can be sterilized between patients, making them safe for those with burns, frostbite and pressure sores. The clients most likely to be treated with a whirlpool are those with problems from the elbows or knees down, including post-traumatic pain, swelling after hand or foot surgery, plantar fasciitis, Achilles tendon rupture, acute muscle spasms, and frostbite. In one hospital study patients who took full-body warm whirlpool baths twice every day for the first few days after major abdominal surgery had significantly less post-operative pain and swelling around

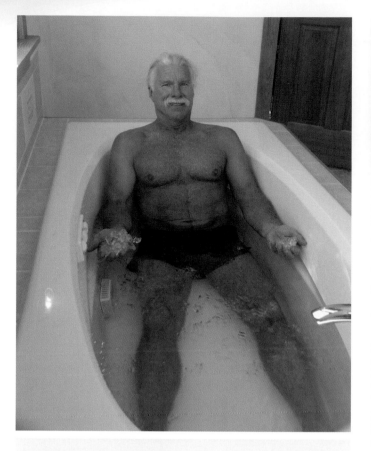

FIGURE 6.18
Athlete after exercise. Ice-water baths have become a popular method of speeding recovery after an intense game or competition, especially when research showed that cold baths and contrast baths, not hot baths, decreased muscle swelling and soreness after a hard workout (Vaile, 2008).

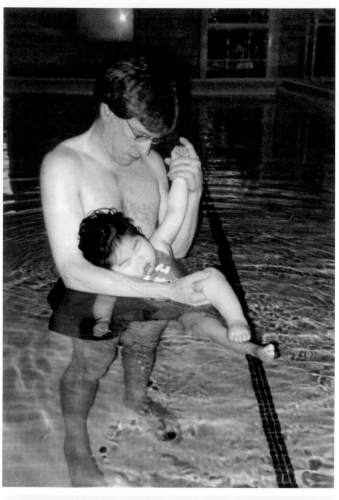

FIGURE 6.19
Kira receiving Watsu treatment. Photo courtesy of Jeff Bisbee.

the surgical site. Researchers felt that their decreased pain was due to the relaxing effect of the bath as well as better movement of trapped anesthesia gases out of the intestines, and the surgical wounds were less inflamed because they were much cleaner than usual (Meeker, 1998). Today, massage therapists are only likely to encounter stainless steel whirlpools if they work at a physical therapy clinic or an athletic training facility.

Watsu

Watsu is a relatively new form of bodywork that is performed in a pool (see Case history 6.5). It combines the effects of traditional Japanese Shiatsu massage therapy, the feeling of being cradled and supported in someone's arms, and the buoyancy, pressure, and soothing sensation of warm water. As seen in Figure 6.19, the therapist stands chest-high in a swimming pool or specially made Watsu pool while the client floats in his or her arms. The therapist performs many of the Shiatsu techniques, including pressure points, rocking movements, and gradual twists and stretches of different parts of the body. The water is kept at a temperature of 93–98°F (34–37°C) because the receiver is barely moving and is not generating any body heat. If the water is cooler, her muscles will begin to tighten and it will be much harder to relax.

| A CLIENT WITH ENCEPHALITIS | CASE HISTORY 6.5 |

BACKGROUND

Kira was an 18-month-old girl who had recently suffered a severe case of viral **encephalitis**. As a result, she was partially paralyzed on one side, and had weakness in some muscles and spasticity in others. Her muscles were so contracted that she often woke in the night crying from pain. If the contractions continued, she would almost certainly develop permanent joint **contractures**.

TREATMENT

Jeff Bisdee, recreational therapist and Watsu practitioner, saw Kira three or four times a week for Watsu sessions. Kira floated in his arms as he manipulated and stretched her tight muscles. Kira often became profoundly relaxed, and often fell asleep. As an added benefit, after just a few sessions she began to sleep through the night. Because her muscles were now looser than before, she was no longer in danger of developing joint contractures.

DISCUSSION QUESTIONS

1. What was the effect of Watsu on Kira's muscles?
2. What caused this effect?

Watsu is given to create deep states of relaxation, to free specific tight muscles, to increase range of motion, and to allow the spine to be moved in ways not possible on land. Improvement is possible in neuromuscular conditions, stress-related disorders, and musculoskeletal pain. Watsu may also bring up strong emotions, elicited by the receiver's being held in a safe and nurturing way. Training and certification is available for therapists who are interested in incorporating this treatment into their practice. For more information, visit the following website: www.watsuinstitute.com.

CHAPTER SUMMARY

In this chapter you have learned about a wide variety of baths. When combined with bodywork, bathing a body part or the entire body in hot, warm, neutral, cold, or alternating hot and cold water, or in melted paraffin, can help meet many clients' needs. When therapeutic substances such as salts, oatmeal or mustard powder are added to the bathwater, bodywork can be even more effective.

And now, as we have added on to the wide variety of treatments you learned about in earlier chapter, you can safely pick and choose water baths when they are suited to your clients' needs and your massage methods. In the chapters ahead, we will continue to learn more water treatments, and learn even more about how to fine-tune them for your own practice and for your clients.

REVIEW QUESTIONS

Short answer

1. Name two baths that can be used to treat arthritis.

2. Name two baths that can be used for a migraine headache.

3. Explain how the additives in a detoxification bath help the body detoxify.

4. Give two examples of baths that can be used for insomnia.

5. Explain why baths are the most efficient way to heat or cool an area.

6. Discuss four different uses for a hot footbath, and explain why this treatment is helpful for each one.

7. Give two examples of conditions when a cold whole-body bath would be preferred to a warm one.

Fill in the blank

8. Because they can be sterilized, stainless steel whirlpools are preferred for clients with _____ or _____.

9. What are two footbaths which are not used to for people with poor arterial circulation and diabetes? _____.

10. A full-body contrast bath is a _____ choice of treatment for clients who are sedentary or fragile.

11. Oatmeal baths are useful for clients with skin _____.

12. Epsom salts baths are helpful for clients with _____, _____, and _____.

13. One way to increase the effectiveness of a contrast bath is to have the client _____.

14. Paraffin baths are helpful before scar tissue massage because they _____.

15. We use grab bars when clients might _____ because they are _____.

References

Altman R, Marcussen KC. Effects of a ginger extract on knee pain in patients with osteoarthritis. Arthritis Rheum 2001; 44(11): 2531–8

Azaria E et al. Magnesium sulfate in obstetrics: current data. J. Gynecol Obstet Bio Reprod 2004; 33: (6 Pt 1): 510–17

Baruch S. An Epitome of Hydrotherapy for Physicians, Architects and Nurses. New York: WB Saunders, 1920, pp. 95–9

Belanger A. Evidence-Based Guide to Therapeutic Physical Agents. Baltimore: Lippincott, Williams and Wilkins, 2002

Bricklin M. Rodale's Encyclopedia of Natural Home Remedies. Emmaus, PA: Rodale Press, 1982

Childs PE. History of Epsom salts. Chemistry in Action 1993; 40: 25

Chiu HY. A feasibility randomized controlled crossover trial of home-based warm footbath to improve sleep in the chronic phase of traumatic brain injury. J Neurosci Nurs 2017; 49(6): 380–5

Ebben MR. The effects of distal limb warming on sleep latency. Int J Behav Med 2006; 13: 221

Fiscus KA. Changes in lower-leg blood flow during warm, cold, and contrast-water therapy. Arch Phys Med Rehabil 2005; 86(7): 1404–10.

Golant A et al. Cold exposure injuries to the extremities. J Am Acad Orthop Surg 2008; 16(12): 704–15

Horay P. Hot Water Therapy. Oakland, Ca: New Harbinger Publications Inc, 1991

Jelinek R. Continuous bath in surgical therapy. J Internatl Coll of Surg; August 1953: 156–60

Karuchi K, Cajochen C, Werth E, Wirz-Justice A. Warm feet promote the rapid onset of sleep. Nature 1999; 401 (6748): 36–7

Li W. Effect of warm water footbath on fatigue, sleep and quality of life in post-stroke patients. Paper presented at 25th International Nursing Research Congress, Hong Kong, July 2014

Liao WC et al. Effect of a warm footbath before bedtime on body temperature and sleep in older adults with good and poor sleep: an experimental crossover trial. Int J Nurs Stud 2013; 50(12): 1607–16

Livingstone SD et al. Heat loss caused by cooling the feet. Aviat Space Environ Med 1995; 66: 232

Meeker J. Whirlpool therapy on post-operative pain and surgical wound healing: an exploration. Patient Education and Counseling 1998; 33: 39–48

Millard O. Under My Thumb. London: Christopher Johnson, 1952

Miwa C et al. Human cardiovasacular responses to a 60-minute bath at 40°C. Environ Med 1994; 38(1): 77–80

Mooventhan A, Nivethitha L. Scientific evidence-based effects of hydrotherapy on various systems of the body. N Am J Med Sci 2014; 6(5): 199–209

Murphy W. Healing the Generations: A History of Physical Therapy and the American Physical Therapy Association, Lyme, CT: Greenwich Publishing Group, 1995, p. 103

Oh PJ, Kim YL. Effectiveness of non-pharmacologic interventions in chemotherapy induced peripheral neuropathy: a systematic review and meta-analysis. J Korean Acad Nurs 2018; 48(2): 123–42

Olszewski WL et al. Flow and composition of leg lymph in normal men during venous stasis, muscular activity and local hyperthermia. Acta Physiol Scand 1977; 99(2): 149–55

Proksch E et al. Bathing in a magnesium-rich dead sea salt solution improves skin barrier function, enhances skin hydration, and reduces inflammation in atopic dry skin. Int. J. Dermatol 2005; 44(2): 151–7

Qualls E. Personal communication with author. Wildwood, GA, 2007

Rashid S et al. Evaluating the efficacy of mobilization techniques in post-traumatic stiff ankle with and without paraffin wax bath. Pak J Med Sci 2013; 29(6): 1406–9

Rayman RJ et al. Cutaneous warming promotes sleep onset. AM J Physiol Regul Integ Comp Physio 2005; 288

Sakula A. Doctor Nehemiah Grew (1641–1712) and the Epsom Salts. Clio Med 1984; 19(1–2): 1–21

Shafeik H, Abdelaziz S, ElSharkawy S, Effect of warm water footbath on fatigue in patients undergoing hemodialysis. International Journal of Nursing Didactics 2018; 8: 26–32

Simons DG, Travell JG, Simons LS. Travell and Simons' Myofascial Pain and Dysfunction: the Trigger Point Manual, Vol 1: Upper Half of Body, 2nd edn. Baltimore, MD: Lippincott, Williams and Wilkins, 1999, pp. 133, 170

Sung E. Effects of bathing and hot footbath on sleep in winter. J Physiol Anthropol Appl Human Sci 2000; 19: 21

Thrash A, Thrash C. Home Remedies: Hydrotherapy, Massage, Charcoal and Other Simple Treatments. Seale, AL: Thrash Publications, 1981, p. 120

Thrash A, Thrash C. Natural Remedies for Hypertension. Seale, AL: New Lifestyle Books, 1998

Vaile J et al. Effect of hydrotherapy on the signs and symptoms of delayed onset muscle soreness. Eur J Plly Physiol 2008; 102: 447–55

Vie K et al. Modulating effects of oatmeal extracts in the sodium lauryl sulfate skin irritancy model. Skin Pharmacology and Applied Skin Physiology 2002; 15: 120–4

Waring R. Absorption of magnesium sulphate (Epsom salts) across the skin. Report for Epsom Salt Council, UK, 2004. www.epsomsaltscoUncil.org/wp,,/report_on_absorption_of_magnesium_sulfate.pdf [Accessed November 2018]

Zemke J et al. Intramuscular temperature response in the human leg to two forms of cryotherapy: ice massage and ice bag. JOSPT 1998; 27(4): 301–7

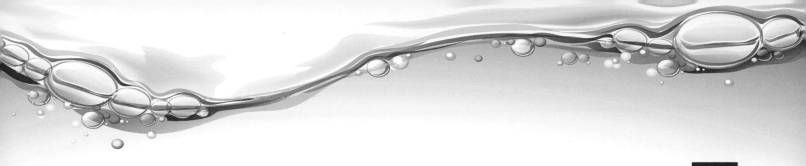

Hot air baths 7

A loud crack and sizzle punctures the darkness and suddenly a wave of sage-scented steam engulfs my face. The heat rushes down my body and I have barely enough time to take a breath before another hornful of water is dumped on the rocks … the leader continues dumping more and more water onto the stones and each burst of steam ratchets up the heat more and more …
I listen to my brothers bare their hearts, addressing in turn the Creator, God, the Father, the Mother, the Great Spirit. Their prayers are beautiful and earnest, and it doesn't occur to me until it's my turn that I have forgotten the heat. Our prayers, the prayers of all my relations, become one in the timeless heart of the **inipi** *(sweat lodge).*

Michael Paul Mason, *Head Cases: Stories of Brain Injury and Its Aftermath*

I was without hope before I began detoxification … until just a few weeks ago I was suffering. It is going to take hard work, but I believe I will be able to regain the ability to fly. The biggest obstacle, the one I saw no way to overcome, is now behind me … to say that my doctors have been amazed by the [sauna treatment] results is putting it mildly.

Sean Donahue, helicopter pilot: testimony before the New York City Council, February 2004

CHAPTER OBJECTIVES

After completing this chapter, the student will be able to:

1. Name and describe the various hot air baths
2. Describe the effects of various hot air baths
3. Explain the contraindications for various hot air baths
4. Describe a variety of applications for hot air baths
5. Give hot air baths using the procedure included with each treatment.

Hot air baths are another ancient and popular hydrotherapy treatment. If clients take a bath before beginning a bodywork session, they will be so comfortably warm that they will not become chilled, their muscles will be warm, relaxed and pliable, any muscle or joint pain will be reduced, and they will feel relaxed. Both dry and wet hot air baths are excellent for insomnia and nervous tension. After a massage, taking a sauna or steam bath leaves clients further relaxed, warmed to the core, and cleansed of all oil or lotions. You can combine saunas and steam baths with some of the other hydrotherapy treatments you have learned: for example, in Chapter 13 you will learn how to combine a sauna or steam bath with a local application of heat to treat an acute lower back spasm.

Some advantages to using hot air baths to warm clients:

- Hot air baths can be turned on with just a flip of a switch, unlike hot compresses, body wraps or many other applications of moist heat.

- Some clients simply prefer the feeling of a hot air bath over a body wrap or hot bath.

- Hot air baths can be used to apply therapeutic substances such as herbs and essential oils.

- You can work with one client while another takes a sauna or steam before or after their bodywork session.

In the past, hot air baths were more expensive and elaborate than many other treatments and so they were used almost exclusively by massage therapists who worked at athletic clubs or spas. Today, however, advances in technology are making them less expensive and more accessible to the massage therapist in private practice. Many massage studios now offer saunas or hot tubs as part of treatment packages which include massage. In this chapter we will discuss the uses and effects of hot air baths, including a classic local hot air bath, steam inhalation.

HOT DRY AIR BATH: THE SAUNA

A sauna is a cabinet or small room where air can be heated to a high temperature. Over the millenia, saunas have been constructed from wood, sod, stone, brick, metal, packcloth, volcanic rock or heavy-duty plastic, and heated with wood, gas, light bulbs, electricity or infra-red rays. Most modern saunas are modelled after the classic Finnish one, which consists of a small wood-paneled room with benches and a gas, electric, infrared or wood-burning stove (Figure 7.1). Cedar, redwood, or white spruce woods are used because they are soft, aromatic and porous, and stay cool to the touch. (Temperatures in far infrared saunas are cooler than in classic saunas, because far infrared rays penetrate and heat human tissue directly, rather than heating the surroundings. Some people prefer the cooler sensation.)

Taking a sauna involves going into a pre-heated room for some minutes. Sauna temperatures are usually 145–200°F (63–93°C), and average about 160°F (71°C). (The World Sauna championships in Finland ended permanently after a finalist died after 6 minutes in a 230°F (110°C) sauna.) Intake and outlet vents help to circulate hot air and keep the humidity to 6–10%: the air is very dry, and the human body can tolerate the high temperatures because sweat evaporates fast and produces an instant cooling effect. In traditional Finnish saunas, dipperfuls of water may occasionally be poured over stones which are placed upon the stove: this produces steam, and a wave of heat and humidity rolls onto the bather. If the sauna is hot enough, however, this steam disappears into the air almost immediately.

Since it causes the client's core temperature to rise, taking a sauna has the same physiological effects as any other whole-body heating treatment. These effects include peripheral vasodilation, increased sweating, increased oxygen consumption and relaxation of skeletal muscles. The heart beats faster and pumps out more blood with each beat. *(Continued on page 182)*

FIGURE 7.1
Sauna. (**A**) Therapist offering water to the client as he enters the sauna. (**B**) Client seated in the sauna.

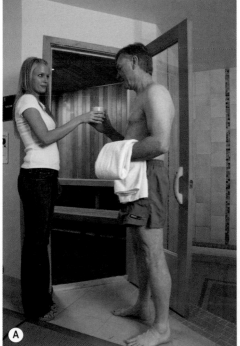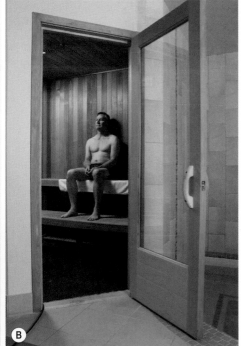

BOX 7.1	POINT OF INTEREST

HEAT MEDICINE: MEDICAL USES OF SAUNA

Emerging evidence suggests that beyond its recreational use, sauna bathing may be linked to several health benefits, including a lower risk of vascular diseases such as high blood pressure, cardiovascular disease, and **neurocognitive diseases** such as Alzheimer's and **vascular dementia**; in nonvascular conditions such as pulmonary diseases; and improvements in arthritis, headache and flu. The beneficial effects of sauna bathing on these outcomes have been linked to its effect on circulatory, cardiovascular and immune functions (Cardiologist Jari Laukkanen, 2018).

Sauna use may have unexpected positive effects on the body. For example:

- Since a study that followed 2300 Finnish men for 20 years showed that lifelong sauna use reduces the risk of fatal heart attacks, other researchers have found that sauna use (and other body heating such as regular hot baths) exercises the circulatory system in many of the same ways as aerobic exercise. As the body heats up, cardiac output increases and arteries stretch to hold the increased blood flow. One study found that cardiac output of sauna-takers increased by 60–70%, about as much as during a brisk walk, with blood being shifted from the internal organs to the skin (Husse, 1977). These effects carry over into everyday life, i.e. after regular sauna use (and in one study when subjects took 5 hot baths a week for 8 weeks), arteries dilate better and become more flexible and blood pressure is lowered (Brunt, 2016; Laukkanen 2015; Laukkanen 2018).

- Recent research has shown that diabetes may be treated partly by saunas or hot baths, as they may promote better control of blood sugar levels.

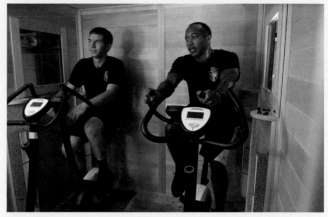

FIGURE 1

Fire station "Decon System" sauna. Immediately after returning to the station after a call, firefighters shower and pedal on the exercycles inside the hot sauna. Photo courtesy of SaunaRay.

Researchers hope to continue studying diabetics who have 15-minute heat exposures (saunas at 150–175°F (65–80°C) or hot tub at 104°F (40°C) three times a week for months (Krause, 2015). Philip Hooper, MD, found regular hot tubs helped Type 2 diabetics lower their blood sugar levels (Hooper, 1999).

- In some kidney diseases where fluid overload is a problem, increased water loss through saunas has been used to help the body reduce edema (Pyrih, 2003).

- Detoxification through increased sweating has been shown to lower blood levels of substances such as heavy metals and pesticides (see Figure 1), and drugs such as cocaine, methamphetamine and opioids. (For more on this, see *Detoxification treatments* on page 243.)

Note: Since research findings may be preliminary, observe all contraindications with clients!

Levels of noradrenaline double after 10 minutes, and remain elevated after a cold plunge and a 15-minute rest. There is a brief rise in blood pressure, which is then followed by a fall in blood pressure as a result of vasodilation. Blood pressure remains lower for at least one hour after a sauna: in one study, the systolic blood pressure of hypertensive subjects was lowered about 35 points (Hannuksela et al., 2001). Just how high the client's body temperature rises will depend upon how hot and how dry the sauna is, how long one stays in, and one's sweating capacity.

Body temperature may rise high enough that the healthy sauna bather can go directly from the sauna to an icy-cold shower, leap into a cold pool or roll in the snow, with no ill-effects from this sudden change of as much as 100°F (38°C) or more. At the South Pole, where temperatures can be extremely cold, the "300° club" has been formed by hardy souls wearing only their boots who run from a 200°F (93°C) sauna to the Pole itself, where the outside temperature is −100°F (−73°C)! The sauna's extreme heat warms the body's tissues so well that they are not damaged during their brief cold exposure, which would otherwise be deadly.

Many holistically-oriented doctors recommend intense body heating at the onset of a viral infection to make it milder or go away entirely. They believe that the higher temperature, like that which occurs with a natural fever, weakens or kills the infectious organism (Doub, 1970). A 1990 study found that individuals who took regular saunas had significantly fewer colds than those who did not (Ernst, 1990).

The body's metabolic rate increases significantly and then afterwards falls to slightly lower than it was beforehand. This is why very frequent saunas or other whole-body heating treatments are not recommended for someone with a hypothyroid condition, in which the metabolic rate is already too low (an occasional sauna is fine, however). Because saunas can cause profuse sweating, dehydration can occur unless sauna-goers drink extra water. Competitive wrestlers are notorious for using saunas to compete in a lower weight class by cutting back on water and then going into a sauna while wearing many layers of clothes and exercising: a wrestler can lose as much as 6 pounds (3 quarts; 2.8 liters) of water in several hours. Some wrestlers have died of dehydration from this dangerous practice. Therapists should be sure to encourage their clients to drink water before, during, and after a sauna. People who normally sweat frequently, such as athletes or those living in hot climates, tend to sweat more profusely, and regular saunas will encourage this as well. Anyone not accustomed to intense heat should be especially vigilant about not staying in too long.

Heat mobilizes toxic substances that linger in fatty tissues, so saunas have long been used for detoxification. For more on saunas and detoxification, see Case history 7.1 and Box 11.1

Below are some directions to give your client before entering the sauna:

- Do not eat for at least an hour before you go in to the sauna and do not drink alcohol beforehand. A combination of dehydration and alcohol consumption is especially dangerous: deaths have occurred when an intoxicated person lost consciousness in the sauna and then died of dehydration (Press, 1991).

- After vigorous exercise, first wait a few minutes so your body cools down before you go in.

- Drink a glass of water before entering the sauna and 1–2 glasses more during and afterwards.

- Stay in for 10–15 minutes, until you are perspiring freely, but do not stay too long. As with a very hot bath, when you have been in too long, you may get lightheaded or dizzy—people have been known to pass out! Leave the sauna immediately if you begin to feel that you are not tolerating the heat well.

- Finish your sauna experience with a shower as cold as you can tolerate it, and finish with one more glass of water.

SNAPSHOT

Air temperature Hot (145–200°F; 63–93°C) with only 6–8% humidity.

Time needed 10–15 minutes in the sauna plus a few minutes for a cool shower after the sauna (the client may do more than one cycle).

Equipment needed thermometer; two bath towels; drinking water; small towel wrung out in cold water to use around the neck for cooling (optional); grab bars.

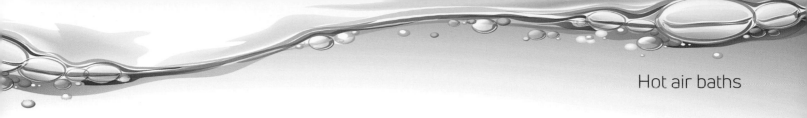

| A RESCUE WORKER BENEFITS FROM SAUNA TREATMENTS | CASE HISTORY 7.1 |

BACKGROUND

In 2001, 33-year-old Sean Donahue (real name used with permission) was a captain in the New York State National Guard. A healthy, highly conditioned athlete who also worked as a computer consultant in lower Manhattan, Captain Donahue was working near the World Trade Center during the attacks of September 11, 2001. He hastened to help out, arriving just as the building's twin towers went down, and he spent the rest of that day and the next searching for and rescuing victims. Everyone present was engulfed in deep smoke and airborne soot made up of such toxic substances as burning jet and diesel fuel, asbestos, benzene, dioxins, mercury, lead, manganese, fiberglass, silicon, and sulfuric acid. Donohue had no special protective clothing except an occasional paper dust mask, and so it was only hours before he began to suffer from breathing difficulties. He returned to his work as a computer consultant but as he walked blocks to his office every day, continued to breathe in small particles from the toxic cloud that had settled over lower Manhattan. Even the air inside his office was foul with soot.

Five days after the September 11 attacks, he experienced near-fatal respiratory distress and had emergency treatment at a local hospital. Over the next year and a half, he developed a variety of health problems, including shortness of breath, chronic cough (the most common health complaint of rescue personnel), sinus pain, severe stomach and chest pain, chronic nausea, vomiting, diarrhea, skin rashes, flashbacks, and an inability to concentrate. He failed a military physical and could no longer pilot an aircraft. By January of 2004 he was taking ten different medications without any noticeable improvement and was considering taking whole-body steroids as a last resort. However, concerned about potential side-effects, he opted to begin the detoxification program offered by the New York City Rescue Workers Detoxification Project.

TREATMENT

Designed to help rescue workers such as police, fire, and medical personnel excrete poisons, the program combined prolonged sweating in a sauna with nutritional supplements that support detoxification (Cecchini, 2006; Root, 2003; Donahue, 2006). Captain Donohue followed the same routine for 33 days: vigorous exercise followed by a 2–5 hour stay in a 140–180°F (60–82°C) sauna bath, with frequent breaks to shower and rehydrate. Detox personnel monitored all participants for heat exhaustion and dehydration. Donohue felt no major difference at first. Although his sweat was never highly highly colored (many rescue workers have had purple, orange, gray, blue, or black sweat), he did notice that his sweat had a very strong odor. Then, after eight or nine days on the program, he began to feel a dramatic improvement. His symptoms began to slowly decrease. For example, at the beginning of the program he was unable walk up a single flight of stairs; a few weeks later he could run three miles. His chronic cough disappeared and he was able to discontinue all his medications. He notes his medical treatment did not change in any way during the time he was in the program. Not only was he able to return to active duty and to pilot aircraft, but today he has no health problems, takes no medications, and runs miles each day. He has gone on to serve in combat zones overseas and to assist in the recovery efforts in New Orleans after Hurricane Katrina, and has been promoted to the rank of major (Donahue, 2006).

Effect Primarily thermal.

Cleanup Launder the used towels. The sauna should be cleaned and sanitized periodically according to the manufacturer's recommendations.

Indications General relaxation; warming of tissue prior to massage, stimulation of circulation; muscle spasms in the neck or back; arthritis pain; pain and joint stiffness in rheumatic disease; preparation for cold treatments; detoxification; onset of a cold or the flu.

Contraindications Systemic or chronic conditions, including cardiovascular problems, diabetes, hepatitis, lymphedema, multiple sclerosis and seizure disorders (note that these contraindications are the same as for any whole-body heating treatment); loss of sensation; great obesity; pregnancy; recent meal (wait at least an hour after eating); inability to tolerate heat; under the influence of alcohol or drugs.

Note Sauna manufacturers usually install a sign on their sauna doors stating that persons in poor health should consult their doctor before taking a sauna. Such a sign can serve as a visual reminder to the client and a reinforcement of the contraindications mentioned above.

Cautions

1. If a client experiences intense itching in a sauna (which is rare), he or she needs only to exit the sauna and the sensation will stop.

2. Frequent saunas are not recommended for those with hypothyroid conditions.

3. Anyone who is at risk for lymphedema due to removal of lymph nodes should avoid saunas altogether.

4. Drug patches should not be worn in a sauna as increased blood flow to the skin means that more of the drug will be absorbed. (For more on this, see Box 2.3.)

Procedure

1. Check with the client to make sure there are no contraindications for the sauna.

2. Explain the use of the sauna to the client and get their consent.

3. Turn on the sauna. It may take 15 minutes for a cold sauna to heat up. In an athletic club or spa, however, many saunas are left on all the time.

4. Have the client take a brief shower and drink a glass of water before entering the sauna (Figure 7.1A).

5. Have the client enter and stay seated for about 10–15 minutes (Figure 7.1B) until he or she begins to perspire or feel too warm. Have the client exit the sauna immediately if he or she starts to feel dizzy, lightheaded, fatigued or too hot. In other words, anytime the heat begins to be too extreme for the client, it is time to get out.

6. When the client leaves the sauna, the next step is a tepid or cool shower followed by resting for a few minutes in the cooler air outside the sauna. The purpose of the shower is to cool down between sauna sessions: if the client does not care to take a cold shower or plunge, use the coolest water that he or she can tolerate.

7. The client can then go back into the sauna room again for another cycle of sweating and cooling. The perspiration and then cooling cycles may be repeated a number of times, but never overdo saunas – 15 minutes is long enough to prepare the person for a massage session.

8. Have the client take a cool shower; then offer him or her drinking water.

HOT WET AIR BATHS: LOCAL AND FULL-BODY STEAM TREATMENTS

Like saunas, steam baths have such a strong appeal that over the centuries they have been made out of whatever materials were at hand, and steam has been created using energy sources such as firewood, coal, gas and electricity (see Box 7.2). Modern steam baths are rooms or small cabinets of different types which usually have electric steam generators that make steam and inject it into the enclosure.

Local steam baths

Cultures all over the world have used local steams for a wide variety of problems (for one example, see Figure 1.3). Medicinal herbs were often added to the water that was used to make the steam.

Local steams not only heated and moistened specific areas, but also used far less water and fuel than heating bigger spaces. Healers devised small containers that could enclose a painful part and then be filled with steam. In Bath, England, doctors used local steam to loosen "stubborn Joints"; in Germany Sebastian Kneipp prescribed foot steams for swollen, cold or diseased feet; while in the US, John Harvey Kellogg used jets of steam for headaches and pain, especially when an area was too painful to be touched. Today's aestheticians and barbers use local steam on the face to warm and moisten skin and to open the pores.

One local steam bath that is still widely used is steam inhalation. An ancient remedy for nasal and chest congestion, inhaling small droplets of hot water liquefies nasal mucus so that it drips out easily, and can have the same effect with congestion in the chest (Saketkhoo, 1978). Steam inhalation moistens, soothes and warms the entire respiratory tract. Blood flow is increased and congestion in the chest is eased. Viruses such as influenza A and the virus that causes COVID-19 thrive in cold dry air, and indoor air is very dry in the winter. Many researchers now recommend breathing very moist air

BOX 7.2	POINT OF INTEREST

WHAT IS A SWEAT LODGE?

A Native American ceremony of prayer, contemplation and purification, the sweat lodge is also a full-fledged steam bath. The ceremony is traditionally used as a ritual preparation before a hunt or community event, and as a way of putting oneself into balance (each tribal nation may have its own traditions). An elder (medicine man) who knows the ceremonies and native language runs the sweat. He is responsible for the mental and emotional state of those involved, and ensures that no one becomes too hot. He gathers about 12 people in the structure, which is usually made of willow branches and covered with animal skins or blankets. A firekeeper heats stones in a fire outside, brings the stones in, and carefully pours water over them to create steam. The temperature inside is hard to regulate, but averages about 150°F (65.5°C), and participants may be inside for one or more rounds.

Each round is roughly 15 or more minutes followed by a cool-down outside. The total time is about 60–90 minutes. A ritual of speaking or prayer may follow. The ceremony concludes with a cool-down, often with a cold dip in nearby creeks or lakes (Bruchac, 1993).

In 2009, a New Age guru James Arthur Ray, who was not Native American was responsible for the heatstroke deaths of three people and an additional 20 people were hospitalized for burns, dehydration, kidney failure, and heatstroke. Ray ran a pseudo-sweat ceremony in Sedona, Arizona, and made a great many mistakes. For example, no one was screened for health problems, the makeshift structure was greatly overcrowded, participants did eight rounds of 15 minutes each, people's complaints of sickness and faintness were ignored, and many became unconscious before the sweat was over. Ray received jail time for his actions (Wikipedia, 2019).

---

in winter to help slow viral spread (Noti, 2013; Sajadi, 2020) Traditionally, many anti-inflammatory and anti-bacterial herbs have been added to the water that was boiled to make steam, and some essential oils have been used to open nasal passages and discourage bacterial growth (Ivker, 2000; Shehata, 2008). A traditional self-care method is to boil water, pour it into a large heavy bowl, place the bowl on a table top, then sit over the bowl with a towel draped over the head so that the steam cannot escape. Steam is inhaled into through the nose and mouth, pulling hot moist air into the nasal passages and bronchial tree.

Massage therapists do not treat the common cold; during a massage session, however, local steam treatments can ease "cradle congestion" – a fullness in the sinuses and puffiness in the face that can occur when clients are in the prone position for an extended period of time. Lying prone may be uncomfortable for clients with allergies or sinus headaches, but breathing steam often makes them far more comfortable. To add steam to the face during a massage, simply place a small steam vaporizer on a low table directly underneath the face cradle. When it is turned on, it emits a fine vapor that wafts up the inside of the cradle to the middle parts of the client's face. This may cause the client's nose to drip, so be sure to provide her with facial tissues.

SNAPSHOT

Air temperature Hot (140°F; 60°C), with 100% humidity.

Time needed 10–15 minutes, as the client is receiving a massage in the prone position.

Equipment needed Small steam unit; low table on which to place the steam unit; disposable tissues; two face towels (one to be placed underneath the steam unit and one for the face cradle); wastebasket for used tissues.

Effect Primarily thermal.

Cleanup Have the client place used tissues in the wastebasket. The steam unit should be cleaned and sanitized periodically, according to the manufacturer's recommendations. Launder used face towels.

Indications Sinus congestion and facial puffiness caused by lying in a prone position on a massage table; sinus congestion from allergies or the sub-acute stage of a cold; sinus headache.

Contraindications Congestive heart failure.

FIGURE 7.2
Steam inhalation treatment on the massage table. (**A**) Placing the small steam unit on the table underneath the face cradle. (**B**) Placing the face towel over the face cradle. (**C**) The client prone upon the table, with his or her face in the face cradle. (**D**) Giving disposable tissues to the client. (**E**) Turning on the steam unit. (**F**) The client wiping off her face with the face towel.

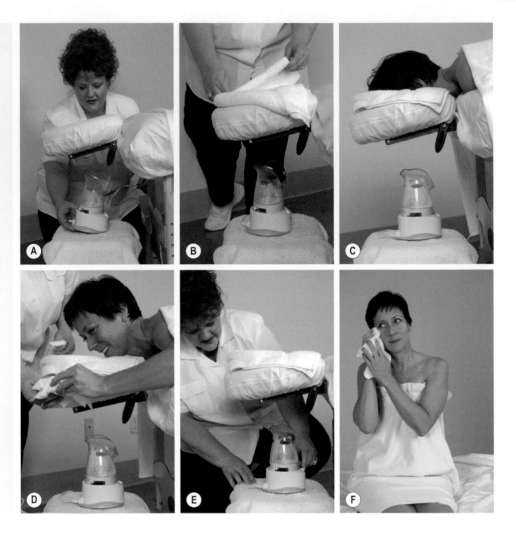

Cautions Some persons with asthma may be uncomfortable breathing hot moist air.

Procedure

1. Check with client to make sure there are no contraindications for the steam unit.

2. Explain the use of the steam unit to the client and get his or her consent.

3. Place a low table underneath the face cradle and cover it with a towel.

4. Place the small steam unit on the table underneath the face cradle (Figure 7.2A).

5. Place the face towel over the face cradle (Figure 7.2B).

6. Have the client lie prone upon the table, face down over the face cradle and steamer (Figure 7.2C).

7. Give the client disposable tissues (Figure 7.2D) and have a wastebasket available.

8. Turn on the steam unit (Figure 7.2E).

9. At the conclusion of the treatment, have the client sit up and wipe off his or her face with the face towel (Figure 7.2F).

Whole-body steam baths

A steam bath is designed to hold hot moist air and one or more bathers. Taking a steam bath involves going into the steam-filled space and remaining there for some minutes. Temperatures range within 105–130°F (40.5–54°C) and the humidity is 100%. This is the real difference between the steam bath and the sauna, where temperatures are much hotter (145–200°F; 63–93°C) and the humidity is lower (about 10%). Steam baths are at a lower temperature because when the air around you is saturated with moisture, your sweat cannot evaporate, so it beads up on your skin but does not cool you. (As noted earlier, breathing very moist air in winter may discourage transmission of influenza and coronaviruses.)

Both the benefits and the dangers of any other whole-body heating treatment apply here: the contraindications for steam treatments are almost exactly the same as those for hot baths, saunas, and even heating body wraps. Steam baths are excellent for relieving musculoskeletal pain of various types.

Many long-time hydrotherapists believe that our muscles become more relaxed with steam than with any other type of heat as moist heat penetrates deeper into the tissues and so heats them more effectively: the effect on skeletal muscles is similar to that of having moist hot packs applied all over the body. Seventh-Day Adventist chiropractor and nurse Louella Doub used steam room treatments for over 50 years as she treated a wide variety of musculoskeletal and other types of ailments. She found the "perfect relaxation" of the muscles achieved through steam was a great aid to successful treatment with both massage and manipulation (Doub, 1970).

You may wonder when a massage therapist would choose to use a steam bath with a client rather than a sauna. Since steam baths will bring the core temperature up more quickly than a sauna, they may be used if treatment time is at a premium. Other reasons to pick a steam treatment over a dry sauna: your client wants to prevent muscle soreness after a workout (moist heat is superior to dry heat for this purpose (Petrofsky, 2013)); you want to expose the client's skin to herbs or essential oils added to steam

water; your client simply likes the sensation of a steam bath more than that of a sauna; your client is getting over a cold but still has a lot of nasal congestion; with a steam canopy, no shower is needed and the client may be quickly washed off using a warm wet towel followed by a dry towel, and then proceed directly to the massage table. Unlike the client who takes a sauna, a shower is not needed.

Head-out steam baths

For clients who enjoy steam heat but dislike breathing hot moist air, one of the many modern head-out versions of steam cabinets would be a good solution. Canopies that fit over a massage table and box-like cabinets in which the client sits upright both leave the client's head out, but "steam" the rest of the body. Another head-out steam treatment can be performed with the hydrotherapy tub pictured in Figure 6.15. The client lies supine on a fitted plate, the tub lid comes down and covers the body except the head, and steam comes up through vents in the bottom of the tub. A **Russian steam bath** is another classic: the client lies on a tiled bench inside a small room with a hole cut for his head. Steam fills the room and bathes the entire body except the head, which protrudes out of the hole.

Steam canopies

A **steam canopy** is suspended over a supine client during a session (Figure 7.3). On the ground below the foot

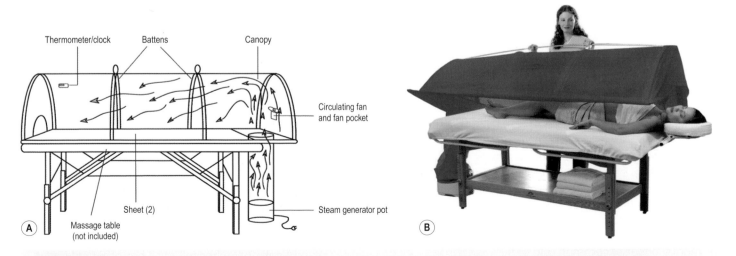

Figure 7.3
Steam canopy. (**A**) View inside the steam canopy. (**B**) Client receiving treatment. Courtesy of Natural Health Technologies, Fairfield, Iowa.

end of the table, a pot of simmering water creates steam, which rises into and fills the canopy. (Herbal teas may also be used.) The client can be completely or partially undressed. A thermal blanket may be laid over the canopy to speed up heating or to retain heat longer. The air temperature inside the canopy may rise as high as 130°F (54°C). Exposure to the hot wet air, if prolonged, will have the same effects as any whole-body heating treatment, as the client's core temperature rises above normal.

This is perhaps the simplest whole-body steam bath to give someone before or after receiving a massage, since the client does not have to leave the table. It is also far less expensive than installing a steam room, and it uses very little electricity and only a few cups of water. If you give the client a salt glow at the beginning of the session and then use the canopy, the client will begin the session even more relaxed and invigorated and his skin will be entirely clean of salt; in total, this helps to greatly deepen the effectiveness of the bodywork.

SNAPSHOT

Air temperature Hot (110–130°F or 43–54°C).

Time needed 15–20 minutes.

Equipment needed thermometer; steam canopy; pot of water to create steam; special sheets and one towel to cover the massage table (these generally come with a steam canopy as a kit); two additional towels to wash and dry the client at the end of the steam bath. Optional: a tray under the steampot to keep the floor dry, and a plastic tub under the table for wet linens.

Effect Primarily thermal.

Cleanup The canopy should be sprayed inside with a natural cleanser recommended by the manufacturer, then stood on end with a clean towel underneath it to air-dry. It must be completely dry before the next use. Launder used sheets and towels, and sanitize the plastic tub if used.

Indications General relaxation; warming of tissue prior to massage; stimulation of circulation; muscle spasms in the neck or back; musculoskeletal pain including gout, osteoarthritis, rheumatoid arthritis, sciatica, acute and chronic low back pain; sprains and fracture sites after a cast has been removed; preparation for cold treatments; onset of common cold or flu.

Contraindications Systemic or chronic conditions, including cardiovascular problems, diabetes if steam treatments are prolonged, hepatitis, lymphedema, multiple sclerosis and seizure disorders (note that these contraindications are the same as for any whole-body heating treatment); loss of sensation; great obesity; pregnancy; recent meal (wait at least an hour after eating); inability to tolerate heat; under the influence of alcohol or drugs.

Cautions

1. Very frequent steam baths are not recommended for hypothyroid conditions.

2. Anyone who is at risk for lymphedema due to removal of lymph nodes should avoid hot or prolonged steam baths (more than 15 minutes).

Procedure

1. Check with the client to make sure there are no contraindications for the steam canopy.

2. Explain the use of the steam canopy to the client and get his or her consent.

3. Cover massage table with special canopy sheets and a large towel, and put the face cradle in place. Put water in the steam generator pot.

4. Offer water to the client just before he or she lies on the table.

5. Have the client lie on the towel-covered massage table, nude or wearing a bathing suit, head resting on the face cradle.

6. Place the steam canopy over the client, with her head projecting through the open end.

7. Wrap a towel around the neck to keep steam from escaping and to ensure the neck does not touch the canopy fabric.

8. Turn on the steam generator pot and put the fan in its inside pocket.

9. Have the client remain in the steam bath for 10–20 minutes, an excellent time to massage the neck and shoulders.

10. Place a cold compress on the client's forehead when she begins to sweat.

11. To finish, remove the canopy and quickly wash the client off with a warm wet towel, then dry the skin briskly with a dry towel, working quickly so that there is no chilling.

12. The towel underneath the client will be damp and should be removed. First, have the client roll onto one side. Next, bunch the towel up against her back and finally have her roll onto her other side over the bunched-up sheet. Then you may easily gather it up and remove it. (For an illustration of how this is done, see *Cold wet sheet wrap*, page 224.)

Alternatively, the client can stand up while you remove the towel, then lie back down upon the table.

13. Cover the client with a dry sheet.

14. Offer water to the client.

15. Now the massage session may begin.

Variation Steam canopy for a diabetic client

A short stay under a steam canopy – 10 minutes or less – is acceptable for diabetics, as it will not significantly raise the core temperature.

Steam cabinets

A steam cabinet is a small outer case or box with a door. It contains a seat for the client, a hole for his or her head to protrude, and a port through which steam can enter (Figure 7.4). The cabinet walls keeps steam from escaping so it surrounds the client's body, except for the head.

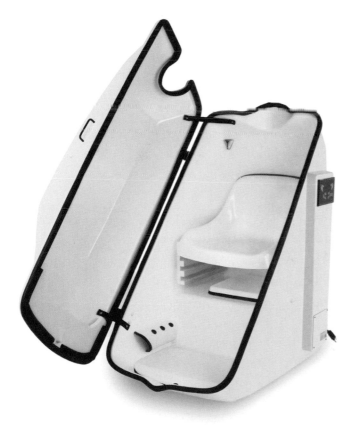

FIGURE 7.4
Steam cabinet. Note the steam generator at the base of the cabinet and the cut-out for the client's head. Photo courtesy of Promolife, Fayetteville, AZ.

SNAPSHOT

Air temperature Hot (110–130°F; 43–54°C), with 100% humidity.

Time needed 10–20 minutes.

Equipment needed Steam cabinet; three towels, to use on the seat, floor, and head opening of the cabinet; washcloth for a cold compress; two additional towels to wash and dry the client at the end of the steam bath; water for the client to drink. A plastic tub under the table is handy for wet linens.

Effect Primarily thermal.

Cleanup Wipe down the walls of cabinet with a natural cleanser recommended by the manufacturer, then dry them. Launder the washcloth and towels, and the plastic tub if used.

Indications General relaxation; warming of tissue prior to massage, stimulation of circulation; muscle spasms in the neck or back; musculoskeletal pain including gout, osteoarthritis, rheumatoid arthritis, sciatica, acute and chronic low back pain; sprains and fracture sites after a cast has been removed; preparation for cold treatments; onset of common cold or flu.

Contraindications Systemic or chronic conditions, including cardiovascular problems, diabetes, hepatitis, lymphedema, multiple sclerosis and seizure disorders (note that these contraindications are the same as for any whole-body heating treatment); loss of sensation; great obesity; pregnancy; recent meal (wait at least an hour after eating); inability to tolerate heat; under the influence of alcohol or drugs.

Cautions

1. Very frequent steam baths are not recommended for hypothyroid conditions.

2. Anyone who is at risk for lymphedema due to removal of lymph nodes should avoid hot or prolonged steam baths (more than 15 minutes).

3. Any water on the floor should be wiped up immediately.

Procedure

1. Check with the client to make sure there are no contraindications for the steam cabinet.

2. Explain the use of the steam cabinet to the client and get his or her consent.

3. Place water in the steam generator pot, with herbal teas or essential oils if desired.

4. Place towels on: (a) the seat itself; (b) over the front of the seat, so that steam will not burn the

back of the legs; and (c) on the floor where the client's feet will rest.

5. Offer water to the client just before he or she enters the cabinet.

6. Have the undressed or partially dressed client sit on the cabinet seat; assist if needed.

7. Wrap a towel around the neck to keep steam from escaping and to ensure that the client's neck does not touch the sides or the opening of the cabinet.

8. Have the client remain in the steam bath for 10–20 minutes.

9. Place a cold compress on the client's forehead when he or she begins to sweat.

10. After 10–20 minutes, assist the client out of the steam cabinet. Now wash the client off with a warm wet towel, then dry the skin briskly with the dry towel. Work quickly so that there is no chilling. A warm shower can be taken if one is available.

11. Have the client lie on the massage table, and cover him with a dry sheet.

12. Offer water to the client.

13. Now the massage session may begin.

Steam rooms

Steam rooms are enclosed rooms with ports through which steam pours in. Unlike head-out canopies or cabinets, the client breathes hot, humid air. Essential oils of eucalyptus or peppermint are sometimes added to steam rooms to help people with sinus congestion.

In a traditional steam room, the floor, walls and benches are tiled. Figure 7.5 shows one which takes advantage of steam from a stream that flows from a hot spring Figure 7.6 shows a traditional tiled style, but newer non-tiled steam rooms are now being constructed in a variety of styles and materials. For example, some steam baths are constructed of molded acrylic, and include built-in seats and a shower. Another type is marketed as a "steam capsule" and has clear plastic walls and a separate plastic chair. Electric steam generators located outside of the room make steam, which is then injected through a vent into the room. Essential oils can be added to special ports. Any bathroom may be turned into a mini-steam room: simply turn on the shower full force with hot water, and sit in the shower stall on a bath chair or, in a very small bathroom, sit on the toilet seat. Stay

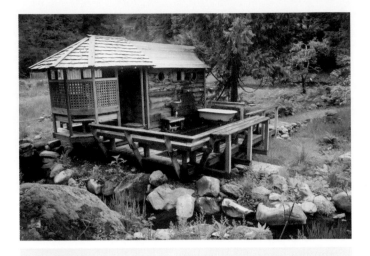

FIGURE 7.5
Natural steam room heated by a hot creek, with a bathtub outside for cold plunges. Photo courtesy of Breitenbush Hot Springs, Oregon, USA.

for about 15 minutes. Many family doctors recommend this for small children who have respiratory problems. (Over time, however, excess moisture in any bathroom may encourage mold.)

Below are some directions to give your clients before the steam room treatment:

- Do not eat for at least an hour before you go in the steam bath.

- After vigorous exercise, let your body cool down for a few minutes before going in.

- Drink a glass of water before the steam bath, and 1–2 glasses more during and after.

- Be aware that wet tile-covered surfaces can be slippery. Take a towel into the steam room to sit on. Then, when you are ready to get out of the steam room, move slowly, using grab bars if needed.

- Stay in for 10–20 minutes, until you are perspiring freely, but before overdoing it. As with a very hot bath, when you have been in too long, you may get lightheaded or dizzy-people have been known to pass out!

- Finish your steam bath experience with a cool or cold shower and another glass of water.

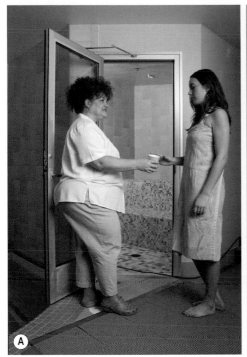
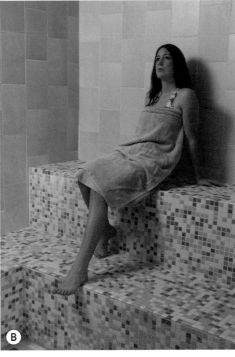

FIGURE 7.6
Steam bath. (**A**) Therapist offering water to the client as she enters the steam bath. (**B**) Client seated in the steam bath.

SNAPSHOT

Air temperature Hot (105–130°F; 40–55°C), with 100% humidity.

Time needed 10–20 minutes, depending upon the client's tolerance.

Equipment needed Air thermometer; bath towel; steam room; water for the client to drink. Grab bars both inside and outside.

Effect Primarily thermal.

Cleanup Clean the steam room according to the manufacturer's instructions. Public steam baths are usually cleaned and sanitized with products recommended by the manufacturer. Dispose of used linens.

Indications General relaxation; warming of tissue prior to massage, stimulation of circulation; muscle spasms in the neck or back; musculoskeletal pain including gout, osteoarthritis, rheumatoid arthritis, sciatica, acute and chronic low back pain; sprains; fracture sites after a cast has been removed; preparation for cold treatments; onset of common cold or flu.

Contraindications Systemic or chronic conditions, including cardiovascular problems, diabetes, hepatitis, lymphedema, multiple sclerosis and seizure disorders (note that these contraindications are the same as for any whole-body heating treatment); loss of sensation; great obesity; pregnancy; recent meal (wait at least an hour after eating); inability to tolerate heat; under the influence of alcohol or drugs.

Cautions

1. Some persons with asthma may be uncomfortable breathing hot moist air.
2. Very frequent steam baths are not recommended for hypothyroid conditions.
3. Anyone who is at risk for lymphedema due to removal of lymph nodes should avoid hot or prolonged steam baths.

Procedure

1. Check with the client to make sure there are no contraindications for the steam room bath.
2. Explain the use of the steam room bath to the client and get her consent.
3. Turn on the steam generator.
4. Have the client take a brief warm shower.
5. Offer her water to drink just before she enters the steam bath (Figure 7.5A).
6. Have the client enter the steam bath and remain for 10–20 minutes (Figure 7.5B).

7. Have the client exit the steam bath and take a cool or cold shower to bring the body temperature down and give a feeling of invigoration.

8. If the client wishes, she may repeat the steam bath–shower cycle.

9. Offer her drinking water.

10. Have her rest following the treatments, perhaps by lying down on the massage table if a massage session is planned.

CHAPTER SUMMARY

Hot air baths are beloved by clients and can greatly deepen the effectiveness of your bodywork. As you learn these hydrotherapy treatments in addition to those you have learned in earlier chapters, and indeed can even begin to combine treatments, your ability to tailor sessions to many different situations will continue to expand.

REVIEW QUESTIONS

Short answer

1. What is the main difference between saunas and steam baths?

2. How does the body respond differently to each?

3. How is blood pressure affected by a sauna?

4. A 70-year-old woman is making a first visit to a luxurious spa with her girlfriends. They each plan to receive a massage and then go into the steam room together. You review her health history and note she has had three minor strokes in the last few years. How do you explain to her that she should not join her friends for the steam bath after her session?

5. Explain the local effects of steam inhalation.

6. Why is congestive heart failure a contra-indication for steam inhalation?

7. Name three reasons to choose a steam bath over a sauna.

Multiple choice

8. Which of these does *not* use steam?
   A. Canopy
   B. Russian bath
   C. Scotch hose
   D. Cabinet

9. Three of the following can occur when a person is in a sauna too long. Which is the exception?
   A. Profuse sweating
   B. Body cooling
   C. More concentrated blood
   D. Exhaustion

10. Which of these is *not* a chemical application?
    A. Medicinal herbs in local steam treatments
    B. Soft aromatic woods of sauna wall
    C. Essential oils of eucalyptus and peppermint in steam room
    D. Herbal teas in crockpot of steam canopy

11. Which of these would sweating *not* cause? all but one:
    A. Dehydration
    B. Release of toxins
    C. Loss of fat
    D. Loss of electrolytes

12. Three of these are contraindications for whole-body heating treatments. Which is not?
    A. Pregnancy
    B. Muscle spasms in neck or back
    C. Cardiovascular problems
    D. Under the influence of alcohol of drugs

13. Which of these is not a reason to choose a steam bath over a sauna?
    A. To prevent muscle soreness after a workout
    B. When you want to expose the client's skin to herbal or essential oils added to steam water
    C. The client prefers the sensation of a steam bath over that of a sauna
    D. When your client is getting over a cold but still has a lot of nasal congestion

Chapter seven

References

Bruchac J. The Native American Sweatlodge: History and Legend. NewYork: Crossing Press, 1993

Brunt VE et al. Passive heat therapy improves endothelial function, arterial stiffness and blood pressure in sedentary humans. J Physiol 2016: 594(18): 5329–42

Cecchini M, Root D, Rachunow J, Gelb P. Chemical exposures at the World Trade Center: use of the Hubbard sauna detoxification regimen to improve the health status of New York City rescue workers exposed to toxicants. Townsend Letter for Doctors and Patients, April 2006, pp. 58–65

Donahue S. Personal communication with author. 10 October 2006

Donahue S. Testimony before New York City Council. From website of New York City Rescue Workers Detoxification Project: www.nydetox.org/results3.htm [Accessed November 2006]

Donahue S. Testimony before the New York City Council, February 2004. www.nydetox.org/results3.htm [Accessed February 2007]

Doub L. Hydrotherapy. Self-published manuscript. Fresno, California, 1970, p. 51

Ernst E, Pecho E, Wirz P, Saradeth T. Regular sauna bathing and the incidence of common colds. Ann Med 1990; 22(4): 225–7

Hannuksela ML, Ellahham S. Benefits and risks of sauna bathing. Am J Mcd 2001; 110(2): 118–26

Hooper PL. Hot-tub therapy for Type 2 Diabetes Mellitus. N England J Med 1999; 341: 924

Husse E. Plasma catchecolamines in Finnish sauna. Ann Clin Res 1977; 9(5): 301–4

Ivker R. Sinus Survival. New York: Putman, 2000

Krause M et al. Heat shock proteins and heat therapy for type 2 diabetes: pros and cons. Curr Opin Clin Nutr Metab Care 2015; 18(4): 374–88

Laukkanen T et al. Association between sauna bathing and fatal cardiovascular and all-cause mortality events. JAMA Intern Med 2015; 175(4): 542–8

Laukkanen T et al. Cardiovascular and other health benefits of sauna bathing: a review of the evidence. Mayo Clin Proc 2018; 93(8): 1111–21

Mason MP. Head Cases: Stories of Brain Injury and Its Aftermath. New York: Farrar and Strauss, 2008

Noti J. High humidity leads to loss of infectious influenza virus from simulated coughs. PLOS ONE, Feb 27, 2013

Petrofsky J. Moist heat or dry heat for delayed onset muscle soreness. J Clin Med RES 2013; 5(6): 416–25

Press E. The health hazards of saunas and spas and how to minimize them. American Journal of Public Health 1991; 41(8): 141–8

Pyrih LA et al. Infrared sweat secretion stimulation as a means of homeostatic correction in patients with kidney dysfunction. Fiziol Zh 2003; 49(2): 25–32

Root D. Downtown medical: a detox program for World Trade Center responders. Fire Engineering, June 2003, pp. 12–18

Saketkhoo K, Januszkiewicz A, Sackner MA. Effects of drinking hot water, cold water, and chicken soup on nasal mucus velocity and nasal airflow resistance. Chest 1978; 74: 408–10

Sajadi M et al. Temperature, Humidity and latitude to predict spread and seasonality of COVID-19 virus. arcj 05. 2020. Available at SSRN: ssrn.com

Shehata M. History of inhalation therapy. Internet Scientific Publications 2008; 9(1) https://en.wikipedia.org/wiki//James_Arthur_Ray_ [Accessed January 2019]

Recommended resources

Iwasaki A. Why is flu more serious in the winter? Yale University, YouTube Video, May 15, 2019

Pollock E. Without the Banya We would Perish: a History of the Russian Bathhouse. An extensive look at the history of the banya or Russian steam bath, and its important place in Russian health, hygiene and culture. Oxford University Press, 2020

www.cyberbohemia.com/sweatWebsite by Mikkel Akkel, the author of SWEAT, a book about his world travels to try different types of whole-body heating treatments. The website contains copious information on this topic.

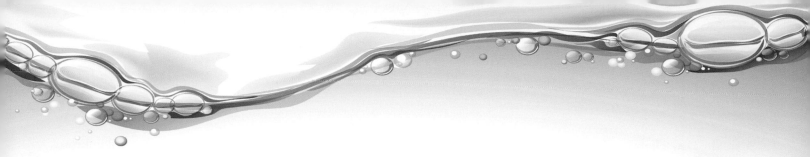

Showers 8

The healing time of practically any fracture can be shortened notably by the use of hydrotherapy as soon as the cast is removed … It eliminates the long periods of weakness, stiffness and partial disability that are commonly the sequel … Sprays that may be given in the shower have a distinct value especially in the later stages of healing. They may be hot or cold or an alternation of both. They may be strong or soft, needle point or of a flooding type. They may be given with a hose by the operator, or they may be manipulated at the shower head or regulated by the patient. The type suitable to the patient's condition and liking must be chosen.

Louella Doub, RN, DC, *Hydrotherapy*

CHAPTER OBJECTIVES

After completing this chapter, the student will be able to:

1. Name and describe different partial-body and whole-body showers
2. Describe the effects of partial-body and whole-body showers
3. Explain the cautions and contraindications for various partial-body and whole-body showers
4. Perform partial-body and whole-body shower treatments using the procedure included with each treatment
5. Give examples of shower additives
6. Give examples of how to use showers for various musculoskeletal problems.

Shower treatments can be applied to the whole body, using one or more showerheads, or to specific areas using handheld sprays. They can be used either before or after massage sessions, and as a home treatment for various musculoskeletal problems. They are useful for cleansing, for stimulating the skin and underlying tissues, and for various thermal treatments. Streams of water striking the skin stimulate pressure receptors and many people

find this sensation pleasant and relaxing, especially with warm water.

Many higher-end spas have specialty showers which are said to be invigorating and relaxing and to prepare the body for massage, so if you work in a spa you may be asked to use them. One example is a "waterworks" treatment, which consists of a hot bath followed by a Swiss shower and Scotch hose (illustrated later, in Box 8.2).

Showers can create different effects, depending upon the water's temperature, how much of the body is treated, the water pressure and how long the shower lasts. For example, a prolonged warm whole-body shower at low pressure (where water just falls like rain) will have a very different effect than a short, icy-cold, high-pressure shower, and a hot shower on the feet will produce a different effect than a cold shower on the scalp. The skin-stimulating effect of a shower can be increased by adding friction, for example by beginning a shower with a dry brushing, or friction under the water with salt or an exfoliating glove. The thermal effects of showers are similar to those of baths, in which local and reflex effects take place due to the application of water at a specific temperature.

This chapter describes a variety of showers and explains how they can be used to complement your massage techniques and benefit your clients. We will also explain how clients will benefit from using showers at home in between sessions. For example, a client who has an acute joint sprain, or who has just had a cast removed, can benefit from using a partial-body shower over the area of concern as many as three times a day.

One disadvantage to showers is that they may use a lot of water and consequently release more chlorine into the air compared to baths. A 10-minute shower will use 60 gallons (230 liters) of water or more, whereas a full hot bath uses only 30 gallons (115 liters). If you are using showers in your practice, you may want to install a shower water filter to eliminate chlorine in the air.

GENERAL CAUTIONS AND SAFETY

To make sure clients do not slip getting into or out of a bathtub or shower, always provide grab bars and a bathmat. Never let water puddle on the floor, and mop up any spills immediately. Be especially vigilant with anyone who is obese, walks with difficulty, or is unsteady on their feet. Clients in wheelchairs can take showers, but may require a transfer to a bath chair, and then a transfer back to their wheelchair.

General precautions to take when performing a shower treatment:

1. Never use showers directly over implanted devices such as cardiac pacemakers, pumps or infusion ports, or over open skin (cuts or wounds). While it is rare for a person to become burned from shower water, it can happen if your water heater's temperature is set too high. It takes less than 2 seconds for skin to burn from contact with 150°F (65°C) water! Most manufacturers recommend that water heaters be set at no higher than 120°F (49°C) and you should make sure this is the case. Those most likely to get a hot-water burn are the elderly, who might not sense water temperature very well or be slow to move away from it, and young children, since they have thinner skin than adults (Emam, 2017).

2. Water temperatures given in these showers should be followed as closely as possible, but always within your client's tolerance: if water seems too hot or too cold, adjust it accordingly. You can explain that when a shower is given over a period of time, toler-

ance to higher or lower temperatures will improve. For example, repeated cold showers make getting in a cold bath more tolerable (Eglin, 2005).

3. Water temperatures should be milder when a client has reduced feeling or numbness, such as can occur with **neuropathy**. Although temperature ranges given here are safe, use milder temperatures at first to determine how the client will react.

4. Keep the bathroom warm at all times and never begin a cold shower with a chilled client.

PARTIAL-BODY SHOWERS

Much like many other local cold or hot treatments, partial-body showers can be used to target specific areas. A prolonged icy-cold shower will cool one knee as much as putting an ice pack on it, and, like contrast leg baths, contrast showers to the legs can greatly increase blood flow. You might also recommend a hand-held shower as a home treatment for this simple reason: when recuperating from an upper extremity issue such as tennis elbow, wrist fracture, thumb tendonitis or carpal tunnel syndrome, carrying tubs full of water is not a good idea. Rather, the client can simply stand in the shower or sit on the side of the bathtub and spray the area of concern. Since it is almost impossible to immerse a knee or hip after joint replacement, or a shoulder after rotator cuff surgery, hot and cold sprays are better at targeting these areas.

Partial-body showers are also helpful in desensitizing areas such as healed fractures when the cast has just been removed, or incisions which are healed but still very sensitive. Over time, a cold shower over an area where there has been a crush injury can make that area less sensitive to cold. This not only makes the body part more comfortable but helps the client tolerate other types of tactile stimulation, such as massage. Shower pressure should never be painful, and must be adjusted to make a sensory impression without discomfort.

Head showers

A shower to the scalp is pictured in Figure 8.1. It can be used to relieve scalp muscle tightness and increase blood flow. It can be performed sitting down in a bathtub,

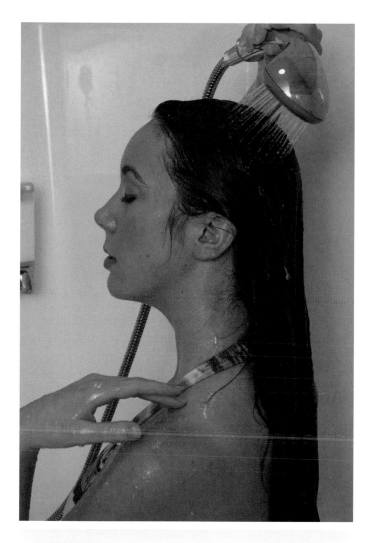

Time needed

- For hot head shower: 2 minutes.
- For short cold head shower: 30 seconds to 2 minutes.
- For long cold head shower: 5–10 minutes.
- For contrast head shower: 10 minutes: three rounds of 2 minutes of hot followed by 30 seconds of cold.

Equipment needed Water thermometer; hand-held shower; towel; bathmat; bathtub or shower stall; grab bars.

Effect Thermal and mechanical.

Cleanup Clean and sanitize the tiled area, tub or sink; launder the used towel and bathmat.

Indications

- For hot head shower: nervous tension; tightness in scalp; poor circulation in scalp.
- For short cold head shower: mental fatigue; poor circulation in scalp; as part of a contrast treatment.
- For long cold head shower: overheated client; migraine headache; tension headache. This encourages constriction of the scalp blood vessels much like an ice pack to the head (taking a long hot whole-body shower while rubbing the scalp with an ice cup has helped some migraine sufferers).
- For contrast head shower: poor circulation in scalp; hematoma on scalp after 24 hours; migraine headache; any other condition in which increased circulation to the scalp is desired.

Contraindications

- For hot head shower: migraine headache; acute bruise or other injury on head.
- For short cold head shower: none.
- For long cold head shower: chilled client.
- For contrast head shower: none.

Procedure

1. Check with the client to make sure there are no contraindications for the head shower.
2. Explain the use of the head shower to the client and get her consent.
3. Place a bathmat in front of the bathtub or shower.
4. Have the client undress or put on a bathing suit or spa wrap.
5. Turn on the water in the shower, check the temperature with a thermometer, and adjust

FIGURE 8.1
Head shower.

standing up in a shower, or with the client's head positioned over a sink (see Case history 8.1 for an example of how a head shower can be helpful). We include directions for giving head showers in a shower stall as well as over a sink.

SNAPSHOT

Temperature

- For hot head shower: 102–110°F (39-43°C).
- For short cold head shower: 55–70°F (13–21°C).
- For long cold head shower: 55–70°F (13–21°C).
- For contrast head shower: 110°F (43°C) alternated with 55°F (13°C).

Chapter eight

BACKGROUND 1

50-year-old Andrew was formerly a professional surfer in sunny Australia. Ten years ago he had multiple skin cancers removed from the top of his head, and a skin graft from his hip used to replace tissue that was removed during the procedure. Four years later, another procedure was performed by a plastic surgeon to stretch Andrew's scalp, using dozens of staples along his hairline to hold the stretched tissue in place. After this, his scalp, his entire head, and his neck felt tight all the time and he had frequent tension headaches. His first massage session with Jim was arranged because he had had a headache for two full days. Jim found Andrew's scalp was extremely tight and there were many areas of restriction around the scars left by the staples.

TREATMENT 1

Jim began by placing a hot pack over Andrew's scalp for 20 minutes while he massaged his neck and shoulders. He then used a combination of Swedish massage, ischemic compression and myofascial release on the head and face. Andrew then exclaimed that his headache was entirely gone, and his scalp felt better than it had since the first surgery. Jim recommended that Andrew relieve tension and increase blood flow by giving his entire scalp a contrast treatment every day. In this case the overhead shower was used so that Andrew could massage his scalp with both hands during the hot phase of the contrast treatment. Andrew still came in for a massage occasionally, but reported that the scalp shower with self-massage was often sufficient to relieve the head and neck tightness and especially helpful when he had a headache in the early stages.

BACKGROUND 2

Katrina, a 62-year-old retired bookkeeper, was diagnosed with multiple sclerosis (MS) twenty years ago. A determined and energetic person, Katrina continued to work and function fairly normally for many years after her diagnosis. As her MS progressed, however, Katrina's muscles became progressively weaker. While she still had full use of her upper extremities, she was not able to move her legs at all, and used a motorized scooter. For this reason, the circulation in her lower extremities was very poor. Her feet were often scraped when she transferred from scooter to bed, and becuase of the poor circulation, the scrapes sometimes became infected and turned into large sores.

TREATMENT 2

Katrina received a massage on a regular basis to release muscle tension, maintain range of motion, and improve local circulation, particularly in her legs. However, because almost all of her waking hours were spent sitting upright in her scooter and her legs were not exercised at all, the improvement in her leg blood flow lasted only a few hours. Her massage therapist suggested trying a daily contrast shower for her legs and feet and her physical therapist agreed.

A contrast shower was easily incorporated into Katrina's daily bath routine. Each morning, her caregiver helped Katrina transfer from her scooter to a bath chair that was placed in her bathtub and she then used a hand-held sprayer to wash herself with warm water. Her massage therapist, taught Katrina how to perform the contrast leg shower at the end of her regular bath, using 3 rounds of hot water followed by cold. After a few days of this routine, the color in Katrina's lower extremities began to improve, and the circulatory effect of the massage lasted much longer. Katrina's legs now stayed warmer, pinker, and more relaxed for a full day after massage, rather than for just a few hours. As an added benefit, although she continued to get scrapes on her feet from transferring, they healed more quickly and no longer became infected.

DISCUSSION QUESTIONS

1. How did the contrast leg shower improve the circulation in Katrina's legs?
2. What other hydrotherapy treatments could have been used to improve her circulation?
3. Why did the therapist recommend contrast showers for Andrew instead of contrast hot and cold packs?
4. What other contrast treatments could have been suggested?

the flow as necessary to reach the desired temperature.

6. Spray the client's head for the desired amount of time. If the client prefers, demonstrate she can spray her head herself.

7. Turn off the water.

8. Have the client towel off and dress quickly to avoid chilling.

Variation Head shower over a sink

1. Check with the client to make sure there are no contraindications for the head shower.

2. Explain the use of the head shower to the client and get his or her consent.

3. Turn on the water in the sink, check the temperature with a thermometer, and adjust the flow as necessary to reach the desired temperature.

4. Place a towel around the client's neck to protect clothing.

5. Have the client stand in front of the sink, lean on the counter, and lower the head so the shower water will end up in the sink, not on the floor.

6. Let the water flow over the client's head for the appropriate time.

7. The client's head and hair should be dried thoroughly.

Chest showers

A shower to the chest, such as that pictured in Figure 8.2, can be used to warm or cool the chest muscles, change local blood flow, and stimulate the skin over the chest muscles. Hot showers relax muscles for easier breathing, while cold showers stimulate breathing. An ice-cold chest shower activates sympathetic nervous system reflexes, causing the client to gasp and breathe more quickly at first, then breathe more deeply by the end of the shower (Keatinge, 1964).

SNAPSHOT

Temperature

- For hot chest shower: 102–115°F (39–46°C).
- For short cold chest shower: 55–70°F (13–21°C).
- For long cold chest shower: 55–70°F (13–21°C).

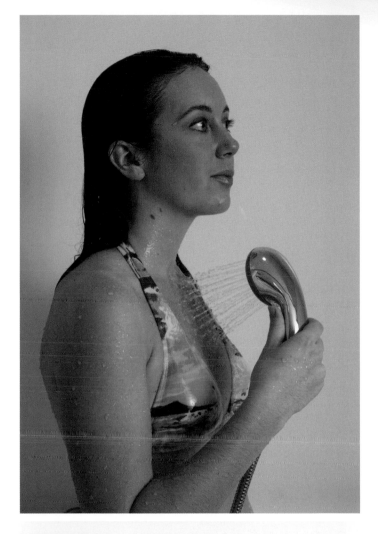

FIGURE 8.2
Chest shower.

- For contrast chest shower: 110°F (43°C) alternated with 55°F (13°C).

Time needed

- For hot chest shower: 5–10 minutes.
- For short cold chest shower: 10–30 seconds.
- For long cold chest shower: 5–10 minutes.
- For contrast chest shower: 10 minutes—three rounds of 2 minutes of hot followed by 30 seconds of cold.

Equipment needed Water thermometer; hand-held shower; towel; bathmat; bathtub or shower stall; grab bars.

Effect Thermal and mechanical.

Cleanup Clean and sanitize the tiled area, tub or sink; launder the used towel and bathmat.

Indications

- For hot chest shower: chronic tightness in chest muscles; soreness as a result of heavy coughing or vigorous exercise such as lifting weights.
- For short cold chest shower: low energy; after heat treatment to chest; as part of a contrast treatment.
- For long cold chest shower: acute rib sprain; acute chest muscle strain; sub-acute rib fracture (with a doctor's permission).
- For contrast chest shower: chest muscles that are strained or chronically tight; sub-acute rib sprain or healed rib fracture; trauma to chest, such as when a car accident causes the driver's sternum to hit the steering wheel or seatbelt compression leads to bruising.

Contraindications

- For hot chest shower: acute injury to chest, such as a muscle strain; cardiac problems; cardiac pacemaker; chilled client.
- For all cold or contrast chest showers: asthma; cardiac problems; cardiac pacemaker; chilled client.

Procedure

1. Check with the client to make sure there are no contraindications for the chest shower.
2. Explain the use of the chest shower to the client and get her consent.
3. Place a bathmat in front of the bathtub or shower.
4. Have the client undress or wear a bathing suit or spa wrap. A towel may be wrapped around the shoulders and upper back to keep them warm.
5. Turn on the water in the shower, check the temperature with a thermometer, and adjust the flow as necessary to reach the desired temperature.
6. Spray the client's chest, including the sides of the ribcage, for the desired amount of time. If the client prefers, demonstrate how she can spray her chest herself.
7. Turn off the water.
8. Have the client towel off and dress quickly to avoid chilling.

Abdominal showers

A shower to the abdomen, such as in Figure 8.3, can be used to warm or cool the abdominal muscles, to change local blood flow, and to stimulate the skin overlying the abdominal muscles. Hot showers relax abdominal muscles and cold showers can stimulate them.

SNAPSHOT

Temperature

- For hot abdominal shower: 102–115°F (39–46°C).
- For short cold abdominal shower: 55–70°F (13–21°C).

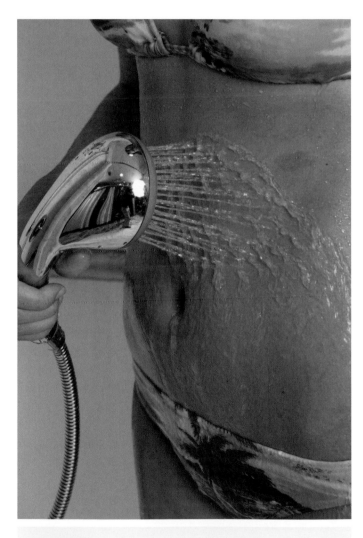

FIGURE 8.3
Abdominal shower.

- For contrast abdominal shower: 115°F (46°C) alternated with 55°F (13°C).

Time needed

- For hot abdominal shower: 5–10 minutes.
- For short cold abdominal shower: 10–30 seconds.
- For contrast abdominal shower: 10 minutes—three rounds of 2 minutes of hot followed by 30 seconds of cold.

Equipment needed Water thermometer; hand-held shower; towel; bathmat; bathtub or shower stall; grab bars.

Effect Thermal and mechanical.

Cleanup Clean and sanitize the tiled area, tub or sink; launder the used towel and bathmat.

Indications

- For hot abdominal shower: chronic tension in abdominal muscles; menstrual pain; to soothe abdominal area at least 24 hours after delivery of a baby.
- For short cold abdominal shower: atonic constipation; general sluggishness.
- For contrast abdominal shower: chronic tension or poor circulation to abdominal muscles; muscle strain.

Contraindications

- For hot abdominal shower: acute injury, such as muscle strain; recent abdominal surgery, except with a doctor's permission.
- For short cold abdominal shower: chilled client.
- For contrast abdominal shower: recent abdominal surgery, unless with permission of the client's doctor; chilled client.

Procedure

1. Check with the client to make sure there are no contraindications for the abdominal shower.
2. Explain the use of the abdominal shower to the client and obtain his or her consent.
3. Place a bathmat in front of the bathtub or shower.
4. Have the client undress or wear a bathing suit or spa wrap. A towel may be wrapped around the upper body for warmth.
5. Turn on the water in the shower, check the temperature with a thermometer, and adjust the flow as necessary to reach the desired temperature.
6. Spray the client's abdominal area for the desired amount of time. If the client prefers, demonstrate

how to spray the abdominal area herself, and allow the client to do it.

7. Turn off the water.
8. Have the client towel off and dress quickly to avoid chilling.

Arm showers

A shower to the arm, such as that pictured in Figure 8.4, can be used to warm or cool the arm muscles, stimulate the skin overlying them and change local blood flow. Hot showers relax the muscles, while cold showers can stimulate them. Although instructions are given for performing the arm shower in a bathtub or shower stall, a deep

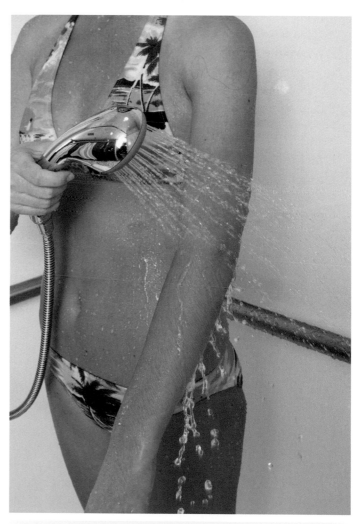

FIGURE 8.4
Arm shower.

201

Chapter eight

sink may be used, depending upon the part of the arm to be sprayed and the length of the client's arm. Although this is not as effective, clients may also stand in a whole-body shower and direct the spray primarily on the arms.

SNAPSHOT

Temperature

- For hot arm shower: 102–115°F (39–46°C).
- For short cold arm shower: 55–70°F (13–21°C).
- For long cold arm shower: 55–70°F (13–21°C).
- For contrast arm shower: 110°F (43°C) alternated with 55°F (13°C).

Time needed

- For hot arm shower: 5–10 minutes.
- For short cold arm shower: 10–30 seconds.
- For long cold arm shower: 5–10 minutes.
- For contrast arm shower: 10 minutes–three rounds of 2 minutes of hot followed by 30 seconds of cold.

Equipment needed Water thermometer; hand-held shower; towel; bathmat; bathtub or shower stall; grab bars.

Effect Thermal and mechanical.

Cleanup Clean and sanitize the tiled area or tub; launder the used towel and bathmat.

Indications

- For hot arm shower: aching or tired arm muscles after a workout or hand-intensive activity such as giving massages or doing carpentry; derivation in migraine headache; preparation for stretching arm muscles; chronic tightness in arm muscles; arthritic pain in shoulder, elbow or wrist.
- For short cold arm shower: aching or fatigued arm muscles; poor circulation in hands or arms; to stimulate tone in a weak muscle before exercises will be performed, as in conditions such as stroke, spinal cord injury or cerebral palsy (for more information, see the ice-cold footbath in Chapter 7).
- For long cold arm shower: aching or fatigued arm muscles; poor circulation in hands or arms. Unlike a long cold application to the chest, where the muscles are quite thin and cool quickly, a long cold shower to the dense muscles of the arms stimulates the circulation.
- For contrast arm shower: aching, fatigued or chronically tight arm muscles; poor circulation in arms and hands; edema of hands caused by pregnancy; hematoma of an arm muscle; muscle strain; joint

sprain after 24 hours; healed hand, wrist or elbow fracture, after cast is removed; osteoarthritis pain; aching or fatigued arm muscles from vigorous exercise; derivation in migraine headache.

Contraindications

- For hot arm shower: lymphedema in the arm; axillary lymph nodes removed; acute joint sprain; acute bruise.
- For short cold arm shower: Raynaud's syndrome.
- For long cold arm shower: Raynaud's syndrome; chilled client.
- For contrast arm shower: lymphedema in the arm; Raynaud's syndrome.

Procedure

1. Check with the client to make sure there are no contraindications for the arm shower.
2. Explain the use of the arm shower to the client and get his or her consent.
3. Place a bathmat in front of the bathtub or shower.
4. Have the client undress or wear a bathing suit or spa wrap.
5. Turn on the water in the shower, check the temperature with a thermometer, and adjust the flow as necessary to reach the desired temperature.
6. Spray the client's arm and hand for the desired amount of time. If the client prefers, demonstrate how she can do it herself.
7. Turn off the water.
8. Have the client towel off and dress quickly to avoid chilling.

Variation Contrast forearm and hand shower using a sink

This "shower" is especially helpful for clients who have repetitive stress injuries of the hands such as carpal tunnel syndrome or tendonitis. It is an excellent self-treatment for anyone who performs heavy work with the hands, and is especially helpful for massage therapists at the end of a day's work. Clients with lymphedema of the arm or Raynaud's syndrome should not try this. Use hot water at 110–115°F (43–46°C) and cold water at 40–70°F (4–21°C).

Procedure

1. Check with the client to make sure there are no contraindications for the forearm and hand shower.
2. Explain the use of the forearm and hand shower to the client and get his or her consent.

3. Turn on the water in the sink, check the temperature with a thermometer, and adjust the flow as necessary to reach the desired temperature.

4. Have the client stand in front of the sink and keep her forearms and hands under the stream of hot water for 2 minutes, all the while moving her arms so that the water stream runs from her hands up to her elbows and back.

5. Turn the water to the maximum coldness that the client can tolerate, then have her continue to move her forearms and hands under the stream of cold water for 30 seconds.

6. Repeat steps 4 and 5.

7. Repeat steps 4 and 5, for a total of three rounds of hot followed by cold.

8. Give the client a towel to briskly dry the forearms and hands.

Leg showers

A leg shower (Figure 8.5) can be used to warm or cool the leg muscles, stimulate the skin overlying them and change local blood flow. As they warm the legs, hot showers relax muscles and increase blood flow, while cold showers stimulate and vasoconstrict. Although instructions are given for performing the leg shower in a bathtub or shower stall, a deep sink can work if the feet alone are sprayed (special leg tubs can be purchased from spa suppliers).

SNAPSHOT

Temperature

- For hot leg shower: 102–115°F (39–46°C).
- For short leg shower: 55–70°F (13–21°C).
- For long cold leg shower: 55–70°F (13–21°C).
- For contrast leg shower: 110°F (43°C) alternated with 55°F (13°C).

Time needed

- For hot leg shower: 5–10 minutes.
- For short cold leg shower: 10–30 seconds.
- For long cold leg shower: 5–10 minutes.
- For contrast leg shower: 10 minutes–three rounds of 2 minutes of hot followed by 30 seconds of cold.

Equipment needed Water thermometer; hand-held shower; towel; bathmat; bathtub or shower stall; grab bars.

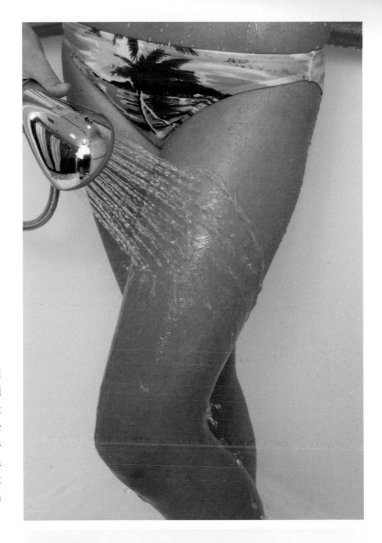

FIGURE 8.5
Leg shower.

Effect Thermal and mechanical.

Cleanup Clean and sanitize the tiled area or tub; launder the used towel and bathmat.

Indications

- For hot leg shower: aching or fatigued leg muscles from vigorous exercise; derivation in migraine headache; preparation for stretching leg muscles; chronic tension in leg muscles; arthritis pain.

- For short cold leg shower: poor circulation in the legs, shown by chronically cold feet and poor healing of injuries; to stimulate tone in a weak muscle before exercises will be performed, as in conditions such as stroke, spinal cord injury or cerebral palsy (for more information, see the ice-cold foot-bath in Chapter 7).

- For long cold leg shower: aching or fatigued leg muscles after vigorous exercise; to prevent delayed-onset muscle soreness after exercise.

- For contrast leg shower: aching or fatigued muscles after vigorous exercise; poor circulation in legs; edema of the legs and feet caused by pregnancy; hematoma of a leg muscle; leg muscle strain; healed fracture of leg bone, after cast is removed; derivation in migraine headache; chronic tension in leg muscles; arthritis pain. (For information on two studies which document the improvement in local circulation brought about by contrast leg showers, see page 253: *Partial-body tonic treatments*.)

Contraindications

- For hot leg shower: joint sprain during the first 24 hours; acute bruise; lymphedema in the leg; inguinal lymph nodes removed; peripheral vascular disease, including diabetes, Buerger's disease, arteriosclerosis of the lower extremities, and decreased feeling or numbness.

- For short cold leg shower: Raynaud's syndrome.

- For long cold leg shower: Raynaud's syndrome; chilled client.

- For contrast leg shower: diabetes, lymphedema in the leg; Raynaud's syndrome.

Procedure

1. Check with the client to make sure there are no contraindications for the leg shower.

2. Explain the use of the leg shower to the client and get her consent.

3. Place a bathmat in front of the bathtub or shower.

4. Have the client undress or put on a bathing suit or spa wrap.

5. Turn on the water in the shower, check the temperature with a thermometer, and adjust the flow as necessary to reach the desired temperature.

6. Spray the client's leg and feet for the desired amount of time. If the client prefers, demonstrate how to do this herself.

7. Turn off the water.

8. Have the client towel off and dress quickly to avoid chilling.

Foot showers

As you can see in Figure 8.6, it is easy to spray the feet. Using cold water on a regular basis can stimulate blood flow to the feet and diminish chronic coldness, or the feet can simply be sprayed with cold water at the end of any whole-body hot shower to prevent congestion of the head.

SNAPSHOT

Temperature for short cold foot shower 55–70°F (13–21°C).

Time needed for short cold foot shower 30 seconds to two minutes.

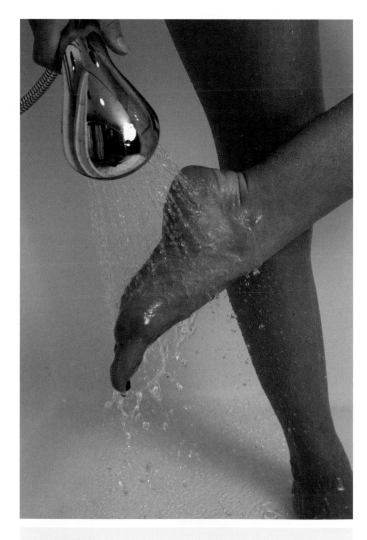

FIGURE 8.6
Foot shower.

Equipment needed Water thermometer; hand-held shower; towel; bathmat; bathtub or shower stall; grab bars.

Effect Thermal and mechanical.

Cleanup Clean and sanitize the tiled area or tub; launder the used towel and bathmat.

Indications Chronically cold feet.

Contraindications Raynaud's syndrome; Chilled client; Menstruation.

Procedure

1. Check with the client to make sure there are no contraindications for the foot shower.

2. Explain the use of the foot shower to the client and get his or her consent.

3. Place a bathmat in front of the bathtub or shower.

4. Have the client remove shoes and socks, then sit on the edge of the bathtub or in the shower on a plastic stool or chair.

5. Turn on the water in the shower, check the temperature with a thermometer, and adjust the flow as necessary to reach the desired temperature.

6. Spray the tops and bottoms of both feet with cold water for 30 seconds to 2 minutes. If the client prefers, demonstrate how she can spray the feet herself, and allow her to do it.

7. Turn off the water, then have the client dry the feet briskly, then don socks and shoes quickly to avoid chilling. She should not step barefoot on the floor.

Variation Cold foot spray to relieve congestion after a whole-body hot shower

After a hot shower, quickly dry the rest of the body, then spray the feet for 30 seconds only. Dry the feet well and put on socks immediately.

Underwater "showers"

As noted in the spa bathtub section in Chapter 5, using jets of water underwater in a special tub is a technique that mimics the effects of hands-on massage (**see** Box 8.2). It is thought to promote lymphatic drainage and is a popular technique in Europe for injuries, edema, sciatica, low back pain, joint contractures, arthritis, scoliosis and various types of paralysis.

BOX 8.1	POINT OF INTEREST

PRIMARY EFFECTS OF SHOWERS

Showers have a wide range of uses in modern medicine due to their primary effects:

Showers can warm or cool tissues

1. After surgeries in the perineal and rectal areas (for childbirth trauma, rectal cancer or hemorrhoids) patients often have pain and muscle spasms in these sensitive areas. Surgeons have recommended sitz baths to ease symptoms in the past, but many now recommend a hot hand-held shower which heats more directly and is therefore more analgesic and anti-spasmodic (Abcarian, 2018). Colonic spasm and pain are common during colonoscopies, but when warm water is introduced during the procedure, spasm, pain, and the need for sedative medication are reduced (Church, 2002).

2. In 2017, Finnish researchers at a chronic pain clinic tested the effects of cold showers for rheumatoid and psoriatic arthritis. A group of 121 patients took 2-minute cold showers twice daily for one week, then filled out pain questionnaires. Compared to another control group who received no showers, the cold shower group had significantly less pain and better quality sleep, and so cold showers are recommended as a safe home treatment option (Hinkka, 2017).

Pressure on tissues using streams of water causes them to deform and spring back, much like hands-on massage

This on-off pressure helps desensitize sensitive area such as sensitive scars and inflamed gums while improving lymph flow. Dental shower flossers use a stream of water to massage and stimulate the gums as well as cleansing them, and are significantly better than string flossing at reducing gum inflammation and bleeding (Barnes, 2005; Rosema, 2011). Known as "underwater showers" (see Box 8.2, Figure 1C), pressure sprays from hoses are used as a lymphatic drainage technique. Usually the trunk is "massaged" first, then any specific areas of lymphedema are treated next.

Specific water streams can clean better than other techniques

For example, a dental water jet (shower flosser) cleanses plaque and bacteria between the gums, and is especially favored by orthodontists for cleaning teeth and appliances (Goyal, 2013). Pressurized water sprays are used to clean steel surgical instruments. Water sprays are also used during routine dental cleanings. After hair transplant surgery, patients use a gentle spray with saline to keep wounds clean and avoid infection; and before all major surgeries, repeated whole body showers with antibacterial soap are considered the best way to keep bacteria counts down and avoid infections.

Moist heat during a shower hydrates tissues

Pediatricians recommend steamy showers to hydrate nasal passages and dry, irritated throats when children are suffering from croup and the common cold. In 2001, Viennese radiologists investigated the use of showers for skin care while a person is undergoing radiotherapy. Previously, standard skin care protocol was to keep the area dry except for a warm-water wash once daily, and to powder the skin as well. Instead, patients were put on a moist skincare program which consisted of cool whole-body showers – including the irradiated skin areas – three times weekly. No soap was used. Dryness of the skin and allergic skin reactions became less common, skin breaks and peeling were clearly reduced, and superinfections were prevented. Patients were more positive about the radiation and tolerated it better (Schratter-Sehn, 2001). By wetting the eyes, an electro-sprayer (warm moist air device) set up near computers helps reduce symptoms of dry eyes in computer workers (Matsumoto, 2006). As noted in the previous chapter, breathing very moist air helps discourage transmission of influenza, COVID-19, and other viruses, and hot showers are now recommended by some scientists (Isawaka, 2019).

Showers are soothing and calming

This effect is helpful for labor and delivery pain (Lee, 2013), postpartum fatigue (Hsieh, 2017), and agitation and aggression in persons with dementia (Sloane, 2004). Cold exposure including cold showers increases release of norepinephrine and beta-endorphins, the "feel-good" molecules, and fights depression (Shevchuk, 2010).

WHOLE-BODY SHOWERS

Whole-body showers such as that pictured in Figure 8.7 are a great addition to bodywork. While these showers can provide many of the same thermal effects as whole-body immersion baths, they are better suited for certain situations. For example, people who are physically disabled, obese, arthritic or have back pain usually find it easier to get in and out of a shower than a bathtub. In addition, showers take less time since there is no waiting while a bathtub is filled; showering can quickly remove massage oil, creams, or other products on the client's skin after a session; and the feeling of water striking the skin is relaxing and soothing. A warm shower can remove the client's topmost layers of tension before a session, or deepen the client's sense of relaxation after the session (see Case history 8.2). After a hot shower or sauna, a cold shower increases levels of cortisol, norepinephrine and other hormones, which may account for not only a prolonged feeling of warmth but mental clarity and mild euphoria. When done over time, these levels become even higher (Kauppinen, 1989). Some physicians even recommend regular contrast showers as part of a program to relieve depression (Kellogg, 1923; Nedley, 2001; Shevchuk, 2008). For more on this, see page 325, *Depression*, and Case history 8.2.

Hot showers

Many clients enjoy the sensation of a hot shower, either before or after a massage session. A hot shower can be

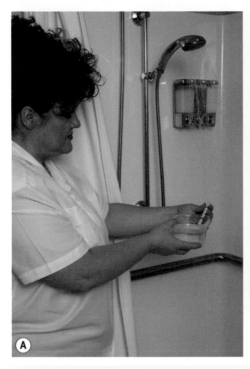 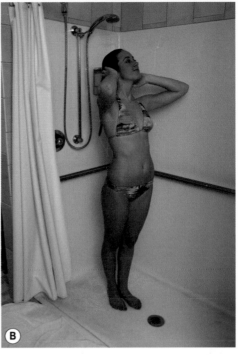

FIGURE 8.7
Whole-body shower. (**A**) Checking the shower water temperature. (**B**) Client in the whole-body shower.

"I HAVEN'T FELT THIS GOOD IN YEARS!" CASE HISTORY 8.2

BACKGROUND

At Wildwood Hospital in Chattanooga, Tennessee, daily contrast showers are given to a wide variety of patients, many hospitalized for serious health problems. Under the direction of the hospital's physicians, patients are given contrast showers whenever possible in order to stimulate their vital functions and speed recovery. Patients also feel better, which gives them motivation to stay on a new regimen (Qualls, 2006). Water temperature and length of showers are carefully tailored to sick patients, so that someone who cannot tolerate cold water may initially receive a mild contrast shower which alternates warm and tepid water. Bath chairs are used if there is any chance that someone might be unsteady on their feet.

TREATMENT

Robert is a former member of a motorcycle gang, now in his mid-fifties, who had a hard-driving partying lifestyle for most of his life. He was hospitalized recently because his health had declined dramatically: he is newly diagnosed with alcoholic **cirrhosis** of the liver and **ascites**, and suffers from abdominal bloating and pain, fatigue, great edema in his legs, loss of appetite, and nausea. He is at the hospital on a lifestyle-change program including diet, exercise and daily contrast showers. He moves slowly down the corridor from his room to the hydrotherapy department, where two male nurses assist him in getting into a gown and entering a multi-jet shower. First he is sprayed with twelve jets of hot water as nurses monitor his response. He does well, so after 2 minutes the water temperature is lowered and for 60 seconds he is sprayed with cool water from all sides. He continues to respond well, so the process is repeated two more times, with the final spray at a much lower temperature than the first one. He dries off, dresses and moves—more quickly now-back towards his room. An observer (the author) asks him how he feels, and a big grin breaks out on his face while he says, "I haven't felt this good in years!"

used to raise the core temperature, which can be useful anytime a client feels cold. One study found that both hot showers and baths raise the core temperature about equally, but since shower water does not completely surround the body, it needs to be 2°F (1°C) hotter than the bath water to do that. For this reason, people typically run their shower water hotter than their bathtub water (Ohnaka, 1995). Blood flow to the skin is increased as the body attempts to maintain the proper core temperature by throwing off excess heat (Charkoudian, 2003). As with other heat applications, hot showers reduce muscle tension and make connective tissue more elastic, both of which are helpful before massage. Shower additives such as Epsom salts, herbs and essential oils can also enhance a hot shower. For more on showers, see Box 8.2.

SNAPSHOT

Water temperature for hot shower Hot (102–110°F; 39–43°C).

Time needed for hot shower 5–10 minutes.

Equipment needed Shower stall with grab bars; water thermometer; bath towel; bathmat; exfoliating glove or luffa if extra stimulation is desired.

Effect Thermal and mechanical.

Cleanup Clean, sanitize and dry the shower, and the bath chair if used. Launder the used towel and bathmat.

Indications When warming and softening of the connective tissue of the upper body is desired before massage; muscle tightness; nervous tension; musculoskeletal pain, including arthritis, gout, dysmenorrhea, back pain, arthritis, neuralgia, muscle spasm, muscle tension, sprains, strains, stiffness, bruises and contusions.

Contraindications Systemic or chronic conditions, including cardiovascular problems, diabetes, hepatitis, lymphedema, multiple sclerosis and seizure disorders, loss of sensation; great obesity; pregnancy; inability to tolerate heat; ingestion of alcohol or drugs; recent meal (wait at least an hour).

Cautions

1. Anyone who is at risk for lymphedema due to removal of lymph nodes should avoid hot showers. Warm showers are fine for this condition.

2. Very frequent hot showers are not recommended for hypothyroid conditions.

3. Since long hot showers may strip the skin of some of its natural oils, moisturize right after a shower (this is easy if the client will be receiving a massage afterwards).

BOX 8.2	POINT OF INTEREST

SPECIALTY SHOWERS

Applying pressurized water to the body through showers, jets, sprays, and pours has long been an important part of traditional hydrotherapy. In Figure 1 (**A**), we see a Scotch hose or percussion douche, a very strong spray of water, applied to the posterior aspect of a man's body. Though there are many other specialized ways of applying water to the body, today's massage therapist is likely to use showers rather than jets, sprays or pours. Besides the standard full-body shower, given with water coming out of one showerhead above the client's head, a number of other showers may be used to perform hydrotherapy treatments. Such specialty equipment is often quite expensive and a waterproof room is needed, so these treatments are generally available

only in spas. In (**B**), we see a tiled shower with extra showerheads on both the ceiling and the walls. A Vichy shower is being given, with the client lying on a special waterproof table. Water showers down from a horizontal pipe that is positioned about 4 feet (120 cm) above the table and has many jets. Vichy showers can be given as hot, warm, cold, or contrast treatments.

In (**C**), lymphatic massage is being done with a special sprayer.

A Swiss shower (**D**) has multiple showerheads mounted in the shower wall at different levels and on all sides of the client, and sprays the entire body from head to toe. Swiss showers may have pipes in all four corners of a shower stall, with 8–16 streams of water coming from each pipe.

Box 8.2 *continued*

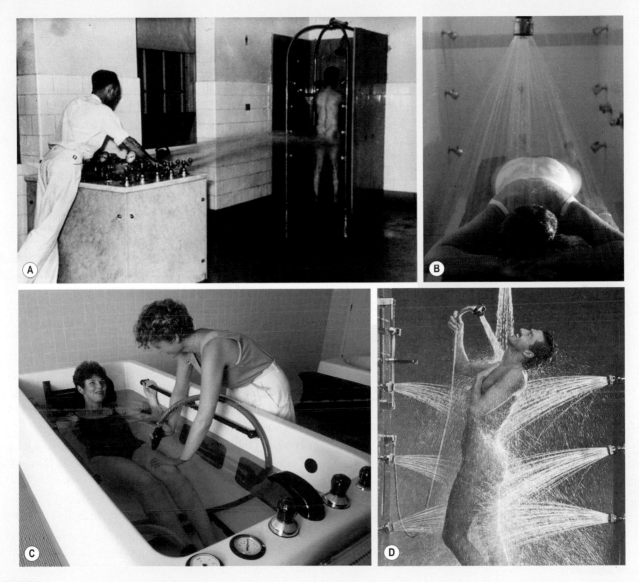

FIGURE 1
(**A**) Scotch hose or percussion douche to the back. Image from the History of Medicine, National Library of Medicine. Sourced from ihm.nlm.nih.gov/images 101447290. (**B**) Vichy shower. Photo courtesy of HEAT Spa Kur Therapy Development, Inc. Bonita, California. (**C**) Therapist administering underwater "showers" with a water hose. Photo courtesy of HEAT Spa Kur Therapy Development, Inc. Bonita, California. (**D**) Swiss shower. Photo courtesy of HEAT Spa Kur Therapy Development, Inc. Bonita, California.

Procedure

1. Check with the client to make sure there are no contraindications for the whole-body shower.

2. Explain the use of the whole-body shower to the client and get his or her consent.

3. Place a bathmat in front of the bathtub or shower.

4. Have the client undress or put on a bathing suit or spa wrap.

5. Turn on the water in the shower, check the temperature with a thermometer (Figure 8.7A), and adjust the flow as necessary to reach the desired temperature.

6. Have the client enter the hot shower (Figure 8.7B).

BOX 8.3 | **POINT OF INTEREST**

SHOWER ADDITIVES

1. Like a salt glow, whole body scrubs can be performed in the shower, using a variety of ingredients such as Epsom salts and powdered charcoal. Commercial products may include gritty ingredients such as cornmeal, ground almonds and coconut shells. Before using these, it is always wise to make sure such additives will not clog the drains or damage the plumbing. Generally, the client takes the scrub into the shower stall, wets down with warm water and applies it, then begins the shower. Absorption is increased when the skin is warm and blood vessels are dilated.

2. Special teabags filled with dried herbs can be placed in special showerheads with compartments for them: when hot water runs through the showerhead, an herbal tea is created which rains down upon the user and also creates aromatic steam.

3. To release essential oils into the air for a warm aromatic steam, add a few drops of an essential oil to a washcloth which is placed at eye level, or flick a few drops directly onto each wall of the shower.

4. Shower tablets, made with essential oils and inert ingredients such as cornstarch, baking soda or arrowroot powder, release essential oils into the air as warm water dissolves the tablet.

---

7. Have the client remain in the water for at least 5 minutes, so that her body is thoroughly warm. If desired, begin with the water temperature at 102°F (39°C), then gradually increase the water temperature to 110°F (43°C).

8. Have the client towel off and dress quickly to avoid chilling.

9. The client may now lie down for a rest or massage session.

Variation Using a hot shower to warm specific muscle areas (suitable for the upper body only)

Many stretching exercises for the upper body can be performed in a shower or bath after the application of hot water has relaxed a chronically tight neck, back, or shoulder muscles. See Chapter 11 for instructions.

Warm showers

Since they are relaxing, gently warming and cleansing, warm showers are suitable for many clients for whom hot showers are contraindicated, including clients with lymphedema and diabetes (Hermann, 1994). There will be a mild vasodilation of the entire skin surface. Rubbing the skin with an exfoliating glove or loofah can stimulate even greater additional vasodilation without using heat. Simply follow the procedure for the hot shower with cooler water (99–102°F; 37–39°C).

Warm showers are contraindicated for those with loss of sensation, great obesity, inability to tolerate heat, ingestion of alcohol or drugs, or having eaten a meal recently (wait at least an hour).

Graduated showers

Graduated showers feature water that is first hot, then gradually lowered in temperature. They are helpful for clients who have just had a hot bath or sauna, but are not hardy enough to tolerate a quick change from hot to cold. Unless they are long-time sauna or steam bath takers, most elderly clients will really dislike such changes! Instead, the temperature change is gradual. The shower begins with the client standing under 102°F (39°C) and then the temperature is raised even further (up to 110°F; 43°C). It is held there for 2 minutes, and then lowered by reducing the water temperature a few degrees at a time, holding that temperature for 1 minute, and continuing until the water temperature has been reduced to 80–85°F (27–29°C).

SNAPSHOT

Water temperature for graduated shower Begins at 102°F (39°C) and ends at 80–85°F (27–29°C).

Time needed for graduated shower 10 minutes.

Equipment needed Shower stall with grab bars; water thermometer; bath towel; bathmat; exfoliating glove or loofah if extra stimulation is desired.

Effect Thermal and mechanical.

Cleanup Clean, sanitize and dry the shower, and the bath chair if used. Launder the used towel and bathmat.

Indications Overheated client; gentle stimulation of the general circulation after a heat treatment.

Contraindications Systemic or chronic conditions, including cardiovascular problems, diabetes, hepatitis, lymphedema, multiple sclerosis, seizure disorders; sedentary or frail person whose blood vessels may not react well to cold; advanced kidney disease; loss of sensation; great obesity; pregnancy; inability to tolerate heat; ingestion of alcohol or drugs; recent meal (wait at least an hour).

Procedure

1. Check with the client to make sure there are no contraindications for the graduated shower.
2. Explain the use of the graduated shower to the client and get his or her consent.
3. Place a bathmat in front of the bathtub or shower.
4. Have the client undress or put on a bathing suit or spa wrap.
5. Turn on the water in the shower, check the temperature with a thermometer, and adjust the flow as necessary to reach 102°F (39°C).
6. Have the client enter the hot shower.
7. Increase the temperature to maximum tolerance, but no hotter than 110°F (43°C).
8. After 2 minutes, decrease the temperature by about 4 degrees.
9. After 1 minute, decrease the temperature by about 4 degrees.
10. Continue decreasing the temperature in the same manner until the water reaches 80–85°F (27–29°C).
11. Have the client towel off and dress quickly to avoid chilling.
12. The client may now lie down for a rest or a massage session.

Neutral shower

A neutral shower can be an effective way for a very tense client to relax before bodywork. According to John Harvey Kellogg, a 3–5-minute shower can produce the same calming effect as a 40–60-minute neutral bath. One scientific study explored the average person's sensitivities to the temperature of shower water and to changes in water temperature. Although a shower at neutral temperature produced no discomfort, most subjects preferred a warmer temperature; and when the shower was made hotter

than neutral, they rated their skin as warmer and the shower more pleasant (Hermann, 1994). This means the client must never be cold before taking a neutral shower and the bathroom must always be warm. In a hypertensive person, a longer neutral shower may lower the systolic blood pressure about 20 points. You may suggest a neutral shower to clients as part of home self-treatment in between massage sessions.

SNAPSHOT

Water temperature Neutral (92–97°F; 33–36°C).

Time needed for neutral shower 5–10 minutes.

Equipment needed Shower stall with grab bar; water thermometer; bath towel; bathmat; exfoliating glove or luffa if extra stimulation is desired.

Effect Thermal and mechanical.

Cleanup Clean, sanitize and dry the shower, and the bath chair if used. Launder the used towel and bathmat.

Procedure

1. Check with the client to make sure there are no contraindications for the neutral shower.
2. Explain the use of the neutral shower to the client and get his or her consent.
3. Place a bathmat in front of the bathtub or shower.
4. Have the client undress or put on a bathing suit or spa wrap.
5. Turn on the water in the shower, check the temperature with a thermometer, and adjust the flow as necessary to reach the desired temperature.
6. Have the client enter the neutral shower.
7. Have the client remain in the water for 5–10 minutes.
8. Have the client towel off and dress quickly to avoid chilling.
9. The client may now lie down for a rest or a massage session.

Cold showers

Along with the short cold bath, the short cold shower is perhaps the most challenging as well as the most rewarding of all hydrotherapy treatments. It was historically one of the hydrotherapist's most important tools in building strength in a weak or ailing person. According to John

Chapter eight

Harvey Kellogg, the shock of a cold shower set up a "perfect cyclone of nerve impulses, stimulated all general metabolic activity and increased the movement of lymphatic fluid". Regular cold showers build tolerance to cold. For example, one experiment began with eighteen subjects new to cold water baths or showers. To begin, they took two 50°F (10°C) cold baths while researchers studied their responses. Then they took six cold showers over a period of four days. On the fifth day when they again took a cold bath at 50°F (10°C), their respiratory and cardiac systems adapted better to the cold (Eglin, 2005). Traditional hydrotherapists always gave the patient a hot footbath, a period under a heat lamp, or a sweating body wrap first: patients even took their showers inside steam rooms to avoid chilling from evaporation and currents of cool air. In any case, the bathroom must always be warm.

Today we can use cold showers to cool overheated clients, to stimulate and tone their muscles and skin, and as a general tonic. Other creative ways to help your clients will soon occur to you; for example, a client with chronically cold and sore feet may try a hot bath followed by a cold shower followed by your hands-on work to address this problem. Unless a person is very hot, cold showers require a certain amount of discipline to endure, yet almost everyone agrees that the feeling of invigoration and warmth that follow a short cold shower is worth the effort.

Never give a cold shower to someone who is chilled: rather than being invigorated, the person will become even colder and certainly won't appreciate your efforts. If there is any question about their core temperature, warm the client first. Cold showers that are longer than 1 minute should not be given without the advice of a doctor. For more on the cold shower as a tonic treatment, see Chapter 11.

SNAPSHOT

Water temperature for cold shower About 55–65°F (13–18°C), ideally as cold as can be tolerated by the client.

Time needed for cold shower 1 minute. A longer shower may cause the client's core temperature to drop too low.

Equipment needed Shower stall with grab bar; water thermometer; bath towel; bathmat; exfoliating glove or loofah if extra stimulation is desired.

Effect Thermal and mechanical.

Cleanup Clean, sanitize and dry the shower, and the bath chair if used. Launder the used towel and bathmat.

Indications Overheated client; inflammatory arthritis; general feelings of lethargy or fatigue although the client has no health problems, such as in jet lag or insomnia; to prevent muscle soreness after vigorous exercise.

Contraindications Chilled person; Raynaud's syndrome; sedentary or frail person whose blood vessels may not react well to cold; very fatigued person; advanced kidney disease; great obesity; and because a brief rise in systolic blood pressure (about 18 points) will occur at the beginning of the shower, cardiovascular disease is contraindicated. Very frequent cold showers are not recommended for hyperthyroid conditions.

Procedure

1. Check with the client to make sure there are no contraindications for the cold shower.

2. Explain the use of the cold shower to the client and get his or her consent.

3. Place a bathmat in front of the bathtub or shower.

4. Have the client undress or put on a bathing suit or spa wrap.

5. Turn on the water in the shower, check the temperature with a thermometer, and adjust the flow as necessary to reach the desired temperature.

6. Have the client enter the cold shower.

7. Have the client remain in the water for 1 minute, towel off and dress quickly to avoid chilling, or lie down for a rest or a massage session.

Contrast showers

A contrast shower shifts back and forth between hot and cold water three times. The client will experience large shifts in blood flow as the body alternately "revs up" to throw off heat during the hot phase and then to conserve heat during the cold phase. Typically, clients who take a contrast shower report that they feel alert, invigorated and warm for a long time, much as clients who take a sauna, steam bath or other hot treatment followed by a cold shower or cold plunge. Athletes favor a contrast shower to prevent post-exercise muscle soreness after workouts, and migraine sufferers use them at the first sign of a headache (Buchman, 1994). Only the hardiest of clients can tolerate the temperature extremes of very hot alternated with very cold, so for a first time, begin with milder temperatures to see how clients react. If a salt glow or dry brushing is performed first the client will experience an even deeper sense of invigoration and wellbeing. This treatment is generally more suitable after a massage session rather than before one, because the client will feel wide awake and stimulated, rather than in the mood to relax.

SNAPSHOT

Water temperature Hot (102–110°F; 39–43°C) alternated with cold (65°F; 19°C or less).

Time needed for contrast shower 10 minutes.

Equipment needed Shower stall with grab bar; water thermometer; bath towel; bathmat; exfoliating glove or loofah if extra stimulation is desired.

Effect Thermal and mechanical.

Cleanup Clean, sanitize and dry the shower, and the bath chair if used. Launder the used towel and bathmat.

Indications Stimulation of blood flow to the skin; general feelings of lethargy or fatigue although the client has no health problems, such as in jet lag and insomnia; prevention of soreness after vigorous exercise; to prevent development of a migraine headache; as a tonic (see Chapter 11); as a finish for other hydrotherapy treatments.

Contraindications Systemic or chronic conditions, including cardiovascular problems, diabetes, hepatitis, lymphedema, advanced kidney disease, multiple sclerosis, seizure disorders; loss of sensation; great obesity; pregnancy; inability to tolerate heat; ingestion of alcohol or drugs; recent meal (wait at least an hour); chilled person; sedentary or frail person whose blood vessels may not react well to cold; very fatigued person. Frequent contrast showers are not recommended for hyperthyroid conditions.

Procedure

1. Check with the client to make sure there are no contraindications for the contrast shower.
2. Explain the use of the contrast shower to the client and get her consent.
3. Place a bathmat in front of the bathtub or shower.
4. Have the client undress or put on a bathing suit or spa wrap.
5. Turn on the water in the shower, check the temperature with a thermometer, and adjust the flow as necessary to reach the desired temperature.
6. Have the client enter the hot shower and remain for 2–5 minutes, until she is thoroughly warmed.
7. Change the water temperature to cold for 30 seconds to 1 minute.
8. Change the water temperature back to hot for 2 minutes.
9. Change the water temperature to cold for 30 seconds to 1 minute.
10. Change the water temperature back to hot for 2 minutes.
11. Change the water temperature to cold for 30 seconds to 1 minute.
12. Have the client towel off and dress quickly to avoid chilling.
13. The client may now lie down for a rest or a massage session, if desired, but often she will feel invigorated, not relaxed, so after a session would be ideal.

CHAPTER SUMMARY

Showers are simple and practical ways to cleanse and stimulate the skin and tissues underneath, incorporate herbs, salts and essential oils into a session, and target specific musculoskeletal problems. Clients enjoy showers and the variety they can bring to sessions, and showers are a great addition to any home self-care program. You can also combine showers with other hydrotherapy treatments: for example, in the next chapter you will learn how to combine a whole-body salt glow with a whole-body shower.

REVIEW QUESTIONS

Short answer

1. How can the mechanical effect of a shower be increased without altering the water temperature or force?

2. Explain how to adjust water pressure for an area that needs extra tactile stimulation.

3. Explain the effects upon the client's circulation of whole-body showers of different temperatures.

4. Describe and explain the effects of a hot chest shower on sore, tight or aching chest muscles.

5. Explain why a contrast arm shower is contraindicated for a client with Raynaud's syndrome.

6. Describe three different methods of incorporating salts, herbs or essential oils into a warm or hot shower.

True/False

7. True/False — Whether they are targeted to a specific area or to the entire body, showers have the same effect.

8. True/False — A hot leg and foot shower can be used to treat a migraine due to its derivative effect.

9. True/False — A cold head shower can be used to treat a migraine headache due to its vasoconstricting effect.

10. True/False — Older clients enjoy very cold showers.

11. True/False — A neutral shower can have the same calming effect as a neutral bath.

12. True/False — A graduated shower consists of hot water alternated with cold water.

13. True/False — Contrast showers make clients relaxed and sleepy.

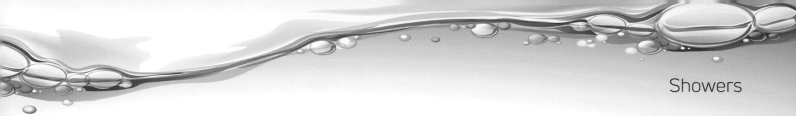

References

Abcarian H. Instead of a sitz bath use a detachable shower head. Dis Colon Rectum 2018 Oct; 61(10)

Barnes CM et al. Comparison of irrigation to floss as an adjunct to tooth brushing: effect on bleeding, gingivitis, and supragingival plaque. J Clin Dent 2005; 16(3): 71–7

Charkoudian N. Skin blood flow in adult human thermoregulation: how it works, when it does not, and why. Mayo Clin Proc. 2003; 78: 603–12

Church JM. Warm water irrigation for dealing with spasm during colonoscopy: simple, inexpensive, and effective. Gastrointest Endosc 2002 Nov; 56(5): 672–4

Eglin KCM. Repeated cold showers as a method of habituating humans to the intial responses to cold water immersion. Eur J Appl Physiol 2005 Mar; 93(5–6): 624–0

Emam A et al. Scald burn injuries caused by showers among the adult population in the southwest region. J Burn Care Res. 2017 Jul/Aug; 38(4)

Goyal CR et al. Evaluation of the plaque removal efficacy of a water flosser compared to string floss in adults after a single use. J Clin Dent 2013; 24(2): 37–42

Hermann C, Candas V, Hoeft A et al. Humans under showers: thermal sensitivity, thermoneutral sensations, and comfort estimates. Physiol Behav 1994 Nov; 56(5): 1003–8

Hinkka H et al. Effects of cold mist shower on patients with inflammatory arthritis: a crossover controlled clinical trial. Scand J. Rheumatol 2017 May; 46(3); 206–9

Hsieh CH et al. Efficacy of warm showers on postpartum fatigue among vaginal-birth Taiwanese women: a quasi-experimental design. Res Theory Nurs Pract. 2017 May 1; 31(2): 96–106

Kaupinnen K et al. Some endocrine responses to sauna, shower and ice water immersion. Arctic Med Res 1989; 48(3): 131–9

Keatinge W et al. Cardiovascular responses to ice cold showers. J Appl Physiol 1964; 19: 1145–50

Kellogg JH. Rational Hydrotherapy. Battle Creek, MI: Modern Medicine Publishing Company, 1923, p. 381

Lee SL et al. Efficacy of warm showers on labor pain and birth experiences during the first labor stage. J Obstet Gynecol Neonatal Nurs 2013; 42(1): 19–28

Doub L. Fresno, CA; 1971, self-published manuscript

Matsumoto Y, Dogru M, Goto E et al. Efficacy of a new warm moist air device on tear functions of patients with simple meibomian gland dysfunction. Cornea 2006; 25: 644–50

Nedley N. Depression: a Way Out. Tulsa, OK: Nedley Publishing, 2001

Ohnaka T, Tochhara Y, Kubo M et al. Physiological responses to standing showers, sitting showers, and sink baths. Appl Human Sci 1995 Sep; 14(5): 235–9

Rosema NA, Hennequin-Hoenderdos NL, Berchier CE et al. The effect of different interdental cleaning devices on gingival bleeding. J Int Acad Periodontol 2011; 13(1): 2–10

Qualls E. Director of Hydrotherapy Department, Wildwood Hospital. Personal communication with the author, 1 December 2006

Schratter-Sehn AU et al. Improvement of skin care during radiotherapy. 2001 Feb; 24(1): 44–6

Shevchuk N. How to Get Smarter. Createspace Publishing, 2010

Shevchuk NA. Adapted cold shower as a potential treatment for depression. Med Hypotheses 2008; 70(5): 995–1001

Sloane PD et al. Effect of person-centered showering and the towel bath on bathing-associated aggression, agitation, and discomfort in nursing home residents with dementia: a randomized, controlled trial. J AM Geriatr Soc 2004 Nov; 52

Recommended resources

Buchman D. The Complete Book of Water Healing. New York; Instant Improvement, Inc. 1994, p. 206

Thrash A. Nature's Healing Practices: A Natural Remedies Encyclopedia. Fort Ogelthorpe, GA: TEACH Services Publishing, 2015

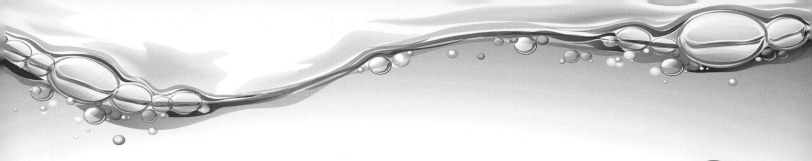

Body wraps 9

The wet sheet pack is one of the most useful of hydrotherapeutic procedures, as it combines at once very powerful effects, great convenience and universality of application, and remarkable flexibility to suit different pathological conditions.

John Harvey Kellogg, *Rational Hydrotherapy*

CHAPTER OBJECTIVES

After completing this chapter, the student will be able to:

1. Describe wet and dry blanket wraps, a cold wet sheet pack, and a leg-only wrap
2. Explain the cautions and contraindications for all wraps
3. Describe the effects of each of four different wraps
4. Perform various wraps, using the procedure included with each treatment
5. Explain how additives may be used with wraps.

Body wraps are a soothing, inexpensive and practical treatment which can deepen the effectiveness of body-work. They can be used for various therapeutic purposes, as they require no elaborate hydrotherapy equipment, are easily incorporated into a massage therapy setting. Although multiple layers need to be assembled, once wraps are in place many clients enjoy the sensations of warmth and snugness (see Box 9.1).

When might you choose to give a wrap? For clients who are chilled or anxious or who need to let go of chronic holding patterns before their hands-on work, a wrap is a great beginning to a session. Elderly clients who are too stiff or too fragile to get in and out of a tub or shower can be cocooned and warmed effectively. To prepare for deep work on the legs, clients can absorb additives for inflammation, pain or relaxation through a leg wrap while

they receive upper body massage. Finally, for those clients who would like to spend quiet time warm and snug as they absorb the full effects of their hands-on work, a wrap is a great ending to a session. Historically, the wet sheet wrap was used for more dire situations such as severe toxicity from drug and alcohol addiction, mental problems and infectious illnesses (for more information, see Box 9.1). It continues to be widely used today by naturopathic doctors.

Simple blanket wraps are common at hot springs resorts, after a warm soak and before massage; while specialized wraps combining various substances are popular in higher-end spas. For our purposes, wrap additives for specific conditions such as fatigue, joint pain, muscle soreness, dry skin and body toxicity are more useful (see Box 9.2).

Although some healthcare professionals may think wraps are old-fashioned, the use of wraps is currently being rediscovered for specific medical situations. For example, heating wraps are used with cancer patients at the Center for Hyperthermia Cancer Treatment at the University of Texas Health Science Center in Houston. Since higher body temperatures can stimulate the immune system and weaken cancer cells, clinical trials are currently testing whether radiation or chemotherapy treatments may be more effective when patients are heated during treatment. At the Center, heat lamps are used to raise core temperatures to 104°F (40°C) during infusions. The patient is then "wrapped like a mummy" in a cotton flannel blanket and a space blanket, while fluid is given intravenously to avoid dehydration. Patients are finally uncovered after six hours, given a complete washing with

| BOX 9.1 | POINT OF INTEREST |

SNUG AS A BUG IN A RUG: THE CALMING EFFECT OF BODY WRAPS

Note: there are exceptions to every rule, so before giving a body wrap always ask your client if he or she is claustrophobic!

Firm pressure applied to both sides of the body at once activates what is known as the **skin pressure-vegetative reflex.** This reflex response results in many signs of relaxation and calming: for example, muscle tone is lower, the heart beats more slowly and there are fewer signs of an overly active sympathetic nervous system. Researchers have found that subjects who had firm pressure applied on both sides of the body startled less in response to loud noises. Not only is firm pressure calming, but the larger the body's surface area is involved, the more calming it is (Takagi, 1955). In the infant massage world, we know that light, tickling strokes are more stimulating to babies than slow, firm compressions. Firm holding and hugging are calming to babies, and they are calmer and sleep better when swaddled (Van Sleuwen, 2007). Older children with sleeping problems often do better inside a snug mummy sleeping bag. Deep pressure stimulation, such as being rolled up in a gym mat, helps to decrease tactile defensiveness and to calm children who are hyperactive or have psychiatric disorders (Ayres, 1981). Autistic children will often seek out deep pressure sensations such as sleeping under heavy or very tightly tucked-in blankets. Scientist Temple Grandin, who has autism, used to crawl under sofa cushions when she was small and have her sister sit on them, and she later invented a "squeeze machine" for autistic people (Grandin, 1992). Therapeutic body wraps are so helpful for autistic children with self-injurious behavior, and for highly anxious mentally ill patients, that they may be used as an alternative to medications for aggressive or irritable behavior (Delion, 2018; Opsommer, 2016). Wraps are such a universally calming intervention that one psychiatrist has proposed everyone learn how to use them, in order to reduce their own stress response when they experience negative emotions (Sato, 2015). As discussed in Chapter 1, wraps were once a common intervention for patients in psychiatric hospitals.

| BOX 9.2 | POINT OF INTEREST |

BODY WRAP ADDITIVES

Over the centuries, countless ingredients have been incorporated into body wraps, including herbal solutions, seawater, essential oils, muds, clays, salts and fatty oils. Foods such as fruits, vegetables, vinegar, seaweeds and honey are always popular additions. Body wraps for cosmetic purposes, such as looking younger, breaking up cellulite, losing weight and improving the skin's appearance are popular at many spas. Since most of these wraps are not intended for musculoskeletal issues and can be very messy and time-consuming they are not really helpful to a bodyworker who is performing therapeutic massage. However, here are examples of a few simple wraps incorporating additives that can be useful for our clients:

- *Aromatherapy wraps:* About 10 drops of essential oil are added to wrap water. A typical wrap for **fibromyalgia** incorporates juniper, camphor and citrus oils.
- *Herbal tea wraps:* About 5 teabags are steeped in very hot water, then this tea is added to wrap water. A typical wrap for relaxation uses chamomile teabags.
- *Wraps from food ingredients:* Powdered foods such as oatmeal, milk, honey or aloe vera gel are added to the wrap water. A typical wrap for dry or irritated skin uses all four ingredients.

warm water, and left to cool until their body temperature returns to normal (US National Library of Medicine, 2006; Wust, 2002; Scott, 2006). Academic centers in other countries are researching similar thermal body wrap treatments for cancer. Princeton University's *Outdoor Action Guide to Hypothermia and Cold Weather Injuries* recommends a different body wrap as the most effective way to treat hypothermia (Curtis, 2019). First, heat sources such as hot water bottles or chemical hot packs are placed over the body's major arteries – at the neck for the carotid, the armpits for the brachial, the groin for the femoral, and the palms of the hands for the arterial arch. Next, the lightly clothed person is completely wrapped in a space blanket so no heat can escape. Blood is warmed as it flows by the warmers inside the pack and then heats the entire body, while the blanket wrap prevents loss of this precious warmth through radiation. Still another use for a wrap is to calm anxious, agitated or aggressive people. Therapeutic body wraps are extremely calming both for severely autistic children with self-injurious behavior and for highly anxious mentally ill patients. A Therapeutic Wrap Study Group in France has concluded that they are an excellent alternative to medications for aggressive or irritable behavior (Delion, 2018). (For a video from this study, see the *Recommended resources* on page 229. See also Box 1.3.)

Four body wraps suitable for massage sessions are included in this chapter: moist and dry blanket wraps, a cold wet sheet wrap, and a legs-only wrap.

MOIST BLANKET WRAPS

As seen in Figure 9.1, this wrap is essentially a hot compress for the entire body (see also Case history 9.1). A cotton blanket wrung out in 110°F (43°C) water is wrapped around the client and covered with more blankets, then external warmers such as hot water bottles or heating pads are applied on the outside of the wrap. First, the client's body is thoroughly warmed with aerobic exercise, heat lamps, a hot footbath, hot shower or other heat treatments. Next, the client gets on the massage table for the wrap. This treatment is commonly used to stimulate circulation, to detoxify, and to help the client relax. The cold mitten friction is a finishing touch which also stimulates circulation and leaves the client feeling refreshed. If a head towel is not used, massage of the head, neck and shoulders can be performed during the wrap.

SNAPSHOT

Wrap water temperature Hot (110°F; 43°C).

Time needed 20–30 minutes.

Equipment needed

1. Two sheets that will be used for massage after the body wrap is finished.
2. Two wool or heavy polar fleece blankets, one space blanket, and one cotton blanket. The cotton blanket can be prepared ahead of time by soaking it in hot water, wringing it out, and keeping it warm in a slow cooker or hot towel cabinet.
3. Body warmers, such as hot water bottles or heating pads.
4. Small bath towel, to wrap around the client's head and/or neck.
5. Large container of water at 110°F (43°C), for wetting the blanket.
6. Bolster, to go under the client's knees.
7. Cup with drinking water and a straw.

Effect Thermal.

Cleanup Launder the wet cotton blanket and the small bath towel. Spray the space blanket with alcohol and leave it to air-dry, then fold it and put it away. Fold and put away the wool blankets. Clean, disinfect and dry the water container.

Indications Chilled client; anxious or emotionally upset client; need for detoxification; chronic muscle or joint pain, especially arthritis, sciatica or gout.

Indications for when the legs alone could be wrapped Discomfort or chronic pain in the legs or feet, such as fibromyalgia; arthritic or neuropathic pain; tired, aching legs; tired, burning feet; cold legs and feet or Raynaud's syndrome; poor leg circulation after a stroke, spinal cord injury, or any client who spends their days in a wheelchair; knee injury such as ligament or meniscal damage, after 48 hours; menstrual pain; derivation for migraine (when used for migraine, cold packs may be used on the back of the neck).

Contraindications

1. Unless performed under the supervision of a doctor, any condition that specifically contraindicates whole-body heating, such as cardiovascular

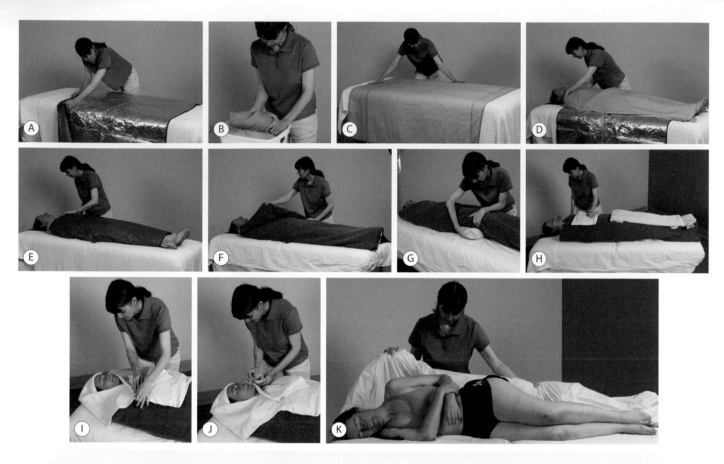

FIGURE 9.1
Moist blanket wrap. (**A**) Preparing the massage table. (**B**) Wringing out hot wet blanket. (**C**) Laying out the hot wet blanket. (**D**) Wrapping the client in the hot wet blanket. (**E**) Wrapping the client in a space blanket. (**F**) Wrapping the client in a wool blanket. (**G**) Placing a bolster under the client's knees. (**H**) Applying external warming devices. (**I**) Draping the head with a towel. (**J**) Offering the client drinking water. (**K**) Removing blankets without having the client get off the table.

problems, diabetes, hepatitis, lymphedema, multiple sclerosis, and seizure disorders.

2. Pregnancy.

3. Ingestion of alcohol and drugs.

4. Claustrophobic client.

Cautions

1. Like other whole-body heating treatments, very frequent wraps are not recommended for hypothyroid conditions.

2. Anyone who is at risk for lymphedema due to removal of lymph nodes should avoid prolonged heating (wrap should be no longer than 15 minutes after the client has begun sweating).

Procedure

1. Check with the client to make sure there are no contraindications for the use of the body wrap.

2. Explain the use of the body wrap to the client and get her consent.

3. Make sure that the client is warm.

4. Cover the massage table with 1 massage sheet, 2 wool blankets and then a space blanket (Figure 9.1A). Reserve the other massage sheet to use when the wrap is finished.

5. Using gloves to protect your hands, soak a cotton blanket in 160°F (71°C) water and wring it out (Figure 9.1B). Now lay it out upon the massage table so it completely covers the space blanket (Figure 9.1C). Work quickly so the blanket does not cool off.

6. Have the nude or partially dressed client lie on the wet blanket, wrap it around her, and tuck the sheet in snugly around her neck so that no air escapes (Figure 9.1D). Next wrap the space blanket over the client's cotton-blanket-covered body (Figure

9.1E) and wrap both wool or polar fleece blankets over that (Figure 9.1F).

7. Place a bolster under the client's knees (Figure 9.1G).

8. Apply one external warmer such as a hot water bottle, heating pad or fomentation to the client's feet. If the client does not warm up quickly, place one over the abdomen as well (Figure 9.1H).

9. Drape her head with a towel (Figure 9.1I) or begin head and shoulder massage.

10. As the client begins to warm up, add a cold compress to her forehead (not pictured).

11. Offer the client drinking water from a cup with a straw (Figure 9.1J).

12. After 20–30 minutes, unwrap the client (remove all the blankets) and, if possible, give a cold mitten friction.

13. The final step is to prepare the therapy table for hands-on work. The wool blankets, space blanket, and wet blanket must all be removed so there is only one dry massage sheet remaining on the massage table. Have the client roll onto one side; then bunch up the sheet and all the blankets up against her back, and then have the client roll onto her other side. To do this, she will have to roll over the bunched-up blankets, but then you may easily gather up all the linens and remove them (Figure 9.1K). Underneath the client there is now one clean massage sheet. Cover the client with the last (reserved) massage sheet, and now the hands-on session may begin. (Another option is to have the client get off the massage table momentarily while you remove the linens.)

Variation 1: Wrap beginning with hot towels to the back

Procedure: With wrap linens on the table and the client prone, apply a series of hot moist towels to the back and massage through them. Now have the client get off the table momentarily, put a hot moist blanket on the table and ask the client to get back on for a full wrap. For directions and contraindications, see *Hot compresses* on page 98.

Variation 2: Leg wrap without additives

Equipment needed: Same as for the whole-body wrap, but the blankets are laid lengthwise, from the hip down; container of hot water; two extra-large bath towels, rather than a wet sheet; three small hand towels, one to cover the client's anterior pelvic area, two for cold mitten friction. Bath towels can be prepared ahead of time by soaking them in hot water, wringing them out, placing them in a bowl, and keeping warm in a slow cooker or hot towel cabinet.

Procedure

1. First heat the legs and feet using a heating pad, hot footbath, heat lamp, etc. The client may take an exfoliating glove or a salt glow mixture into the shower and do just the legs before treatment.

2. Spread wrappings on table as for whole-body wrap. Have the client lie on the table, and cover the pelvic area with a small hand towel. Wring out two large bath towels in hot water.

3. Ask the client to roll onto one hip, slide one hot towel under the other leg, and center it so that the middle of the towel is directly under the back of the leg. Now have the client lie back on it; then wrap it snugly over the leg and foot so that these are entirely covered. Cover with the space blanket and the two wool or polar fleece blankets.

4. Working quickly, repeat with the other leg. Pull the blankets up to cover the entire top of the legs.

5. Massage of the upper body can be done during the wrap.

6. After 20–30 minutes, remove the blankets and towels and, if possible, finish with a cold mitten friction.

Variation 3: Leg wraps with additives

Anti-inflammatory leg wrap: This wrap is for any type of leg pain or discomfort, as well as for poor circulation in the legs. Simply add ingredients to wrap water and follow the basic sequence for a leg wrap (see Figure 13.4). Perform the basic leg wrap, but add the following ingredients to 2.25 quarts (2.25 liters) hot water:

- 1½ cups baking soda
- ⅓ cup lemon juice
- ⅓ cup aloe vera gel.

Mix aloe vera gel and baking soda with one half of the hot water, and stir well to dissolve the soda completely, then add the lemon juice and remaining hot water and stir again. After the wrap, perform a cold mitten friction or the client can shower: ingredients should be washed off.

Honey and herb leg wrap for arthritic pain or dry skin: Add the following ingredients to 2.25 quarts (2.25 liters) hot water:

Chapter nine

BACKGROUND

Roberta was a healthy 62-year-old woman who had suffered from **fibromyalgia** for many years. She had been involved in a motor vehicle accident the day before and was bruised, sore over her entire body except her head, and emotionally upset. When she visited the emergency department at her hospital after the accident, Roberta was told she had no fractures or other major injuries. The next day she visited her daughter's therapist to have her first-ever massage session.

TREATMENT

As the massage therapist began to take Roberta's health history, Roberta said she was cold, so he immediately gave her a hot footbath at 102°F (39°C). Roberta exclaimed that it was much too hot, so he added cold water until it was 99°F (37°C). As Roberta answered his questions, the therapist began to suspect that she was not only bruised from yesterday's accident, but hypersensitive to touch as well. Roberta acknowledged that she could not tolerate very hot or cold water, loose threads in her socks, tags in her clothing or any kind of wool next to her skin; she could only tolerate very soft fabrics and disliked touch of any kind on her abdomen and feet.

The therapist decided that massage would likely be more stressful than relaxing to Roberta, especially when she was bruised and sore. He chose instead to perform a moist blanket wrap. He soaked a cotton blanket in warm water with a high concentration of Epsom salts (1 cup (240 ml) Epsom salts to 4 cups (1 liter) water), then he laid it on the massage table and used it to wrap Roberta snugly, adding more blankets on top.

Then, while Roberta was relaxing in the wrap, he performed very gentle massage of her head and neck as well as energetic techniques. Roberta became not only comfortably warm but deeply relaxed. When she was dressed again at the end of the session, she told the therapist that she felt much better emotionally, and "It doesn't hurt so much when I move."

DISCUSSION QUESTIONS

1. How did the moist blanket wrap relieve Rebecca's pain?

2. Why did the therapist use Epsom salts water for the wrap?

3. What other additives could have been mixed with the wrap water?

4. What other hydrotherapy treatments would have been appropriate for this client's needs?

- ⅛ cup honey
- 4oz (120 ml) tincture of any herb that is recommended for arthritis.

After the wrap, remove the mixture on the skin. Either perform a cold mitten friction or the client can shower.

DRY SHEET WRAPS

The **dry sheet wrap** consists of two blankets and one sheet, with various warmers placed on the outside of the wrap. It is excellent for warming a cold client before a session or providing a warm environment in which to relax afterwards. As seen in Figure 9.2, the client is simply wrapped snugly so that body heat is trapped, and then warmers are added. In water-cure institutions, patients would often receive a morning body wrap while still in bed. First a large cloth bag containing warm steamed herbs was placed on one part of the patient's body and then he or she was wrapped in a dry sheet and a blanket and left to relax. Kneipp health resorts continue this practice today.

Although it is possible to overheat a client if this treatment is prolonged, this is unlikely; however, if the client begins to sweat, apply a cold compress to the forehead.

SNAPSHOT

Temperature Warm – trapped body heat and external body warmers warm the person through the blankets.

Time needed 10 minutes or more, depending on the client's core temperature.

Equipment needed Two blankets; three sheets; warming device such as a hot water bottle, hydrocollator pack or heating pad; small bath towel to wrap around the neck; bolster for the client's knees.

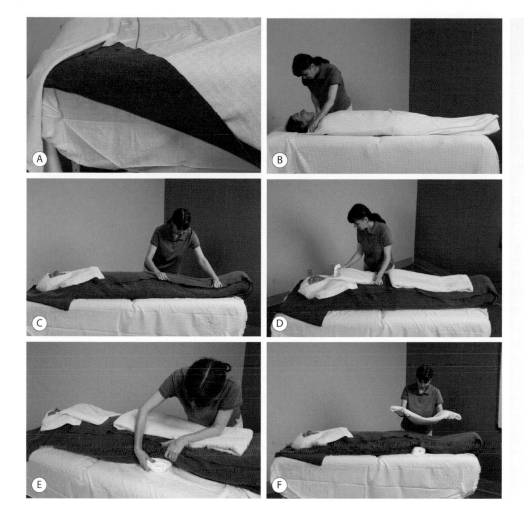

FIGURE 9.2
Dry sheet wrap. (**A**) Preparing the table. (**B**) Wrapping the client in the dry sheet. (**C**) Wrapping the client in the blankets. (**D**) Placing the warming devices. (**E**) Placing a bolster under the knees. (**F**) Removing the warming devices.

Indications Chilled or emotionally upset client.

Contraindications Claustrophobia; lack of feeling in the legs; because body warmers will be applied to the legs and the skin cannot be directly monitored, any compromised circulation to the lower extremities, including arteriosclerosis of the legs, Buerger's disease, or diabetes.

Procedure

1. Check with the client to make sure there are no contraindications for the use of the body wrap.

2. Explain the use of the body wrap to the client and get her consent.

3. Cover the massage table with one massage sheet. Lay two wool blankets on top of that, and top with another dry sheet (reserve the fourth sheet to cover the client with at the conclusion of the body wrap). Place the small bath towel at the head of the table (Figure 9.2A).

4. Have the client get on the table so that she is lying on the sheet, then wrap her in it. Tuck the sheet in snugly around the client's neck so that no air escapes (Figure 9.2B).

5. Next wrap the blankets over the client's sheet-covered body (Figure 9.2C).

6. Place a small bath towel around the head and neck, and warming devices such as fomentations, hot water bottles, hydrocollator packs and electric heating pads on the client's legs. Add one over the chest if the client is very cold (Figure 9.2D).

7. Place a bolster under the client's knees (Figure 9.2E).

8. After 10 minutes or more, check to make sure the client is thoroughly warm. If so, remove the warmers, sheets and blankets (Figure 9.2F), then, if desired, perform a cold mitten friction.

9. The client may now receive a massage. However, you want only one dry sheet remaining on the

massage table. The wool blankets and the sheet that were covering the client must all be removed. Have the client roll onto one side, bunch the sheet and both blankets up against her back, and then have her roll onto her other side. To do this, she will have to roll over the bunched-up blankets, but then you may easily gather up all the linens and remove them (Figure 9.1K). There is now one clean massage sheet under the client. Cover her with the reserved massage sheet, and now the massage session may begin. Another option is to have the client get off the massage table momentarily while you remove all the blankets.

Variation: Seated wrap with hot footbath

For instructions for hot footbaths, see page 145; observe all contraindications.

1. Have the client sit in a large deep chair with blankets draped as in a dry sheet wrap.
2. Now wrap the client in a clean sheet.
3. Bring the hot footbath to the client and set it on a towel, then the client can put his feet in the water.
4. Wrap a small towel around the client's neck to prevent body heat escaping and to catch sweat.
5. Wrap the blankets one at a time around the client, enclosing the footbath as well. Care is needed to keep the blankets out of the water.
6. Continue the treatment for 15–20 minutes, massaging the head, neck and shoulders if desired. Use a cold cloth on the face if the client is sweating.
7. Move the linens away from the footbath, pour cold water over the client's feet, dry them well, and put on thick, warm socks.
8. Unwrap the client, who can now move to the massage table: and bodywork can begin.

COLD WET SHEET WRAPS

Over the centuries many people have noticed that wrapping a person in cold linens and then covering him or her with blankets leads to profuse sweating. For example, in 1697, English doctor Sir John Floyer, author of *The History of Hot and Cold Bathing*, advised sportsmen who wanted their jockeys to lose weight to "Dip the rider's shirt in cold water; and after it is put on very wet, lay the person in warm blankets to sweat him violently, and he will after lose a considerable weight" (Floyer, 1923). Vincent Priessnitz (1801–1851) invented the formal use of the cold wet sheet wrap, in which the client was wrapped in one wet sheet and a few blankets and left for varying amounts of time.

This treatment was a staple, first of the water cure and then of classic naturopathic medicine. Different stages of the wet sheet pack were used for various conditions: stage one for fever, weakness and as a tonic for convalescents; stage two for mental illness, anxiety, nervousness and insomnia; stage three for pneumonia, digestive problems and congestion of internal organs; and stage four was used for infectious illnesses such as bronchitis and influenza, toxic states, and drug and alcohol addictions. One 1878 case report relates the helpful effect of a cold sheet pack on an alcoholic suffering from severe alcohol withdrawal symptoms, which included seizures and other major problems (Delion, 2018). Partial wraps were also popular: cold wet hip and leg packs treated arthritic or injured lower extremities and acute menstrual pain, and heating trunk packs were used for all manner of digestive disturbances.

For today's massage therapist, the **cold wet sheet wrap** (Figure 9.3), in which the client is wrapped in a cold wet sheet and two blankets, can be an effective method of manipulating the client's core temperature without expensive or elaborate hydrotherapy equipment. Therapeutic substances such as herbal preparations, salts, or essential oils can also be incorporated by mixing them with the water in which the sheet is soaked.

The first stage of the wet sheet wrap has a cooling effect, since the client is surrounded by a sheet which was soaked in very cold water before being wrung out (for this reason, this method was once used to reduce fevers). The cold is a strong stimulus to the cold receptors on the surface of the skin and, as always, the body protects itself against a drop in the core temperature. Skin blood vessels constrict powerfully and then dilate, and increased blood to the skin creates a burst of heat (core temperature increases about 0.4°F or 0.2°C). The wrappings trap the burst of heat and this leads to a quick rise in core temperature. Within about 5 minutes, the client's trapped body heat has warmed the wrap, so the client is neither hot nor cold. This second stage has a calming effect similar to that of a neutral bath.

After another 15 minutes, the client's trapped body heat has continued to raise the core temperature from neutral to hot. This is the third stage. If they continue

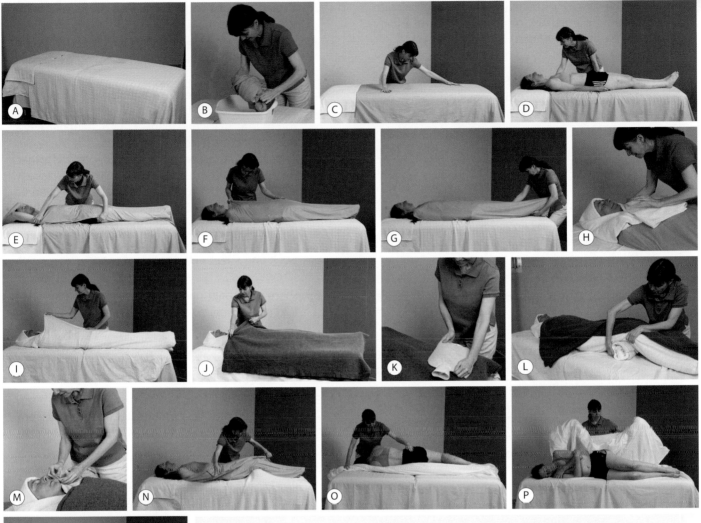

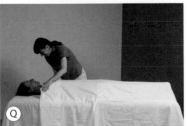

FIGURE 9.3
Cold wet sheet wrap. (**A**) Preparing the table. (**B**) Wringing out the cold sheet. (**C**) Placing the cold sheet upon the blanket. (**D**) The client lying supine on the sheet. (**E**) Wrapping the client's body except the arms. (**F**) Wrapping the entire body including the arms. (**G**) Tucking the bottom of the sheet snugly under the feet. (**H**) Placing the small bath towel around the head and neck. (**I**) Tucking the blanket on the table around the client. (**J**) Applying the second blanket to the client. (**K**) Placing a hot water bottle over the feet. (**L**) Placing a bolster underneath the client's knees. (**M**) Offering the client water. (**N**) Removing the wet sheet. (**O**) With the client rolled onto one side, bunching up the sheet and both blankets up against the back. (**P**) Removing the linens. (**Q**) Covering the client with the reserved massage sheet.

in the wrap, they eventually become warmer still, and sweat profusely. This is the fourth stage, and is better used as a detoxification procedure under the supervision of a doctor than as a treatment performed in a massage session.

SNAPSHOT

Water temperature Cold (60–70°F; 15–21°C).

Time needed Approximately 5 minutes or more for the first stage, 15 minutes or more for the second or neutral stage, 30 minutes for the heating phase, and 1–2 hours for the sweating stage. (Times are approximate because some clients will be able to generate body heat more easily than others.)

Equipment needed

1. Water thermometer.

2. Plastic sheet to cover the massage table; one cotton blanket; one wool or polar fleece blanket.

3. One sheet which will be wrung out in cold water; two sheets which will be used for massage after the body wrap is finished.

4. One small bath towel, to wrap around the neck.

5. Large container of water at 60–70°F (15–21°C), for wetting the sheet.

6. Warming device such as a hot water bottle or hot footbath.

7. Bolster to go under the client's knees.

8. Cup with drinking water and a straw.

Effect: Thermal.

Cleanup: Launder the wet sheet, both blankets, and the small bath towel. Clean, disinfect, and dry the water container. Dispose of the plastic sheet or clean it as you would a space blanket.

Indications Cooling and tonifying (first stage); sedative for a nervous or emotionally upset client and helps to reduce insomnia (second and third stages); warming (third stage); detoxification/sweating treatment (fourth stage).

Contraindications Claustrophobic person; chilled client; ingestion of alcohol and drugs; any skin problem that is aggravated by excess moisture; when the wrap is taken to the third and fourth stages, any condition that specifically contraindicates whole-body heating will be contraindicated, including pregnancy, cardiovascular problems, diabetes, hepatitis, lymphedema, multiple sclerosis and seizure disorders, unless treatments are specifically prescribed by a doctor.

Cautions

1. Very frequent sweating wraps are not recommended for hypothyroid conditions.

2. Anyone who is at risk of lymphedema due to removal of lymph nodes should avoid prolonged sweating in wraps (no longer than 15 minutes once the sweating stage is reached).

Procedure

1. Check with the client to make sure there are no contraindications for the use of the body wrap.

2. Explain the use of the body wrap to the client and get her consent.

3. Make sure that the client is quite warm, giving a hot footbath or other type of warming treatment if necessary.

4. Cover the massage table with one dry massage sheet, and cover that with a plastic sheet. On top of that place one blanket, with its upper edge about 8 inches (20 cm) from the head of the table. The edge of the blanket should hang down farther on the far side of the table than on the side closest to you. Place the small bath towel at the head of the table (Figure 9.3A). Reserve the second blanket for step 13 and the second massage sheet for step 19.

5. Soak one sheet in the cold water and wring it out (Figure 9.3B).

6. Place the sheet upon the blanket, with its upper end slightly below the upper edge of the blanket (Figure 9.3C).

7. Have the client lie supine upon the sheet, with the shoulders about 3 inches (8 cm) below the top of the sheet (Figure 9.3D).

8. Have the client hold her arms up while you wrap one side of the sheet around her body (away from yourself) and tuck it in under the opposite side (Figure 9.3E).

9. Now have the client lower her arms. Wrap the opposite side of the sheet around her body (you will be bringing the sheet toward yourself) and tuck it in (Figure 9.3F).

10. Tuck the bottom of the sheet snugly under the feet (Figure 9.3G).

11. Place the small bath towel around the head and neck to protect the client's neck and keep out cold air (Figure 9.3H).

12. Draw the shorter side of the blanket over the body and tuck it in, and then do the same with the wider side (Figure 9.3I).

13. Lay the second blanket over the client and tuck it in (Figure 9.3J).

14. Place a hot water bottle, hydrocollator pack or other warming device on the feet to speed warming (Figure 9.3K).

15. Place a bolster underneath the client's knees (Figure 9.3L).

16. Offer the client a sip of water from a cup with a straw, as needed (Figure 9.3M).

17. When the client has reached the desired stage – neutral, hot, or sweating – remove the blankets and the wet sheet (Figure 9.3N).

18. When the pack has been removed, give the client a cold mitten friction (see Figure 10.2).

19. Now the client may receive a massage. However, you want only one dry massage sheet remaining on the massage table. The blankets and wet sheet must all be removed. Have the client roll onto one side, then bunch up the sheet and both blankets against her back (Figure 9.3O), and then have her roll onto her other side. To do this, she will have to roll over the bunched-up blankets, but then you may easily gather up all the linens and remove them (Figure 9.3P). Another option is to have the client get off the massage table momentarily while you do this. Now there is only one clean massage sheet underneath the client. Cover the client with the reserved massage sheet (Figure 9.3Q). Now the massage session may begin.

CHAPTER SUMMARY

In this chapter you have learned about another useful and versatile treatment, the body wrap. When one has been properly done, clients will feel soothed, relaxed and comfortably warm afterwards. You may perform these wraps in your office without expensive equipment, and in other places such as at your clients' homes. Body wraps may also be combined with other treatments such as hot compresses before a wrap, or a cold mitten friction afterwards. Additives such as herbs and essential oils can also be incorporated with ease.

Chapter nine

REVIEW QUESTIONS

Multiple choice

1. The first stage of the wet sheet pack is:

   A. Cooling

   B. Relaxing

   C. Useful in detoxification

2. Blankets are used in body wraps for all but one of the reasons below. Which is the exception?

   A. To keep the massage table dry

   B. To prevent claustrophobia

   C. To trap body heat

   D. To give clients an enclosed sensation

3. All but one of these can be added to wrap water for a chemical effect. Which is the exception?

   A. Oatmeal

   B. Sand

   C. Essential oil

   D. Herb tea

4. Body wraps may be combined with all but one of these. Which is the exception?

   A. Mustard plaster

   B. Ice packs

   C. Sauna

   D. Hot compresses

5. For which of these would a A moist wrap *not* be appropriate?

   A. Chilled client

   B. Hypersensitive client

   C. Overheated client

   D. Resting client

Fill in the blank

6. Heating body wraps may be used for patients with cancer because they _____ the immune system and weaken _____.

7. The _____ wrap and the _____ wrap may be used for detoxification.

8. The moist blanket wrap is used for a general _____ and for chronic _____ or _____ pain.

9. The first stage of the cold wet sheet wrap has a _____ effect.

10. The second stage of the cold wet sheet wrap has a _____ effect.

Short answer

11. Give two examples of when a cold application would be indicated with a body wrap.

12. Give three examples of wrap additives, and explain how to add them to a wrap.

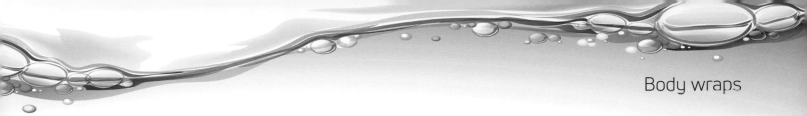

References

Ayres R. Sensory Integration and the Child. Los Angeles, CA: Western Psychological Services, 1981

Curtis R. The outdoor action guide to hypothermia and cold weather injuries. https://www.princeton.edu/~oa/safety/hypocold.shtml [Accessed March 2019]

Delion P et al. Therapeutic body wraps for treatment of severe injurious behaviour in children with autism spectrum disorder (ASD): a A 3-month randomized controlled feasibility study. PLoS ONE 2018; 13(6): e0198726

Floyer J, quoted in Kellogg JH. Rational Hydrotherapy. Battle Creek, MI: Modern Medicine Publishing Company, 1923, p. 28

Grandin T. Calming effects of deep touch pressure in patients with autistic disorder, college students, and animals. J Child Adolesc Psych 2(1) 1992

Kellogg JH. Rational Hydrotherapy. Battle Creek, MI: Modern Medicine Publishing Company, 1923

Opsommer E et al. Therapeutic body wraps in Swiss public adult acute inpatient wards. A retrospective descriptive cohort study. J Psychiatr Mental Health Nurs, 2016 Apr; 23(3–4): 207–16

Sato W. Inhibition of emotion-related autonomic arousal by skin pressure. Springer Plus 2015(4): 294

Scott G. Interview with the author. University of Texas Medical Center, 1 December 2006

Takagi. Skin pressure-vegetative reflex. Acta Med Bio 4, 1955(3): 31–57

US National Library of Medicine. www.clinicaltrials.gov/ct/gvi/show/NCT00178802 [Accessed 1 December 2006]

Van Sleuwen B et al. Swaddling: a systematic review. Pediatrics 2007 Oct; 120(4): 1097–106

Wust P et al. Hyperthermia in combined treatment of cancer. Lancet Oncol 2002; 3: 487–97

Recommended resources

Delion P et al. Therapeutic body wrap video demo, 2018 http://doi.org/10.5281/zenodo.1157306

Peterson S. Hydrotherapy in the Home. Loveland, CO: Eden Valley Institute Press, 1973

Shorter E. From Paralysis to Fatigue: A History of Psychosomatic Illness in the Modern Era. New York: Free Press, 1992

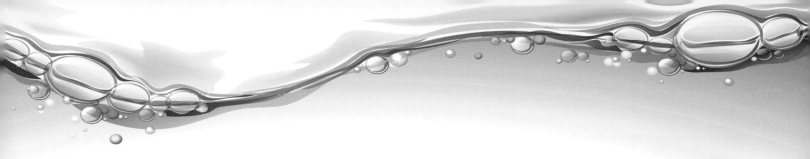

Friction treatments 10

Use a rough brush to vigorously brush down the patient's entire body … this has the same effect as an underwater massage and stimulates the capillaries. It removes congestions and any unpleasant feeling of constriction will disappear.

Alfred Vogel, *The Nature Doctor*

CHAPTER OBJECTIVES

After completing this chapter, the student will be able to:

1. Name and describe various friction treatments
2. Describe the effects of various friction treatments
3. Explain the indications, cautions and contraindications for friction treatments
4. Perform friction treatments using the procedure described here.

Like massage, friction treatments make use of the body's own self-healing mechanisms. Anytime the skin surface is vigorously frictioned, underlying blood vessels dilate, so if the skin has been cut or otherwise injured, extra oxygen and nutrients are available for healing. Early hydrotherapists recognized that not only was the skin a living, vital organ with many important functions, but frictioning helped increase the effect of other hydrotherapy treatments. For example, to reduce temperatures, feverish patients were doused with cold water and rubbed vigorously at the same time. Perhaps this was not the most enjoyable treatment, but as blood vessels dilated with warm blood, the skin radiated more heat, and cold penetrated more deeply. As this approach can stimulate the respiratory system and ease discomfort, pneumonia was treated with hot fomentations over the chest, alternated with cold mitten frictions. To rouse patients with drug overdoses out of

their stupors, the patients were covered with wet icy-cold sheets and frictioned vigorously, and then again with hot sheets. In the pre-antibiotic days when patients might take many days or weeks to recuperate from an illness, patients received daily cold mitten frictions to strengthen their constitutions, while salt glows were developed for patients who were too weak to handle even those, and dry brushing became a classic method of gradually strengthening the immune system (Kellogg, 1923).

As shown in Figure 10.1, treatments, which are loved and used around the world, make use of various local materials. Such treatments include mitts made of animal hair, raw silk, rough rayon, terrycloth or coarse plant material; gritty materials such as Epsom salts or sand mixed with oils; dried sponges or luffas; natural bristle brushes, various types of leaves combined with soaps, and whisks made of bundles of dried twigs; and in Native American sweat lodges, deer ribs were used to friction the skin.

Today, you can use frictions to stimulate function in a particular area, provide enjoyable sensations to your clients, and melt top layers of tension before you begin hands-on work. Frictions are often used for cosmetic purposes, since they exfoliate (remove the top layer of dead skin cells), and are thought to improve absorption of beauty products. Frictions can also work with other hydrotherapy treatments: for example, a classic arthritis treatment combines a hot Epsom salts bath with frictioning of painful joints (see Chapter 13).

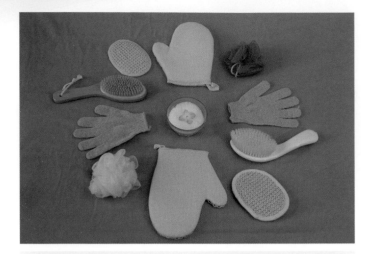

FIGURE 10.1
Friction treatments around the world use a variety of local materials.

Three distinct friction treatments are included in this chapter: cold mitten friction, salt glows and dry brushing. We also include a back treatment that incorporates hot towels, frictions and bodywork for a supremely relaxing session. You will learn not only how to perform these treatments, but how to use them appropriately in your massage practice.

COLD MITTEN FRICTION

This is undoubtedly one of the finest hydrotherapy measures known for stimulating the circulation in the skin … the cold mitten friction is better than any tonic one can take from a bottle.

Stella Peterson, *Hydrotherapy in the Home*

This friction treatment is performed with a coarse terrycloth mitt or washcloth that has been dipped in cold water. Each part of the body is uncovered and frictioned separately, while the rest of the body remains covered and warm. This simple but powerful treatment can be given to "finish" a whole-body heating treatment, and it is also helpful for clients who are bedridden and not receiving any circulatory stimulation through movement. It is the only friction treatment that has both thermal and mechanical effects. As you will learn in the next chapter, regular applications of cold act as a form of exercise for the small muscles that dilate and constrict skin blood vessels, and water temperature can be gradually lowered as the blood vessels react more strongly.

Never begin this treatment in a cold room or with a chilled client. Even though the cold cloth will give a brief "shock" to the client, it stimulates cold receptors on the surface of the skin. The body creates a burst of heat and once the area is frictioned, dried and covered, the client will have a comfortable feeling of warmth.

As with other applications of cold given to a warm client, the cold receptors on the surface of the skin are stimulated, and the body creates a burst of heat there. The area is also stimulated by brisk drying, and covering it helps retains the heat produced by the body. For a client who is too hot after a heating treatment such as a hot shower, see the variation at the end of the instructions.

SNAPSHOT

Water temperature 50–60°F (10–15.5°C). The colder the water, the greater the reaction. If repeated on a regular basis, colder water will gradually become more tolerable.

Time needed 5–10 minutes.

Equipment needed Water thermometer; two sheets; washable blanket; container for water; 2 quarts (2 liters) of water; two or more towels; one or two friction mitts, made from coarse toweling or luffa. A coarse terrycloth washcloth wrapped around the hand may also be used.

Effect Thermal and mechanical.

Cleanup Clean, disinfect and dry the water container; launder the mitts or washcloths.

Indications Poor capacity of skin blood vessels of the skin to react to cold; skin stimulation, particularly for individuals who are sedentary, bedridden or wheelchair-using, or who have reduced sensation; overheated clients; sensory stimulation.

Contraindications Open, infected, damaged or sunburned skin, eczema, fungal infections such as ringworm or athlete's foot, skin rashes, skin that has just been shaved, advanced varicose veins.

Procedure

1. Check with the client to make sure there are no contraindications for the use of the cold mitten friction.

2. Explain the use of the cold mitten friction to the client and get her consent.

3. Make sure that the client is warm, giving a hot footbath or other type of warming treatment if necessary.

4. The client should wear minimal or no clothing, and lie on top of one sheet and under a second sheet and a blanket. For the treatment to be effective, only one part of the body will be exposed to cold at a time, and the rest of the body should be covered and warm. In order to make this a comfortable treatment, each area must be frictioned, dried, and then covered without getting the bottom sheet damp.

5. Expose one arm, and slide a towel underneath the arm all the way up to the shoulder. Dip the friction mitt in the cold water, wring it out, and begin frictioning the arm (Figure 10.2A). Use light to moderate pressure and a brisk back-and-forth motion, so that the client's skin is strongly stimulated. Move from the fingers to the top of the shoulder and back again. The skin should become pink; if not, repeat the frictioning. The more water that is left in the mitts the greater the reaction will be; in any case, the client should not become dripping wet.

6. Remove the mitt from your hand and dry the arm briskly with a dry towel (Figure 10.2B). Remove the first towel from under the client's arm, and place the arm back on the bottom sheet, which should be dry, and under the top sheet and blanket.

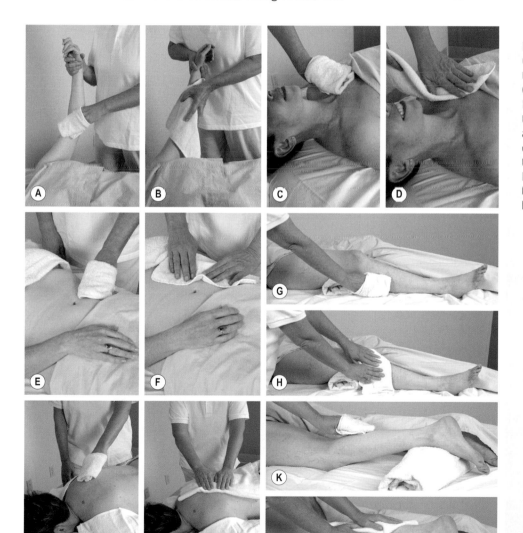

FIGURE 10.2
Cold mitten friction. (**A**) Frictioning the arm. (**B**) Drying the arm. (**C**) Frictioning the chest. (**D**) Drying the chest. (**E**) Frictioning the abdomen. (**F**) Drying the abdomen. (**G**) Frictioning the front of the leg. (**H**) Drying the front of the leg. (**I**) Frictioning the back. (**J**) Drying the back. (**K**) Frictioning the back of the leg. (**L**) Drying the back of the leg.

7. Repeat steps 5 and 6 with the client's other arm.

8. Now uncover the chest.

9. Dip the mitts in cold water and wring them out. Do not have them dripping wet or water will run down the client's chest and wet the bottom sheet.

10. Ask the client to inhale deeply as you apply friction with the mitts. Move up the middle of the chest, across the shoulders, down the sides of the torso, and back to the midline (Figure 10.2C). In a female client, do not apply friction over the breasts.

11. Remove the mitt from your hand and briskly dry the chest with a dry towel (Figure 10.2D). Cover the chest with a towel so it will stay warm as you friction the abdomen.

12. Dip the mitts in cold water and wring them out. Do not have them dripping wet or water will run down the client's abdomen and wet the bottom sheet.

13. Uncover and friction the client's abdomen (Figure 10.2E).

14. Remove the mitt from your hand and briskly dry the client's abdomen with a dry towel (Figure 10.2F). Now cover both chest and abdomen with the top sheet and blanket.

15. Repeat this procedure with the fronts of both legs, placing a towel under the leg before frictioning and then removing it after drying the leg (Figures 10.2G and H).

16. Have the client roll over into the prone position, and friction the back in the same manner (Figure 10.2I). Do not have the mitts dripping wet or water will run down the client's back and wet the bottom sheet.

17. Remove the mitts from your hands, dry the back briskly, and then cover it with the top sheet and blanket (Figure 10.2J).

18. Friction the backs of the legs in the same manner, placing a towel under each leg before frictioning it, and removing the towel afterwards (Figures 10.2K and L).

19. The client will be warmed and relaxed, and a massage may now be performed if desired. If you have followed the directions correctly, both sheets will be dry.

Variation Cooling friction suitable for an overheated client
Simply use plenty of colder water (32–50°F; 0–10°C) and leave the client uncovered throughout the treatment.

SALT GLOWS

This friction treatment uses moistened Epsom salts rather than a washcloth or brush. During a salt glow, the skin turns pink or "glows" due to vasodilation. Salt glows were originally developed for patients who were too weak to tolerate cold mitten frictions, but today so many people find them enjoyable that they are used not only to increase blood flow to the skin, but as a pampering treatment.

Of particular importance to the massage therapist, the salt glow prepares the client's tissues for massage: the circulation will be much improved, the superficial muscles will be more relaxed, and the client will have a pleasant feeling of euphoria.

General tips on performing salt glows

1. Salt is drying to the skin, so always apply some type of emollient lotion or oil to the client's skin afterwards. If a massage is to be performed after the salt glow, then the massage oil, cream or lotion will serve this purpose.

2. Be careful not to irritate the client's skin. Salt crystals have sharp edges and can feel unpleasant if too much pressure is used.

3. Do not use table salt, which may contain anti-caking agents, bleach and other unwanted chemicals. Coarser salts are better and give a greater reaction. Sea salt, kosher salt, pickling salt, Epsom salts, and Dead Sea salts are all good choices. The skin will absorb only a small amount of the chemicals in the wetted salt since these are on the skin for such a brief time.

4. Salt glows can be varied by adding whole or ground herbs, clays, honey, creams or essential oils.

5. Salt glows can also be varied by changing the water temperature: in vigorous clients, very cold water will cause a stronger reaction.

6. It is important to use good body mechanics. Follow directions carefully so you are not working in awkward positions.

Partial-body salt glows

Partial-body salt glows are a convenient prelude to massage of a specific area and are greatly enjoyed by clients for the sensory stimulation they provide, including for some the nurturing sense of being washed like a child.

With care, they can be given on a massage table with little mess. Instead of the client sitting on a stool in a bathtub, as for a whole-body salt glow, the client lies on a towel on the massage table. At the end of the salt glow, the towel will likely contain salt crystals, and can be removed so that the client is lying on clean dry sheets (as seen in Figure 9.1).

SNAPSHOT

"World's best back massage" how to combine frictions, hot compresses, and hands-on work.

Water temperature Pleasantly warm for salt glow – about 95–100°F (35–38°C) and cold (50–60°F; 10–15°C) for cold mitten friction.

Time needed 10 minutes, right before you perform a back massage.

Equipment needed

1. Water thermometer.
2. One hot and one cold bowl of water.
3. A few tablespoons of Epsom salts in a small container (exfoliation gloves and a pump bottle of liquid soap may be used instead of Epsom salts and water).
4. Three washcloths.
5. One large bath towel.
6. Slow cooker with four thick hand towels, hot and ready to use (see page 98 for instructions). Thin towels do not retain heat and make for an unsatisfying experience. Herbal tea or essential oils may be added to the water for the towels and massage tools.

Cleanup Clean and sanitize the containers; launder used linens; cleanse and sanitize the back roller or other massage tools. A plastic tub placed under the table may be used to dispose of linens during the session.

Effect Mechanical from both types of friction, thermal from hot compresses and cold mitten friction.

Indications Local muscle tension, poor local circulation, stress reduction, sensory stimulation.

Contraindications Open, infected, damaged or sunburned skin, eczema, fungal infections such as ringworm or athlete's foot, skin rashes, skin that has just been shaved, advanced varicose veins.

Procedure

1. Place all three containers, washcloths, the slow cooker and the back roller or other massage tools close at hand – a rolling cart is best for this – so you will not have to break the flow of the session to get what you need.
2. Place a bath-sized towel so that it will lie under the client from shoulders to hips.
3. Drip just enough water onto the container of salt so that the granules clump together (Figure 10.3A).
4. Gently wet the back with a washcloth dipped in warm water (Figure 10.3B).
5. Now scoop about one tablespoon of the moistened salt onto your hands and spread it on the back. Use more salt if needed. (If exfoliation gloves are used, add liquid soap to them and work up a thick lather.) Use a brisk upward movement with one hand while making a brisk downward movement with the other hand, like a friction massage stroke. Friction the entire back a few times (Figure 10.3C) and continue for 2–3 minutes, depending on the size of the client.
6. Use the warm wet washcloth to gently wash off the salt or soap lather, and then place the washcloth in the plastic tub (Figure 10.3D).
7. Now remove one hot towel from the slow cooker and mold it over the entire back, especially over the top of the shoulders. Massage over the hot towel, kneading the neck and shoulders and performing pressure points, compressions, skin rolling, etc. (Figure 10.3E).
8. After that hot towel has cooled, add a fresh hot one on top of it and flip them so the cooler one is now on top (Figure 10.3F).
9. Massage over both towels using a back roller or other massage tools (Figure 10.3G).
10. Remove both towels, add a new hot towel, massage through it briefly and then remove it; then apply massage oil and begin whole back strokes (Figure 10.3H).
11. At the end of the hands-on work, take the fourth hot towel from the cooker, place it on the client's back and massage through it briefly. Then, while the last of the heat is seeping into the back, soak a washcloth in cold water, wring it out well, and finish with a brief friction of the entire back (Figure 10.3I).

Whole-body salt glows

In this treatment, the entire body is frictioned one area at a time and the client is rinsed off (see Case history 10.1).

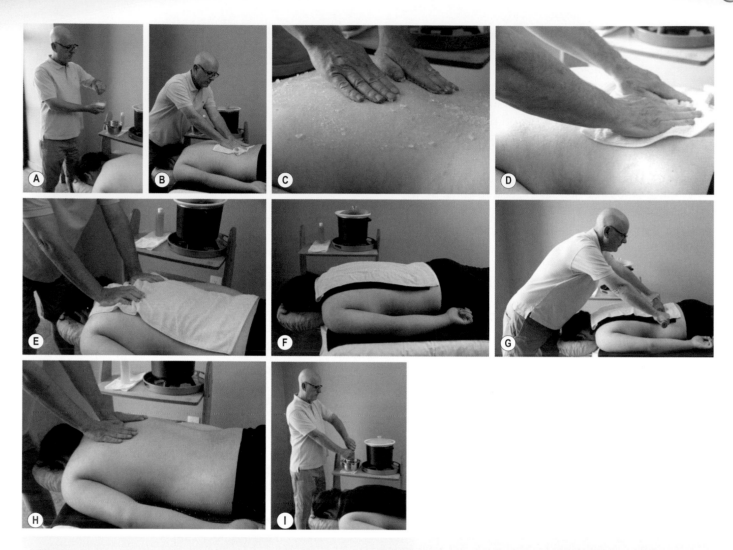

FIGURE 10.3

"World's best back massage." How to combine frictions, hot compresses, and hands-on work. (**A**) Dripping water over the Epsom salts. (**B**) Wetting the back with a washcloth dipped in warm water. (**C**) Frictioning the entire back. (**D**) Using the warm wet washcloth to gently wash off the salt. (The washcloth is then placed in the plastic tub.) (**E**) Massaging over the hot towel, kneading the neck and shoulders, and performing pressure points, compressions, skin rolling, etc. (**F**) After the hot towel has cooled, adding a new one on top of it and flipping them so the cooler one is now on top. (**G**) Massaging over both towels using a back roller or other massage tools. (**H**) Whole-back strokes using massage oil. (**I**) The last hot towel on the client's back as the cold washcloth is being prepared.

Make sure that there is no salt remaining on the client's skin at the end.

SNAPSHOT

Indications Poor circulation, stimulation of sweat glands before a whole-body heating treatment such as a sauna or steam bath, stimulation of the skin and muscles before massage.

Contraindications Open, infected, damaged or sunburned skin; eczema; fungal infections such as ringworm or athlete's foot; skin rashes; skin that has just been shaved; advanced varicose veins.

Water temperature Pleasantly warm: about 95–100°F (35–38°C).

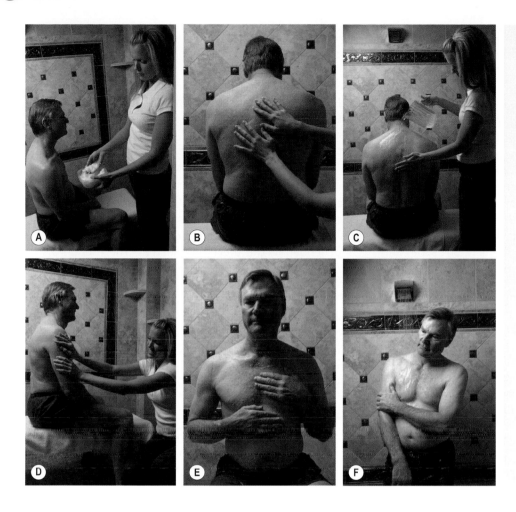

FIGURE 10.4
Whole-body salt glow. (**A**) Scooping out moistened salt for the salt glow. (**B**) Frictioning the back using the moistened salt. (**C**) Washing the salt off the back. (**D**) Frictioning the arm and leg on one side. (**E**) The client frictioning the chest and abdomen. (**F**) The client rinsing the salt off the chest and abdomen.

Time needed 15 minutes.

Equipment needed Bathtub with grab bars; plastic stool, plastic bench, or bath chair; pitcher; two bath towels; water thermometer; 1–2 cups of Epsom salts, moistened with just enough water so that the grains clump together (too much water will dissolve the salt).

Effect Primarily mechanical.

Cleanup Clean and sanitize the tub, flushing the drain with extra water. (Table salt or sea salt can corrode pipes, whereas Epsom salts do not.) Launder used linens.

Procedure

1. Check with the client to make sure there are no contraindications for the use of the salt glow.

2. Explain the use of the salt glow to the client and get his consent.

3. Place a plastic stool, plastic bench or bath chair in the bathtub or tiled area, and cover it with a towel. Here we demonstrate the salt glow in a large shower stall, but if a bathtub is used, fill it with enough warm water to cover the client's ankles.

4. Have the client undress and sit on the stool, bench, or bath chair. The client may wear a bathing suit or disposable underwear, but this will reduce the amount of skin that can be frictioned.

5. Add a little water to the container of salt, enough to make the grains clump together but not enough to dissolve the granules.

6. Pour warm water over the client's back. Now take a handful of the salt in your hands and put it on his back (Figure 10.4A). Using a back-and-forth motion, rub briskly but gently. Cover the entire back from top to bottom (Figure 10.4B). The trick is to use enough friction that the skin glows pink and the client enjoys the sensation, without having an overly abrasive effect. Use more salt if needed. When the client's back is thoroughly pink, use the pitcher to pour warm water over his back and rinse off the salt completely

Chapter ten

A WHOLE-BODY SALT GLOW FOR STIMULATION	CASE HISTORY 10.1

BACKGROUND

Alfredo was a 62-year-old osteopath who was generally in excellent health. He exercised regularly, was careful about his diet, and received massage therapy once a month to relieve muscle tightness and post-exercise soreness. However, ten days before this session, he had had surgery to remove a large benign tumor behind one eye, and he had been recuperating at home ever since. The surgery was successful and his recuperation was going fine, but Alfredo was still not feeling well. The entire experience had been emotionally stressful, and he still felt very tense. Since he was still not supposed to exercise, he also felt lethargic. Alfredo hoped that massage could address both of these problems.

TREATMENT

The massage therapist visited Alfredo at his home. Although there was considerable bruising in his mid-face, Alfredo looked well otherwise. After discussion, the therapist considered what hydrotherapy treatments might be beneficial to Alfredo along with his massage. Something relaxing and gently stimulating seemed to be ideal. Treatments on the head would have a tendency to affect blood flow there and were clearly contraindicated. Alfredo's doctor did not want him to exercise for at least four more days, and so very hot or cold treatments that could move blood around the body were also contraindicated. While a neutral bath would have been a relaxing treatment, it is specifically designed to decrease stimulation, and so it was not suitable either. The therapist finally decided to perform a whole-body salt glow with warm (102°F; 39°C) water.

Alfredo then sat in his bathtub on a plastic stool covered with towels, with warm water up to his ankles. His entire body was frictioned using Epsom salts, just as described in the preceding section. The friction of the salt upon the skin felt pleasantly stimulating to him, and shortly after the salt glow began, he happily told the therapist, "My skin needed this!" After the salt glow was over, Alfredo showered briefly to remove all traces of salt, then moved to the massage table. As he lay down and the therapist prepared to begin the massage session, Alfredo said he felt more alive and more relaxed already.

DISCUSSION QUESTIONS

1. Why would treatments on the head that would affect blood flow have been contraindicated?

2. What other hydrotherapy treatments might have been suitable in this situation?

(Figure 10.4C). If at any time the friction begins to feel irritating to the client, stop and wash the salt off immediately.

7. After the back has been frictioned and rinsed, you are ready to continue with the legs and the arms. Apply salt to the arm and leg that are facing you (Figure 10.4D), friction them and rinse the salt off. Now have the client stand up, turn 180 degrees and sit down again. He should use the provided grab bars to prevent slipping. The other arm and leg are now facing you. Apply salt to them and friction them just as you did with the first arm and leg.

8. Friction of the torso and abdomen comes next, but because the skin of the abdomen and chest is usually more sensitive, let the client do this himself (Figure 10.4E).

9. Either pour water over the torso and abdomen to rinse off the salt or, if a shower is available, the client can use that (Figure 10.4F).

10. Have the client dry himself briskly with a towel, and then lie down on the massage table for a session. If he is not going to receive a massage, his skin should be moisturized with cream or lotion.

DRY BRUSHING

Beginning with the feet and finishing with the back, the entire body is brushed without using water or lubricants. As with other frictions, brushing stimulates the skin and the nerves, blood vessels and lymphatic vessels underneath it, making it the perfect complement to the sensory stimulation of hands-on techniques. Dry brushing is also

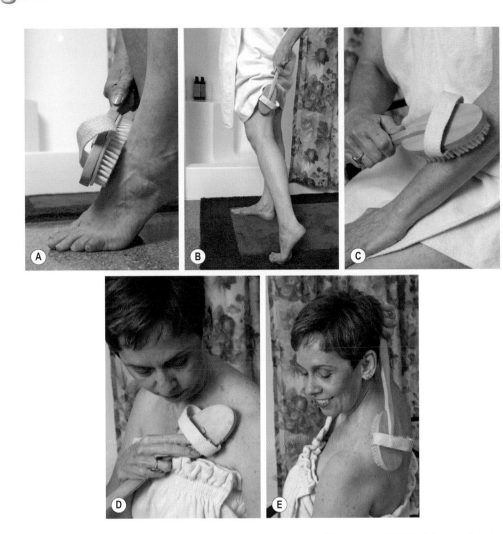

FIGURE 10.5
Dry brushing. (**A**) Dry brushing the foot. (**B**) Dry brushing the leg. (**C**) Dry brushing the forearm. (**D**) Dry brushing the chest. (**E**) Dry brushing the back.

an excellent self-care treatment (see Figure 10.5). Use a natural fiber brush since nylon or synthetic fiber brushes are often too sharp and may damage the skin.

Wilbarger Brushing Therapy is very similar to the technique you will learn, and is given specifically to help the nervous system. Developed by an occupational therapist for parents to use with their children, it consists of long sweeping strokes on bare skin with a soft-bristled brush. Parents generally begin a Wilbarger Program by brushing the whole body every two hours during the day. This technique is recommended for children who are autistic, tactilely defensive, highly anxious, or hyperactive, or who have poor motor co-ordination. In these cases, the child's central nervous system is thought to be immature and the brushing stimulates sensory nerves to such an extent that neurological pathways become better developed and many issues disappear. Parents also find it helpful for their child's anxiety and insomnia (Wilbarger,

2002). Many old-time hydrotherapists also recommended brushing for neurological problems, anxiety and tics.

SNAPSHOT

Time needed 5–10 minutes.

Equipment needed A soft natural-bristle brush, loofah sponge, or coarse bath glove. A softer brush should be used with clients who are new to this treatment; then, when the skin has become less sensitive, a coarser brush may be used.

Effect Mechanical.

Cleanup When a brush has been used during a session, wash it thoroughly with soap and hot water, then spray it with alcohol and air-dry it before storing it. When a client is brushing herself daily, her brush should be washed regularly with soap and hot water, and then thoroughly air-dried.

Indications General conditioning; skin stimulation, particularly for individuals who are sedentary, bedridden, or wheelchair-using, or who have reduced sensation; stimulation of blood vessels and lymphatic vessels underneath the skin.

Contraindications Open, infected, damaged or sunburned skin; eczema; fungal infections such as ringworm or athlete's foot; skin rashes; skin that has just been shaved; advanced varicose veins.

Procedure

1. Begin brushing by brushing one entire foot (Figure 10.5A) and leg (Figure 10.5B), starting with the sole of the foot and working up the leg. Brush vigorously in circular motions, keeping the brush in contact with the skin. Use the maximum pressure that is comfortable; over time, the skin will tolerate more pressure. Go more slowly and lightly over sensitive areas. If you wish, you may use a warm compress as each area is brushed.

2. Repeat on the other foot and leg.
3. Brush one arm (Figure 10.5C), starting with the hand and working up to the shoulder.
4. Repeat on the other arm.
5. Brush the abdomen and chest (Figure 10.5D) with strokes moving towards the heart.
6. Brush the entire back (Figure 10.5E) and the posterior surface of the legs.
7. Brush the neck, using slower and lighter pressure. Do not brush the face.
8. Take a shower of any desired length: all that is necessary is a brief shower to cleanse the skin, but a contrast shower enhances the tonifying effect of the brushing. Or you may finish each area by applying a hot compress.
9. Towel off vigorously.
10. Moisturize the skin with an appropriate oil or lotion.

CHAPTER SUMMARY

This chapter has discussed three classic friction treatments that may be used to advantage by massage therapists, using rough wet washcloths, moistened salt, or dry brushes. You have also learned a treatment which combines frictions and hot compresses with hands-on treatments. Frictions are easy to perform, are enjoyed by massage clients, and complement hands-on massage techniques. They are simple to integrate into your massage sessions, and to combine with other hydrotherapy treatments if you like, and you can also share them with your clients as a home treatment.

REVIEW QUESTIONS

Short answer

1. The salt glow was originally seen as an alternative to what other friction treatment?

2. Why was the salt glow substituted for this treatment?

3. Explain the stimulating effect of a cold mitten friction.

4. Name two ways to vary the effects of a salt glow.

5. Why would a contrast shower add to the tonifying effect of dry brushing?

6. Name one neutral-temperature treatment from this chapter and one from a previous chapter.

Multiple choice

7. When performing a salt glow, which would you use? use one:

   A. Slightly moistened salt

   B. Dry salt

   C. A 20% salt solution

   D. Salt water

8. Which is not an effect of a friction treatment?

   A. Sensory stimulation

   B. Dilation of surface blood vessels

   C. Skin exfoliation

   D. Removal of wrinkles

9. Salt glows can be varied by using all these additives but one. Which is the exception?

   A. Whole and ground herbs

   B. Pebbles

   C. Creams

   D. Essential oils

10. Which of these does a cold mitten friction *not* use?

    A. Sea salt or Epsom salts

    B. Terrycloth mitts

    C. Natural fiber brush

    D. Soapy water

11. Local salt glows are contraindicated for all but one:

    A. Eczema

    B. Fungal infections

    C. Poor local circulation

    D. Ice stroking

    E. Sunburned skin

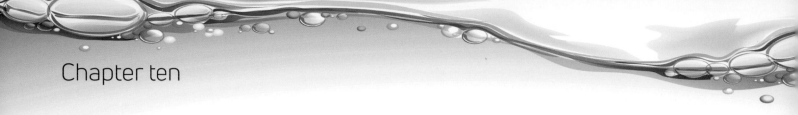

Chapter ten

References

Kellogg JH. Rational Hydrotherapy. Battle Creek, MI: Modern Medicine Publishing Company, 1923

Peterson S. Hydrotherapy in the Home Made Easy. New York: Professional Health Media Services, 1974

Vogel A. The Nature Doctor. New York; Keats Publishing, Inc., 1952

Wilbarger P. Wilbarger approach to treating sensory defensiveness and clinical application of the sensory diet. In Bundy AC, Murray EA, Lane S (eds). Sensory Integration: Theory and Practice, 2nd edn. Philadelphia, PA: FA Davis, 2002

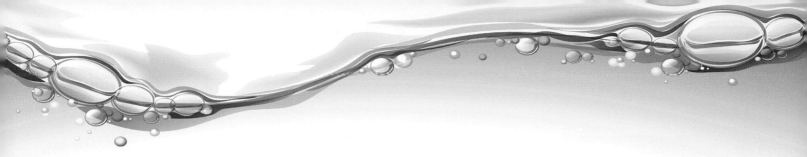

Hydrotherapy self-treatments for health and wellness 11

The various applications of water tend to remove the roots of the disease; they are able to dissolve the morbid matters in the blood, to evacuate what is dissolved, to make the cleansed blood circulate rightly again, finally to harden the enfeebled organism.

Sebastian Kneipp, *My Water Cure*, 1897

CHAPTER OBJECTIVES

After completing this chapter, the student will be able to:

1. Describe three different detoxification treatments and explain how they work
2. Define and explain body hardening
3. Give specific examples of body hardening treatments
4. Describe and perform tonic hydrotherapy treatments that are given to the whole body
5. Describe and perform tonic hydrotherapy treatments that are given to just one part of the body
6. Describe self-care treatments for the professional massage therapist.

As we have seen throughout this book, hydrotherapy can be an excellent adjunct to massage. It can also promote general health and wellness, while helping your clients see faster and better results from their massage sessions. Various treatments described in this chapter can stimulate the body's functions, increase local circulation, eliminate toxins and even help prevent repetitive strain injury. Tonic treatments are traditional in many cultures; most need to be performed on a regular basis (see Figure 11.1). These can be woven into the work you do with your clients, if you give them the self-treatment instruction sheets in Appendix A and then check in on

how well the treatments are working. This chapter also highlights an effective treatment for lead poisoning: although unusually time-consuming by today's standards, this technique helps us understand how we can use water treatments to assist the body's own self-healing powers. It also explains the usefulness of close observation of the client when carrying out treatments and how, with patience and persistence, simple-looking techniques can be very effective.

DETOXIFICATION TREATMENTS

Detoxification treatments use the body's own self-healing processes either to excrete **toxins** or to prevent their build-up. Toxins from the external environment may be swallowed, inhaled, or absorbed through the skin, while metabolic wastes such as urea and lactic acid are produced by normal body processes. Chemicals to which we humans were never exposed until recently are now found at low levels in numerous items we use all the time, from cookware, clothing, children's toys and personal-care products to electronics, furniture and building materials. Many popular cosmetics contain petroleum derivatives, dyes, preservatives and synthetic fragrances, while our drinking water is frequently contaminated with antidepressants, painkillers and other prescription medications (Malkan, 2007; Sinclair, 2012). Because we take in so many of these chemicals, toxic or not, our bodies have been likened to molecular sponges. Children are the most at risk of contamination, so much so that some toxicologists now advise women to go on detoxification programs before pregnancy. Mother's milk concentrates pollutants

Chapter eleven

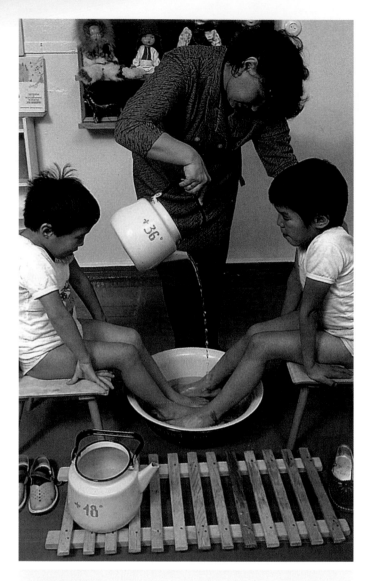

FIGURE 11.1
Just south of the Arctic circle, where winter temperatures may go as low as −50°F (−45°C), Chukotka children receive contrast footbaths to train their bodies to tolerate cold. Photo courtesy Mark Wexler.

stored in fat and passes them on to the next generation. For example, synthetic fragrances and sunscreens a mother applies to her skin can be found first in her breastmilk and then in the bloodstream of her nursing baby. Pollutants such as heavy metals, some pesticides, phthalates and fire-retardant chemicals are found in everyone's bloodstream and contribute to chronic issues.

After centuries of trial and error, observant humans have found ingenious ways to eliminate toxins. Three traditional hydrotherapy treatments that are used for this purpose are whole-body heating, bathing in water with chemical additives, and deep-water bathing.

Whole-body heating

Sweating is stimulated by any hydrotherapy treatment that raises the core temperature, and, as discussed in Box 11.1, many toxic chemicals can be excreted in sweat. These include both recreational and prescription drugs – everything from nicotine to antibiotics (Hoigy, 1995; Hoigy, 2000; Liberty, 2004; Saito, 2004). Metabolic wastes such as urea and lactic acid can be sweated out as well. One dramatic example of detoxification using sweating is the sauna treatment used with sickened rescue workers who were at the World Trade Center in New York City soon after the attack on September 11, 2001. Massive amounts of concrete, asbestos building materials, drywall, plastics, steel, office furnishings and thousands of computers were first pulverized and then incinerated, while diesel and jet fuel burned in great clouds overhead. There was an enormous release of toxic substances into the air, including asbestos, benzene, dioxins, mercury, manganese, lead, **polychlorinated biphenyls** (PCBs), fiberglass, silicon, sulfuric acid and other chemicals. Rescue workers absorbed complex mixtures of the poisons through their skin or by inhaling smoke and soot. Soon after the event, many of the rescue workers began to develop persistent health problems: most common were respiratory ailments such as asthma, bronchitis and sinus problems, digestive tract problems such as gastroesophageal reflux disease and severe stomach pain, and emotional changes such as depression. Mainstream medical treatment was often not effective, and so hundreds of the rescue workers tried the sauna program, with good results. The process lasted a full month and began each day with aerobic exercise to heat the body, followed by a stay of two or more hours in a 140–180°F (60–82°C) sauna (Figure 11.2 shows two New York City firefighters in the sauna). Rescue workers exited the sauna, showered and then went back in the sauna again a few more times: this prevented overheating and washed off excreted substances before they could be reabsorbed by the skin. Towels used to wipe off their chemical-laden sweat were stained a variety of unusual colors including orange, blue, green and black. (One such towel is shown in Figure 11.3, being held up by the firefighter who used it. When a sample of the towel was cut off and sent for analysis, tests showed the man's sweat had high levels of

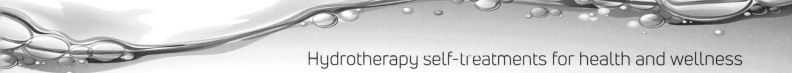

toxic heavy metals, especially manganese, which had been a component of the building's steel girders.) Afterwards, the great majority of sauna-takers needed less medication and had fewer sick days, and their vestibular and neurologic function was much improved. Blood samples were taken before and after the saunas, and revealed greatly reduced levels of polychlorinated biphenyls (PCBs), improved thyroid function, and more normal cholesterol levels (New York Detox and Drug Rehab, 2006; Dahlgren, 2007). Not just the 9/11 rescue workers but all US firefighters now have more cancers than American citizens as a whole, and their chance of having lung cancer and leukemia increases with the amount of time they spend at fires (Li, 2012; NIOSH, 2016). Today, the smoke and soot they are exposed to is far higher in cancer-causing chemicals than in the past – the

more synthetic materials there are in the burning building, the more carcinogens in the smoke. Their firefighting gear and any exposed skin can become coated with carcinogenic compounds and a hot environment greatly increases skin absorption. To address this concern, many US and Canadian fire departments have now incorporated saunas into their departments. When firefighters return from a call, they shower, put on gym clothes, then pedal on a stationary bicycle inside the sauna to work up a sweat, and then shower again. Many find their bodies no longer have the "fire smell" that used to come off their bodies for up to a week after a call (McKay, 2018). Police officers with major health problems stemming from methamphetamine exposure at work have also benefited from sauna therapy (Ross, 2012).

BOX 11.1	POINT OF INTEREST

SWEATING: A HYDROTHERAPY TREATMENT FOR DETOXIFICATION

Many external substances are obviously toxic and can cause significant health issues. For example, arsenic can cause lowered immunity, some types of cancer, and poor respiratory or cardiovascular function; while lead can cause slow growth, hyperactivity and learning problems in children, and muscle and joint pain, anemia, infertility, immune system problems, hypertension and kidney problems. More than half of the lead-related deaths in the US each year are due to the effects of hypertension on the heart (Lanphear, 2017, 2018; WHO, 2018). In large amounts, both arsenic and lead can be fatal.

The toxins that individuals are exposed to often depend upon where they live. Some naturally occurring chemicals can contaminate the water or food supply. For example, if you live where the bedrock contains high levels of arsenic, your groundwater will also have high levels of arsenic. If you live where there are human activities such as farming or mining there may be different toxins. Just living close to a copper smelter or a mercury mine can expose one to high levels of copper or mercury in one's soil, water or air, while a person who lives in a farming area is more likely to be exposed to pesticides, and a resident of an urban area could be exposed to heavy metals

associated with chronic illness, such as cadmium, chromium or mercury (Alloway, 2005). Children can also accumulate toxins during fetal life – chemicals that a woman has accumulated in her body, such as dioxins and PCBs, can affect a baby from conception onwards.

Although the primary effect of sweating is to help cool the body, it can also eliminate many of the toxins discussed above. When a hot person perspires profusely, toxins are mobilized from fat tissues into the sweat. When a person's other channels of excretion (such as the lungs or kidneys) are not functioning properly, many other toxins may leave the body via the sweat. For example, if a person has long-standing kidney disease, the sweat glands will adapt by excreting more of the wastes the kidney cannot. Because the detoxifying action of sweat can be so powerful, the skin is sometimes referred to as the "third kidney," and the sweat glands as "miniature nephrons."

Environmental toxins which are associated with chronic illness and can be excreted in the sweat include:

1. Pesticides, including organochlorine pesticides
2. Persistent flame retardants and bisphenol-A (BPA; Sears, 2012)

Box 11.1 *continued*

3. Phthalates and polychlorinated biphenyls (PCBs), which are used to manufacture plastics (Genius, 2011)

4. Dioxins (Genius, 2011)

5. Heavy metals such as cadmium, aluminum, lead, mercury, copper and nickel (Sunderman, 1974; Sears, 2012)

6. Illicit drugs, including methamphetamine, amphetamine and cocaine, which can be detected in sweat within two hours (Barnes, 2008; Ross, 2012)

Mercury is a striking example of a dangerous toxin that can be excreted in sweat. Mercury poisoning generally has its most devastating effects on the central nervous system, but it is also toxic to other body systems. Women exposed during pregnancy are more likely to have children with neurological and immune system problems. Mercury can be absorbed by breathing vapor, having it directly upon your skin, or eating contaminated food.

Ideally mercury is simply excreted through the urine and feces, but for hundreds of years sweating treatments have been used to help rid the body of large amounts. In Almaden, Spain, site of the world's largest mercury mine, saunas have been used since 1752 to detoxify mine workers suffering from acute exposure (Figure 1). In 1978, toxicologist William Stopford used daily saunas (Figure 2) at 160–180°F (71–82°C) to successfully detoxify a man who had been exposed to high levels of mercury and was very sick. As his mercury levels dropped, the patient's health improved (Stopford, 1979).

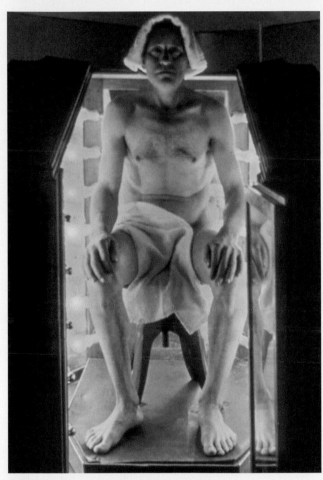

FIGURE 1
Mercury miner in a "hot box" at the world's oldest and largest mercury mine, in Almaden, Spain, 1972. Miners who are sick from mercury vapors have used the mine hospital's sauna for hundreds of years: at Spain's colonial mercury mines they were sent away to hotter climes to work and sweat. Note: a "hot box" is normally closed when the person is in it, but in the photo the door is open so you can see the light bulbs that are being used to heat it. Photograph courtesy of Bob Madden.

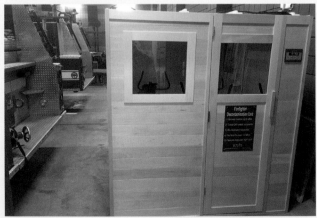

FIGURE 2
Fire Station Decontamination Unit, 2019: stationary bicycles can be seen inside the sauna. Photo: Rodney Palmer, courtesy of SaunaRay.

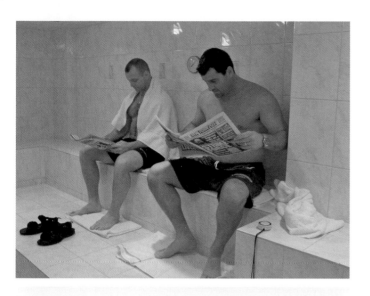

FIGURE 11.2
Using saunas for detoxification. Sauna treatment of two New York City firefighters exposed to toxins at the World Trade Center Site, 2001. Photograph courtesy of New York City Rescue Workers Detoxification Project.

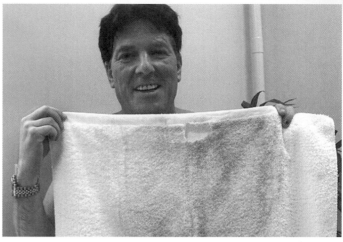

FIGURE 11.3
Sweat excreted by one firefighter. As seen in the photograph, a small piece of this towel was removed so the man's sweat could be analyzed; tests found that it contained high levels of manganese and other heavy metals. Manganese was one of the components of the steel girders of the Twin Towers of the World Trade Center and found in the toxic dust afterwards. Manganese toxicity can lead to cognitive problems and a type of Parkinson's disease. Photograph courtesy of New York City Rescue Workers Detoxification Project.

At the same time that it detoxifies through sweating, whole-body heating also shifts toxic substances out of fatty tissues. The core temperature rises, blood flow increases, and toxic chemicals stored in the tissues are picked up and returned to the bloodstream. When that blood flows through the liver, the toxins are broken down and excreted in the person's urine, bile and feces. The case of a patient treated by Jozeph Krop is a good example of this process. She had been exposed to a variety of toxic chemicals in her work at an appliance factory and suffered from asthma, irritable bowel syndrome, fibromyalgia, chronic urinary tract infections and many other health problems. Initial blood tests detected three highly toxic **solvents**. After one week of daily 150°F (66°C) saunas, tests showed that the levels of the original three solvents were lower, but three additional solvents were now circulating in her bloodstream. Finally, after more saunas, none of the six solvents was found in her blood tests. While she felt sicker than usual during the detox process, her health improved dramatically afterwards (Krop, 1998). Other patients with toxic exposures have been sauna-treated with similar results (Tretjak, 1990; Schnare, 1984; Kilburn, 1989; Rhea, 1997; Ross, 2012).

TREATMENT

SAUNA

Cross-reference

See Chapter 8.

Duration and frequency

15–30 minute sessions two or three times a week.

Cautions

1. To avoid dehydration, be sure to drink a cup of water before entering the sauna and 1–2 cups more during and after the sauna.

2. Do not take more than 2 or 3 saunas a week; too many heating treatments can actually be weakening to the system due to water and electrolyte losses.

3. Take only 10–15 minute saunas until you are used to taking them. Leave the sauna immediately if not tolerating the heat well, i.e. feeling lightheaded or weak.

Special instructions

Shower each time you leave the sauna.

Baths with detoxifying additives

Warm baths with special additives are another traditional hydrotherapy treatment that may be used for detoxification (see Case history 11.1). Baking soda, sea salt, Epsom salts, activated charcoal or powdered seaweed are used here. When used with a bath, these additives may have the effect of neutralizing or absorbing toxins (see pages 114, 167, 168 and 171). For example, seaweed has the ability to remove not only heavy metals such as arsenic from the body, but do the same for toxic compounds in municipal wastewater; while charcoal is used worldwide to adsorb hundreds of substances, including drugs and toxins that are swallowed. Other uses for charcoal include capturing mercury emissions, radioactive substances at nuclear power plants, and toxins in sewage treatment plants. Charcoal is used in filters to purify air and water as well (Bhattacharva, 2017; Bilal, 2018; Dinsley, 2005; Schechter, 1990).

A CHARCOAL BATH FOR DETOXIFICATION **CASE HISTORY 11.1**

BACKGROUND

Ustes, a healthy 26-year-old welder, became acutely sick after inhaling fumes from galvanized metal, which contained zinc oxide (a metal known to damage the kidneys and prevent them from functioning correctly). Blood tests showed high levels of waste products that are normally removed by the kidneys, and he was scheduled to begin dialysis in a matter of days.

TREATMENT

Calvin Thrash, MD, put Ustes on a healthy diet and exercise program: however, his main treatment was a daily whole-body charcoal bath, combined with a charcoal poultice over the kidney area each night. His blood tests showed steady drops in waste products after one week, and by the end of three weeks his blood chemistry was near normal. Ten years later, he had remained healthy, and he never did have to undergo dialysis (Dinsley, 2005).

BOX 11.2   **POINT OF INTEREST**

REPEATED BATHING GETS THE LEAD OUT!

Lead poisoning has been around for a long time, at least since the Roman Empire. This useful but highly toxic metal can accumulate over time, injures many body systems, and is particularly harmful to young children. Sources of environmental contamination include mining, manufacture of lead-acid car batteries, recycling of products that contain lead, and the continued use of leaded paint and gasoline in some countries. As consumers, we are also exposed to lead in many of the objects we use every day, and in our drinking water if it is carried in lead pipes. As recently as 2014, a lead-caused public health crisis began when the city of Flint, Michigan, began to draw its water from an extremely polluted river. Lead began to leach from water pipes into the city water supply, which doubled the number of children with elevated blood levels, while fertility rates fell and fetal deaths tripled. Long-term effects are expected to be seen for decades or longer (Hanna-Attisha, 2018).

The Industrial Revolution created not only a massive demand for the metal but widespread lead poisoning. Huge numbers of people were exposed through their jobs as painters, plumbers, potters, glass workers and miners. The most common beverages (cider, rum and wine) were contaminated by lead equipment when they were made, had lead added to them as a preservative, were stored in lead-lined casks, or were drunk from pewter tankards. Ludwig van Beethoven's deafness and many other chronic health problems came mainly from drinking contaminated wine and from treatment with medicines such as lead paste poultices (Martin Mai, 2007). In the late 1700s, Bath Hospital in Bath, England, was full of young men suffering from lead-induced paralysis, known as the 'lead palsy'. (Hundreds of case

Box 11.2 *continued*

histories from Bath doctors were published, beginning in the 1600s.) Acute lead exposure can affect the peripheral nervous system, especially motor nerves, and these sad individuals could be seen dragging themselves around the wards, their arms hanging limply at their sides, some unable to feed or dress themselves. Patients with painful lead-induced gout were also common at Bath. While the standard treatment for lead palsy and lead gout was purges and opiates, spa therapy showed itself to be far more effective for these two conditions.

The usual regimen was three long baths a week for 24 weeks, and daily drinking of copious amounts of Bath water. Bathers were required to sit in alcoves along the pool's walls so they could be immersed up to their necks for two hours or more. Records show at least half of lead palsy patients were completely cured and the rest had obvious benefit. Gout sufferers improved too: as their urination increased and lead was flushed, their joint swelling and pain decreased. Without knowing the exact mechanisms, but simply though trial and error and close observation, Bath doctors had come up with a very effective treatment for lead poisoning (Rolls, 2012).

Over the centuries, different theories were advanced to explain Bath's therapeutic success: from getting rid of excess humors, to dissolving overly thick body fluids, to minerals in the Bath water penetrating the skin and having a therapeutic effect on internal organs, to simple warming of the patients. It was not until 1986 that it became clear how lead was flushed by bathing.

How did the baths work?

1. Seated baths created greater water pressure on the lower body than the upper body (known as **hydrostatic pressure**). Then, the pressure squeezed blood up into the trunk, like toothpaste squeezed from the bottom up, which increased the blood volume and hence the blood pressure there.

2. Nerve endings in the arterial walls (called **baroceptors**) relayed the rise in pressure to the brain.

3. The brain stimulated the kidneys to release more urine in order to decrease blood volume and lower blood pressure. Patients, who were already urinating more since they had drunk so much water, then urinated even more.

4. Researchers finally worked out that during the second hour of a seated bath, lead begins to be excreted by the kidneys at almost five times the normal rate (Heywood, 1986). The treatment would cause only a small amount of lead to be lost per bath, but over time a great deal of the metal was gradually removed from the body. The patient's lead palsy (paralysis) was either gone or greatly improved, and gout symptoms greatly relieved. (Doctors had figured out that sufferers from other types of paralysis not connected to lead, such as that from strokes, brain damage or disc injuries, did not improve very much.)

TREATMENT

BATHS WITH DETOXIFYING ADDITIVES

Cross-reference

See Chapter 6.

Duration and frequency

20–30 minute baths two or three times a week.

continued

TREATMENT *continued*

Cautions

1. To avoid dehydration, be sure to drink a cup of water before entering the bath, and 1–2 cups more during and after the bath.

2. Leave the bath immediately if not tolerating the heat well, i.e. feeling nauseated or tired. If you feel light-headed or weak, let the water out of the tub and sit there while your body cools down and until you feel normal again.

continued

Special instructions

1. Below are five different recipes for a detoxifying bath:

   - 1 cup of sea salt, 1 cup of Epsom salts, and 1½ cups of baking soda.
   - 2 cups of sea salt and 1½ cups of baking soda.
   - 4 cups of Epsom salts.
   - ¼–½ cup of powdered charcoal.
   - ¼–½ cup of powdered dried seaweed.

2. Shower off right after the bath, to clean the skin of any toxins that have been excreted.

TONIC HYDROTHERAPY TREATMENTS

Tonic hydrotherapy treatments stimulate body functions, increase physical vigor, decrease fatigue and give a sense of well-being. Exposing yourself to extremes of hot and cold or exercise in order to strengthen the body is sometimes called "body hardening." Many of the early hydrotherapists relied heavily upon cold treatments to treat chronic illness, using baths, showers, wet sheet wraps and walking in snow or morning dew. Local treatments such as contrast baths were popular for stimulating function in specific areas.

As discussed in Chapter 2, the body senses both extreme cold and extreme heat as potential threats to the core temperature and reacts defensively. First whole-body cold exposures cause the sympathetic nervous system to rev up; next skin blood vessels constrict, shivering begins, and many other processes work together to increase internal heat production. If you tend to react weakly to cold, repeated exposure can train your blood vessels to contract more strongly, or if your thyroid is underactive, this can stimulate its function. Repeated exposure to whole-body heating treatments also conditions the blood vessels to react more strongly, and sweat glands to produce more fluid. Tonic treatments for individual areas of the body have similar effects.

In summary, below is a list of key points to remember about tonic hydrotherapy treatments:

1. They can have powerful short-term effects, particularly upon the circulatory system. They are the perfect complement to the circulation-enhancing effects of bodywork.

2. These effects are not permanent, and so they need to be done on a regular basis.

3. Although anyone can benefit from these tonic treatments, those with weak constitutions, low energy and endurance, and poor resistance to infections can benefit the most.

4. Anyone not accustomed to extremes of heat or cold should begin with a milder treatment and gradually increase (or decrease) the water temperature. (In 1894, world-famous hydrotherapist Sebastian Kneipp travelled to Rome to treat the ailing Pope Leo XIII, and immediately started the frail old man's treatment with an ice-cold bath: Kneipp was sent straight home!) Ask your client to stop any treatment immediately if they have a bad reaction such as feeling nauseated or light-headed.

5. It is important to observe the contraindications given with each treatment, as some of these treatments can be a significant challenge to the body's adaptive powers.

6. Tonic treatments provide different sensations. Some are soothing and relaxing, such as saunas and warm baths, while others are more invigorating, such as contrast treatments and cold showers. As such, they complement the relaxing and/or invigorating sensations that our clients get from bodywork.

7. These tonic treatments have long histories of continuous use in many cultures for a good reason – try them, use them safely, and see for yourself what effect they have.

Whole-body tonic treatments

Studies suggest these treatments have several benefits, including improving mood, boosting immunity, affecting basal metabolic rate, increasing tolerance to both cold and heat, and stimulating healthy functioning of blood vessels.

- Exposure to both extreme cold and extreme heat causes increased numbers of white blood cells. Thus, people who take either contrast showers or saunas

CONTRAST SHOWERS INCREASE RESISTANCE TO THE COMMON COLD   CASE HISTORY 11.2

BACKGROUND

Edzard Ernst, a professor of medicine at the Hanover Medical School in Munich, Germany, investigated the effect of contrast showers on the common cold. Ernst selected contrast showers because he wanted to find a simple, practical and inexpensive therapy that could be performed in anyone's home. 25 people participated by taking regular contrast showers, while a similar group of 25 people acted as controls and took no contrast showers. Their average age was 28 years old. Whenever any of the 50 participants had a cold, blood samples were taken to confirm the diagnosis, and each person also kept a diary of their cold symptoms during the six months of the study.

TREATMENT

In one study, 25 people gave themselves contrast showers five times a week for six months, for a total of 137 showers. Another 25 people were controls and didn't take the showers. Subjects were gradually introduced to the entire procedure: hot showers (96–104°F; 36–40°C) always lasted 5 minutes, but cold showers were limited to the arms and legs at first, then became very brief whole-body ones, and finally the cold showers became longer and colder, until they lasted 2 minutes at 52–65°F (11–18°C).

After six months, Dr. Ernst examined blood samples and the cold diaries from both groups. He found that the shower group had significantly fewer colds and that those colds were milder and shorter. It took about three months for this improvement to show up, suggesting that the showers had gradually strengthened their immune systems. It was possible that the improvement might have been even greater if the experiment had continued for more than six months (Ernst, 1990).

---

on a regular basis have fewer colds, while regular swimming in very cold water significantly increases concentrations of plasma interleukin, leukocytes and monocytes in the blood (Dugue, 2000; Ernst, 1990). See Case history 11.2, which investigates the relationship between contrast showers and greater immunity.

- A short intense exposure to whole-body cold stimulates heat production, raises the basal metabolic rate and reduces fatigue. Subjects who were immersed in 75°F (24°C) water up to their necks for 90 minutes had three times their original metabolic rate (Leblanc, 1975). Similar results have come from studies with experimental animals and people who work in cold temperatures (Tikuisis, 2000; Radomski, 1982). One 1998 study investigated the effect of cold baths on blood cholesterol levels. Using 68 patients with high numbers, blood samples were taken before and after three months of regular cold baths. Not only did patients have a higher metabolic rate, they also produced more **noradrenaline** and thyroid hormone than before and their cholesterol levels were significantly lower. Low levels of thyroid hormones are associated with chronic feelings of coldness (DeLorenzo, 1998; DeLorenzo, 1999).

One scientist reviewed eight studies of cold showers and found that cold water can reduce fatigue in patients with fibromyalgia, multiple sclerosis, and rheumatoid arthritis (Shevchuk, 2010). For more on cold immersion and depression, see Chapter 13.

- Many people who take regular contrast showers feel warmer in the winter than those who do not. After repeated short stays in intensely cold air or cold water, the same is true (Leppaluoto, 2001; Smith, 2004). One study looked at how well men who had been exposed to cold fared when they moved to a cold climate. Before travelling, the men took very cold baths for three weeks. Tests showed their sympathetic nervous systems were more active than before, and they had higher basal metabolic rates and increased body temperature. Only then did they travel to the Arctic and stay for 16 days, along with another group of men who had not taken any cold baths. Those in the cold bath group tolerated the −80°F (−62°C) weather much better than the non-bath group (Hannuksela, 2001).

- Regular whole-body heat exposures increase tolerance. When winter ends and summer begins, the body quickly adjusts from the task of keeping itself warm in winter to the task of keeping cool in summer.

Chapter eleven

Within two weeks of hotter weather, remarkable adaptations are made: sweating begins sooner, people sweat more, less salt is lost in our sweat, and metabolic rates become lower. In the same way, someone who takes regular saunas also sweats more when he or she is exposed to heat, begins sweating sooner, and so has a better tolerance (Ogilvie, 1972). The blood vessels and heart also become better at adapting to intense heat: the person's heart rate does not increase as much in the sauna, blood vessels actually dilate and constrict better, and over a period of time there is often a significant decrease in systolic blood pressure. Some researchers now advocate using saunas to treat conditions in which patients suffer from poorly functioning blood vessels (Masuda, 2004; Biro, 2003; Hooper, 1999; Kihara, 2004). However, more research is needed before this can be safely recommended.

Below are a number of tonic whole-body treatments that you can recommend to your clients. Each of the treatments below are also used as specific tonics for the immune system.

TREATMENT

CONTRAST SHOWER

Cross-reference

See Chapter 8.

Duration and frequency

Take a 2-minute hot shower followed by a 1-minute cold shower and do this three times, for a total time of 9 minutes. Perform once daily.

TREATMENT

CONTRAST COLD-WATER TREADING

Cross-reference

See Chapter 6.

Duration and frequency

Alternate a 30-second hot footbath followed by cold water marching for 10 seconds. Do this ten times,

continued

TREATMENT *continued*

for a total time of about 6 minutes. Perform once daily.

Special instructions

The client will need to prepare a hot footbath and also fill a bathtub half-full of cold water. Then perform ten rounds of immersing the feet in the hot footbath for 30 seconds, then carefully transferring to the cold bathtub to march in place for 10 seconds.

Cautions

The client needs to be very careful that he or she does not slip while transferring from the hot water to the cold and back again. A mat or a towel that does not slip should be placed under the hot footbath, and a grab bar is recommended.

TREATMENT

COLD SHOWER

Cross-reference

See Chapter 8.

Duration and frequency

Total time in the shower is 1 minute. Perform once daily.

TREATMENT

WHOLE-BODY SALT GLOW

Cross-reference

See Chapter 10.

Duration and frequency

Total time for the salt glow is about 10 minutes. Perform one to three times per week.

Special instructions

Finish by moisturizing the skin.

TREATMENT

COLD MITTEN FRICTION

Cross-reference

See Chapter 10.

Duration and frequency

Total time for the cold mitten friction is about 10 minutes. Perform daily.

TREATMENT

BATH WITH VASODILATING ADDITIVES

Cross-reference

See Chapter 6.

Duration and frequency

Total time for the bath is 20 minutes. Take the bath two or three times weekly.

Special instructions

1. Add 5 tablespoons (75 ml) of either powdered ginger or ground mustard seed to the water, or add 2 teaspoons of cayenne pepper (10ml). Begin with slightly less than these amounts, since some people's skin may be extra sensitive, then increase as needed.

2. Finish the bath with a 1-minute cold shower, making it as cold as can possibly be tolerated.

3. Drink water before and after the bath.

TREATMENT

DRY BRUSHING

Cross-reference

See Chapter 10.

Duration and frequency

Total time for dry brushing is 5–10 minutes. Perform daily.

TREATMENT

SAUNA

Cross-reference

See Chapter 7.

Duration and frequency

Take 15–30 minute saunas two or three times per week.

Cautions

1. To avoid dehydration, be sure to drink a cup of water before entering the sauna, and a total of 1–2 cups more during and after the sauna.

2. Do not take more than two or three saunas a week; too many heating treatments can actually be weakening to the system due to water and electrolyte losses.

3. Until accustomed to taking saunas, stay in only 10–15 minutes. Leave the sauna immediately if not tolerating the heat well, i.e. feeling light-headed or weak.

4. Take a shower at the end of the sauna for 1 minute, making it as cold as can be tolerated.

Partial-body tonic treatments

Tonic treatments for individual areas of the body actually condition blood vessels so they contract faster and with more force. Common signs of poor local circulation include tissue which is cold to the touch, puffy, pale, or seems cold to the client, and many poorly healing scrapes, cuts or other wounds. Many studies have found improvements in the body's response to hot and cold temperatures with the following tonic treatments. For example, when the hands are regularly immersed in cold water, their arterioles begin to contract faster and more strongly (Ogilvie, 1972). When people with Raynaud's syndrome are exposed to cold temperatures, the arterioles in their hands tend to spasm, leading to greatly decreased blood flow to the tissues, discomfort and, in extreme cases, tissue damage. But regular hot hand soaks can train their arterioles to dilate when they would normally constrict. Three different experiments found that by having patients regularly immerse their hands in hot hand baths as they sit in a very cold room, their response to cold becomes more normal. At the end of each experiment, their hands were 3–6°F warmer, even when they were out in the cold air (Jobe, 1982; 1985; 1986).

By alternating maximum vasodilation with maximum vasoconstriction, contrast treatments provide even greater stimulation. These fluctuations in local blood flow can be helpful for many circulatory issues (Fiscus, 2005; Rudovsky, 1977). For example, patients with varicose veins who received alternating hot and cold showers to the legs for 25 days experienced significant improvement in the circulation to their legs. In people with advanced varicose veins, blood tends to pool in their lower legs and cause an increase in leg and ankle circumference; in this case, however, the volume of blood and the circumference in the lower legs and ankles was significantly reduced by this contrast treatment. More important to the patients, they had significantly less leg discomfort and pain (Saradeth, 1991).

The muscles of the person's arterial walls generally function better for some time after a series of contrast treatments is over. For example, contrast leg showers were used with a group of elderly patients with **intermittent claudication,** a condition where there is reduced blood flow to the legs. When someone with this condition tries to walk, there is not enough blood flow and oxygen to the leg muscles and the legs hurt. Everyone in this study received a 25-minute contrast treatment to the legs every other day for three weeks, for a total of ten treatments. They sat in shower chairs while alternating streams of hot and cold water flowed over their legs and feet. Immediately after the experiment and one month later, there was a significant increase in everyone's leg/foot blood pressure. Three quarters of the patients could walk longer before their legs hurt, and they had less pain overall. A year later, some of them still had higher leg blood pressure and less pain when walking, indicating that their blood vessels were still functioning better (Elmstadthl, 1995). Doctors at modern Seventh-Day Adventist hospitals frequently prescribe contrast treatments with leg whirlpools to speed healing of ankle sprains, plantar fasciitis, poorly healing foot and leg wounds (such as varicose and diabetic ulcers), and other conditions.

Tonic treatments for poor local circulation

Below are a number of partial-body tonic treatments that you can use with your clients.

TREATMENT

LOCAL CONTRAST BATH FOR THE HAND, ARM, FOOT OR LEG

Cross-reference

See Chapter 6.

Duration and frequency

Begin by immersing the part in hot water (104–110°F; 40–43°C) for 3 minutes followed by cold water (55°F; 13°C) for 1 minute. Perform 3–6 rounds, ending with cold. Perform the contrast bath daily.

Special instructions

If desired, add vasodilating herbs to the hot water: use one teaspoon (5g) of ginger, mustard powder, or cayenne, and add this to 1 gallon (4 liters) of the hot water.

TREATMENT

LOCAL CONTRAST SHOWERS FOR THE HAND, ARM, FOOT, KNEE OR LEG

Cross-reference

See Chapter 8.

Duration and frequency

Using a hand-held shower, spray hot water on small areas such as the feet for 3 minutes, but longer (up to 5 minutes) for larger, denser areas such as the thighs. Alternate with 1 minute of cold water, and perform a total of 3–6 rounds. Use the contrast shower daily.

Special instructions

The client may sit on the side of a bathtub rather than stand in the shower.

TREATMENT

LOCAL COLD FOOT SHOWER

Cross-reference

See Chapter 8.

continued

TREATMENT *continued*

Duration and frequency

Spray the tops and bottoms of both feet with cold water for 30 seconds to 2 minutes, and use this shower one or two times daily.

Special instructions

1. Make sure you are warm before performing this shower.
2. At the end of the shower, do not step barefoot on the bathroom floor. Dry your feet briskly, then quickly don socks to avoid chilling.

Tonic treatments for the digestive system

Local treatments improve blood flow to the digestive organs and can stimulate tone in sluggish conditions such as atonic constipation.

TREATMENT

LOCAL CONTRAST APPLICATION OVER THE ABDOMEN

Cross-reference

See Chapters 4 and 5.

Duration and frequency

Place large hot compresses, hot fomentations or hydrocollator packs over the entire abdomen for 3–5 minutes; follow that with a brisk cold mitten friction for 30 seconds; and perform a total of three or more rounds. Perform daily.

Special instructions

1. This treatment is contraindicated during pregnancy.
2. This treatment is sometimes given as a liver tonic, done over the upper abdomen only. Follow with a whole-body contrast shower if possible.

Tonic treatments for the eyes

Improving the circulation over the eyes can relieve eyestrain and eye fatigue, as well as give the client's eyes a very refreshed feeling. Especially helpful for those who work at a computer.

TREATMENT

CONTRAST APPLICATIONS USING HOT AND COLD COMPRESSES OR HOT AND COLD GEL PACKS

Cross-reference

See Chapters 4 and 5.

Duration and frequency

Use 2 minutes of hot compresses followed by 30 seconds of cold compresses and repeat three times. Perform daily.

Tonic treatments for skeletal muscles

Because muscle strength is temporarily increased by cold applications, they can be helpful before workouts. For example, a 30-minute leg bath at 54°F (12°C) increases the maximum lifting strength of the legs and delays muscular fatigue, and improved circulation can last up to 6 hours. This effect is due to the combination of both hydrostatic pressure and cold (Menetrier, 2014). Acute heat exposure has the opposite effect on skeletal muscles: after 30 minutes in a hot sauna, muscular endurance in both the leg press and the bench press is significantly decreased (Hedley, 2002). To take advantage of the muscle-stimulating effect, use water as cold as can be tolerated, and submerge the part in the water for at least 5 minutes.

TREATMENT

PARTIAL-BODY COLD BATH

Cross-reference

See Chapter 6.

Duration and frequency

5 minutes. Perform before vigorous exercise.

Special instructions

1. Make sure you are warm before taking the cold bath.
2. Finish by drying the part briskly; then dress, and begin exercise immediately.

TREATMENT

PARTIAL-BODY COLD BATH FOR WEAK OR SPASTIC MUSCLES

Cross-reference

See Chapter 6.

Duration and frequency

The hand, arm, foot or leg is immersed in 35°F (2°C) water for 3 seconds and removed for 30 seconds, and this is repeated six times. Use once daily as a tonic, or whenever the weak or spastic muscles are going to be exercised.

Special instructions

1. Make sure the client is warm before using the cold bath.
2. Instead of a cold bath, a body part can be wrapped in an ice pack made with crushed ice for 10 minutes.

Tonic treatments for the respiratory system

Local treatments improve blood flow to the chest muscles and lungs and make breathing easier.

TREATMENT

LOCAL CONTRAST APPLICATION OVER THE CHEST

Cross-reference

See Chapters 4 and 5.

Duration and frequency

Place large hot compresses, hot fomentations or hydro-collator packs over the entire chest for 3–5 minutes. Be sure to place the heat so that it covers the sides of the chest as well as the front. Next perform a cold mitten friction over the entire chest for 30 seconds. Repeat for a total of three or more rounds. Perform once daily.

TREATMENT

HEAT-TRAPPING COMPRESS TO THE CHEST

Cross-reference

See Chapter 5, Box 5.3.

continued

TREATMENT *continued*

Duration and frequency

The compress is best left on all night. Perform 3–5 times a week.

Special instructions (for the client)

1. Make sure you are warm before applying the compress.
2. Dip a cotton T-shirt in water as cold as can be tolerated, even adding ice to the water if possible.
3. Put the T-shirt on.
4. Take a large plastic trash bag and cut holes for your arms and head.
5. Put the plastic bag on over the T-shirt.
6. Put a dry shirt or sweater on over the plastic bag.
7. Leave on all night, or, if it is uncomfortably warm, for at least 1 hour.
8. Remove and give a cold mitten friction to your chest and as far around the back as you can reach.
9. Dry yourself well and dress warmly.

Tonic treatments for the anterior cervical muscles and throat

A contrast treatment to the throat is especially helpful if the anterior muscles are extremely tight, which can happen if someone has strained the area by singing or coughing a lot (Figure 11.4).

TREATMENT

LOCAL CONTRAST APPLICATION OVER THE THROAT

Cross-reference

See Chapter 5 and Box 6.1.

Duration and frequency

Place a hot compress, moist heating pad or small hot water bottle over the throat for 3–5 minutes. Next place a cold compress over the throat for 1 minute, as shown in Figure 11.4, or perform a gentle cold mitten friction over the throat for 30 seconds. Repeat for a total of three or more rounds.

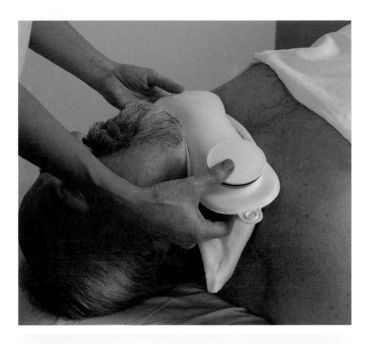

FIGURE 11.4
Throat ice bag.

Tonic treatments for the skin

Tonic treatments for the skin increase circulation and nutrition to the skin and stimulate the nerves.

TREATMENT

CONTRAST SHOWER

Cross-reference
See Chapter 8.

Duration and frequency
Three rounds of a 2-minute hot shower followed by a 1-minute cold shower, for a total time of 9 minutes. Perform once daily.

TREATMENT

WHOLE-BODY SALT GLOW

Cross-reference
See page 235, *Whole-body salt glows.*

continued

TREATMENT *continued*

Duration and frequency
Total time for the salt glow is about 10 minutes. Perform one to three times per week.

Special instructions
Moisturize the skin well afterwards.

TREATMENT

DRY BRUSHING

Cross-reference
See Chapter 10.

Duration and frequency
Total time for dry brushing is 5–10 minutes. Perform daily.

SELF-CARE TREATMENTS FOR THE MASSAGE THERAPIST

Because massage therapist work with their hands and arms intensively – not only for prolonged periods of time, but often while using great pressure – they are particularly at risk of having some type of **repetitive strain injury (RSI).** Even the most conscientious massage therapist, mindful of proper posture and use of the body, and careful to take breaks or rest between massage sessions, must be constantly vigilant to avoid this occupational hazard.

RSIs can affect any of the structures that are involved in massage, such as muscles, tendons, joints, nerves or bursae. Work that requires repetitive bending and twisting of the hand is especially correlated with hand – wrist arthritis (Dillon, 2002).

Our tissues need to be both strong and flexible to avoid injury. Below are a number of local hydrotherapy treatments that can help prevent RSI by stimulating circulation in the upper extremities, making stretching easier, releasing chronic muscle tightness, and maintaining normal range of motion. They can make all the difference between minor injuries that heal quickly and long-lasting ones.

Chapter eleven

Local treatments for the hands, forearms and upper body

Use these when your hands, arms, or other parts of your upper body are aching or tired, or you want to stimulate blood flow between or after sessions.

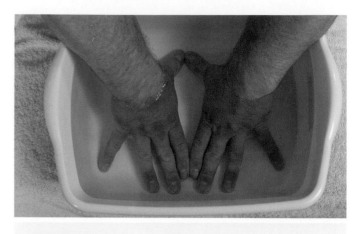

FIGURE 11.5
Epsom salts hand baths with stretching of hand muscles.

TREATMENT

CONTRAST HAND BATHS OR FOREARM BATHS

Cross-reference

See Chapter 6.

Duration and frequency

Three rounds of immersing the hands in hot water for 2 minutes, then immersing the hands in cold water for 1 minute, for a total of 9 minutes. This treatment can be performed as many times as needed during the day, especially before or after performing massage. A shorter version can be easily done when washing your hands after a session.

Special instructions

Contrast baths are an excellent preparation for stretching of the hand and wrist muscles.

TREATMENT

ICED COMPRESS USING GLOVES FOR TIRED, ACHING OR INFLAMED HANDS

Cross-reference

See Chapter 5.

Duration and frequency

10 minutes. This treatment can be performed as many times as needed during the day, especially before or after sessions.

Special instructions

Soak a pair of thin cotton or wool gloves in water, wring them out, and place in a zip-closure bag in the freezer. They will be very cold and stiff when taken out of the freezer: simply run a little cold water over them and then wring them gently so that they are flexible enough to slip on your hands.

TREATMENT

EPSOM SALTS HAND BATH

Cross-reference

See Chapter 6.

Duration and frequency

10–20 minutes. Use anytime the hands feel inflamed or cold.

Special instructions

1. Finish with a brief cold-water dip and dry your hands briskly.
2. As shown in Figure 11.5, the hand and wrist muscles may be stretched while your hands are in the water.

TREATMENT

ICE PACKS AND ICE-WATER BATHS

Cross-reference

See Chapter 6.

Duration and frequency

10–20 minutes. This treatment can be performed as many as three times during a day, especially before or after performing massage.

TREATMENT

PARAFFIN HAND BATH
FOLLOWED BY A SHORT COLD WATER BATH

Cross-reference

See Chapter 6.

Duration and frequency

15 minutes. May be repeated as often as three times daily.

Special instructions

After the hands have been dipped and covered, wait 10 minutes. Remove paraffin, dip your hands in cold water for half a minute, and perform stretching exercises for the hand and wrist muscles.

TREATMENT

HEAT-TRAPPING COMPRESS
FOR THE HANDS OR ARMS

Cross-reference

See Appendix A, page 372.

Duration and frequency

The compress should ideally be left on all night, but at least for 1 hour. It can be used every night if needed.

Stretching and range of motion exercises in a hot shower

A hot shower is an excellent place to stretch the muscles of the upper body, not only because stretching is easier when muscles and fascia are warm, but also because it is a convenient way to add stretching to your daily routine. Prevent slips by using grab bars and placing non-slip tape on your shower floor. You can do the following sequence in about 10 minutes. When you first get in the shower, you can perform gentle range of motion exercises while the hot water warms your tissues. To learn more about stretching in hot water anywhere, see *Hot Water Therapy* by Patrick Horay.

TREATMENT

RANGE OF MOTION EXERCISES

Special instructions

1. Slowly trace the letters of the alphabet with your nose. As you form each letter, you will be making many subtle movements that help free all the joints of the cervical spine. Trace all 26 letters.

2. Roll the shoulders up, back, down and forward to make a circular movement, ten times. Now roll the shoulders in the opposite direction: up, forward, down, and then back to form a circle in the opposite direction, ten times.

3. Straighten the arm, then alternate fully pronating and fully supinating the palm, ten times.

4. Make circles with the wrists in a clockwise direction ten times, then in a counter-clockwise direction ten times.

TREATMENT

UPPER BODY STRETCHES

Hold each area directly under the hot spray, then perform each stretch gently and until you feel a mild tension. Never stretch to the point of pain.

Special instructions

1. Lifting your chin towards the ceiling, turn your head to one side to stretch the front of the neck (Figure 11.6). Hold for 15 seconds; then repeat on the opposite side.

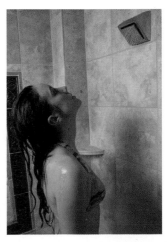

FIGURE 11.6
Front of neck stretch.

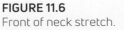

continued

TREATMENT *continued*

2. Tucking your chin to your chest, stretch the back of the neck (Figure 11.7). Hold for 30 seconds.

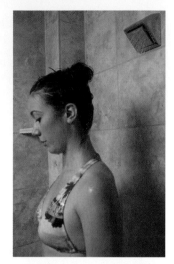

FIGURE 11.7
Back of neck stretch (tucking the chin).

3. Placing one hand over your head and onto the opposite ear, gently stretch the upper trapezius (Figure 11.8). Hold for 15 seconds; then repeat on the opposite side.

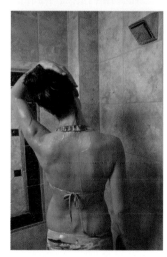

FIGURE 11.8
Trapezius stretch.

4. Extend your upper arm to stretch the bicep (Figure 11.9). Hold for 15 seconds; then repeat on the opposite side.

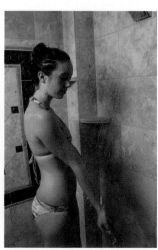

FIGURE 11.9
Biceps stretch.

TREATMENT *continued*

5. Bend your arm, then, with your elbow pointed towards the ceiling, touch your scapula. This stretches the triceps. At the same time, with your other arm, bring your hand back behind you and try to touch that same scapula. This stretches the anterior shoulder muscles of the other arm (Figure 11.10). Hold for 15 seconds; then repeat on the opposite side.

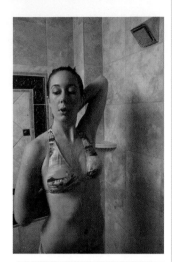

FIGURE 11.10
One hand up, one hand down (stretches the triceps and the front of the shoulder at the same time).

6. Cross your arms behind your back and bring your shoulders back until you feel a mild tension in the pectoral muscles (Figure 11.11). Hold that stretch for 15 seconds; then repeat on the opposite side.

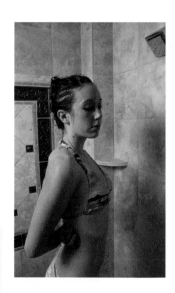

FIGURE 11.11
Pectoral muscle stretch.

TREATMENT *continued*

7. Lean to the side until you feel a stretch along the side of the torso but not down into the side of the leg (Figure 11.12). Hold for 15 seconds; then repeat on the opposite side.

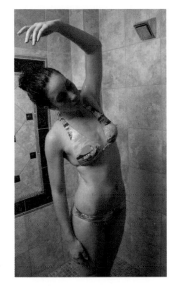

FIGURE 11.12
Side-of-torso stretch.

8. Twist the spine (Figure 11.13). Hold for 15 seconds; then repeat on the opposite side.

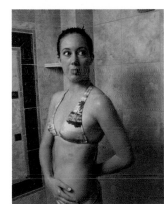

FIGURE 11.13
Spinal twisting stretch.

9. Bring the wrist back and, holding it with your other hand, gently stretch the wrist flexor muscles (Figure 11.14). Hold for 15 seconds; then repeat on the opposite side.

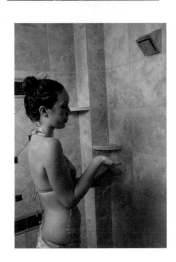

FIGURE 11.14
Wrist flexors stretch.

TREATMENT *continued*

10. Bring the wrist down and, holding it with your other hand, gently stretch the wrist extensor muscles (Figure 11.15). Hold for 15 seconds; then repeat on the opposite side.

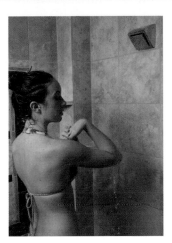

FIGURE 11.15
Wrist extensors stretch.

11. Place the tips of your fingers together, bring the palms towards each other and gently stretch the fingers (Figure 11.16). Hold for 30 seconds.

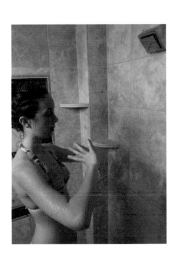

FIGURE 11.16
Fingers stretch.

12. Now that your shoulder is thoroughly warm, extend your arm up and "walk" your fingers up the shower wall as high as possible without pain (not pictured). Next, rest there for a few seconds and then try to gently move a tiny bit higher; then walk down again. Repeat ten times.

Special considerations

With any condition that contra-indicates local heat, such as an acute whiplash injury, the affected part should not be exposed to hot water for long periods of time.

Increasing joint range of motion through swimming

Swimming is an excellent way to retain and increase range of motion and stay fit at the same time. Participating in water fitness classes, swimming laps, or simply moving for pure enjoyment in the water can be a fun way to keep your body healthier and your tissues more supple.

CHAPTER SUMMARY

In this chapter, you have learned how many hydrotherapy treatments can be used to promote health and wellness, including classic detoxification treatments, tonic treatments which stimulate the body's functions, and treatments to help you keep your upper extremities healthy. Using hydrotherapy treatments as self-care can also help your clients get faster and better results from their massage treatment. In our final two chapters, we will explore how you can also use hydrotherapy in conjunction with massage to help a wide range of clients with many specific issues.

REVIEW QUESTIONS

Multiple choice

1. A short exposure to whole-body cold does all but one of these. Which is the exception?

A. Heightens the body's activities

B. Stimulates the body to try to keep warm

C. Is relaxing

D. Increases the body's basal metabolic rate

2. A person who takes regular saunas experiences:

A. Feelings of warmth and relaxation

B. Decrease in systolic blood pressure

C. Loss of fluid and electrolytes

D. All of the above

3. Massage therapists are prone to repetitive strain injury if they do which of the following:

A. Take frequent breaks between massages

B. Have good body mechanics

C. Use their hands improperly

D. Have their table at the proper height

4. Detoxifying bath additives work in all but one of these ways. Which is the exception?

A. Neutralizing toxins

B. Withdrawing toxins from the body

C. Enhancing the body's ability to detoxify

D. Changing kidney function

5. All but one statement about tonic treatments is correct. Which one is false?

A. Stimulate local function

B. Must be done regularly

C. Don't need to be adjusted for weak or frail clients

D. Provide different sensations

Fill in the blanks

6. Stretching should be performed _____ and never to the point of _____.

7. When a local area is exposed to cold over a period of time, the blood vessels are able to contract _____ and _____.

8. This occurs because the _____ of the vessels are _____ to increase their contractions.

9. When toxins are _____ in the body they can contribute to _____ or chronic _____ health.

10. Symptoms of poor local circulation include _____ hands and feet and poorly healing _____ and _____.

11. Flushing lead out of the body with repeated baths worked because of a combination of _____ drinking and _____ pressure.

Chapter eleven

References

Alloway B, Davies B. Essentials of Medical Geology: Impacts of the Natural Environment on Public Health. Burlington, MA: Elsevier, 2005

Barnes A et al. Excretion of methamphetamine and amphetamine in human sweat following controlled oral methamphetamine administration. Clin Chem 2008; 54(1): 172–80

Bhattacharva S. Medicinal plants and natural products in amelioration of arsenic toxicity. Pharm Biol 2017 (1): 349–54

Bilal M et al. Biosorption: an interplay between marine algae and potentially toxic elements. Mar Drugs 2018; 16(2)

Biro S et al. Clinical implications of thermal therapy in lifestyle-related diseases. Experimental Biology and Medicine 2003; 228: 1245–9

Dahlgren J et al. Persistent organic pollutants in 9/11 rescue workers: reduction following detoxification. Chemosphere 2007, Jan 16

DeLorenzo F et al. Haeomodynamic responses and changes of haemostatic risk factors in cold-adapted humans. QJ Med 1999(92) 509–13

DeLorenzo F, Sharma V, Scully M, Kakkar VV. Central cooling effects in patients with hypercholesterolemia. Clinical Science 1998(95): 213–18

Dillon C, Petersen M, Tanaka S. Self-reported hand and wrist arthritis and occupation: data from the US National Health Interview Survey Occupational Health Supplement. American Journal of Industrial Medicine 2002; 42(4): 318–27

Dinsley J. Charcoal Remedies. Coldwater, MI: Gatekeepers Books, 2005

Dugue B. Adaptation related to cytokines in man: effects of regular swimming in cold water. Clin Physiol 2000; 20(2): 114–21

Elmstadhl S et al. Hydrotherapy of patients with intermittent claudication: a novel approach to improve systolic blood pressure and reduce symptoms. Int Angiol 1995; 14(4): 3899–94

Ernst E. Prevention of common colds by hydrotherapy. Physiotherapy 1990; 76(4): 207–10

Ernst E et al. Regular sauna bathing and the incidence of common colds. Ann Med 1990; 22(4): 225–7

Fiscus KA. Changes in lower-leg blood flow during war, cold, and contrast water therapy. Arch Phys Med Rehabil 2005; 86: 1404

Genius S. Induced sweating appears to be a potential method for elimination of many toxic elements from the human body. Arch Environ Contam Toxicol 2011; 61(2): 344–57

Hanna-Attisha M. What the Eyes Don't See. New York, NY: Random House 2018

Hannuksela M, Ellahham S. Benefits and risks of sauna bathing. American Journal of Medicine 2001; 110: 118–26

Hedley AM et al. The effects of acute heat exposure on muscular strength, muscular endurance, and muscular power in the euhydrated athlete. J Strength Cond Res 2002; 16(3): 353–8

Heywood et al. Effect of immersion on urinary lead secretion. BR J Industrial Med, 1986; 43: 713–15

Hoigy N. Ciprofloxacin in sweat and antibiotic resistance. The Copenhagen Study Group on Antibiotics in Sweat. Lancet 1995; 4: 346

Hoigy N et al. Excretion of β-lactam antibiotics in sweat: a neglected mechanism of antibiotic resistance? Antimicrobial Agents and Chemotherapy 2000; 2855–7 (44): 10

Hooper P. Hot tub for diabetes. New England J. of Medicine 1999; 341(12): 924–5

Jobe JB et al. Induced vasodilation as a home treatment for Raynaud's disease. J Rheumatol 1985; 12(5): 953–6

Jobe JB, Sampson JB, Roberts DE, Beetham WP Jr. Induced vasodilation as treatment for Raynaud's disease. Ann Intern Med 1982; 97(5): 706–9

Jobe JB, Sampson JB, Roberts DE, Kelly JA. Comparison of behavioral treatments for Raynaud's disease. J Behav Med 1986; 9(1): 89–96

Kihara T et al. Effects of repeated sauna treatment on ventricular arrhythmias in patients with chronic heart failure. Circulation Journal 2004; 69: 1146–51

Kilburn KH et al. Neurobehavioral dysfunction in firemen exposed to polychlorinated biphenyls (PCBs): possible improvement after detoxification. Arch Environ Health 1989; 44: 345–50

Kneipp S. My Water Cure. Edinburgh: William Blackwood and Sons, 1897

Krop J. Chemical sensitivity after intoxication at work with solvents: response to sauna therapy. J. Altern Complement Med 1998; 4(1): 77–86

Lanphear B. Still treating lead poisoning after all these years. Pediatrics 2017 (2): 140

Lanphear B et al. Low-level lead exposure and mortality in US adults: a population-based cohort study. The Lancet Public Health 2018 (3): 4

LeBlanc J et al. Autonomic nervous system and adaptation to cold in man. J Applied Physiology 1975; 39(2): 181–6

Leppaluoto J, Korhonen I, Hassi J. Habituation of thermal sensations, skin temperatures and norepinephrine in men exposed to cold air. J. Applied Physiology 2001; (4)90: 1121–8

Li J. Association between World Trade Center exposure and excess cancer risk. JAMA 2012(23): 308

Liberty HJ, Johnson BD, Fortner N. Detecting cocaine use through sweat testing: multilevel modelling of sweat patch length of wear data. J Anal Toxicol 2004; 28(8): 667–73

Malkan S. Not Just a Pretty Face: The Ugly Side of the Beauty Industry. Gabriola, Canada: New Society Pub, 2007

Martin Mai F. Diagnosing Genius. Ottawa: Institute of Intergovernmental Relations, 2007

Masuda A et al. Regular sauna use reduces oxidative stress. Japanese Heart Journal 2004; 45: 297–303

McKay J. US Fire departments are turning to detox saunas to fight off the cancer threat – but are they effective? CTIF 8 April 2018

Menetrier T. Changes in femoral artery blood flow during thermoneutral, cold, and contrast-water therapy. Journal of Sports Medicine and Physical Fitness, January 2014

National Institute for Occupational Safety and Health (NIOSH). Findings from a Study of Cancer among U.S. Fire Fighters 2016: www.cdc.gov/niosh/pgms/worknotify/pdfs/ff-cancer-factsheet-final.pdf

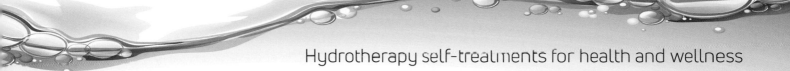

New York Detox and Drug Rehab. www.nydetox.org [Accessed November 2006]

Ogilvie R. Benefits and risks of sauna bathing. Hypertension Canada 2003; 74: 7

Putman J. Quicksilver and slow death. National Geographic, October 1972: 507–27

Radomski MW. Hormone response of normal and intermittent cold-preadapted humans to continuous cold. *J. Applied Physiology* 1982; 53: 610–16

Rhea W. Chemical Sensitivity: Tools of Diagnosis and Methods of Treatment, Volume 4. Boca Raton, FL: Lewis Press, 1997

Rolls R. Diseased, Douched and Doctored. London, England: London Publishing Partnership, 2012

Ross G. Methamphetamine exposure and chronic illness in police officers: significant improvement with sauna-based detoxification therapy. Toxicol Ind Health 2012 (8): 758–68

Rudofsky G et al. Changes of venous hemodynamics by thermic stimuli. Med Klin 1977; 72(40): 1639–44

Saito T et al. Validated gas chromatographic-negative ion chemical ionization mass spectrometric method for delta(9)-tetrahydrocannabinol in sweat patches. Clin Chem 2004; 50(11): 2083–90

Saradeth B et al. A single blind, randomized, controlled trial of hydrotherapy for varicose veins. Vasa 1991; 20(2): 147–52

Schechter S. Fighting Radiation and Chemical Pollutants with Food, Herbs and Vitamins. Escondido, CA: Vitality Ink, 1990

Schnare D, Ben M, Shields M. Body burden reductions of PCBs, PBBs and chlorinated pesticides in human subjects. Ambio 1984; 13(5–6): 378–80

Sears M. Arsenic, cadmium, lead, and mercury in sweat: a systematic review. J Environ Public Health 2012, February 22

Shevchuk NA. The anti-fatigue effect of moderate cooling. In: Svoboda E, ed. Chronic Fatigue Syndrome: Symptoms, Causes and Prevention. Nova Science Publishers, 2010

Sinclair M. Environmental costs of pain management: pharmaceuticals versus physical therapies. Integrative Medicine, Oct/Nov 2012

Smith E et al. Thermal sensation and comfort in women exposed repeatedly to whole-body cryotherapy and winter swimming in ice cold water. Physiol Behav 2004; 82(4): 691–5

Stopford W. Industrial exposure to mercury. In The Biogeochemistry of Mercury in the Environment. New York: Elsevier/North Holland Biomedical Press, 1979, pp. 375, 381

Sunderman FW. Excretion of copper in sweat of patients with Wilson's disease during sauna bathing. Ann Clinic Lab Sci 1974(4): 407

Tikuisis P et al. Comparison of thermoregulatory responses between men and women immersed in cold water. J Appl Physiol 2000; 89(4): 1403–11

Tretjak Z, Shields M, Beckmann S. PCB reduction and clinical improvement by detoxification: an unexploited approach. Human and Experimental Toxicology 1990 (9): 235–44

World Health Organization 2018. Lead poisoning and health. www.who.int/news-room/fact-sheets/detail/lead-poisoning-and-health [Accessed March 2019]

Recommended resources

Geurts C. Local cold acclimation of the hand impairs thermal responses of the fingers without improving hand neuromuscular function. Acta Physiol Scand 2005; 183: 117–29

Horay P. Hot Water Therapy. Oakland, CA: New Harbinger Publications, 1991

Merendez N. The history of the Almaden Mine Hospital. Quad Int Stor Med Sanita 1996; 3(2): 51–69

Theobald JL, Mycyk MB. Iron and heavy metals. In: Walls RM, Hockberger RS, Gausche-Hill M, eds. Rosen's Emergency Medicine: Concepts and Clinical Practice, 9th edn. Philadelphia, PA: Elsevier, 2018

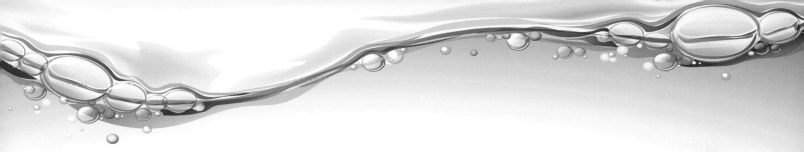

Hydrotherapy and massage for musculoskeletal injuries 12

Maybe you lifted something heavy or swung a golf club a little too enthusiastically; now you're flat on your back wishing for something–anything–to end the agony. The bad news is that unless you have a major injury or disc problem, your doctor may not be able to do much for you other than prescribe some pain medication and advise you to rest … Applying an ice pack to the painful area within 24 hours of the injury can keep inflammation and discomfort to a minimum. Ice does one thing–it decreases the nerve's ability to conduct a painful stimulus, but if more than 24 hours have passed since the injury occurred, ice will not reduce pain and inflammation. After that time, heat can ease pain and increase the elasticity of the muscles by about 10 percent.

John Renner, *The Home Remedies Handbook*

CHAPTER OBJECTIVES

After completing this chapter the student will be able to:

1. Explain the most common types of musculoskeletal injuries and their causes
2. Describe the inflammatory process
3. Explain the rationale for using hydrotherapy to treat the injuries in this chapter
4. Explain the difference between hydrotherapy treatments for new injuries and those for older ones
5. Explain how hydrotherapy and massage work together to treat specific injuries
6. List five common injuries and the appropriate hydrotherapy treatments for each.

Musculoskeletal problems from recent or poorly healed old injuries are common in people of all ages. They are one of the main reasons clients seek bodywork, so it is vitally important that massage therapists have many tools at their disposal to help heal them. This chapter explains how hydrotherapy can be one of our best tools for this purpose.

There are a few main types of injuries in the US. Traumatic injuries result in 27 million visits to hospital emergency departments each year, and are the leading cause of death in people under 45 years old (Centers for Disease Control and Prevention, 2019). Sports injuries are common in children and adults, and one in 10 people will develop a repetitive strain injury during their lifetime (Simon, 2000). Recent injuries can cause swelling, pain, stiffness and muscle guarding. Massage therapy can help to relieve those symptoms and promote complete healing by increasing local circulation, reducing muscle tension, and relieving muscle spasm and pain (see Case history 12.1). Older, poorly healed injuries may feature myofascial restriction, active trigger points, and painful or restricted movement. When compensations develop, this may only make things worse (for specific examples of the long-term effects of poorly healed injuries, see Box 12.1). Massage therapy can address these issues as well, by reducing muscle tension and pain, releasing fascial restrictions, softening excess scar tissue, and helping clients avoid dysfunctional movement habits. Hydrotherapy treatments can work together with massage to make this happen.

TYPES OF INJURIES
Traumatic injuries

Physical trauma can cause bruises, muscle strains, fractures, sprains, dislocations, torn cartilage, back injuries and even amputations. Falls and car crashes

---

BOX 12.1   POINT OF INTEREST

POORLY-HEALED INJURIES CAN HAVE LONG-TERM EFFECTS ON THE BODY

Traumatic injuries that are not properly healed can lead to long-lasting physical problems. Each of the examples below highlights the importance of proper healing.

Injuries from accidents

At eight years of age, massage therapist Genie Martin fell 20 feet out of a tree, striking branches on the way down and hitting her head hard enough to be knocked unconscious. She stopped breathing, lost consciousness and had to be given artificial respiration. As she tells it, "My life was given back to me, though I was not aware of it for many hours. And when I did become aware of it, I no longer wanted it. Pain, here-to-fore unknown to me except for little hurts, was now my constant companion. A more nagging, convulsive, ruthless and demanding companion I had never known about in all my small life. Pain kept me awake at night – made my head ache with every move–burned my chest with fire, so much that I squeezed my arms tightly around to smother the flames." From that time on, Martin carried tremendous tightness and fear in her chest, persistent chest pain when she was anxious, and a continual fear of recurring pain. As an adult, she slept with her arms so tightly gripped over her chest that sometimes when she woke they were numb. While receiving bodywork, she had to make a tremendous effort to stop her arms from springing protectively over her chest. It was not until decades later when she began receiving bodywork that she finally began to heal from the emotional and physical effects of the injury (Martin, 1985).

Sports injuries

Football great Joe Namath was injured numerous times in his career, suffering bruises, muscle strains and ruptures, dislocations, sprains, torn cartilage, torn ligaments, fractures and concussions. Namath frequently played even when he was suffering from new, unhealed injuries. This not only increased the chances of making the original injuries worse, but also made it more likely that another nearby body part would be injured as well. He began to suffer severe ongoing knee pain as early as age 20, was diagnosed with osteoarthritis at age 23, developed bursitis and severe swelling in both knees by age 24, and underwent many surgeries on his knees in an attempt to repair extensive damage. His physical problems forced him to retire at age 34, but he continued to pay the price for playing with poorly healed injuries: by age 37 he had developed severe osteoarthritis in his fingers and spine, and had double knee replacement at age 47. Brain scans in his 60s showed residual brain damage from concussions and he suffered from pain in many areas of his body (Krieger, 2004).

Unequal limb lengths

Leg length inequality can have many causes, including trauma. One leg bone may actually be shorter than the leg bone on the other side, but often it is soft tissue imbalances that cause this condition. For example, trigger points in the quadratus lumborum muscle are often activated by trauma from a motor vehicle accident, which can lead to the person holding one leg in a posture that makes it functionally shorter. If they remain untreated, secondary trigger points can occur in nearby muscles, a lumbar scoliosis may be created, and the normal lumbar curve may be flattened. Over time these imbalances can cause an uneven gait and pain in the back, hip or knee, and may possibly lead to osteoarthritis and pain in the hip joint of the longer leg, or the spine, or both (Simons, Travell and Simons, 1999).

---

are the most common traumatic injuries, but bicycle crashes, accidents while operating machinery, fires, recreational accidents and violence cause many more. On the job, traumatic injuries can include sprains, strains, muscle tears, dislocations, fractures and disc herniations.

Sports injuries

Sports injuries may be acute, such as a muscle strain, fracture or dislocation. However, they can also be chronic in nature. Table 12.1 shows injuries that can develop from specific sports.

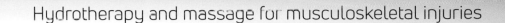

Sport	Acute injuries	Overuse injuries
American football	Traumatic brain injury Adductor strain (groin pull) Hip joint labral tear Torn knee ligaments	Rotator cuff tears Shin splints Muscle strains
Baseball	Knee meniscal injury Shoulder dislocation	Biceps tendonitis Ulnar collateral ligament, labral and rotator cuff tears Muscle strains
Basketball	Ankle sprains Meniscal tears	Achilles tendonitis Quadriceps tendonitis
Climbing	Bruising and fractures from falls	Finger flexor tendon rupture
Competitive swimming	Concussions from flip turns	Rotator cuff tendonitis Medial collateral ligament strain (breaststroker's knee) Calcaneal stress fractures from flip turns
Distance running	Ankle sprains Gastrocnemius strains	Iliotibial band syndrome Metatarsal stress fractures Shin splints
Kayaking	Shoulder dislocation	Wrist, shoulder, elbow tendonitis
Mountain biking	Upper extremity fractures	Sciatica Quadriceps tendonitis Iliotibial band syndrome
Skateboarding	Head trauma Wrist fractures and sprains	Plantar fasciitis Achilles tendonitis
Skiing	Tibial fractures Torn knee ligaments	Shoulder sprain Knee ligament injuries Skier's thumb
Snowboarding	Shoulder dislocations Clavicle/ humeral fractures Lumbar compression fractures	Rotator cuff tears Back muscle strains
Soccer	Traumatic brain injury Knee ligament tears Ankle sprains	Adductor strain (groin pull) Quadriceps tendonitis Hamstring strains
Surfing	Head injuries from being struck by board	Back and shoulder muscle strain from paddling

TABLE 12.1 Sports injuries – acute or overuse?

How athletic overuse injuries occur:

1. Athletes do not warm up properly or stop when they are tired, or they perform stunts that are beyond their skill level.

2. Athletes make sudden changes in their training routines, rather than increasing their activity gradually.

3. Most athletes have been highly active for many years and accumulated multiple issues stemming from poorly healed injuries, such as overly tight muscles, myofascial adhesions, muscle imbalances, or joints that are loose, twisted or poorly aligned. These problems make it more likely that the athlete will develop an overuse injury. Athletes benefit from being treated with hydrotherapy and massage before a smaller injury progresses to become a major one, such as a torn ligament leading to arthritis or a toe fracture progressing to hammertoe.

Chapter twelve

Extreme sports injuries

Since extreme sports involve greater speed, heights and risk than traditional sports, they also lead to many injuries. Orthopedic injuries are very common, including lumbar compression fractures. Trauma to the head and neck (such as bruises, strains, sprains, fractures, and brain injuries), is involved in more than 10% of all extreme sport injuries. Skateboard crashes cause more head and neck trauma than any other sport; mountain bikers' falls over the handlebars lead to head injuries and upper extremity fractures; and snowboarders' falls upon outstretched hands result in many broken and sprained shoulders, clavicles and wrists (Halpern, 2003; Laver, 2017).

Repetitive stress injuries

These injuries are caused by the physical stress of performing the same movements for many hours, particularly if the person is in an awkward position, performs heavy lifting, or has to use great force. Any repetitive activity with the hands–from typing to playing a musical instrument–can chronically overload and harm the hand, arm and shoulder muscles (Passan, 2016). The workstations we are expected to use can be a major factor as well. For example, a massage table or computer desk at the wrong height may cause you to slump forward and this can lead to upper back and neck strain and a chronic forward-head posture, which can even lead to a cervical disc herniation. Chronic tendonitis is perhaps the most common injury of this type.

HYDROTHERAPY AND MUSCULOSKELETAL INJURIES

It is important that injured clients have medical treatment to make sure that their injuries are properly diagnosed and that your treatment is approved by a doctor. That done, you can treat them whether their injury is acute or chronic. As shown in Box 12.2, hydrotherapy techniques can greatly accelerate healing of acute injuries.

BOX 12.2	POINT OF INTEREST

HYDROTHERAPY AND MASSAGE WORK TOGETHER TO HEAL ATHLETIC INJURIES

Football injury

When Corby Jones suffered a significant toe sprain in the University of Missouri's football game against North Western on October 3, 1998, the clock began ticking for the Missouri sports medicine staff. The staff had seven days to improve Jones's condition and keep him in football-playing shape so that he could take the field next Saturday at Iowa State. Rex Sharp, MU's head athletic trainer, knew the pressure was on to heal the ailing digit. Sharp treated Jones for 10 hours a day, heating the injury in the whirlpool, running him a rehabilitation pool with a current, having him ride a stationary bike and exercise on a stair stepper. Sharp coated Jones' toe in a paraffin bath and treated the toe with ultrasound and massage. "We did everything we could, but on Friday I still did not know whether he'd be able to play," Sharp said. Jones did play Saturday, in an MU win – 9 for 15 passing for 176 yards and two touchdowns, along with one rushing touchdown. "When people come to a football game, all they see are the players running out on the field," Sharp said. "Then they go home. They have no idea of what goes on all week long" (Vilelle, 1999).

Mountain-biking injury

Rosario, a 28-year-old mountain biker, limped in slowly and painfully for a session, and a dark purple hematoma could be seen which covered most of her left thigh. Two days before, she had launched herself off a high jump, landed off-center, and crashed with her entire weight onto her left side. Her leg was extremely painful but her bike was too damaged to ride, so she then had to walk a long way out. Her left hip and her back were still hurting, and her lateral thigh was very sensitive to the touch. The therapist considered

continued

BOX 12.2 *continued*

hydrotherapy options, including an Epsom salts compress, charcoal pack, castor oil pack, or applications of hot or cold. She finally opted for a contrast treatment using a moist heating pad and a cold gel pack. First Rosario lay on the treatment table on her right side, bruised leg up. The therapist put a thin moist cloth on the lateral thigh from hip to knee, and added a large heating pad on top of that. She placed a long thin gel pack in a bowl of ice water, then began massaging Rosario's entire back. After three minutes she stopped massage briefly, switched the cold gel pack for the heating pad, then went back to massage. She repeated this hot-followed-by-cold procedure five times while she massaged Rosario's entire back. Once the final cold gel pack was removed, the bruise was now lighter in color, since the improved circulation had carried away

some of the blood which had leaked into her tissues. The therapist was then able to massage around the bruise, which was far less painful and continued to feel better. For the last few minutes, Rosario lay on her back and the therapist massaged her other leg and hip. Once back on her feet, Rosario's pain was greatly reduced and her back felt looser and more comfortable as well. The therapist explained to her that she could use an Epsom salts bath, a cold half bath, contrast gel packs, or a contrast spray on the thigh at least twice a day, and follow that with a heat-trapping compress or castor oil pack at night, and adding self-massage whenever possible. The treatments would help prevent long-term problems such as adhesions in the muscles and fascia of her left leg and possible compensations such as a permanent limp.

Hydrotherapy and pain from injuries

The application of heat or cold to relieve the pain of acute or chronic inflammatory disorders has been used for centuries, and is still a method without peer in the area of pain control. No other method is so effective, so safe and easy, and so free from side effects and expense.

Agatha and Calvin Thrash, *Home Remedies: Hydrotherapy, Massage, Charcoal and other Simple Treatments*

When it is properly used, hydrotherapy relieves much of the short-term discomfort and pain of recent musculoskeletal injuries and speeds healing, just as massage does. Heat relaxes muscles and slows conduction of pain messages to the brain. In one study, researchers found that local heat applied over the palm could even relieve the pain of a mild electric shock (On et al., 1997). Heat wraps that are worn continuously over a period of hours may relieve both neck and low back pain better than ibuprofen or acetaminophen (Mayer, 2006). Cold applications, on the other hand, relieve pain by overriding or bypassing pain messages to the brain. Contrast treatments work by combining the advantages of both hot and cold alone: heat alone vasodilates but also brings fluid to an area, while cold numbs but cuts down on blood flow. When used alternately, blood flow is stimulated and swelling is decreased at the same time. When myofascial work or breaking up of old adhesions is necessary, heat

applications relax and warm soft tissues, making deep work more tolerable, while a warm Epsom salts bath after a session of deep bodywork prevents post-treatment soreness.

Hydrotherapy and inflammation

As shown in Figure 12.1, injuries are almost always accompanied by inflammation. Because massage therapists work with many clients who have both recent and old injuries, and injured tissues are always inflamed at first, it is important to understand this process (see Box 12.3 for more about the stages of inflammation). First, musculoskeletal trauma is generally treated with cold applications for the first 24 hours, while blood vessels seal off and stop any remaining bleeding (cold causes local blood vessels to constrict, which reduces bleeding and inflammation). Since cold treatments continue to reduce blood flow to the injured area, contrast applications are now recommended after that time. Various anti-inflammatory medications may also be used at this stage of an injury, but recent research indicates that they can actually delay or inhibit healing (Hauser, 2019). A contrast treatment followed by suitable hands-on techniques can be used in all later stages of healing. Herbal preparations for inflammation can be helpful as well, and for centuries have been added to hydrotherapy treatments for injuries.

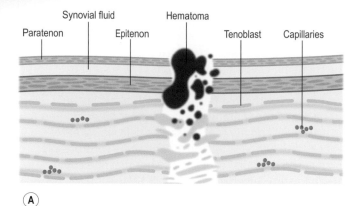

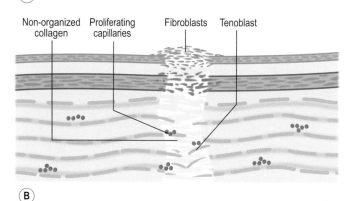

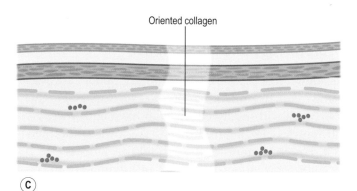

FIGURE 12.1
Tendon healing. (**A**) Acute phase of repair of a torn tendon. (**B**) Sub-acute phase of repair of a torn tendon. (**C**) Healed tendon. Reprinted with permission from Bucholz RW, Heckman JD. Rockwood and Greens Fractures in Adults, 5th edn. Baltimore, MD: Lippincott, Williams and Wilkins, 2001.

In his 1978 *Sports Medicine Book*, Gabe Mirkin coined the acronym **RICE** for the four elements which became the standard of care for soft tissue injuries such as sprains, fractures and muscle strains: Rest, Ice, Compression and Elevation. Ice was supposed to combat inflammation, and inflammation was not regarded as helpful in the healing process. Athletes were supposed to apply ice frequently, over many days or weeks. Coaches, physicians, physical therapists and the lay public have recommended and followed the **RICE** guidelines for decades, but as more research has been done, it has become clear that ice has been overused. Cold does reduce swelling, and if there are microscopic tears in tissues that are leaking blood, cold helps them seal off. However, it also restricts blood flow for long periods of time, and researchers have now learned a lot about blood flow, the use of ice, and the role of inflammation in healing. To repair damage from injuries, the body requires many different chemicals (including proteins) and new cells: because ice reduces blood flow, it also reduces the supply of the chemicals and cells needed for repair (Adie, 2012; Howatson, 2003; Martin, 2002; Thienpoint, 2014; Watkins, 2014). Dr. Mirkin eventually reversed his position on ice, stating, "It now appears that both ice and complete rest may delay healing, instead of helping" (Mirkin, 2015).

The best role for ice in injury rehabilitation is to use ice massage or an ice-water bath to numb a specific area, enabling an athlete to perform light rehabilitation exercises for a few minutes while the numbness lasts. Heavy exercises can cause the athlete to re-injure themselves, so this must be done carefully (Sidhy, 2008). This technique is called cryokinetics, and should be supervised by a physical therapist. Ice is also helpful in decreasing pain after therapy or strenuous activities, and before stretching a contracture in its early stage.

Hydrotherapy and scar tissue

Combining hydrotherapy and bodywork can help scars heal with appropriate scar tissue. After the first, acute phase of an injury, cells that produce collagen fibers form scar tissue around the injury to knit the damaged area back together. At the beginning, these collagen fibers don't have any direction or grain (Figure 12.2A), and if they are not treated, they tend to adhere or stick to fascia, muscles or other tissues. However, scar tissue is not elastic, and where a muscle can snap back after being stretched, scar tissue may tear.

Many chronic musculoskeletal problems can result from thick, adhered, or poorly aligned scar tissue. For

THE BODY HEALS THROUGH INFLAMMATION

Inflammation is the body's defensive response to injury. Its four main signs are redness, swelling, heat and pain. What happens when the body sustains an injury in which a lot of force is applied to an area? A shoulder dislocation is a good example; the force that pops the bone out causes the ligaments that hold the humeral head in place to be overstretched or torn, and the labrum, rotator cuff muscles and nearby arteries may also be injured.

As seen in Figure 12.1A, the body responds to injury with many clever protective strategies. In less than one second, local blood vessels constrict to prevent blood loss. Soon afterwards, local capillaries dilate greatly, and as they open wide the area is flooded with fresh blood. Fibrin and blood platelets collect in the blood vessels near the injury and gradually close off the damaged vessels. (Heat should not be applied until the capillaries have sealed and have stopped leaking, which usually requires a maximum of 24 hours). At the same time, damaged tissues activate the entire inflammatory process, including stimulating the flow of white blood cells. (Blood flow to the area now increases. However, with many vessels wide open, the blood actually flows more slowly, and this allows more **macrophages** to get into the area.) Their job is to remove debris from dead cells and to feast on bacteria, which prevents the spread of infection to other parts of the body. As blood vessels leak even more fluid into the tissues, this puts pressure on sensitive nerve endings. Now you have the classic signs of inflammation—redness, heat, swelling, and pain. Extreme inflammation can limit movement, as well.

In the subacute phase, as seen in Figure 12.1B, tissues are beginning to heal; ruptured small blood vessels have closed; white blood cells are cleaning up debris; blood flow has returned to its normal state; and cells which produce collagen fibers are forming scar tissue around the injury to knit the damaged area back together.

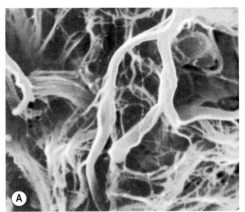
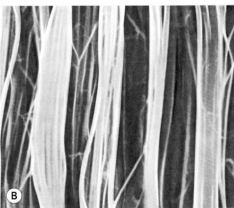

FIGURE 12.2
Ligament fiber organization.
(**A**) Incompletely healed ligament with disorganized fibers.
(**B**) Fully healed ligament with well-organized fibers.
Reprinted with permission from Archer M. Therapeutic Massage in Athletics, page 104. Baltimore, MD: Lippincott, Williams and Wilkins; 2004, Figure 6.4.

example, a poorly healed wrist injury can lead to fascial restriction all the way up the arm to the shoulder. Once pain relief has been achieved with contrast treatments and massage, gentle exercise promotes this optimum healing: the injured part will heal the best when the person moves it actively but gently, ensuring that scar tissue fibers are properly aligned and that tissues are pliable and not adhered (Figure 12.2B).

Chapter twelve

Amputations

Due to increasing rates of diabetes in the Western world, amputations are an injury you are likely to encounter among your clients. Of the almost 100,000 amputations performed in the US in 2017, 88% were due to diabetes (Geiss, 2019). Amputations are performed when it would be dangerous to leave that part of the body attached because of life-threatening infections, irreversible damage to local blood vessels, or tissue that is damaged beyond hope of repair. (Musculoskeletal trauma or cancer can also lead to amputations.) Advanced diabetics require these amputations when even small foot wounds that are infected don't heal well. An infection that spreads from the foot to the rest of the person's body could be fatal.

Hydrotherapy can be a helpful treatment for clients with amputated limbs, in particular when the stump is sensitive to the touch or circulation is poor. Hydrotherapy is an excellent way to improve the client's tolerance for tactile stimulation, to improve circulation, to soften adhesions, and to begin the massage experience in a soothing, relaxing way. Warm whirlpools may be used for this purpose and sometimes to relieve phantom limb pain. Moist hot pack applications before massage can help relieve discomfort and tension in muscles in other parts of the body, such as the back or an extremity, which are compensating for the missing part. For example, with one leg amputated above the knee, compensations may cause muscle tightening and discomfort at the hip directly above the stump, the entire other leg, and/or in the back. Ice massage may relieve phantom limb pain as it slows nerve conduction. Regular, gentle self-massage on a daily basis can be helpful for the client.

Below are four hydrotherapy treatments that are useful for treating clients with amputations.

TREATMENT

CONTRAST TREATMENT OF AN AMPUTATION STUMP

The contrast treatment may be extended to the entire extremity by using a larger hot pack or multiple ones.

continued

TREATMENT *continued*

A moist hot pack alone can be used, but will not stimulate the circulation as much as a contrast treatment.

Duration and frequency

10–12 minutes. This may be performed as many as three times daily.

Cautions

If the stump is sensitive, temperatures may need to be less extreme: ask the client to tell you what feels right. For clients with diabetes, use hydrocollator packs covered with extra towels so packs are warm, not hot, on the skin. Moist heating pads should not be on a high setting.

Procedure

1. Apply a moist heating pad or hydrocollator pack to the amputation stump for 3 minutes while massaging the rest of the extremity.

2. Wring out a washcloth in ice water and rub the stump for 30 seconds, or perform ice massage for 1 minute. Brisk rubbing will help desensitize sensitive tissues.

3. Repeat steps 1 and 2 two more times, for a total of three rounds.

TREATMENT

CONTRAST PARTIAL SHOWER

Cross-reference

See Chapter 8.

Duration and frequency

10–12 minutes. May be performed three or four times daily.

Cautions

Use water no hotter than 102°F (39°C) for diabetics, and stop if the client is uncomfortable.

Procedure

1. Spray the amputation stump with hot water for 2 minutes.

2. Spray the stump with cold water for 30 seconds.

3. Repeat steps 1 and 2 two more times, for a total of three rounds.

TREATMENT

WHIRLPOOL BATH
FOR AN AMPUTATION STUMP

Cross-reference

See Chapter 6.

Duration and frequency

15–20 minutes. This may be performed before a massage session.

Special instructions

Water can be warm to hot (98–105°F; 37–41°C), whatever is comfortable. Diabetics should receive whirlpool baths no hotter than 102°F (39°C).

TREATMENT

ICE MASSAGE FOR PHANTOM LIMB PAIN

Cross-reference

See Chapter 5.

Duration and frequency

8–10 minutes. This may be performed before a massage session.

Special instructions

Inform the client that the cold will be intense, and ask for feedback as you apply the ice. It is OK to apply ice directly over the incision.

Bursitis

This injury can stem from trauma, overuse, and sometimes even from arthritis. Unaccustomed activities such as reaching overhead to paint a ceiling can provoke bursitis – in that case, of the shoulder. Tight, short muscles running across a joint may put pressure on the nearby bursae and cause them to become inflamed. Seen most often in the shoulder, bursitis can occur at many other joints.

Acute bursitis

Acute bursitis is extremely painful, but if someone stops moving due to the pain, adhesions between the joint capsule and the bone, known as **adhesive capsulitis**, can develop and make things even worse. Our goals are to relieve pain, to prevent adhesions from forming and to help keep the joint mobile. Massage is contra indicated on or near an acutely inflamed bursa. A good initial strategy is to apply a hydrotherapy treatment on the area with the bursitis, while you perform massage techniques on other parts of the body. Which treatment should you choose? For some clients, cold applications relieve pain better than heat, but for others, cold may cause their muscles to spasm. (You may ask a client to experiment under a shower at home before a session. This is also an excellent opportunity to perform gentle stretching and range of motion exercises in the shower, as shown in Chapter 11.) If both hot and cold work well, you may use a contrast treatment, which is the most effective in reducing inflammation.

The following treatments can be performed over any joint with an inflamed – bursa – here we use the shoulder as an example.

TREATMENT

UPPER HALF-BODY PACK

Cross-reference

See Chapter 4.

Duration

30 minutes.

Cautions

All fomentations should be well covered with towels, so there is no risk of burning the client.

Special instructions

This treatment can fit into a massage session well if you perform massage on the other parts of the body while the client is in the half-body pack, and then remove the pack and perform massage to address the shoulder.

Procedure

1. Place two fomentations (or a flat plastic water bottle filled with warm water) on the massage table so that they will cover the area from neck to waistline. Have the client lie on them, and then place one more hot fomentation over the front of the shoulder. Now proceed with massage of other areas of the body.

continued

275

Chapter twelve

TREATMENT *continued*

2. After 15 minutes, replace the cooled fomentation of the front of the shoulder with a fresh one and continue massage.

3. After another 15 minutes, remove all fomentations, then briefly friction the shoulder and the back with a washcloth dipped in cold water.

4. Dry the shoulder well. Massage, stretching or gentle range of motion exercises can be done at this time.

TREATMENT

LOCAL SALT GLOW
FOLLOWED BY APPLICATION OF CASTOR OIL AND HEAT-TRAPPING COMPRESS

Cross-reference

See Chapters 4 and 10.

Duration and frequency

20 minutes, then the compress may be left on for 1–8 hours. May be performed daily.

Cautions

- Massage is contra indicated in acute bursitis, so do not perform massage techniques directly over the joint.
- Wrap the compress snugly, but not tight enough to cut off the local circulation.

Special instructions

This treatment may be performed at the very beginning of a massage session, but will be more effective if the heat-trapping compress is left on overnight. After you have demonstrated it to a client during a session, it can then be used at home.

Procedure

1. Apply moist heat over the joint for 10 minutes.
2. Perform a salt glow with Epsom salts over the joint.
3. Gently rub a generous amount of castor oil into the skin over the joint.
4. Apply a heat-trapping compress over the joint, and leave it in place for 1–8 hours.
5. Gentle range of motion exercises may be safely performed after the compress has been removed.

TREATMENT

COLD APPLICATIONS

Cross-reference

See Chapter 5.

Duration and frequency

15 minutes. Can be performed every 1–3 hours.

Special instructions

An ice-water compress or ice pack can be used instead of ice massage: if so, place it over the shoulder joint for 20 minutes. By alternating a cold treatment with hands-on bodywork that improves circulation, ice can be used without being overdone. Herbal teas or essential oils can be added to water for ice massage.

Procedure

1. Perform ice massage over the shoulder joint for about 5 minutes, then take the ice off for 1 minute.
2. Massage around the painful area during this rest period.
3. Repeat step 1 twice more, for a total of three rounds of hot followed by cold.
4. The client may now perform gentle range of motion exercises.

TREATMENT

CONTRAST TREATMENT
FOR THE SHOULDER JOINT

Cross-reference

See Chapters 4 and 5.

Duration and frequency

10–15 minutes. This contrast treatment can be performed up to four times daily.

Procedure

1. Place moist heat over the joint, as hot as can be tolerated. Leave on for 3 minutes.
2. Place an ice pack, ice-cold compress or cold gel pack over the joint for 1 minute.

continued

TREATMENT *continued*

3. Repeat steps 1 and 2 twice, for a total of three rounds of hot followed by cold.
4. The client may now perform gentle range of motion exercises.

Sub-acute bursitis

At this stage, the client can benefit from deep heating treatments such as paraffin baths, hot moist applications, castor oil packs or mustard plasters. Used prior to hands-on techniques, these help to release chronic tension and myofascial compensations. Some clients find relief by applying a pain-relieving balm, then covering that with plastic wrap and an athletic bandage and applying external heat.

TREATMENT

HOT MOIST APPLICATIONS

Cross-reference

See Chapter 4.

Duration and frequency

30 minutes. Use before or during a massage session.

Special instructions

Vasodilating herbs such as mustard, ginger or cayenne may be added to the water for the compress.

Procedure

1. Apply a moist heating pad, hot fomentation or hot compress over the joint for 30 minutes. If desired, first rub a generous amount of castor oil around the joint and then cover it with plastic.
2. If the compress cools, switch to another hot fomentation or compress so that you can keep constant heat on the area.
3. Finish with a 1-minute cold application (ice compress or ice massage) over the joint.

TREATMENT

PARAFFIN BATH

Cross-reference

See Chapter 6.

Duration and frequency

15 minutes. Use before or during a massage session.

Special instructions

Joints that cannot be immersed in paraffin may be warmed with a hot moist application for at least 1 minute, and then painted with paraffin.

Procedure

1. Immerse the joint in warm water for at least 1 minute, then dry it briskly.
2. Dip the joint at least six times in hot paraffin, and cover it well to retain the heat.
3. Massage elsewhere while the heat seeps into the area.
4. Wait at least 10–20 minutes before removing the paraffin and beginning local massage and exercise.

Carpal tunnel syndrome

This common and painful condition occurs when overworked, swollen tendons in the wrist put pressure on the median nerve where it passes through the carpal tunnel. Symptoms of this nerve compression include tingling, pain or numbness in the forearms, wrists, or hands. This overuse injury can be caused by many repetitions of the same movement in activities such as typing, playing a musical instrument, operating a machine or performing massage. Treatment includes setting up a better workplace that is ergonomically correct, stopping the activity altogether for a time, and rehabilitation. Hydrotherapy treatments ease pain and facilitate massage and exercise. Robert Simon, MD a specialist in repetitive strain injuries, believes that local contrast baths are the most effective home treatment for reducing pain. He also recommends that anytime the client does the activity that caused the problem, she or he should first warm their hands by soaking them in warm water or wrapping them in a hot moist towel (Simon, 2000). A patient of Agatha

Chapter twelve

Thrash completely healed her carpal tunnel by wrapping an electric heating pad with a towel and pinning it carefully to form a kind of splint for her wrist and lower arm, then slept with it on at night while also wearing gloves to keep her hands warm (Thrash and Thrash, 1981). The therapist should consult with the client's doctor or physical therapist before doing hands-on work.

TREATMENT

HOT HAND SOAK

Cross-reference

See Chapter 6.

Duration and frequency

12–15 minutes. Use before a massage session, and as many as three or four times daily in between sessions. A flat plastic water bottle filled with warm water may also be used to warm the hands (see Figure 13.2).

Procedure

1. This hot soak can be performed three or four times a day.
2. Soak the hand in water as hot as can be tolerated (approximately 110°F or 43°C) for 12–15 minutes. Vasodilating herbs can be added to the water.
3. Have the client exercise the hand or stretch the hand muscles during this time.
4. Immerse the hand in water as cold as can be tolerated (approximately 55°F or 13°C) for 5 seconds.
5. Dry the hands briskly.

TREATMENT

CONTRAST HAND BATH

Cross-reference

See Chapter 6.

Duration and frequency

10 minutes. Can be performed daily as a home treatment.

continued

TREATMENT *continued*

Special instructions

Gentle, non-painful movements performed while the hands are in the water will further increase local circulation. Clients may also use a hand-held shower attachment to perform a contrast treatment: spray one limb at a time, moving up and down the entire arm from shoulder to fingertips. Charcoal, anti-inflammatory herbs or herbal pain relievers may be added to the water.

Procedure

1. Immerse the hands in hot water (approximately 110°F or 43°C) for 2 minutes.
2. Immerse the hands in cold water (approximately 55°F or 13°C) for 1 minute.
3. Repeat steps 1 and 2 twice, for a total of three rounds.

TREATMENT

ICE MASSAGE FOLLOWED BY EXERCISE

Cross-reference

See Chapter 5.

Duration and frequency

3–8 minutes, before exercise and hands-on massage. Use this treatment only once per day.

Special Instructions

This treatment helps reduce fluid around the ligament that covers the carpal tunnel, thus reducing pressure on the median nerve. Herbal teas or essential oils can be added to the water for the ice massage.

Procedure

1. Using an ice cup or cube, gently massage the hand, wrist, and arm up to the elbow, especially over the painful area.
2. Stop as soon as the area is numb.
3. Allow time for the client's hands and wrists to warm, then perform gentle exercises, as prescribed by the doctor or physical therapist.

Cartilage tears

An amazingly tough and resilient structure, articular cartilage helps to protect joints from the stresses placed on them during various activities. However, it can be damaged by a one-time trauma such as a shoulder dislocation that tears the glenoid labrum, an ankle sprain that shreds the talar cartilage, or the heavy impact of a car accident that tears the hip labrum. Cartilage is also more likely to be torn if has become weakened by repeated microtrauma, such as might occur in a construction worker's knee or a professional swimmer's shoulder. Here we use the knee joint as an example of combining hydrotherapy and bodywork to help such injuries heal. (You will see many clients in your practice who have a history of a meniscal cartilage tear. For example, more than half of patients older than 65 years have a degenerative meniscus tear, and obese clients are even more at risk.)

The knee's meniscal cartilage helps to protect the joint from the stresses placed on it during walking, running, bending and twisting. Still, a forceful twist or hyperflexion of the knee can cause the end of the femur to grind into the top of the tibia, possibly pinching, cracking or tearing the meniscus. Sports that require pivoting and sudden stops, like tennis, basketball and golf, or contact sports, like football and hockey, are especially hard on the knees. Because meniscus fibers are interwoven with ligaments that surround the knee, tears of the collateral and cruciate ligaments may contribute to its problems. Often a meniscus tear is associated with a previously torn cruciate ligament which did not heal completely: for example, in one study, 10% of patients who waited for months to have surgery to reconstruct their ACL had a meniscal tear during that time (De Roeck, 2003). Left untreated, a meniscus tear can cause even more damage, hasten the onset of osteoarthritis, and lead to other knee problems. Treatment for a torn meniscus often begins conservatively.

Acute stage

Treatment for a cartilage tear must be approved by the client's doctor. The swelling within the knee joint from a torn meniscus usually takes a few hours to develop: as fluid accumulates within the enclosed area of the knee joint, it may be difficult and painful to fully extend or straighten the knee. For this reason, ice is generally used in the first 24 hours, applied three or four times while the knee is elevated. Crutches and a leg cuff may be needed to enable walking without pain and to protect the knee from unnecessary bending and twisting. Nonsteroidal anti-inflammatory drugs, such as ibuprofen, may also be prescribed, but there are many questions about whether they actually impair long-term healing (Patel, 2011).

Sub-acute stage

Contrast treatments can begin after 24–48 hours, helping to reduce irritation and inflammation around the knee, while cold applications can be used before gentle exercise or after any activity that makes the area sore. You can add anti-inflammatory herbs to these treatments. For instructions, review the contrast treatment for the knee in the dislocation section and ice massage procedure in the section on *Carpal tunnel syndrome* (page 277). The client's doctor will usually prescribe rest, followed by physical therapy consisting of gentle movement and muscle-strengthening exercises; this may be as effective as surgery (Katzm, 2013; Stensrud, 2015). Massage of the leg (but not the knee itself) may assist with lymphatic drainage and blood flow in the entire leg, and may reduce pain from nearby spasming muscles. Structural work is helpful for alignment problems that may have brought on the injury. Manual therapy may help heal tears as well, but requires special training and a doctor's approval (Hudson, 2016). Prolotherapy injections can also help the tissue to heal (Hauser, 2010).

As healing continues, combine castor oil packs, put on at the beginning of a session, with hands-on work, and the client may use the castor oil pack or a heat-trapping compress nightly as homework between sessions.

Dislocations

This injury occurs when great force wrenches a joint apart. For example, in a shoulder dislocation, the head of the humerus is forced completely out of the glenoid fossa (Figure 12.3 shows an anterior dislocation). Tissues around and inside the joint–muscles, ligaments, blood vessels, bursae or nerves–may be torn or bruised at the same time. If these other injuries are not healed, they can cause problems later in life, including repeated

Chapter twelve

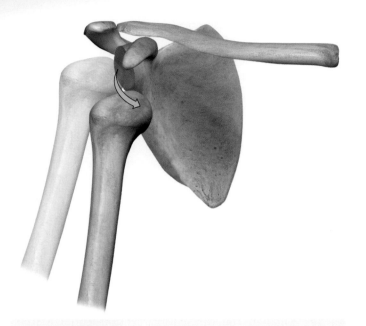

FIGURE 12.3
Subglenoid shoulder dislocation.

dislocations, so complete healing is important. Some of the damage may not show up right away: for example, a rotator cuff muscle may be slightly torn in a shoulder dislocation, but not progress to a full-thickness tear until years later, while joints with poorly healed ligaments are far more likely to develop osteoarthritis as clients age. The standard treatment for a dislocated joint is to put the bones back into position as quickly as possible, to immobilize the joint for a time, and then to begin exercises to strengthen muscles and increase range of motion. Clients are usually told to rest the area for the first 2 weeks, but it will take 3–4 months for the joint to heal completely. Although immobilization of the injured joint is necessary at first, it can also lead to activation of trigger points, contractures and stiff joints. Dislocations can be intensely painful and lead to chronic muscle guarding.

Ice is used as a first-aid measure, but after 24 hours contrast treatments (proximal) to the injury can be used to ease discomfort, to decrease swelling and muscle spasm, and to improve local circulation. Treatments to the uninjured joint on the opposite side can be used to improve circulation in the injured joint through the **contralateral reflex effect**. Early on, gentle circulatory massage

around the joint can be combined with those treatments, and the combination will enhance circulation, ease muscle spasm, and help the client relax more than either one alone. Once the shoulder is no longer immobilized, massage therapists can use warm or contrast treatments directly over the dislocated joint, encourage gentle exercise of the extremity in a warm tub or whirlpool, and encourage a nightly heat-trapping compress or castor oil pack. Massage can prevent muscular guarding by treating trigger points and releasing fascial restriction; all this can help prevent scar tissue build-up in the soft tissues around the joint and will be helpful for years to come. Here, we use the knee to illustrate hydrotherapy treatments, but these treatments may be used with any dislocated joint.

TREATMENT

CONTRAST TREATMENT OVER A RECENTLY DISLOCATED KNEE JOINT

Cross-reference

See Chapters 4 and 5.

Duration and frequency

15 minutes, to be performed before or during a massage session, and up to two or three times daily as a home treatment.

Cautions

Do not put pressure on the joint when performing this contrast treatment.

Special instructions

1. Another way to perform this treatment is to use hot and cold applications at the same time, for the same intervals, so that heat and cold are applied over and under the knee at the same time and then switched every 3 minutes. Do this three or more times.

2. Using a hand-held shower and alternating between very hot and very cold water is another helpful variation. To perform this at home, the client can sit on the side of a tub on top of a towel. There should be a grab bar available.

3. A contrast treatment over the same joint on the non-injured side of the body with alternating hot and cold can be used to create a reflex vasodilation

continued

TREATMENT *continued*

(**the contralateral reflex effect**) on the injured side.

Procedure

1. Have the client lie supine on the table. Extra pillows may be needed to support painful areas and for comfort.

2. Apply a hot fomentation, hot compress or other moist heat around the joint for 3 minutes.

3. Apply an ice pack or cold gel pack over the knee (Figure 12.4), or perform ice massage over the joint for 1 minute.

Repeat steps 1 and 2 twice, for a total of three rounds of hot followed by cold.

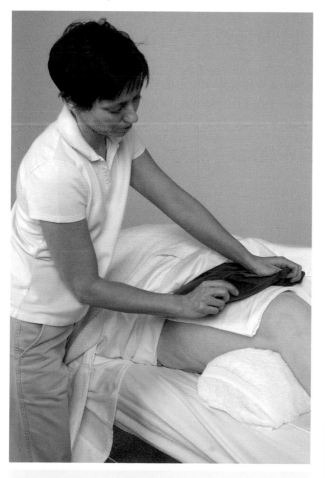

FIGURE 12.4
Applying a cold gel pack to the knee.

Exhaustion from over-exercising

Assuming that the client's doctor has ruled out any other problems that could cause fatigue, hydrotherapy techniques can be used to help rejuvenate and invigorate the client. Here we present three hydrotherapy treatments, two of which are especially effective in reviving an exhausted person because cold increases serotonin levels and stimulates the adrenals (Shevchuk, 2007). Cold mitten friction is a classic treatment for fatigue, especially if followed by massage. The contrast shower is also a time-tested technique. A short hot shower stimulates the circulation and the metabolism, as does a short cold shower. By alternating the two showers, the person who is exhausted can be reinvigorated. (Many high-end spas feature a warm soak followed by contrast sprays and promote this as an anti-fatigue treatment.) Next, even a short massage, using a mechanical massager, tapotement or other stimulating techniques, can complement the shower. The final classic treatment is a hot mustard bath, long used to relieve fatigue.

TREATMENT

COLD MITTEN FRICTION OR SALT GLOW

Cross-reference

See Chapter 10 for full instructions.

Duration and frequency

15–20 minutes. Use before or during a massage session.

Cautions

Do not perform this treatment in a cold room, or with a client who is chilled.

TREATMENT

CONTRAST SHOWER

Cross-reference

See Chapter 8 for full instructions.

Duration and frequency

10–15 minutes. Use before a massage session.

continued

TREATMENT *continued*

Special instructions

For extra skin stimulation, the client may also use soap and exfoliating gloves in the shower.

Procedure

1. Have the client take a short hot shower (2 minutes) followed by a short cold shower (1 minute). Both should be as extreme as the client can tolerate.
2. Repeat both hot and cold showers 2–5 times.

TREATMENT

MUSTARD BATH

Cross-reference

See Chapter 6 for full instructions.

Duration and frequency

15–20 minutes. Use before an invigorating massage session.

Procedure

Fill the tub. Have the client soak for 15–20 minutes, rinse off the bathwater and dry, and then go directly to the treatment table.

Fractures

Fractures can range from a single small crack (stress fracture) all the way to a thorough shattering that leaves a bone like a jigsaw puzzle (complex fracture; see Case history 12.1), so treatments may vary. Sometimes a standard cast will be sufficient to repair a fracture, but in other cases hardware such as pins, screws or metal plates may be required (see Figure 12.5A). Medications may affect bone healing; for example, **NSAIDS** are commonly used for pain, but by suppressing inflammation they disrupt the normal cycle of bone growth and resorption, and may slow or stop the healing of fractures (Cohen, 2006; Nwadinigwe, 2007). By reducing pain and inflammation, your treatment may be an alternative to these medications. Many fractures can be treated effectively with a cast, whereas others, such as a broken rib, cannot be put in a cast at all. Some hydrotherapy treatments are possible with a doctor's approval while the cast is still on. A contrast treatment directly to a limb with a cast, or to the opposite side using the **contralateral reflex effect**, can be used to improve the circulation. Using this approach, blood flow in the uninjured side will be doubled, while that in the casted side will increase by about 25%.

After a broken bone has healed and the cast has been removed, nearby muscles are usually stiff and weak, and there may be great soreness and edema in the tissues around the fracture site. There may also be contractures after a joint has been immobilized. Early on, these contractures can be treated by using ice packs on the shortened muscles for 20 minutes, then stretching them. The pain and trauma of the injury and its aftermath may have caused significant muscle guarding as well. At this time, hydrotherapy combined with massage can improve circulation of blood and lymph, ease soreness and pain, prevent adhesions, and reinvigorate an area that has suffered from a general lack of use during healing. Addressing muscle tension with massage can prevent chronic muscle tightness. For example, a rib fracture can be very painful, since breathing causes a constant grating of sensitive bone ends. Breathing shallowly to avoid discomfort can activate trigger points: unless these are treated, a lifelong habit of muscle guarding may begin (Aftimos, 1989). Contrast treatments are helpful at every stage of healing, while whirlpools can be used to soften dead skin, reduce stiffness and edema and improve local circulation. Pool therapy improves muscle strength, helps free fibrous adhesions and improves range of motion. Massage therapist Meir Schneider has even devised a pool therapy contrast treatment: while exercising in a warm pool, simply get out every 15 minutes and take a short cold shower (Schneider, 2007).

TREATMENT

CONTRAST TREATMENT OF A FRACTURE IN A WATERPROOF CAST OR KEPT COMPLETELY DRY USING PLASTIC BAGS

This treatment should be performed only with a doctor's approval.

Use a standard contrast bath and follow that with massage above and below the cast.

continued

TREATMENT *continued*

Cross-reference

See Chapter 6.

Duration and frequency

10–15 minutes. Perform before or during a massage session.

Special instructions

Alternating heat and cold can be used on the uninjured side to create a reflex vasodilation on the injured side. For example, if the left ankle is in a cast, perform a contrast treatment on the right ankle.

Cautions

It is vital to keep the cast absolutely dry by putting the entire extremity into a large plastic bag, and covering that with another plastic bag.

Procedure

1. Immerse the fractured part in hot water (approximately 110°F; 43°C) for 3 minutes, then switch and immerse it in cold water (approximately 55°F; 13°C) for 1 minute.
2. Repeat steps 1 and 2 twice, for a total of three rounds.

TREATMENT

CONTRAST SHOWER TREATMENT AFTER CAST REMOVAL

Contrast treatments using baths, showers or compresses are all effective, but using a hand-held shower attachment is ideal, because it stimulates the skin and superficial nerves even more than the strictly thermal ones, and thus helps to desensitize tender tissues.

Cross-reference

See Case history 8.1; see also *Contrast showers* on page 212.

Duration and frequency

10–15 minutes. Perform before a massage session, or as a home treatment: it may be performed two or three times daily. Clients may add extra stimulation by using exfoliating gloves and soap over and around the fracture site while in the shower.

continued

TREATMENT *continued*

Procedure

1. Spray the area with water, as hot as can be tolerated, for 2 minutes.
2. Spray the area with water, as cold as can be tolerated, for 30 seconds.
3. Repeat steps 1 and 2 twice more, for a total of three rounds of hot followed by cold.

TREATMENT

ICE PACKS FOR AN EARLY CONTRACTURE (THE JOINT IS OVERLY FLEXED OR EXTENDED DUE TO IMMOBILIZATION)

Cross-reference

See Chapter 5.

Duration and frequency

1. Use as soon as the cast is removed, if possible.
2. Apply directly over the shortened muscles for 20 minutes, then begin stretching and massage.

Cautions

Do not overuse ice, and monitor for frostbite.

TREATMENT

PARAFFIN BATH FOR JOINT STIFFNESS AFTER CAST REMOVAL

Cross-reference

For full instructions, see *Paraffin baths* on page 160.

Duration and frequency

10–15 minutes. Perform before a massage session.

Special instructions

The client's muscles and ligaments will be far more elastic right after the paraffin has been removed, so this is the ideal time for massage, therapeutic exercises, and stretching (Petrofsky, 2013).

COMBINING WATER TREATMENTS AND MASSAGE TO TREAT TWO COMPLEX FRACTURES

CASE HISTORY 12.1

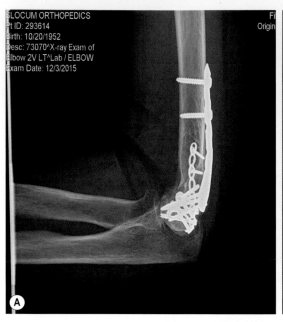

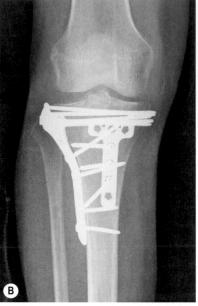

FIGURE 12.5
Complex fracture after surgical repair. (**A**) This elbow fracture was repaired with many screws, pins, and a metal plate. Courtesy MaryBetts Sinclair. (**B**) X-ray of Alexander's repaired right tibiofibular fracture. Courtesy MaryBetts Sinclair.

BACKGROUND 1

Maria Jesus, a healthy 60-year-old massage therapist, tripped and fell while backpacking, cracking her left radius and shattering her medial epicondyle into seven fragments. The elbow was surgically repaired with much hardware, and placed in a cast (see Figure 12.5A). She was told that it was unlikely she would ever be able to fully extend her arm or supinate her hand, and there was little or no likelihood she could ever do massage again. When her cast was first removed her elbow was frozen at a 90-degree angle and hurt with even moderate degrees of extension, her shoulder was rolled forward and down, her arm was very weak, and the surgical scar was large and thick.

TREATMENT 1

Maria Jesus used her forty years of bodywork experience to intensively treat her injury. She began hydrotherapy the day her arm was out of the cast: she used ice or heat to control pain, then wrapped her elbow every night with either a heat-trapping compress or a castor oil pack. She began daily exercise as best she could in a warm pool. When she showered afterwards, she used the hot spray to warm her scar, then did self-massage to stretch it. As she became stronger she swam laps in a cold pool and went through an upper body stretching routine in a warm pool. She received massage at least once a week, massaged her arm herself, and worked diligently at her physical therapy. If her arm hurt after therapy she used ice massage or a heating pad instead of pain medications. She gradually regained nearly full range of motion in her elbow and shoulder, her arm became stronger, the scar became supple and almost invisible, and five months later she resumed practicing massage. Her physical therapist told her, "Your progress is amazing – I never thought you would make it this far!"

TREATMENT 2

A 35-year-old schoolteacher and outdoorsman, Alexander fell 17 feet off a ladder and shattered his right proximal tibia and fibula, as well as his left ankle, which were repaired during a long operation (see Figure 12.5B). Since his doctor had told him not to put any weight on his feet for 90 days, he used a wheelchair during the day.

continued

COMBINING WATER TREATMENTS AND MASSAGE TO TREAT TWO COMPLEX FRACTURES

A few weeks after surgery he was recovering well and his pain was controlled with medication, but his right lower leg had a very uncomfortable sensation he described as being "like a block of wood," especially at night, and both legs twitched constantly, making it difficult to sleep.

TREATMENT 2

A massage therapist saw Alexander at home, beginning with a contrast treatment with Epsom salts. This had been approved by Alexander's doctor. Wearing shorts, Alexander transferred from his wheelchair to a plastic stool placed in the bathtub, and the tub was then filled with 104°F (40°C) water to which 2 cups of Epsom salts were added. Alexander's wife filled a tall plastic garbage can with a full bag of ice and then added cold water. Alexander soaked in the hot water for 20 minutes to fully dilate all the blood vessels in his legs and feet, while the therapist sat on a chair next to him and massaged his calves and feet. With help from his wife, Alexander then swung around to put his legs in the cold water for 60 seconds, returned to the hot water for 3 minutes, went back to the cold for 60 seconds, then did one more round. He transferred back to his wheelchair and rolled back to his bed, where he received a gentle Swedish massage of the legs and feet. Although he was sensitive to touch and slightly apprehensive before the bodywork, afterwards he felt tremendous relief from the discomfort in his legs and feet and was able to get a good night's sleep for the first time since his accident. Alexander was seen weekly for a total of 10 weeks, and each time he felt great relief from his discomfort. The "wooden" sensation in his legs began to decrease, he was able to cut back on his pain medication, and he worked hard at his physical therapy. One year later, he presented the massage therapist with a photograph of himself on the summit of an 11-thousand-foot peak and told her, "You are the reason I could do this!"

Iliotibial band disorders

This chronic condition occurs in long-distance runners, bicyclists, and other athletes who squat repeatedly. It is more likely to develop in athletes with poor body mechanics, tight muscles, poor training habits, and structural problems such as leg-length discrepancy, a tilted pelvis or bowed legs. Foam rolling, stretching and hands-on techniques which treat the hamstrings and iliotibial band are known to be helpful (Winslow, 2014). Moist heat before bodywork and finishing with 1 minute of ice massage will make tissue more receptive to deeper work.

TREATMENT

HOT TOWEL ROLL MASSAGE OVER LATERAL THIGH

Cross-reference

See Chapter 4.

continued

TREATMENT *continued*

Duration and frequency

15 minutes; perform during a massage session.

Procedure

1. With the client in a side-lying position, apply a hot towel roll and perform compressions, gliding strokes and stretches on the lateral thigh.
2. Finish with a brief cold-water rub or ice massage if desired.

Knee injuries in the sub-acute stage

Knee injuries such as muscle strains, torn cartilages and sprains are common in many sports. The following treatment helps the client to relax the entire limb and encourages healing.

Chapter twelve

WHOLE-BODY HEATING
FOLLOWED BY MOIST HEAT TO THE KNEE

Cross-reference

See *Fomentations* on page 92; *Whole-body baths* (page 162), *Hot wet air baths: local and full-body steam treatments* (page 184), and *Hot dry air bath: the sauna* (page 180).

Duration and frequency

45 minutes. The client takes a tub bath, steam bath or sauna just before the session, then goes directly to the massage table for the application of local heat to the knee.

Cautions

Obtain a doctor's approval for this treatment.

Procedure

1. Have the client take a whole-body steam bath, sauna or full hot bath for 15 minutes, dry off and go directly to the treatment table. Avoid chilling.

2. Wrap a hot fomentation snugly around the entire knee, and leave it on for 30 minutes. A moist heating pad on a low or medium setting may be used instead. Monitor both carefully to avoid burning.

3. Remove the heat and give a brief ice massage or cold mitten friction to the knee and the tissues around it, then begin massage.

Muscle strains

This injury occurs when muscle fibers are stretched beyond their elastic limits. The deltoid and biceps are some of the most frequently strained upper extremity muscles, while groin pulls and torn hamstrings are common in the lower extremity, and the muscles of the chest and back can be strained by heavy lifting as well as in sports. Severe vomiting during an intestinal flu or violent coughing from a cold can also cause muscle strains. Among athletes, muscle strains are often caused by not warming up adequately, workouts that are too intensive, continuing to use an injured muscle, and forcing a tight muscle beyond its normal length while stretching. Muscle strains are classified as mild, moderate, or severe by the amount of damage that is done. In mild strains only a few fibers are involved and there is minor discomfort, no loss in strength, and normal range of motion. In moderate strains, 10–50% of the muscle fibers are torn and there is more pain, swelling, and some weakness. Fortunately, severe muscle strains are much rarer: they involve 50–100% of the muscle fibers and cause much more pain and weakness.

Many muscle strains are one-time events, such as a back muscle strain while lifting a single heavy object, but even more are caused by repeated overuse of muscles. As the body tries to heal the strain, scar tissue fibers that form within and around the injured muscle can eventually lead to the muscle tearing easily when it is stressed again. Rehabilitation for muscle strains focuses on helping to restore the muscle to its normal flexibility, endurance, and strength. This is done through stopping the problem activity that strained the muscle, treating inflammation, and performing carefully applied therapeutic exercises. Then, when pain begins to go away, exercise may be cautiously resumed. Hydrotherapy and appropriate massage techniques can help the muscle heal without adhesions and with full mobility. Pool exercise is a handy way to stay limber and get gentle exercise while recovering. Most strains heal in 4–6 weeks.

ICE MASSAGE
OF A STRAINED MUSCLE

Ice massage may be performed in the first 24 hours after a muscle strain.

Cross-reference

See Chapter 5.

Duration and frequency

5–10 minutes. Perform during a massage session, or as a home treatment, two or three times daily.

Special instructions

Using the ice, gently massage the muscle and well around it. Herbal teas or essential oils can be added to the water for ice massage.

TREATMENT

CASTOR OIL PACK

Cross-reference

See Chapter 4.

Duration and frequency

30 minutes or longer, before or during a massage session. The client may use castor oil packs as a home treatment, especially at night.

Special instructions

Apply the castor oil pack directly over the strained muscle for at least 30 minutes.

TREATMENT

HOT MOIST APPLICATION

Use hot fomentations, moist compresses, or local baths or showers for moist heat. Hot rolled towels or a heat lamp over a thin damp towel are excellent for a back muscle strain. Paraffin baths may be used for strained muscles in the hands, forearms, lower legs or feet. Follow the hot application with a short (1 minute) treatment such as ice massage over the muscle, a cold compress or an ice-water bath. Vasodilating and anti-inflammatory herbs or essential oils can be added to all of the treatments.

Cross-reference

See Chapter 4.

Duration and frequency

20 minutes, before or during a massage session.

Special instructions

You can also perform ischemic compression or gentle stretching while the client's strained muscle is immersed in hot water.

TREATMENT

CONTRAST TREATMENT

Virtually any combination of hot and cold may also be used, such as alternating hot and cold compresses, partial baths, and alternating hot and cold sprays using hand-held shower attachments—variations are limited only by what you have in your office.

Cross-reference

See Chapters 4, 5, 6 and 8.

Duration

15 minutes.

Procedure

1. Using a moist heating pad or hydrocollator pack, apply heat to the strained muscle for 3 minutes; then apply cold with an ice cup or cold gel pack, or use a cold mitten friction. If you use contrast baths, you can also perform ischemic compression or gentle stretching while the client's strained muscle is immersed in hot water.

2. Repeat hot and cold two more times, for a total of three changes.

TREATMENT

MUSTARD PLASTER

Cross-reference

See Chapter 4.

Duration and frequency

20 minutes. Perform during a massage session.

Procedure

1. Place the mustard plaster over the muscle that has been strained, and cover it with a small sheet of plastic, a small towel and a heat source.

2. Leave the plaster on for 20 minutes while you massage elsewhere, and monitor the client's skin carefully to avoid burning.

3. Wipe off the client's skin to remove all traces of mustard.

4. Begin massage of the strained muscle.

Chapter twelve

TREATMENT

TREATMENT

STEAM BATH FOLLOWED BY BRIEF COLD

The steam bath may be given in a steam room, individual cabinet or canopy. Afterwards, perform ice massage on the strained muscle and well around it for 1 minute.

Cross-reference

For ice massage, see page 128: *Ice massage performed four different ways*. For steam baths, see page 184: *Hot wet air baths: local and full-body steam treatments*.

Duration and frequency

20–25 minutes. The client can take the steam bath directly before a massage session.

Muscle soreness

Strenuous exercise can cause microscopic muscle tears, swelling and soreness. The pain is greatest two or three days later, and can last as long as a week.

It can often be prevented by warming up and stretching before exercise, and cooling down and stretching afterwards. If suddenly athletes make their workouts more frequent or intense rather than building up gradually, they will likely have sore muscles as well. However, it is not always possible to avoid soreness: for example, violent coughing during an illness can cause soreness in the intercostal, pectoral and diaphragm muscles. Also, traumatic falls or other accidents often leave tissues sore (see Case history 12.2). Cold and contrast baths relieve muscle soreness and edema, whereas hot baths do not (Vaile, 2008). Epsom salts baths, cold whirlpools, partial-body contrast showers, contrast compresses using Epsom salts, and gentle circulatory massage all increase blood flow to sore muscles all relieve swelling and pain, and help the muscles repair themselves (Simon, 2000; Thomas, 1977). Many dedicated distance runners take cold lower-leg whirlpools after long runs; peripheral blood vessels are constricted, blood flows to deeper vessels, and soreness in the deeper leg muscles is avoided (Menetrier, 2014). Heat-trapping compresses can also soothe muscle aches and pains (see Appendix A for instructions).

TREATMENT

CONTRAST PARTIAL-BODY SHOWER

Cross-reference

See Chapter 8.

Duration and frequency

15 minutes. Perform before a massage session, or the client may perform this as a home treatment three or four times daily.

Cautions

1. Pain in a joint might indicate a torn cartilage or ligaments: the client should see a doctor.
2. Inform clients that they can stay active even with muscle soreness, but if their neck or back aches, they should switch to a low-impact activity that won't further aggravate the area.

Procedure

1. Using a hand-held shower attachment, spray the sore area for 5 minutes with water that is as hot as the client can tolerate, and alternate that with 1 minute of cold water. Perform a total of three or more rounds.
2. Have the client dry off and begin massage.

   For full instructions and contraindications, see partial-body shower section in Chapter 4.

TREATMENT

EPSOM SALTS BATH

Cross-reference

See Chapter 6.

Duration and frequency

20 minutes. Perform before a massage session, or the client may perform this as a home treatment three or four times daily. If there is no time before a session for this treatment, Epsom salts may also be used to make a cold compress over the sore area instead.

continued

TREATMENT *continued*

Anti-inflammatory herbs or essential oils may be added to the water as well. Alternating hot and cold compresses using water containing Epsom salts can be employed during a session.

Procedure

1. Add 2 pounds (1kg) Epsom salts to a full tub of water at 98–104°F (37–40°C). Anti-inflammatory herbs or essential oils may be added to the water as well.

2. Have the client soak in the tub for 20 minutes.

Plantar fasciitis

Inflamed plantar fascia often cause great pain from the heel to the base of the toes. Plantar fasciitis is really an overuse syndrome. Conditions which put more strain of the plantar fascia include high arches, tight or weak calf muscles, flat or inflexible feet, obesity, shoes that are too narrow or rigid, and, for runners, suddenly increasing the distance or intensity of their workouts. Mainstream treatment for this condition includes icing; stretching and strengthening exercises; and wearing better-fitting shoes, and possibly arch supports. If these conservative measures don't work, injections of cortisone into the fascia are sometimes used, but rupture of the Achilles tendon or plantar fascia may result (Melvin, 2015).

You can help this condition heal by combining hydrotherapy treatments with hands-on massage techniques. Self-ice massage with a frozen water bottle or a cold gel pack on the sole can prepare the client's tender, inflamed tissues for massage, and contrast treatments can relieve inflammation and promote healing. Bodywork can help heal this injury at its most basic level: (1) by addressing tightness in the gastrocnemius and soleus, which pull on the arch and can distort it so that it can't support the same weight; or (2) by treating postural problems such as pelvic rotations or leg length inequality. For permanent healing, the real causes of this injury must be addressed.

MUSCLE SORENESS AND BRUISES AFTER A FALL FROM A TREE

CASE HISTORY 12.2

BACKGROUND:

Eleven-year-old David climbed a tall tree, then fell at least 15 feet (4.5 meters), slamming into a few large branches before he hit the ground. He immediately felt severe back pain and soon an enormous bruise formed across his entire back. He was examined by his family doctor who ruled out fractures and other serious injuries. Although this was welcome news, David was in a lot of pain, and he felt stiff and sore whenever he tried to move or even take a deep breath. At home he rested quietly and his mother began applying ice packs, at intervals of 20 minutes on and 20 minutes off, throughout the day. Despite this, three days later his body still felt stiff and sore, so his mother scheduled a massage for him.

TREATMENT

Although the therapist felt that massage was likely to relieve much of David's discomfort, she was not sure he could tolerate being touched, and therefore she suggested warm baths with two pounds of Epsom salts in the tub each time. The next day, David's mother called to say that three Epsom salts baths had relieved much of his pain, so he was willing to come in after school for a massage. During the session, the therapist planned to use contrast compresses on the remaining sore areas and even over David's bruise, to make massage more tolerable for him.

DISCUSSION QUESTIONS:

1. Why didn't the ice packs have a better effect on David's pain?

2. What made the Epsom salts bath effective?

3. Why would alternate compresses be appropriate during the massage session?

4. What is another treatment that could be helpful?

TREATMENT

SELF-MASSAGE
USING AN ICE-FILLED SODA BOTTLE

Cross-reference

See Chapter 5.

Duration and frequency

10 minutes. Perform before a massage session; as a home treatment it can be performed two or three times daily.

Special instructions

1. The client may use small cold stones instead. Cool 20 smooth stones; then lay a towel on the floor, add the stones, and tread gently on them. Using the toes, pick the stones up one by one and drop them into a bowl.

2. If tissues are too tender for self-massage with the cold bottle, begin bodywork with the client in the prone position, and gently lay a cold gel packs or compresses over each sole. Leave on for 5–10 minutes and repeat at the end of the session.

Procedure

1. Fill a 20-ounce plastic soft drink bottle with water and freeze it.

2. Have the client roll his or her feet back and forth over the bottle. Rather than leaning his or her entire body weight onto the bottle, the client should use just enough pressure to gently stretch the muscles, tendons and fascia.

3. Begin massage.

TREATMENT

CONTRAST FOOTBATH

Cross-reference

See Chapter 6.

Special instructions

Gentle movements performed during the footbath will further increase local circulation.

continued

TREATMENT *continued*

Duration and frequency

15 minutes. Perform before or during a massage session; as a home treatment it can be performed two or three times daily.

Procedure

1. Fill two deep buckets or washtubs with water up to mid-calf level, one at 110°F (43°C) and the other at 50°F (10°C). Anti-inflammatory herbs or essential oils can be added to the water.

2. Put both feet in the hot water for 3 minutes, then in the cold water for 30 seconds.

3. Repeat steps 2 and 3 twice more, for a total of three rounds of hot followed by cold.

Rotator cuff tears

The rotator cuff muscles surround the shoulder joint and help to keep the humeral head in place by controlling its internal and external rotation. Of the four muscles, the supraspinatus is the most commonly torn. Tears are most often caused by repetitive strain, but any previous trauma such as a shoulder dislocation may cause one of the tendons to be torn even before that. Most rotator cuff tears occur in people 40 years of age or older, who may already have tendons which are weak, contain thick adhesions or have simply degenerated from chronic overuse. However, direct trauma–such as an anterior shoulder dislocation, a fall onto an outstretched hand, or a humeral fracture–can cause tears even in younger people. Throwing a baseball or serving in volleyball or tennis can also cause rotator cuff tears. The famous baseball pitcher Dizzy Dean tore his rotator cuff muscles by pitching with a broken toe: since he could not push off on his injured foot, this increased the load on his shoulder and led to a career-ending injury. In roughly half of all cases, surgery is not necessary. Small rotator cuff tears are treated by using a sling, hot or cold treatments, massage, acupuncture and gentle exercises to maintain and even increase the range of motion. If the tear does not heal properly, the tendon may become thick, scarred and chronically inflamed, while the overlying bursae are constantly irritated. It is particularly important that the client regain full range of motion as soon as possible, so that a frozen shoulder (**adhesive capsulitis**) does not develop. Larger rotator cuff tears often require surgery.

Nonsteroidal anti-inflammatory drugs are commonly pre-scribed after rotator cuff repairs, but they can impair bone formation and tendon-to-bone healing (Cohen, 2006).

Hydrotherapy treatments can help address the inflam-mation that so often accompanies rotator cuff tears and relax the muscles around the shoulder joint. Ice massage can numb the shoulder temporarily so that gentle range of motion exercises can be performed. Hands-on tech-niques can treat many aspects of this problem, from mus-cle guarding to pain to inflammation.

Note: Obtain a doctor's approval before treating rota-tor cuff injuries.

TREATMENT

ICE MASSAGE

Cross-reference

See Chapter 5.

Duration and frequency

8–10 minutes. Perform during a massage session, or the client may perform this as a home treatment two or three times daily. Herbal teas or essential oils can be added to the water for the ice massage.

Procedure

1. Massage with the ice, over the length of the torn muscle and well around it, for 8–10 minutes.
2. Let the area warm up briefly, then have the client perform very gentle shoulder range of motion ex-ercises. Follow these with massage.

TREATMENT

CONTRAST TREATMENTS

Cross-reference

See Chapters 4–8.

Duration and frequency

15 minutes. Perform during a massage session.

Special instructions

Besides the specific hot and cold methods used here, you can also try alternating hot and cold compresses,

continued

TREATMENT *continued*

or a hot fomentation, castor oil pack or mustard plas-ter, followed by ice massage or alternating hot and cold sprays. See earlier directions for each treatment.

Procedure

1. Apply a moist heating pad or hydrocollator pack to the entire shoulder joint, front and back, for 3 minutes. If necessary, use two moist heat sourc-es to cover the entire joint, and monitor the client carefully for burning while you massage related areas.
2. Wring out a washcloth in ice water, then rub the warmed area briskly for 30 seconds, or do ice massage for 1 minute.
3. Repeat steps 1 and 2 twice more, for a total of three rounds.
4. Begin massage.

TREATMENT

STEAM BATH FOLLOWED BY BRIEF COLD TO THE TORN MUSCLE

The steam bath can be done using a steam room, a canopy or an individual cabinet. At the end of the steam bath, perform ice massage on the strained muscle and well around it for 1 minute, then begin hands-on techniques.

Cross-reference

See Chapter 4 for ice massage and Chapter 6 for steam baths.

Duration and frequency

20–25 minutes. Perform before a massage session.

Scar tissue

If the surgery [to remove old adhesions] is followed each morning and evening with large abdominal steam packs, adhesions rarely form again, no matter how extensive they were before surgery. The hydrotherapy generates such good circulation, relief of pain, relaxation of the tissues and activity of the phagocytes, it inhibits more adhesions.

Louella Doub, *Hydrotherapy*

Chapter twelve

Scar tissue is made of collagen fibers that the body makes to replace damaged or destroyed cells. It is denser than normal tissue because the fibers grow together to form a thick, firm scar. Unfortunately, scar tissue fibers also form without a definite orientation or grain – rather like a mat – and fascia may bind around them unless they become aligned (see Figure 12.2A). Over a period of about one year, scars begin to soften and fade somewhat and old wounds are as supple as they will ever be without outside intervention. Sometimes the skin or superficial fascia shrinks over a tight area, leading to restrictions and adhesions. There are often trigger points in the scar itself which can cause burning, prickling, or lightning-like jabs of pain. In deeper tissues, such as muscles, scar tissue can cause problems because it is less elastic than muscle and tears more easily when stretched.

Massage techniques soften scar tissue by loosening restricting fibers and adhesions and producing a more parallel fiber arrangement: pain is decreased and the appearance of scars are improved (AMTA, 2018). A few weeks after surgery is the ideal time for massage to make its unique healing contribution, for scar tissue is formed but still moldable. When healed, the scar should have a springy end-feel and an elastic quality.

Concentrated moist heat helps to soften and relax the fibers in and around the scar, so techniques such as cross-fiber friction are then more effective and less uncomfortable. As mentioned in Chapter 5, using a paraffin bath before stretching scar tissue has yielded significant, measurable increases in ease of movement.

HEAT AND MASSAGE FOR OLD AND NEW SCARS	CASE HISTORY 12.3

BACKGROUND 1: OLD SCAR

Justina is a 20-year-old massage student who was born three months premature, weighing only two pounds. She had open heart surgery when she was four days old and has a long J-shaped scar which wraps around the left side of her ribcage. The scar is very restricted, is painful to the touch, and hurts whenever anything bumps into it. She and her class instructor, Helena Tolis, decide to treat the scar.

TREATMENT 1

Helena begins by draping a hot fomentation over the area while Justina is in a side-lying position. She massages other areas of the body for 20 minutes, and then takes off the fomentation to find that Justina's scar is not only less sensitive, but also less taut. Helena begins by treating it with 30 minutes of various scar tissue release methods, including skin rolling, stretching in a variety of directions, and digital pressure. Justina's pain level is quite high at first, but by the end of the session it has decreased modestly, and the scar is more supple. The treatment for the next three sessions is similar, beginning each time with 20 minutes of heat but, since the scar is no longer as sensitive, massage is performed for 60 minutes each time. By the end of the last session the scar is almost painless and non-

adhered. Each treatment has been made much easier by the application of heat, and Justina is extremely pleased, since, as she tells Helena, "I thought it would hurt for the rest of my life."

BACKGROUND 2: NEW SCAR

Marnie was a 40-year-old graphic designer with no previous health problems. Four months ago she underwent an extensive surgery for **neurofibromatosis:** doctors removed a 3.15 inch (8cm) non-cancerous tumor, which had grown into the right side of her neck, and the entire right levator scapulae muscle was removed as well. Next, radiation treatments had caused burns to her neck and to the inside of her mouth, so it still hurt to swallow. Her neck felt very stiff, her right scapular area was so painful she could not sleep at night, and the right side of her neck felt "as hard as a rock." Her stress level was off the charts due to health and money worries, physical pain and poor sleep. She was wary of massage because she had experienced so much discomfort and pain; indeed she had come only because her radiation oncologist felt that the scar, which was at C4 level, was in danger of solidifying and permanently restricting her movements. Her physical therapist had approved gentle massage and moderate heat.

continued

HEAT AND MASSAGE FOR OLD AND NEW SCARS

TREATMENT 2

The entire right side of Marnie's neck looked and felt extremely swollen. The therapist thought through hydrotherapy options: ice massage, while it would have reduced the inflammation, would likely have been uncomfortable and hard to tolerate, thus adding to Marnie's stress. Due to its derivative effect, a hot footbath would have decreased congestion and been comforting as well, but would not directly address her neck issues. The therapist decided to use warm compresses for a first session.

The session began with Marnie lying face up, breathing shallowly, and with her body drawn up and tense. The therapist began by placing a large warm compress on her upper chest, then covering it with a small sheet of plastic and a dry towel. Marnie sighed happily when the moist heat was placed on her chest and her body began to unclench. The therapist used gentle cranial holds for 5 minutes, replaced the first compress with a warmer one, and Marnie relaxed a little more. The therapist massaged her upper back from underneath, being careful to avoid the anterior neck. After 5 minutes she switched compresses once more, then continued massage. After 15 minutes more she removed the last compress, dried the area with a soft cloth, and performed 5 minutes of gentle effleurage strokes on Marnie's upper chest. Now, 20 minutes into the treatment, Marnie's jaw and neck looked less puffy, she felt less pressure on her right lateral neck, and when she touched it exclaimed in amazement at how much softer it felt.

She was also much more relaxed and the massage session proceeded on the upper back, neck, shoulders and face. The therapist chose not to massage the scar itself until she had learned how Marnie responded to this first session. For homework, the therapist suggested Marnie stand in a shower and let warm water flow over her upper chest, while gently massaging and tapping the area, in order to relieve pressure and pain in her neck and throat.

Marnie relaxed more readily at the next session; there was a marked reduction of swelling in her face and anterior neck after the warm compresses and bodywork, and she felt a wonderful sense of relief. This time the therapist was able to perform very gentle scar tissue release, and Marnie tolerated it well. She was seen a total of six times, and the therapist was eventually able to perform many techniques that addressed the scar, edema, shoulder muscle imbalance and chronic tension. Marnie also did gentle self-massage in the warm shower at least once a day, and followed through on physical therapy. Her scar healed without adhesions and was supple and pain-free.

DISCUSSION QUESTIONS:

1. What are two other derivative techniques that could have been used?
2. Why did the therapist select this particular technique?

TREATMENT

MOIST HEAT APPLICATION

Apply a hot water bottle, a moist heating pad, or a hot compress or hydrocollator pack to the area for 10–15 minutes before massage, until the tissue is thoroughly warm.

Cross-reference

See Chapter 4.

Duration and frequency

10–15 minutes. Use during a massage session.

TREATMENT

PARAFFIN BATH FOR SCARS ON THE ELBOWS, WRISTS, HANDS, ANKLES OR FEET

Cross-reference

See Chapter 6.

Duration and frequency

20 minutes. Use during a massage session. Perform a standard paraffin bath treatment before hands-on work. For a hard-to-dip part of the body, paraffin may be painted on instead.

TREATMENT

LOCAL WHIRLPOOL

Before massage, have the client immerse the body part in warm water (98–105°F; 37–41°C) for 15–20 minutes. Stretching and gentle exercises may be performed in the water if desired.

Cross-reference

See Chapter 6.

Duration and frequency

15–20 minutes. Use before a massage session.

Shin splints

Shin splints is a catch-all term for aching, pain and inflammation along the anterior or medial border of the tibia. The basic cause of this injury is running or dancing on hard surfaces, combined with tight calf muscles, weak anterior tibial muscles, and poor foot alignment. Muscle fibers absorb the impact and then become inflamed, and exercise becomes painful. Untreated shin splints may progress to stress fractures or **lower leg compartment syndrome**. Treatments for mild shin splints include stopping the activity for a time and wrapping the area, and then light stretching, exercising in a warm pool, contrast treatments followed by simple exercises, and possibly arch supports. Ice massage can relieve pain, while contrast treatments can dramatically reduce inflammation and can relieve pain – ideally, deep frictioning and massage can be done right afterwards. Clients should be evaluated by a doctor before treatment.

TREATMENT

CONTRAST BATH TREATMENT OF THE LOWER LEG

Cross-reference

See Chapter 5 or the contrast bath in the section on *Plantar fasciitis* in this chapter (page 289).

TREATMENT

ICE MASSAGE OF THE LOWER LEG

Perform a standard ice massage treatment over the anterior and medial tibia for 8–10 minutes, moving the ice from below the knee to the ankle; then begin hands-on massage. Herbal teas or essential oils can be added to water for ice massage.

Cross-reference

See Chapter 5.

Duration and frequency

8–10 minutes. Perform during a massage session, or the client may perform this as a home treatment two or three times daily.

Sprains

Sprains are classified by the percentage of ligament fibers that are torn. First degree tears involve only a few fibers and thus minor swelling, pain, and loss of function. Second degree tears involve many more fibers and modest swelling, diffuse tenderness, and loss of stability. Third degree tears are actual ruptures, when the ligament tears completely off the bone. All sprains feature at least a small amount of blood and fluid leaking into the tissues around the joint, and activation of trigger points in the ligaments and the joint capsule, so sprains *hurt* – sometimes a lot.

When the bone, ligaments, and surrounding muscles are healthy, a joint is stable and free of pain. However, ligaments are more likely to tear if they are too short. For example, if you pronate when you walk, the ligaments on the outside of the ankle tend to get shorter while the ones on the inside of your ankle are stretched. According to podiatrist Gary Null, "Under these conditions, all it takes is one moment of sudden pressure for the too-taut ligaments to rip." To avoid ankle sprains, pronators need to stretch their feet and ankles to lengthen too-short ligaments, and to wear an ankle brace during athletic activity to stabilize the joint (Null, 2000). Ligaments are more flexible when they are warm, so warming up before exercise is an important preventive measure (Petrofsky, 2013).

Unless injured ligaments are completely healed, the joint may re-sprain easily: as many as one third of all sprained ankles will sprain again within a few years

(Van Rijn, 2008). Unstable joints are also more likely to develop arthritis – for example, damage to an anterior cruciate ligament makes that knee far more likely to develop osteoarthritis (Bailey, 2017; Hill, 2001). For this reason, it is important for sprains to heal completely and no matter how mild or severe the sprain is, the ligaments must be supported and protected during their healing process. The standard treatment for first degree sprains is ice, additional support such as braces or taping, compression and elevation. Second degree sprains are treated with additional support, crutches and isometric exercises. Third degree sprains are treated with a rigid cast, and sometimes with surgery to reattach the ligament in its proper place, followed by strengthening and stretching exercises once the cast has been removed.

Adding hydrotherapy treatments and massage to the standard treatment greatly increases comfort and speeds healing. Massage therapist should obtain the doctor's approval before treating an acute sprain. Ice packs or ice massage can be applied during the first 24 hours, and then contrast treatments help reduce joint swelling and pain. For sprains of the shoulder and spine, use hot packs followed by ice massage. Mild sprains without swelling are sometimes treated by a heating compress left on overnight. For old, poorly healed ankle sprains, use the deep heat of a paraffin bath to ease joint stiffness, and follow that with massage.

Bodywork is helpful for sprains in the subacute phase: various techniques can reduce pain and swelling and relax tight or spasmed muscles. Massage of the area can also prevent chronic muscular guarding caused by trauma and pain. (For an example of how musculoskeletal pain can lead to this problem, see Box 12.1.)

TREATMENT

ICE PACKS TO AN ACUTELY SPRAINED JOINT

Cross-reference

See Chapter 5.

Duration and frequency

Apply for 20 minutes once every 3–4 hours for the first 24 hours.

Cautions

Do not overuse ice, and monitor for frostbite.

TREATMENT

LOCAL EPSOM SALTS BATH

Use this for sub-acute sprains. Gentle range of motion exercises may be performed during the bath.

Cross-reference

See Chapter 6.

Duration and frequency

20 minutes. Perform before a massage session, or the client may perform this as a home treatment three or four times daily.

Special instructions

The water should cover a large area around the sprained joint: for an ankle sprain, the water should be at mid-calf level. Gentle, non-painful movements can be carefully performed while the part is in the water.

Procedure

1. Add one cup of Epsom salts per gallon to a container of water at 98–104°F (37–40°C). Anti-inflammatory herbs or essential oils can also be added.

2. Have the client soak the sprained part in the tub for 15–20 minutes. Dry the part and begin massage.

TREATMENT

HEAT-TRAPPING COMPRESS

Heat-trapping compresses may be used for sub-acute sprains of the foot, ankle, knee, shoulder, elbow, wrist or hand, and provide a mild prolonged warmth.

Cross-reference

See Appendix A.

Duration and frequency

1–8 hours. This can be used daily, at any stage of healing.

Special instructions

At the end of a massage session, the massage therapist may assist the client in applying a heat-trapping compress which will keep the sprained joint warm for a few hours or even overnight.

Chapter twelve

TREATMENT

CONTRAST ANKLE AND FOOT BATH

This treatment may be done on many joints, but here we discuss the ankle since it is the most commonly sprained joint.

Cross-reference

See Chapter 6; or use the procedure given in *Plantar fasciitis*, page 289.

TREATMENT

PARAFFIN BATH FOR AN OLD, POORLY HEALED SPRAIN, USING THE WRIST AS AN EXAMPLE

Cross-reference

See Chapter 6.

Duration and frequency

10–15 minutes. Perform before a massage session, or the client may perform this daily as a home treatment. Paraffin can also be painted over any joint.

Procedure

1. Soak the client's hand and wrist in warm or hot water (98–110°F; 37–44°C) for 1 minute or longer, then dip it in paraffin 6–10 times.

2. Wrap the area to keep it warm, then leave the paraffin on for at least 10 minutes while you massage elsewhere.

3. Remove the paraffin and proceed with massage, stretching, or range of motion exercises.

Spinal cord injuries

Most spinal cord injuries happen to young men, and the majority are caused by motor vehicle accidents, falls, or some type of violence (Figure 12.6 shows a spinal cord injury at the T12 level). Sensation and movement may be partially or completely lost below the level of the injury. Massage is helpful in addressing a range of problems associated with spinal cord injuries, including chronic emotional stress, chronic pain, scoliosis, constipation, lack of sensory stimulation, and overuse of some parts of the body coupled with underuse of other parts.

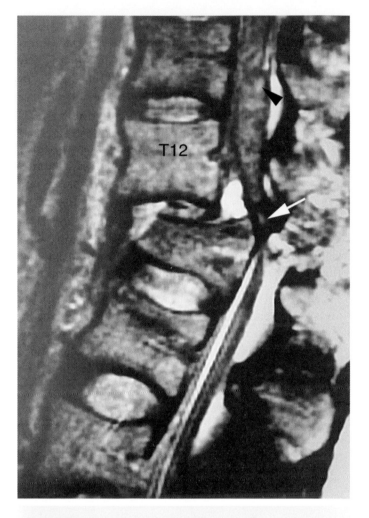

FIGURE 12.6

A crushing blow caused this spinal cord injury at the T12 level. Reprinted with permission from Yochum TR, Rowe LJ. Essentials of Skeletal Radiology, 2nd edn. Baltimore, MD: Lippincott, Williams and Wilkins; 1996, 1:398, Figure 6.38.

Combining hydrotherapy and bodywork will be far more effective than using either modality alone. Advantages of this approach:

1. Applications of moist heat can relax the person and prepare their tissues for massage.

2. Contrast applications can help stimulate blood flow in the legs, which is usually poor due to a lack of movement.

3. Cold footbaths can reduce the body temperature up to 4°F (2°C) when a client is in danger of becoming overheated on a hot day, common in this condition.

4. Before strengthening exercises, cold immersions can stimulate muscle tone for about 20 minutes.

5. Hydrotherapy treatments can be an important source of sensory stimulation.

6. Pool therapy is a wonderful way for a person with a spinal cord injury to exercise without fighting gravity, to improve the circulation as a whole, and to decrease muscle spasms (Kesiktas, 2004).

All hydrotherapy applications must be very carefully monitored since paralyzed areas are sometimes numb. Observe and feel the client's skin more often than usual to prevent burns from hot applications or frostbite from cold applications. Begin by using milder temperatures until you see how the client responds.

Massage therapists should obtain a doctor's permission before working with persons with recent spinal cord injuries.

TREATMENT

MOIST HEAT APPLICATION

Cross reference

See Chapter 4.

Duration and frequency

10 minutes on each body area that will be massaged. Perform during a massage session.

Cautions

Do not let the client become overheated. If this should occur, either remove the moist heat or apply cold (such as a cold compress or gel pack) on another part of the body.

Special instructions

Apply a warm compress or a hydrocollator pack to a single body area for 10 minutes before it. Then, while you massage the warmed area, move the moist heat to the part of the body that will be massaged next.

TREATMENT

CONTRAST TREATMENT FOR SENSORY STIMULATION

Cross-reference

See Chapters 4 and 5.

continued

TREATMENT *continued*

Duration and frequency

12 minutes. Perform during a massage session.

Procedure

1. Apply a warm compress or a hydrocollator pack to one area for 10 minutes.

2. Take it off and place an ice pack or a washcloth wrung out in cold water over the same area, and leave it on for 2 minutes. An Epsom salts glow or exfoliating gloves wrung out in cold water can add even more sensory stimulation.

TREATMENT

COLD WATER IMMERSION AND EXERCISE FOR WEAK OR SPASTIC MUSCLES

After the cold immersion, have the client perform strengthening exercises or even contract his muscles while you provide resistance.

Cross-reference

See Chapter 6.

Duration and frequency

5–10 minutes. Perform during a massage session, and repeat during the session if desired.

Cautions

Monitor the client carefully to make sure he does not become over-tired.

Special instructions

If a body part cannot be immersed, wrap it in an iced compress or crushed ice wrapped in wet towels. Check to make sure that the client is comfortably warm before using any cold application.

Procedure

1. Massage the weak or spastic part for 2–5 minutes.

2. Fill a large container with water and crushed or cube ice for a final temperature of 35–40°F (2–4°C).

3. Warn the client that the part will be dipped in cold water.

4. Immerse the part in the water for 3 seconds.

TREATMENT *continued*

5. Take the part out of the water and have the client perform exercises for 30 seconds. If he becomes fatigued, stop the exercises until after the next cold water immersion.

6. Repeat steps 4 and 5 twice more, for a total of three rounds of cold immersion followed by exercises.

7. Massage the weak or spastic part for 2–5 minutes.

Surgical trauma

Ice is a good local anesthetic and can help reduce pain around your incision during the first 24 hours after surgery. Don't use this treatment after the first 24 hours, though, it can delay wound healing. Next, use a heating pad or hot-water bottle, which keeps the muscles around the incision from becoming too stiff.

Lee Swanstrom, MD, in Renner, *The Home Remedies Handbook*

As helpful and necessary as surgeries are, the body reacts to them as if they were threats. The sympathetic nervous system is activated, inflammation is set in action, and post-surgical pain can be significant. The client may experience pain from any stretching or manipulation that needed to be done during the surgery, and sometimes if he or she needed to be in an unusual position for hours, this too causes pain. Stress and anxiety may accompany the entire experience. How can a massage therapist help in this situation? With doctor's OK, hydrotherapy and massage can begin after just a short time, to relieve inflammation, pain and emotional stress, and help the wound heal. They are helpful at all stages of rehabilitation. Here are some examples:

1. Ice packs in the first 24 hours help reduce use of pain medications and do not harm the wound (Master, 2014).

2. Contrast treatments over incisions may begin after 24–48 hours with the doctor's approval. For example, at Wildwood Hospital in Chattanooga, Tennessee, hot fomentations alternated with ice packs are prescribed to speed healing and reduce pain. Staff visit each patient's room to perform contrast treatments until patients are strong enough to walk to the hydrotherapy department. Incisions are covered with a sheet of plastic to keep them dry and then hot and cold are applied.

3. Soothing general massage while the patient is still hospitalized may help ease pain, anxiety and edema: studies have confirmed this in patients with thoracic, cardiac, breast cancer, lumbar spine and joint replacement surgeries (AMTA, 2018). Simple additions such as heating pads, warm moist towels or salt glows in a patient's bed can be deeply soothing.

4. A hot or contrast footbath may relieve postoperative swelling (see Case history 12.4).

5. Ice massage can be used if clients have overdone their exercises or been on their feet too long.

6. Clients with joint replacements normally have mild to moderate swelling for 3–6 months after surgery: once it is safe, baths with Epsom salts or anti-inflammatory herbs or essential oils can precede massage and be used as a home treatment by the client.

7. Heat before massage can prevent adhesions and improve suppleness and the appearance of scars of scars (see Case history 12.3).

8. In the later stages of rehabilitation, swimming in warm water can loosen muscles and increase range of motion.

Tailbone trauma

This painful injury occurs when a backward fall onto the buttocks causes the coccyx to be bruised, broken or dislocated. Doctors generally begin treatment with ice applications over the coccyx, anti-inflammatory medication and possibly a cortisone injection. After the first acutely painful stage has abated, massage is safe and helpful, but therapists should obtain specific training to work with tailbone trauma. Chiropractors and osteopaths may treat this condition by correcting the position of the coccyx. Ice may be used over the coccyx during the first 24 hours, while applying heat to the gluteals at the same time. After that, switch to a carefully applied contrast treatment directly over the coccyx. To relieve tension and increase blood flow, the client can also sit in a warm bathtub for 15 minutes three times a day, while

RELIEVING POST-OPERATIVE PAIN AND SWELLING WITH A HOT FOOTBATH AND MASSAGE

BACKGROUND

Sarah was a 54-year-old schoolteacher who had been physically active all her life, but she was also hypermobile and prone to musculoskeletal pain for that reason. She had seen a massage therapist many times for muscle spasms, injuries, and stress. She had recently undergone right shoulder surgery to repair a torn labrum and degenerated supraspinatus muscle, and in addition one end of her clavicle had been also removed. One week post-op, she returned to the doctor because she was concerned about increasing pain and swelling of her right upper extremity. Her doctor determined that all was normal, and prescribed physical therapy in about four weeks.

TREATMENT

Her massage therapist then visited her at her home and found Sarah was miserable: she felt cold (her house was cold), she was constipated from the narcotic pain medication, and she had severe shoulder pain (after stopping the narcotic because of the constipation). She wore a sling and did not want to lie down.

Since Sarah would have to be seated, felt cold, and her shoulder was swollen, the therapist decided to offer her a hot foot soak along with his hands-on treatment. Sarah's husband assisted with a tub and hot water, and once her feet were soaking, she began to feel warmer almost immediately. The therapist then proceeded to perform gentle lymphatic massage on Sarah's upper body for about 30 minutes, all the while avoiding the operated area and anything that might pull on her stitches. Her husband added more water to the footbath to keep it at 106°F (41°C). Before the session was finished, Sarah exclaimed at how much her shoulder swelling and pain had decreased. The combination of gentle lymphatic massage along with the warming and derivative effect of the hot footbath was an unbeatable combination.

DISCUSSION QUESTIONS

1. What could have been added to the hot footbath to increase its effect?

2. Discuss other hydrotherapy treatments that could have been combined with the massage.

---

keeping weight off the coccyx. If the condition has become chronic, pelvic floor physical therapy can also be effective. Low impact aerobic activity can help bring nutrients to the area.

TREATMENT

CONTRAST TREATMENT OVER THE COCCYX

Cross-reference

See Chapters 5 and 6.

Duration and frequency

About 15 minutes. Use 3–5 times daily.

Special instructions

Do not put any pressure on the tailbone when applying compresses. Massage elsewhere while the compresses are on.

continued

TREATMENT *continued*

Special instructions

Anti-inflammatory herbs may be added to the compress water.

Procedure

Apply a hot compress over the coccyx for 3 minutes, then switch to a cold compress for 1 minute. Repeat three times, for a total of four rounds of hot followed by cold.

Tendonitis

Tendonitis is a common overuse injury which can be set in motion at sports or at work. Massage therapists are prone to tendonitis because their work often involves the repetitive use of a few muscles for long periods of time, sometimes while applying great pressure; patellar tendonitis develops from sports that involve a lot of jumping, such as basketball; and wrist tendonitis can develop from computer work.

The injury begins with small tendon tears which cause pain, inflammation, and possibly a build-up of scar tissue; if the overuse continues, a vicious cycle may develop as the tendon heals and then tears again. The standard medical treatment for tendonitis is rest, ice, wrapping or taping the area, stretching or strengthening exercises, and anti-inflammatory medications. Steroid injections are sometimes used, but they greatly increase the risk of tendon rupture. Many, but not all, clients will get better and can gradually return to the sport or activity that led to the problem. To prevent the vicious cycle discussed above, this injury must be completely healed. Contrast treatments and ice massage promote healing and combine well with cross-fiber friction and other massage techniques.

Although the treatments below may be used on any tendon, here we demonstrate how to use them for elbow tendonitis.

Inflammation in this area can take the form of either (A) medial epicondylitis or "golfer's elbow" or (B) lateral epicondylitis or "tennis elbow." The first is caused by overuse of the forearm flexor muscles, the second by overuse of the forearm extensor muscles. Treatment is basically the same for both conditions: in the acute phase, the arm is rested and sometimes splinted in a position that relieves tension on the tendons. Anti-inflammatory medications may be prescribed, although some experts believe that these actually delay the healing process, and this makes hydrotherapy and bodywork the preferred treatment (Constantinescu, 2019). To preserve muscle tone and flexibility, strengthening exercises may begin after one week of rest. Ice is used to ease inflammation and relieve pain, but if overused the tendon may heal poorly. When ice massage is alternated with bodywork the client gets the benefit of cold without blood flow being reduced. In the first, acute phase of tendonitis, contrast treatments may be used two or three times daily to relieve inflammation, and lymphatic drainage and gentle transverse friction techniques are appropriate. Local salt glows followed by castor oil and a heating compress may be applied during a massage session, or used by the client at night. In the sub-acute phase, therapy as above

may continue, except that vigorous circulatory massage and deep transverse friction techniques are now more appropriate. Note that massage therapists should obtain the doctor's approval before treating a client with acute tendonitis.

TREATMENT

CONTRAST BATH TREATMENT FOR EPICONDYLITIS

Contrast baths are used here, but hydrocollator packs and ice massage may be used instead.

Cross-reference

See Chapter 6.

Duration and frequency

15 minutes. Perform during a massage session, or the client may perform this as a home treatment two or three times daily.

Special instructions

Gentle, non-painful movements performed while the elbow is in the water will further increase local circulation.

Procedure

1. Fill two deep buckets or washtubs with water, one at 110°F (44°C) and the other at 50°F (10°C). The tendon and an area at least 6 inches (15cm) around it should be covered by the water.

2. Soak the elbow in the hot water for 3 minutes, then in the cold water for 30 seconds.

3. Repeat steps 1 and 2 three more times, for a total of four rounds of hot followed by cold.

4. Dry briskly and begin massage.

TREATMENT

ICE MASSAGE OF INFLAMED TENDONS AT THE ELBOW

Cross-reference

See Chapter 5.

continued

TREATMENT *continued*

Duration and frequency
8–10 minutes, before or after gentle therapeutic exercise or massage.

Special instructions
Perform the ice massage on the tendon and 6 inches (15cm) around it. Herbal teas or essential oils can be added to the water for ice massage.

TREATMENT

LOCAL SALT GLOW FOLLOWED BY A CASTOR OIL PACK OR A HEAT-TRAPPING COMPRESS ON INFLAMED TENDONS AT THE ELBOW

Cross-reference
See Chapters 4 and 10.

Duration
30 minutes or longer

Cautions
Do not wrap the joint so tightly that you cut off circulation.

Special instructions
1. Apply at the beginning of a massage session, remove after 30 minutes, and then perform massage over and at least 6 inches (15cm) around the inflamed tendon.
2. If the client is using this as a home treatment, he or she may leave the heating pad on over the castor oil pack for about one hour, monitoring the skin for burns; then remove the heating pad, apply the heating compress, and leave that on overnight.

Procedure
1. Using Epsom salts, perform a local salt glow over the muscle and tendon and about 6 inches (15cm) around it.
2. Choose A or B:
   (A) Rub a liberal amount of castor oil over and around the tendon, then cover the castor oil-coated skin with a piece of thin plastic and

continued

TREATMENT *continued*

   put a heating pad over that. Leave in place for 30 minutes or more while you massage other parts of the body.
   (B) Put a heat-trapping compress over the area. Remove it after 30 minutes and proceed with massage.

TREATMENT

PARAFFIN DIP FOR ELBOW TENDONITIS IN THE SUB-ACUTE STAGE

Cross-reference
See Chapter 6.

Duration and frequency
15 minutes. Apply before beginning a massage session.

Procedure
1. Immerse the elbow in warm water for at least 1 minute, then dip it in the paraffin at least six times and wrap it well to keep it warm.
2. After unwrapping the area, apply either a cold mitten friction or a brief dip in cold water, then begin massage.

Tired, aching feet

Foot-strenuous activities such as hiking, distance running, basketball, soccer or ballet often lead to tired aching feet. Hydrotherapy is frequently used by competitive runners to ease muscular fatigue and rejuvenate muscles, and massage can bring great relief as well. An athlete can receive both during a rest break and then go back on the field rejuvenated. Cold stimulates muscles, so they are stronger after a contrast or cold bath but not after a hot bath (Earr, 2002; Vaile, 2008).

TREATMENT

CONTRAST FOOTBATH OR COLD FOOTBATH

Cross-reference

See Chapter 6.

Duration and frequency

10–20 minutes. Perform before or during a massage session, and as a home treatment it can be performed two or three times daily.

Special instructions

1. Many runners find a cold footbath very refreshing; simply follow the procedure below, but use only one footbath, make it as cold as can be tolerated, and have the client soak for just 10 minutes. Another option is to have the client sit in a half bath of cold water for 10 minutes.

2. Epsom salts, charcoal, powdered ginger or mustard or anti-inflammatory herbs or essential oils can be added to the hot footbath.

Procedure

1. Fill two deep buckets or washtubs with water, one at 110°F (44°C) and the other at 50°F (10°C). Put both feet in the hot water for 3 minutes, then put both feet in the cold water for 30 seconds.

2. Repeat step 1 twice, for a total of three rounds of hot followed by cold.

TREATMENT

LOCAL SALT GLOW AND WARM FOOTBATH

Cross-reference

See Chapters 6 and 10.

Duration

5–10 minutes.

Special instructions

This technique may be performed with the client supine. Simply put a towel at the foot end of the table to protect the linens, then have the client bend her knees and place her feet in the footbath.

continued

TREATMENT *continued*

Procedure

1. Place a large towel on the floor.

2. Have the client sit in a chair. Lay a towel on the floor and put the footbath of warm water (98–105°F; 37–41°C) on top of the towel.

3. Have the client soak her feet in the footbath for 2 minutes.

4. Take one of the client's feet out of the footbath, and using a small amount of Epsom salts, perform a salt glow on one foot. Either hold the client's foot over the footbath while you do this, or lay her foot on the towel next to it.

5. Now place the client's foot back in the warm footbath and repeat with her second foot.

6. Pour clean water over both feet and then move the footbath off the towel entirely, dry the feet and begin massage. Or, have the supine client soak for a full 20 minutes to absorb the other ingredients in the water.

Traumatic brain injuries

Falls, motor vehicle accidents, sports injuries and being hit on the head are the main causes of traumatic brain injury (TBI). The large mechanical forces involved may damage not only the brain but the bones and soft tissues of the head, spine and other areas. As a result, sufferers sometimes develop chronic problems such as headaches, neck pain, face and scalp muscle tension, vision problems, upper back or shoulder stiffness, poor balance and back pain (Denton, 1996). Massage therapist Dianne Keanne has treated many people with TBI and has found that they often have scar tissue and other soft tissue dysfunction around the cervical spine (Keanne, 2004). In her book *Brainlash: Maximize Your Recovery From Mild Brain Injury*, Dr. Gail Denton explains how Swedish massage and craniosacral therapy, helped her recover from her own brain injury (Denton, 1996).

During the early stages of rehabilitating from a TBI, massage may be used to release tension, decrease headaches, stimulate circulation, prevent muscular atrophy, and maintain joint range of motion. Early contractures may be treated with ice packs followed by massage (Burns, 2015). (See *Ice packs for an early contracture*, page 283.) Craniosacral therapy may be needed, because head trauma can cause misalignment of the cranial bones (Nerman, 2000). Heat or contrast applications can be used before massage and stretching; ice massage helps ease bruises or trauma elsewhere in the body; and a hot footbath may be helpful for post-concussion headaches. As time goes on, hydrotherapy treatments and massage are no luxury but a source of deep comfort. Later, swimming in a warm water pool can strengthen muscles and help with flexibility.

The standard treatment for a post-concussive headache is medication and/or physical therapy. It is not always clear whether pain stems from the brain injury or from trauma to the neck and skull. Many of these headaches are worst in the initial weeks after a concussion and gradually go away, but some become chronic. Old-time hydrotherapists used hot footbaths for traumatic headaches and some TBI sufferers say these do relieve pain. As long as the client is receiving treatment for such headaches from a medical doctor, you may safely use a hot footbath plus an ice pack to the back of the neck during a massage session, and the client may try this at home. Refer to directions in the section on migraine headache, Chapter 13.

Whiplash

The single best movement I have found for healing an injured or painful neck is swimming in warm water using a mask and snorkel so you don't have to turn your head excessively ... the buoyancy of the water helps relax strained muscles and fascia and moving through the water provides a gentle traction between the smaller head and larger shoulders.

Maud Nerman, DO

Because many people suffer from the consequences of poorly healed whiplash injuries, you will often see clients with this problem. This common injury is caused by head-on collisions, falls, and rear-end collisions. It occurs when the head and neck are abruptly snapped forward-and-back (as seen in Figure 12.7), forcing the neck into hyperextension and hyperflexion. Clients may have had some or all of the following problems:

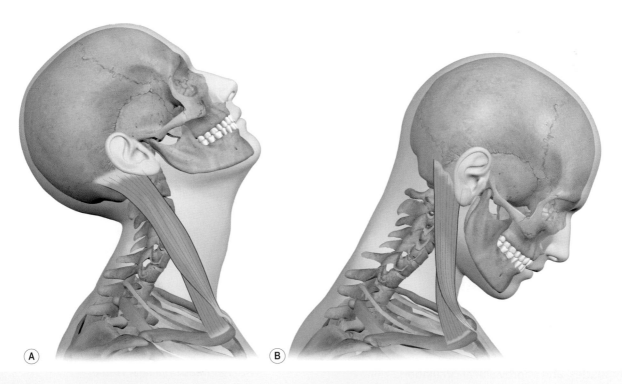

FIGURE 12.7
Whiplash: hyperextension **(A)** and hyperflexion **(B)** of the head and neck.

1. Muscles around the cervical spine, especially the sternocleidomastoid, scalenes and splenius cervicis, may be strained or torn.

2. The anterior and posterior longitudinal ligaments, which hold the cervical vertebrae together snugly, may be sprained or torn, resulting in problems with neck alignment and spinal nerves.

3. The cervical vertebrae or their cartilaginous discs may be damaged.

Depending on the amount of force involved, this injury can result in chronic neck pain, poorly healed scar tissue, ongoing muscle spasms in neck muscles as they contract to splint unstable joints, active trigger points, and problems with misaligned cervical vertebrae. In 15–40% of those with acute neck pain, the pain will become chronic (Schofferman, 2007). Whiplash injuries are serious and require a doctor's ongoing care.

As detailed in Case history 12.5, hydrotherapy treatments can reduce pain and inflammation as well as increase local circulation, and help prepare the client's soft tissues before massage. Physical therapy professor Charles Thomas recommends first alternating ice massage around the entire neck with a heat-trapping compress, then switching to a combination of contrast treatments, gentle warm water exercise, and gentle massage after 24 hours (Thomas, 1977). Maud Nerman, DO, uses osteopathic manipulation to relax muscular and fascial restrictions in whiplash cases (Nerman, 2014). Flotation tank therapy has also relieved chronic whiplash-related neck pain (Edebol, 2008). Many types of bodywork can help heal whiplash injuries, from gentle craniosacral techniques to deeper muscle techniques, and hydrotherapy will improve outcomes. (Before treating recent whiplashes, massage therapists should obtain the doctor's approval.)

TREATMENT

NECK EXERCISE PERFORMED IN A HOT SHOWER

This exercise will gently release warm and relax tight neck muscles, and improve local circulation.

continued

TREATMENT *continued*

Cross-reference

See Chapter 11, Hot shower stretching exercises.

Duration and frequency

5–10 minutes. Perform at the beginning of a massage session; or, if used as a home treatment, may be performed two or three times daily.

Special instructions

Remind the client, if necessary, that this exercise is for gently limbering the neck: it is not a workout, and must not be done if it causes pain.

Procedure

1. Have the client step into a hot shower and let the water beat on her neck for at least 3 minutes to thoroughly warm the cervical muscles.

2. While the hot water continues to beat on her neck muscles, she can draw the letters of the alphabet with her nose one by one as a range of motion exercise.

3. Have the client towel off and dress quickly to avoid chilling. She may now lie down for a rest or a massage session.

TREATMENT

CONTRAST TREATMENT FOR THE NECK

Cross-reference

See Chapters 4 and 5.

Duration and frequency

15 minutes. Perform at the beginning of a massage session; or, if used as a home treatment, may be performed three or four times daily.

Special instructions

A contrast treatment may be performed in the shower, using a hand-held shower attachment and the same intervals of hot and cold.

Procedure

1. Have the client lie prone upon the massage table, with her head on a face cradle.

continued

TREATMENT *continued*

2. Apply a moist heating pad, hot compress or heated gel pack to the back of the neck for 3 minutes. Wrap it around to the front of the neck as far as possible, but do not cover the carotid arteries.

3. Wring out a washcloth in ice water and rub the warmed area for 30 seconds, or perform ice massage for 1 minute instead.

4. Repeat hot and cold twice more, for a total of three rounds.

5. Dry the client's skin and begin hands-on massage.

TREATMENT

FULL HOT BATH WITH GENTLE MOVEMENTS

Cross-reference

See Chapter 6.

Duration and frequency

15-20 minutes. Perform before a massage session.

Cautions

This treatment should not be taken by those with high blood pressure or heart problems.

continued

TREATMENT *continued*

Special instructions

Gentle painless movements while in the tub help relieve pain and spasms and improve circulation.

Procedure

1. Fill the bathtub with hot water (102–110°F; 39–43°C), then place a rolled-up towel or bath pillow behind the client's neck so the neck is in a comfortable position. For a headache, also apply a cold compress to the back of the neck.

2. The client should remain in the tub for 15 minutes or longer, depending upon tolerance. During the last few minutes, have him sit upright and perform gentle slow painless neck movements.

3. Have the client sit on the side of the bathtub on a towel, and then perform a cold mitten friction on the neck and upper back and shoulders. If he is feeling lightheaded, he should continue sitting on the side of the tub until he has thoroughly cooled off and the sensation has passed.

4. The client can now dry off and go directly to the massage table for treatment. To ensure complete relaxation of the neck muscles, you may add a 10-minute hot application followed by a short cold rub directly on the back of the neck, as soon the client lies down on the massage table.

HYDROTHERAPY AND MASSAGE FOR A SUB-ACUTE WHIPLASH INJURY **CASE HISTORY 12.5**

BACKGROUND

Dimitri was a 32-year-old landscaper with no history of back or neck injuries. However, one day as he waited at a stop light his car was struck from behind by a car traveling at 30 miles (48km) per hour. Within two hours after the accident, his neck began to hurt. The pain gradually increased and his right arm and leg felt tingly and numb, so he went to a hospital right away. Fractures were ruled out, but he was given a cervical collar as well as medications for muscle spasm, inflammation and pain. By the next day his paraspinal muscles from T10 to C1 were hypersensitive to light touch, and even light pressure on suboccipital and scalene muscle trigger points caused severe referred pain in his head. His family doctor then prescribed physical therapy plus massage therapy twice a week for four weeks.

TREATMENT

Session 1

Six days later, Dimitri entered the massage therapist's office wearing his cervical collar and still experiencing moderate to severe neck pain and nerve sensations. The session began with hot compresses alternated with ice

continued

massage applied to the back of his neck and his upper back. Dimitri stated that this made his neck feel better. Next he was treated with gentle cranial holds, followed by fingertip kneading and petrissage on his entire back, upper chest and neck. The massage therapist explained how Dimitri could perform contrast treatments to the upper back and neck in the shower.

Sessions 2–8

These sessions were similar to the first. Dimitri's neck pain began to gradually lessen. He was diligent about doing his physical therapy exercises, performed shower contrast treatments each day, and came for massage sessions twice a week. Each session began with the same contrast treatment while the therapist massaged Dimitri's arms, followed by a hot compress on his lower back while she massaged his upper back, followed once more by a hot compress to his upper back while she massaged his lower back. She finished the treatment with one minute of ice massage on his entire spine.

Although he had occasional setbacks caused by forgetting to wear his cervical collar or practicing his physical therapy exercises too vigorously, by his eighth massage session Dimitri had little or no neck pain, he had normal range of motion in his neck, his upper back muscles were noticeably less hypertonic and swollen than before, and pressure on trigger points produced less pain. He would continue to receive physical therapy and use contrast treatments at home for any residual pain and stiffness in his neck. He stood an excellent chance of having no long-term problems from his injury.

DISCUSSION QUESTIONS

1. Why did the massage therapist recommend shower contrast treatments at home, rather than hot showers or cold showers alone?

2. Why did the massage therapist use heat followed by hands-on massage followed by heat again?

3. Name another anti-inflammatory treatment that could have been used at the beginning of Dimitri's treatment.

BOX 12.4	POINT OF INTEREST

HERBS USED WITH HYDROTHERAPY FOR INJURIES

For centuries, the herbs below have been combined with hydrotherapy treatments to treat a number of injury-related problems. These include soreness, aching, and inflammation; muscle spasms; poor local circulation; and wounds. Massage therapists who regularly use herbal preparations in their compresses, baths, fomentations, water for ice massage, and other water treatments feel that the herbs deepen the effectiveness of their hands-on techniques (Treasure, 2004).

Herbs for muscle soreness, aching, and inflammation

Herb	Bruise	Edema	Eye inflammation	Ligament tear	Muscle aching	Muscle soreness	Plantar fasciitis	Sinus inflammation	Sprain	Strain
Arnica	✓	✓		✓					✓	
Calendula	✓									✓
Chamomile			✓					✓		
Comfrey							✓			
St John's wort	✓				✓	✓				
Witch hazel	✓				✓	✓				

BOX 12.4 *continued*

Herbs for muscle spasms and muscle tightness

Herb	Muscular cramps	Flu aches and pains	Rheumatic pain	Sleep aid and relaxant	Spasmodic asthma
Blackhaw	✓				
Chamomile	✓	✓		✓	
Cramp bark	✓				
Ginger	✓	✓			
Lavender			✓	✓	
Lobelia					✓
Mullein					✓

Herbs which treat injuries by improving local circulation

Herb	Fibrositis	Fracture (delayed union)	Frozen shoulder	Low back pain	Migraine	Muscle strain	Poor circulation	Rotator cuff tear
Cayenne					✓		✓	
Ginger	✓	✓	✓	✓	✓	✓	✓	✓
Mustard			✓	✓	✓			✓

Herbs for wounds

Herb	Delayed union of fractures	Damaged joints and muscles	Pulled tendons
Arnica		✓	
Comfrey	✓	✓	✓
St John's wort		✓	

CHAPTER SUMMARY

In this chapter, you have learned about many of the most common injuries you will see in your practice, and how to target each one with hydrotherapy and massage. Because helping injured clients is one of our primary tasks as therapists, the information in this chapter will prove invaluable in your practice.

REVIEW QUESTIONS

Fill in the blanks

1. Mustard plasters provide intense local heat, and can be used for _____ , _____ and _____.

2. Muscle soreness after exercise can be treated using _____ baths.

3. A cold leg bath relieves muscle fatigue, shifting blood flow from _____ to _____.

4. Sprains are injuries to _____, while strains are injuries to _____.

5. A cold water immersion bath is given to someone with a spinal cord injury to stimulate _____.

Essay

6. Run your fingernail quickly and firmly down the length of your forearm, and watch as first a white line appears, a few seconds after that a red streak appears, and then a distinct ridge forms along the red streak. What does this tell you about the inflammation reaction to possible injury?

7. Name three treatments that can be used for a shoulder dislocation after 24 hours.

8. Give two examples of long-term consequences of poorly healed injuries.

Multiple choice

9. Which of the following is *not* an inflammatory condition?
   A. Bursitis
   B. Epicondylitis
   C. Exhaustion after exercise
   D. Plantar fasciitis

10. Which of the following would *not* benefit from a contrast treatment?
    A. Sprains
    B. Scar tissue
    C. Amputation
    D. Plantar fasciitis

11. Which of these treatments is *not* appropriate for acute bursitis?
    A. Upper half-body pack
    B. Paraffin bath
    C. Contrast treatment
    D. Ice massage

12. When scar tissue is formed improperly, which of the following results?
    A. Arthritis
    B. Swelling
    C. Hematoma
    D. Adhesion

13. Which of these is *not* a sign of inflammation?
    A. Redness
    B. Cool skin
    C. Swelling
    D. Pain

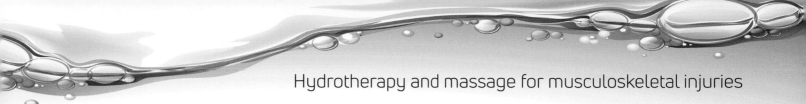

References

Adie S. Cryotherapy following total knee replacement. Cochrane Database Syst Rev 2012 Sep 12

Aftimos S. Myofascial pain in children. New Zealand Medical Journal 1989; August 23: 440–1

AMTA. Massage Therapy in Integrative Care and Pain Management. Evanston, IL: American Massage Therapy Association, 2018

Bailey JR et al. Surgical management and treatment of the anterior cruciate ligament/medial collateral ligament injured knee. Clin Sports Med 2017; 36(1): 87–103

Burns S. Concussion treatment using massage techniques: a case study. Int J Ther Massage Bodywork 2015; 8(2): 12–17

Caring Medical. Rest Ice Compression Elevation; Rice Therapy and Price Therapy. https://www.caringmedical.com/prolotherapy-news/rest-ice-compression-elevation-rice-therapy/ [Accessed: March 2020]

Centers for Disease Control and Prevention. www.cdc.gov/injury.wisgars/index [Accessed March 2019]

Cohen DB. Indomethacin and celecoxib impair rotator cuff tendon-to-bone healing. Am J Sports Med 2006; 34(3): 362–9

Constantinescu DS. Effects of perioperative nonsteroidal anti-inflammatory drug administration on soft tissue healing: a systematic review of clinical outcomes after sports medicine orthopaedic surgery procedures. Orthop J Sports Med 2019; 16: 7(4)

De Roeck NJ. Meniscal tears sustained awaiting anterior cruciate ligament reconstruction. Injury 2003; 34(5): 343–5

Denton G. Brainlash: Maximize Your Recovery from Mild Brain Injury. Niwot, CO: Attention Span Books, 1996

Earr T et al. The effects of therapeutic massage on delayed onset muscle soreness and muscle function following downhill walking. J Sci Med Sport 2002; 5(4): 297–306

Edebol J. Chronic whiplash-associated disorders and their treatment using flotation-REST (restricted environmental stimulation technique). Qual Health Res 2008; 18(4): 480–8

Geiss L et al. Resurgence of diabetes-related nontraumatic lower-extremity amputation in the young and middle-aged adult US population. Diabetes Care 2019; 42(1): 50–4

Halpern B. Knee Crisis Handbook. New York: Rodale Pub, 2003

Hauser R. www.caringmedical.com/ice-why we do not recommend it, Accessed April 2019

Hauser R. Case for utilizing prolotherapy for first-line treatment for meniscal pathologies. Journal of Prolotherapy 2010; 2(3): 416–37

Hill C et al. Knee effusions, popliteal cysts, and synovial thickening: association with knee osteoarthritis. J Rheumatol 2001; 28; 1330–7

Howatson G, Van Someren KA. Ice massage. Effects on exercise-induced muscle damage. J Sports Med Fitness 2003; 43(4): 500–5

Hudson R. An alternative approach to the treatment of meniscal pathologies: a case series analysis of the Mulligan Concept "Squeeze" Technique. Int J Sports Phys Ther 2016; 11(4): 564–74

Katzm J et al. Surgery versus physical therapy for a meniscal tear and osteoarthritis. N Engl J Med 2013; 368(18): 1675–84

Keanne D. Personal communication with the author. September 2012

Kesiktas N et al. The use of hydrotherapy for the management of spasticity. Neurorehabilitation and Neural Repair 2004; 18(4): 268–73

Krieger M. Namath: A Biography. New York: Viking, 2004

Laver L. Injuries in Extreme Sports. J Ortho Surg Res 2017; 12: 59

Martin G. Trauma and recall in massage: a personal experience. Massage Therapy Journal 1985: 35–6

Martin SS. Does cryotherapy affect intraarticular temperature after knee arthroscopy? Clin Orthop Relat Res 2002; 400: 184–9

Master V. Ice packs reduce post-operative pain. J Am Coll Surg 2014; 219(3): 480–9

Mayer JM, Mooney V, Matheson LN et al. Continuous low-level heat wrap therapy for the prevention and early phase treatment of delayed-onset muscle soreness of the low back: a randomized controlled trial. Arch Phys Med Rehabil 2006; 87(10)

Melvin TJ. Primary care management of plantar fasciitis. W V Med J 2015 Nov-Dec; 111(6): 28–32

Menetrier T. Changes in femoral artery blood flow during thermo-neutral, cold, and contrast-water therapy. Journal of Sports Medicine and Physical Fitness, January 2014

Mirkin G. Why Ice Delays Recovery. http://drmirkin.com/fitness/why-ice-delays-recovery.html 2015

Mirkin G, Hoffman M. The Sports Medicine Book. New York City: Little Brown & Co, 1978

Nerman M. Healing Pain and Injury. Pt Richmond, CA: Bay Tree Publishing, 2014

Null G, Robins T. How to Keep Your Feet and Legs Healthy for a Lifetime. New York: Four Walls, Eight Windows, 2000

Nwadinigwe CU. Effects of cyclooxygenase inhibitors on bone and cartilage metabolism: a review. Niger J Med 2007, Oct–Dec; 16(4): 290–4

On AY et al. Local heat effect on sympathetic skin responses after pain of electrical stimulus. Arch Phys Med Rehabil 1997; 78(11): 1196–9

Passan J. The Arm. New York: Harper Collins, 2016

Patel D, Adrian B. Do NSAIDS impair the healing of musculoskeletal Injuries? Rheumatology Network 2011, June 07; 28

Petrofsky R. Effect of heat and cold on tendon flexibility and force to flex the human knee. Med Sci Monitor 2013; 19: 661–7

Renner J. The Home Remedies Handbook. Lincolnwood, IL Illinois: Publications International, 1993

Schneider M. Movement for Self-Healing. Tiburon, CA: New World Library, 2004

Schofferman J. Chronic whiplash and whiplash-associated disorders: an evidence-based approach. J Am Acad Orthop Surg 2007 Oct; 15(10): 596–606

Shevchuk NA. Possible use of repeated cold stress for reducing fatigue in chronic fatigue syndrome: a hypothesis. Behav Brain Funct 2007, Oct 24; (3) 55

Sidhy, A et al. Dabbing the skin surface dry during ice massage augments rate of temperature drop. Int J Exerc Sci 2008, Jan 15; 1(1)

Simon R. Repetitive Strain Injury Handbook. New York: Henry Holt, 2000

Simons DG, Travell JG, Simons LS. Travell and Simons' Myofascial Pain and Dysfunction: the Trigger Point Manual, Vol 1: Upper Half of Body, 2nd edn. Baltimore, MD: Lippincott, Williams and Wilkins, 1999

Stensrud S. Effect of exercise therapy compared with arthroscopic surgery on knee muscle strength and functional performance in middle-aged patients with degenerative meniscus tears: a 3-month follow-up of a randomized controlled trial. Am J Phys Med Rehabil 2015; 94(6): 460–73

Thienpoint E. Does advanced cryotherapy reduce pain and narcotic consumption after knee arthroplasty? Clinical Orthopaedics and Related Research 2014; 472(11): 3417–23

Thomas C. Simple Water Treatments for the Home. Loma Linda, CA: Loma Linda University School of Health, 1977

Thrash A, Thrash C. Home Remedies: Hydrotherapy, Massage, Charcoal and other Simple Treatments. Seale, AL: Thrash Publications, 1981, p. 60

Treasure J. MNIMH, AHG, Course notes from class: herbs and massage. Eugene, Oregon, 2004, Feb 28

Vaile J. Effect of hydrotherapy on the signs and symptoms of delayed onset muscle soreness. Eur J Appl Physiol 2008 Mar; 102(4): 447–55

Van Rijn R. What is the clinical course of acute ankle sprains? A systematic literature review. American J Med, 2008; 121(4): 324–31

Vilelle L. Heal Thyself–With Help. Columbia Daily Tribune, June 16, 1999

Watkins A. Ice packs reduce postoperative midline pain and narcotic use: a randomized, controlled trial. J Am Coll Surg 2014 Sep; 219(3): 511–17

Winslow J. Treatment of lateral knee pain using soft tissue mobilization in 4 female triathletes. Int J of Ther Massage and Bodywork 2014; 7(3): 25–31

Recommended resources

Benjamin B. Listen to Your Pain: The Active Person's Guide to Understanding, Identifying, and Treating Pain and Injury. New York: Penguin Books, 2007

Buchman D. The Complete Book of Water Healing. New York: Instant Improvement, Inc., 1994

Hauser H. Prolo Your Pain Away: Curing Chronic Pain with Prolotherapy, 4th ed. Oak Park, IL Illinois: Beulah Land Press, 2017

Mole T. Cold forced open-water swimming: a natural intervention to improve postoperative pain and mobilization outcomes? BMJ Case Reports, 2018

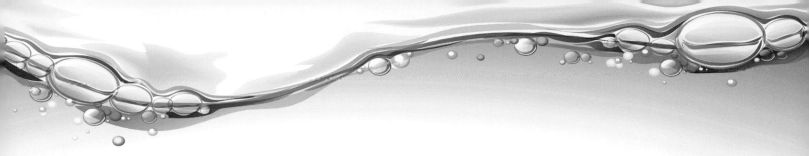

Hydrotherapy and massage for non-injury conditions 13

You know that not even a physician can claim that he heals you; he cannot heal the smallest cut on your finger, but your own body processes can. All you and I, or a physician, can do is to provide conditions or supplies that will assist the body to heal itself.

Jeanne Keller, *Healing with Water*

Once we have mastered the principles, mechanisms and procedures of the various hydrotherapy treatments, we will then attempt to integrate hydrotherapy into a comprehensive approach to a wide variety of medical conditions both acute and chronic.

Wade Boyle and André Saine, *Lectures in Naturopathic Hydrotherapy*

CHAPTER OBJECTIVES

After completing this chapter, the student will be able to:

1. Describe the most common types of chronic pain
2. Name at least one risk factor for developing osteoarthritis, diabetes, peripheral neuropathy and chronic venous insufficiency
3. Explain how either hot or cold applications can relieve pain
4. Explain the rationale for combining hydrotherapy treatments with bodywork for three non-painful presented conditions in this chapter
5. Describe hydrotherapy and massage combinations for three painful conditions discussed in this chapter
6. Describe cold treatments for pain, contracted tissue, and lymphatic congestion
7. Describe three uses for steam treatments mentioned in the chapter, and explain why they are effective.

In this final chapter you will learn about hydrotherapy treatments you can combine with bodywork to help clients with a variety of problems and conditions. Chronic musculoskeletal pain is surprisingly widespread, with arthritis, spine and back problems, and headaches at the top of the list (Hardt, 2008). Many of the other conditions discussed that do not involve pain such as asthma, constipation, depression, insomnia, psoriasis and terminal illness, are also hard on clients and challenging to treat: your hydrotherapy know-how will add another tool for these conditions.

HYDROTHERAPY AND PAIN

In both ancient and modern times, musculoskeletal pain has been a challenge and sometimes a great puzzle to healers. At least three quarters of elderly people report chronic pain that impacts their quality of life and ability to function normally. Osteoarthritis is their most common painful condition (Zhang, 2010). In 2008, 3 million Americans had gout, 5 million had fibromyalgia, roughly 7 million had carpal tunnel syndrome, and 27 million had osteoarthritis. In addition, in the three months leading up to the survey, 30 million people had neck pain and 59 million had low back pain (Lawrence, 2008). In 2016, an estimated 20% of US adults had chronic pain (they hurt most days) and 8% had high-impact chronic pain (that limited activities and work on most days) (Dahlhamer, 2016). According to physiatrist William Nagler, "The vast majority of all physicians are primary care doctors, and studies have shown that pain accounts for the majority of calls or visits to them. In fact, pain is the central element in most patient-physician interactions" (Goldberg, 1997). Although they often do not deal with what is causing the pain and have negative side-effects, pain medications are often the first strategy for patients rather than counseling, nutrition, physical therapy, massage or hydrotherapy. This has made them the single most prescribed type of medication in the US (Graedon, 2008). Since over half of all Americans take at least four medications regularly, dangerous interactions can also result.

Common medications for pain include:

1. Nonsteroidal anti-inflammatories such as ibuprofen, naproxen and celecoxib are used to reduce inflammation and mild-to-moderate pain. Prescription-strength NSAIDs are effective for relief of chronic musculoskeletal pain and inflammation in conditions such as rheumatoid arthritis (RA) or for short-term relief of minor aches and pains such as headache, toothache, backache, menstrual cramps, common cold, and muscular aches. High doses or long-term use of non-steroidal anti-inflammatory

medications can cause intestinal bleeding, heartburn, kidney failure, heart attack, ulcers, and stroke.

2. Opioid medications such as oxycodone, hydromorphone, oxycodone/acetaminophen and codeine were once used primarily for cancer patients suffering from severe pain, and for people who needed a strong pain medication for a few days after an injury or operation. However, because opioids were marketed as being safe for chronic pain, overconsumption of opioids and overdoses became epidemic throughout the USA. The pain medications triggered drowsiness, nausea, vomiting, constipation, addiction, and overdoses. From 1999 to 2017, almost 218,000 Americans died from overdoses related to prescription opioids, 72,000 Americans in 2017 alone (CDC, 2017).

In many studies, massage has reduced chronic pain for a wide variety of medical conditions and acute situations

---

BOX 13.1	POINT OF INTEREST

WATER MAKES AN IMPACT

Below are two hydrotherapy treatments that use the stimulating effect of water on the skin to alleviate chronic conditions. Sadly, because they require specialized equipment and (in the case of the continuous bath) extended periods of time, neither of these treatments is practical for today's massage therapist. Nevertheless, we can learn a valuable lesson from their use about how profoundly stimulation with water can affect the nervous system.

The continuous bath

This was an ingenious extension of the soothing and pain-relieving abilities of warm and neutral baths. The patient was placed on a hammock suspended in a bathtub and warm water ran over his or her body for hours at a time. Like the Trager Method, which employs gentle rocking, the soft feel of water running over the skin created a constant flow of relaxing nerve impulses and produced a calming effect. Continuous baths were once widely used to calm restless, agitated, or combative patients, to lower high blood pressure, to relieve the pain, spasm, burning sensation and tremors of Parkinson's disease, and to treat chronic

musculoskeletal pain. Massage was often given at the end of the bath. Continuous baths were safe and had virtually no contraindications.

The percussion douche

This is a spray of water at high pressure which is directed against some part of the body. A hot or cold spray blasting the skin has a very different effect than the gentle soothing impact of a continuous bath and was used for something quite different. A percussion douche stimulated the sympathetic nervous system, decreased local congestion, and relieved pain. It was widely used in the days of the water-cure to relieve symptoms of neuralgia, rheumatic joint pain, sciatica, chronic low back pain, and migraine headaches. For example, in treating sciatica, the high-pressure stream of water would spray from the foot up the leg, along the path of the sciatic nerve up to the lumbar area, and then back down to the heel again. For chronic low back pain, the spray would begin at the heel and move up the back of the leg to the lower back, middle back, upper back, and neck and back again. For extra stimulation, the client was sprayed with hot water followed by cold. Massage was often given after this procedure was finished (Thrash, 2015).

such as injuries, post-operative pain, and terminal illness. Tremendous suffering could be saved if massage were used as a first resort for pain (AMTA, 2018). Environmental pollution from the manufacture and use of pain medications is another large and growing problem which could also be avoided with non-drug therapies for pain (Sinclair, 2012).

Here are just a few examples where non-drug treatments could be tried as a first resort:

1. Repeated saunas decrease pain in patients with fibromyalgia (Masuda, 2005),

2. Fomentations applied on both the front and the back of a painful limb can reduce pain.

3. Ice massage can numb painful areas and relieve muscle spasm and sciatica pain.

4. Neutral baths are helpful for almost any condition that causes generalized pain, such as widespread arthritis, chronic low back pain, fibromyalgia, stroke, spastic cerebral palsy, spinal cord injury or post-polio pain.

5. Both Watsu sessions and warm water exercise benefit many painful chronic conditions by improving range of motion and soothing chronic tension.

6. Occupational therapy for **complex regional pain syndrome** helps to decrease pain and skin hypersensitivity through contrast baths that gradually increase the temperature difference between hot and cold; vigorous scrubbing with a brush; and tapping, massage, and vibration (Perez, 2010).

More research is badly needed on the use of these safe and effective ways to treat chronic pain and other non-injury-related conditions.

ADHESIVE CAPSULITIS OF THE SHOULDER JOINT (FROZEN SHOULDER)

This problem begins when a person avoids moving a painful shoulder. The original pain may have come from inflamed or torn rotator cuff muscles, bursitis, post-mastectomy pain, a shoulder fracture or dislocation, over-immobilizing a minor injury, a pinched cervical nerve, or even trigger points from a heart attack. Unfortunately, as when any joint is not moved, its surrounding muscles eventually weaken and the person moves it less and less. Eventually, adhesions develop as the superior part of the joint capsule shrinks and adheres to both the bicipital tendon and the head of the humerus. Ligaments may

shorten as well. The end result is greatly reduced range of motion and pain with either active or passive movement: even simple actions such as bathing and dressing may be excruciating.

The frozen shoulder can be reversed with careful rehabilitation – including bodywork, stretching and strengthening – but progress is slow and persistence is needed.

Deep friction, trigger point and myofascial release techniques are all helpful treatments for a frozen shoulder. First, however, adding deep heat from hot packs or mustard plasters before hands-on work helps the surrounding muscles relax and makes scar tissue easier to stretch. Ice massage helps by numbing the shoulder before gentle range of motion exercises are performed. As a home treatment, clients can use moist heat every day to speed healing.

TREATMENT

MOIST HEAT APPLICATION TO THE SHOULDER

Cross-reference

Chapter 4.

Duration and frequency

20 minutes. Perform during a massage session, or as a home treatment before stretching exercises, two or three times daily.

Special instructions

1. Hot compresses may be substituted for fomentations. A hydrocollator pack may be used on the top of the shoulder, but not on the underside: use a flat plastic hot water bottle instead.

2. It may be easier to drape your hot application around the shoulder with the client side-lying with the affected shoulder up. Use pillows as needed for comfort and to keep the cervical spine straight.

Procedure

1. Apply two fomentations, one on the underside of the arm and one on its top surface, so that the shoulder joint is sandwiched between them. Monitor carefully to avoid burning.

2. Wait 20 minutes, then remove fomentations and begin massage, range of motion exercises and stretching.

TREATMENT

MUSTARD PLASTER APPLICATION

Cross-reference

See Chapter 4.

Duration and frequency

20 minutes. Perform during a massage session, or as a home treatment before stretching exercises, two or three times daily.

Procedure

1. Apply the mustard plaster over the top of the shoulder joint and tuck it around to the back. Monitor carefully to avoid burning.

2. Wait 20 minutes, then remove the plaster and begin massage, range of motion exercises and stretching.

TREATMENT

ICE MASSAGE OR ICE PACK APPLICATION TO THE SHOULDER

Cross-reference

Chapter 5.

Duration and frequency

5–8 minutes for ice massage or 10 minutes for an ice pack. Perform during a massage session.

Procedure

1. Perform ice massage around the shoulder joint for 5–8 minutes or apply an ice pack for 10 minutes.

2. The client may now perform gentle range of motion exercises.

ARTHRITIS

Arthritis is the single most common cause of chronic pain. According to pharmacist Joel Graedon, author of *Best Choices from the People's Pharmacy*, "One in three adults is afflicted with some form of arthritis. If you think that's a lot of folks, you ain't seen nothing yet. Aging baby boomers are about to discover up close and personal what it's like to suffer from chronic inflammation" (Graedon, 2008). Many massage therapists will see clients with arthritis in their practices, and for this reason, gout, osteo- and rheumatoid arthritis are discussed at length in this section. Most clients will already have discovered that applications of hot water such as hot baths and showers are a great way to relieve their pain, and many use heating pads for this purpose as well.

Gout

This form of inflammatory arthritis develops in people who have high levels of uric acid in their blood. The acid can form needle-like crystals in a joint and cause sudden, severe episodes of pain, tenderness, redness, warmth and swelling. Acute gout happens when something (such as a night of drinking) causes uric acid levels to spike, or jostles the crystals that have formed in the knee, ankle, and big toe joints, causing swelling and excruciating pain (90% of sufferers are men). The sufferer's symptoms normally ease after a few days and will likely go away in a week to 10 days.

Standard medical treatment focuses on medications to treat pain and inflammation, dietary changes, weight loss and occasional aspiration of fluid from affected joints. (As explained in Box 11.2, if lead poisoning is a factor, repeated spa bathing is helpful.)

Hydrotherapy can help: either hot or cold applications may relieve pain, while contrast applications can relieve swelling. Since sometimes sufferers can't tolerate even the slight weight of a cloth on their skin, baths of water or paraffin are often the best treatment. Contrast baths may also force blood flow into less accessible, hard-to-reach joints and break up crystalline deposits of uric acid. Agatha Thrash, MD, used compresses or foot soaks containing charcoal for acute pain, plus a daily paraffin bath for maintenance. Massage is contraindicated for gouty areas, but, as always, is helpful for general relaxation. Acute attacks of gout are very painful, and a client who has suffered one may welcome relaxing touch.

TREATMENT

COLD APPLICATIONS
(COLD COMPRESS OR ICE PACK)

Cross-reference

See Chapter 5.

Duration and frequency

20 minutes. Apply during a massage session.

Procedure

1. Apply a cold wet compress or an ice pack covered with a thin cloth to the skin for 20 minutes.

TREATMENT

HOT FOOTBATH

Cross-reference

See Chapter 6.

Duration and frequency

20 minutes. Perform during a massage session.

Procedure

1. Rest the client's feet in the hot footbath while he is either seated or supine on the therapy table.

2. Massage of other parts of the body may proceed at this time.

3. After 20 minutes, remove the client's feet, dry them gently and continue massage.

TREATMENT

CONTRAST FOOTBATH

Cross-reference

See Chapter 6.

Duration

10 minutes. Anti-inflammatory oils and herbs are sometimes added to footbaths.

continued

TREATMENT *continued*

Procedure

1. Fill two deep buckets or washtubs with water, one at 110°F (43°C) and the other at 50°F (10°C).

2. Put both feet in the hot water for 3 minutes.

3. Put both feet in the cold water for 30 seconds.

4. Repeat steps 2 and 3 at least two more times, for a total of three rounds, or more if desired.

Osteoarthritis (OA)

The remedy of first choice for the pain and stiffness of both kinds of arthritis is castor oil packs. Castor oil provides stimulating warmth to the cold, over-mineralized joints of the osteoarthritis sufferer, but also has an anti-inflammatory and detoxifying effect for the swollen joints of the rheumatoid arthritis sufferer.

Thomas Cowan, *The Fourfold Path to Healing*

Osteoarthritis (also known as degenerative joint disease) is the most common form of arthritis. It affects the majority of people over 55 years old, and becomes even more common as people age (D'Ambrosia, 2005). The arthritic process begins when the cartilage covering joint surfaces begins to break down, and then rough bony surfaces rubbing together leads to stiff, painful, and hard-to-move joints (Figure 13.1A shows osteoarthritis of the hand). The most common joints to develop this condition are the hard-working finger joints and weight-bearing joints such as the spine, knee and hip. Factors that can contribute to the development of osteoarthritis include: tight, tense muscles which increase wear and tear on the joint; nutritional deficiencies; heredity; the aging process; chronically loose joints; heavy work; playing a sport that repeatedly stresses one particular joint; and, finally, traumatic injuries (Roach, 1994). As discussed in Chapter 12, poorly healed injuries such as cartilage tears, dislocations, and sprains which result in joint instability can lead to arthritis. Traumatic injuries are responsible for over 15% of all osteoarthritis of the hip, knee or ankle (Kujala, 1995; Brown, 2006). (Figure 13.1B shows osteoarthritis which developed one year after a traumatic injury.) Since extra pounds put more pressure on weight-bearing joints, being

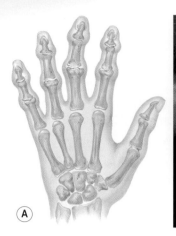

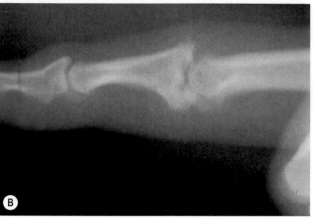

FIGURE 13.1
Osteoarthritis. (**A**) Osteoarthritis of the hand. Asset provided by Anatomical Chart Co. (**B**) Osteoarthritis caused by injury. One year after a traumatic injury, significant osteoarthritis has developed in the middle phalanx of this index finger. Reprinted with permission from Strickland, JW, Graham, TJ. Master Techniques in Orthopedic Surgery: The Hand, 2nd edn. Philadelphia: Lippincott, Williams and Wilkins; 2005, Figure 5.5.

overweight is a definite risk factor. If a person already has arthritis, gaining more weight causes even more problems for his or her joints. Losing even a few pounds can go a long way toward reducing the pressure on the knees or other weight-bearing joints. A 10- to 15-pound (4–7kg) weight loss in obese young people can translate to a much lower risk of osteoarthritis later in their lives.

Chronic arthritis sufferers have stiff, painful joints, sometimes to the point of disability. For example, many older people with advanced arthritis are so stiff that they cannot get in or out of a bathtub and even walking is difficult and slow. Standard medical treatment for osteoarthritis includes medications to reduce pain and inflammation, weight loss, low-impact exercise to keep joints flexible without stressing them, and physical therapy. Joint replacement surgery is often a last resort, but after surgery a high proportion of sufferers still end up with a significantly painful joint (Beswick, 2012).

OA patients need to put their painful joint through its full range of motion at least three times a day. Those who cannot exercise due to muscle weakness or imbalance benefit from gentle movement therapies such as the Feldenkrais and Alexander techniques, warm water exercise, and soft tissue massage (Figure 13.2 shows arthritic hands surrounded by warmth). **Prolotherapy**, the injection of natural substances at the exact site of a ligament injury to repair damage, may also be an effective treatment for osteoarthritis.

Many patients with arthritis prefer to avoid medications and their many side-effects. According to

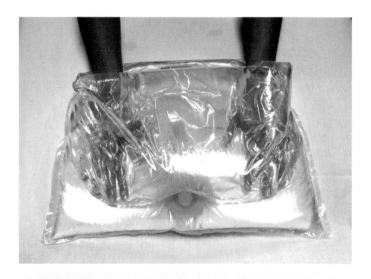

FIGURE 13.2
The warm water inside the water bottle completely surrounds the osteoarthritic hand and wrist joints. Photo courtesy of Fomentek Company, Fayetteville, AR.

pharmacist Joel Graedon, "We now know that most of the medications used for arthritis can have potentially serious side effects. We are caught in a classic double-bind. Without something to control inflammation, pain limits our activities which is not good for our health. Take the medicine, however, and we risk all sorts of complications, from high blood pressure to heart attacks and strokes. Some popular anti-inflammatory drugs may even make our arthritis worse" (Graedon, 2008). Many hydrotherapy treatments, such as warm baths, compresses and cold packs, give short-lived pain relief, but if they are performed regularly the pain relief can last much longer, especially when combined with bodywork. According to rheumatologist Kevin McKown, "I have patients who tell me that for short-term pain relief for their hands and feet, they prefer a paraffin bath to taking an anti-inflammatory pill such as ibuprofen. The heated wax eases stiff, achy joints by relaxing muscles and bringing blood to the area" (Renner, 1993).

Before a massage session, a hydrotherapy treatment will ready the person's tissues by increasing circulation, making tissue more stretchable, and relaxing the muscles. Applications of heat are particularly effective in relieving muscle spasm, although for some people cold works better. You and your clients may need to experiment with both heat and cold to find out which works better for them. Cold may be effective for clients who experience sharper and more penetrating pain, rather than the dull pain which is more common. Contrast treatments can temporarily relieve pain and increase joint flexibility. Massage techniques which address muscle tension and increase local circulation are very helpful for reducing the joint pain, stiffness, and restricted range of motion caused by osteoarthritis, especially if they incorporate active-isolated stretching (Perlman, 2006).

Whole-body treatments for osteoarthritis in multiple areas

For a client who has a great deal of pain, use 15–20 minute hot tub baths, saunas or steam baths followed by full body massage. A steam canopy can be a great help for clients who walk with difficulty and cannot get in and out of a bathtub. The client needs only to get on the table before the session begins, and can stay there until the end. At home, another option is for clients to use a shower bench or chair so they can take a long warm (not hot) shower. Any seat they use in the shower should be approved by the client's doctor or physical therapists to make sure it is safe.

Partial-body treatments for osteoarthritis in specific areas

Many hydrotherapy treatments may be applied to specific arthritic joints. Begin a course of treatment with three

sessions the first week, two sessions the second week, and one the third week. Then skip one week, do one session the following week, then skip two weeks and do one session the next week. Thus, you can gradually decrease the frequency to one session per month. As a follow-up between sessions, clients should take a daily hot shower for morning stiffness, take a hot sea salt bath two or three times a week, or, if they have access to a hot tub, take a 15–20 minute soak several times a week, and perform gentle exercises while in the warm water.

Partial-body treatments for osteoarthritis in specific areas

Many hydrotherapy treatments may be applied to just one specific arthritic joint. Hot applications are soothing, effective, and an excellent preparation for hands-on massage. A mustard plaster, for example, can be put on at the beginning of a session, and removed after 15–30 minutes to perform massage on that area. A paraffin bath may be used at the beginning of a session and the paraffin removed 20 minutes later, immediately before massaging the painful part. Hot packs of various types may be applied over joints for 20 minutes before massage. In many cultures, herbs with anti-inflammatory action, such as ginger, are added to water for compresses and other applications (Mashadhi, 2013). Cold applications may relieve sharp pain. Follow-up between sessions could include daily use of one of these treatments, along with gentle exercise. Here is a full list of treatments to try:

1. Mustard plaster over a joint (see Chapter 4).
2. Hands inside a flat plastic hot water bottle (see Chapter 4 and Figure 13.2).
3. Contrast bath of the joint, combined with gentle, non-painful movements (see Chapter 6).
4. Warm castor oil pack (see Chapter 4).
5. Hot compress to a painful joint, incorporating anti-inflammatory herbs such as ginger (see Chapter 4).
6. Moist heating pad over a joint (see Chapter 4).
7. Heat lamp over a joint (see Chapter 4).
8. Charcoal pack over a joint (see Chapter 4).
9. Paraffin bath for painful or stiff joints in the hands or feet (see Chapter 6).

Chapter thirteen

Rheumatoid arthritis

Rheumatoid arthritis (RA) is an autoimmune disease that primarily affects connective tissue. The synovial membranes that normally protect and lubricate joints become inflamed, leading to arthritis involving many joints, especially those of the hands and feet. Sufferers experience pain, swelling, and stiffness in these joints, as well as a loss of range of motion and, over time, deformity. Figure 13.3 shows the joints of one affected hand. Pronounced morning stiffness, fatigue and malaise are also common. Severe sensitivities to allergens such as corn and wheat may also affect the course of this disease. Standard medical treatment for rheumatoid arthritis usually consists of medications to relieve pain and swelling, physical therapy exercises to develop strength and joint mobility, medications which affect the immune system, and even corticosteroid injections. A last option is surgery to rebuild damaged tendons, remove portions of affected synovial membranes, or replace the entire joint. Many patients with RA prefer to avoid medications with their many side-effects, and regular hydrotherapy may help them do this. In one study, researchers found that sufferers who took saunas on a regular basis had less pain and easier movement (Oosterveld, 2009). Hot showers relieve morning stiffness, as do warm packs before exercising; while alternating heating pads and ice packs decreases inflammation and reduces pain. Since therapeutic massage also reduces pain and fatigue, the effect of combining them will be greater than either one alone (Field, 1997; Gok, 2016). For example, a massage therapist who has a sauna available could have her clients with RA use it before or after their massage session, and use contrast treatments during the session. However, when a client is in a flare, her joints will appear warm to the touch and red. **Do not massage or apply heat until the flare is over.**

Whole-body treatments for rheumatoid arthritis in multiple areas

For a client who has pain in more than one area of the body, a whole-body heating treatment can help relieve pain and prepare his or her tissues for massage. Simply help the client into a warm or hot tub bath, shower, sauna or steam bath: after 20 minutes help him or her out and onto the massage table, and begin bodywork. Or rotate a hot application from one area to another, leaving it on each area for 5–10 minutes. As a follow-up between sessions, clients may take a daily hot bath or shower and perform gentle exercises while in the water. For full instructions and contraindications for full-body heating treatments, see the sections on each in Chapters 6, 7 and 8.

Partial-body treatments for rheumatoid arthritis in specific areas

See *Partial-body treatments for osteoarthritis in specific areas* on page 317.

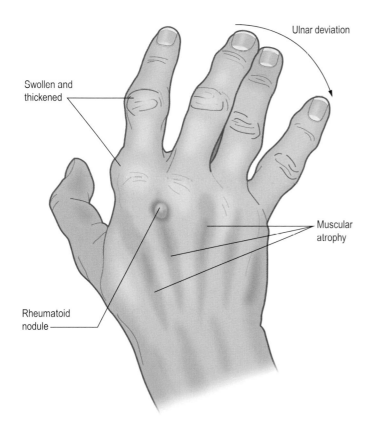

FIGURE 13.3
Rheumatoid arthritis.

Ulnar deviation

Swollen and thickened

Muscular atrophy

Rheumatoid nodule

ASTHMA

This chronic disease is an allergic disorder that can be compounded by emotional stress. It is so common that about 1 in 12 people in the US and EU have asthma (Global Asthma Network, 2018). Standard treatments for asthma consist of avoiding allergens, using inhaled corticosteroid and other medications, doing active breathing exercises, and improving general fitness. As discussed in the section on *Chronic tension in the respiratory muscles* (page 322), a variety of bodywork techniques can help free breathing by releasing emotional stress, relieving chest wall and neck stiffness, improving chest range of motion, and simply helping clients feel better (Field, 1998; Malinski, 1995; Sinclair, 2004; Witt, 1986). Using moist heat in various forms can add to these benefits by improving local circulation, deepening respiration, and warming and loosening trunk muscles. For example, first using moist heat to the trunk followed by a cold mitten friction starts the bodywork off with warmed tissues and a more relaxed, comfortable client (for instructions, see the contrast treatment on page 323). Breathing warm moist air in a steamy shower or steam bath, or even having your client inhale steam on the treatment table, can also be helpful. Not everyone with asthma will enjoy a steam room, so be sure to check in with your client first and never allow your clients to step into a cold draft when exiting a steam room. The combination of hot compresses made with ginger tea, followed by bodywork with massage oil containing ginger, is a traditional Chinese treatment for asthma (for instructions, see *Hot compresses* on page 98).

BELL'S PALSY

Viral meningitis or the herpes simplex virus can cause Bell's palsy, when inflammation puts pressure on the 7th cranial nerve. Then this condition comes on without warning and not only paralyzes the muscles on one side of the face, but causes dull head and neck pain. This condition can also be emotionally stressful because of how the face looks. Depending on how much the nerve is affected, the facial muscles usually recover their strength within one to two months, but sometimes the paralyzed muscles shorten instead, and contractures can develop.

Because most people heal on their own, mainstream treatment is often conservative, including watchful waiting, facial exercises, and sometimes steroid medication to control swelling. Because the client cannot move the muscles, massage is a great intervention which can help to keep facial muscles elastic, prevent contractures and stimulate local circulation. Hydrotherapy treatments will help your massage achieve its goals of relieving pain, easing tension, improving circulation and lessening stress. For example, heat to the face can ease tension and pain before massage: use hot compresses to the face or a castor oil pack. Or have your client take a shower before a session, letting the warm stream wash over the affected muscles, and massaging the scalp vigorously while shampooing the hair (all of these can also be used as home treatments). You can also use the contrast treatment in the section on chronic tension in the facial muscles in this chapter to stimulate the tissues and increase blood flow.

CANCER

Having cancer can be both emotionally and physically stressful and clients can experience a wide variety of unpleasant symptoms. For example, when clients are taking chemotherapy they may experience skin problems, nausea, vomiting, fatigue, constipation, and edema; radiation treatment can cause burns and other skin issues; medical treatments may invasive and painful; and always there is fear of what will come next. It is no wonder if the cancer sufferer experiences anxiety, insomnia, a new, more negative body image, and often a sense of isolation. As massage therapists, our gentle and attentive hands do much to soothe aches and pains and ease stress. At Memorial Sloan-Kettering Cancer Center, 1290 cancer patients received bodywork over a three-year period, and it reduced their stress/anxiety, nausea, depression, pain and fatigue by about 50% (Cassileth, 2004). Patients also enjoy bodywork when it is given during an infusion of chemotherapy medication (Robison, 2016). Neutral and warm baths, warm footbaths, and warm compresses to the spine are also very effective (Patricolo, 2017; Jacobs, 2016; Yang, 2010). (For a real-life example of how much they helped a woman with cancer, see Case history 3.1.) It is important to get the doctor's go-ahead for any hydrotherapy treatment given to patients who are currently in treatment.

According to oncology massage expert Gail McDonald, if the client's cancer is years in the past and a clean bill of health has been given, the session can be approached in exactly the same manner as a client who has never had cancer (McDonald, 2014). Your medical history should be careful and thorough to rule out any long-lasting symptoms that might contraindicate a hydrotherapy treatment. Mild treatments such as warm compresses, floating in a warm pool, neutral baths, body wraps taken to a warm stage, and flat plastic water bottles with warm (not hot) water are suitable. As with bodywork, err on the side of caution until you see how your client responds. (See the section on *Peripheral neuropathy* (page 352) for hydrotherapy and massage for this chemotherapy-related condition.) Some practitioners have used heating treatments after chemotherapy to detoxify their clients, and although little research exists, one 2002 study found that people who had gone through a regimen of steam treatments decreased the levels of PCBs and pesticides in their bloodstreams (Fagan, 2002). Certainly, many clients with cancer will ask you about this. (See Chapter 11 for more on detoxification with whole-body heat.)

Safety note

During radiation treatment, the skin is more sensitive and should be treated with care. Rubbing or massaging the treated area is contraindicated, and you should also avoid extreme hot and cold temperatures to the skin such as heating pads, hot water bottles or ice packs.

CHRONIC TENSION IN SPECIFIC BODY AREAS

Helping clients release tension in areas that are chronically tense is one of the massage therapist's most helpful skills. Using hydrotherapy treatments before hands-on work helps release tension, making tissues more relaxed and pliable and more receptive to deeper work. Here we give three specific procedures for combining them with massage, but of course but there are many other areas of the body where these treatments can be effective.

Chronic tension in the facial muscles

It is a rare person who does not have chronic tension in his or her facial muscles. Emotional stress can play a big part, but so can many other issues in a person's life. Here are some examples:

- Tension in the forehead and around the eyes can come from eye muscle problems such as a "lazy eye"; many hours of looking at a computer, cell-phone, or book with small print; light sensitivity; or straining to see because of eye diseases or poorly prescribed or fitted lenses.

- Tension around the nose can begin with a broken nose or other facial trauma; chronic sinus problems; or exposure to nasal irritants such as polluted air or cigarette smoke.

- Tension in the mouth, jaw and throat muscles can originate with trauma to the mouth or teeth; painful dental work; poorly aligned teeth; swallowing difficulties such as sore throats; or overusing the voice.

Massage is an effective way to release tension in the facial muscles, and moist heat can soothe, relax and warm them beforehand. Simply help the client begin to relax on the table, apply the moist heat, massage another part of the client's body for some minutes, then remove the heat and begin massage. A hot towel cabinet which contains pre-warmed towels is very convenient for this treatment, but small, thin cloths cool off too fast to be effective. For an example of using moist heat and massage for tension in the facial muscles, see Case histories 13.1 and 13.4.

TREATMENT

MOIST HEAT ON THE FACIAL MUSCLES

Cross-reference

See Chapter 4.

Duration

10 minutes.

Caution

Facial skin is thinner than the skin on many other parts of the body, and should be monitored carefully for burning.

Procedure

1. Apply moist heat (hot water compresses, a warm gel pack over a moist washcloth, mini-fomentation) over the area for 2 minutes. Massage elsewhere on the client's body at this time.

continued

TREATMENT *continued*

2. Apply a new warm cloth and leave it on for 2 minutes.
3. Repeat steps 1 and 2, for a total of 8–10 minutes of heat over the area.
4. Apply a cloth wrung out in ice water or perform ice massage for 30 seconds.
5. Begin massage of the facial muscles.

Chronic tension in the abdominal muscles

Holding chronic tension in the abdominal muscles is very common. This habit can begin early in life: for example, one third to one half of those who have stress-related abdominal pain as children will continue to suffer with it when they are adults (Wasserman, 1988). It may begin with a physical trauma, such as being punched in the stomach or falling onto bicycle handlebars, with a painful digestive condition such as irritable bowel syndrome, or with restricting scar tissue after abdominal surgery.

Many clients who know they will benefit from hands-on work still feel quite tentative about being touched here. A few minutes of relaxing moist heat can remove superficial tension and give light sensory stimulation, and thus prepare them for touch in a vulnerable area. Here we use a moist heating pad because it drapes well over body curves and is lightweight, which generally feels more comfortable over the abdomen.

RELEASING MUSCLE TENSION WITH A SIMPLE TREATMENT **CASE HISTORY 13.1**

BACKGROUND

84-year-old Steve had had many major challenges in recent years. He was seriously injured in a motor vehicle accident, he underwent quadruple-bypass surgery, he began to suffer from macular degeneration, and then his wife passed away.

A whole-body Swedish massage session once every two weeks helped ease his many aches and pains, stimulate his circulation, and meet his need for touch. One particular issue was the eyestrain caused by his macular degeneration: Steve was now very light-sensitive and continually tensed his forehead, eye and neck muscles as he squinted and strained to see.

TREATMENT

First, the massage therapist closed the curtains in the therapy room to eliminate the outside light. With Steve's doctor's permission, she tried adding moist heat to Steve's massage session for the first time. Using a small towel soaked in hot water, she wrung it out and laid it gently over his eyes. Since elderly people have thinner skin and could be burned more easily, she checked with him to make sure the cloth was not too hot. She then proceeded to massage Steve's neck and shoulders while applying a new hot cloth every 2 minutes. Normally Steve enjoyed chatting with her during the entire session, but this time something different occurred. He stopped talking and settled down completely after only a minute or so, and after the fifth hot cloth was applied, he let out a deep sigh and said, "My eyes haven't felt this relaxed in years."

Two minutes later, the therapist removed the cloth, wrung out a washcloth in cold water and laid that over his eyes for 30 seconds, then gently dried the area. As she began to massage Steve's forehead and around his eyes, she could see that his skin was pink and could feel that the tissues under her fingers were warmer and more elastic than usual. The top layer of tension that normally required some minutes of massage to release had already gone.

DISCUSSION QUESTIONS

1. Name three reasons why the application of a cloth over the eyes was helpful.
2. Why did the therapist finish the session with a cold washcloth?

TREATMENT

MOIST HEATING PAD FOLLOWED BY MASSAGE

Cross-reference

Chapter 4.

Duration and frequency

10–20 minutes. Perform during a massage session.

Special instructions

A warm (not hot) gel pack wrapped in a moist cloth, or a castor oil pack, a hot compress or a flat plastic water bottle, may be substituted for the moist heating pad (shown later, in Figure 13.6). As a home treatment, a nightly castor oil pack may also be used.

Procedure

1. With the client supine, apply a moist heating pad on a medium setting while massaging another part of the body. Monitor carefully for burning.

2. After 10–20 minutes, remove the heat and begin massage of the abdomen.

Chronic tension in the respiratory muscles

Chronic respiratory problems such as asthma or emphysema can cause a great deal of tension in the muscles involved in breathing, including not only the diaphragm and intercostals, but the scalene, serratus anterior, pectorals, subclavius and thoracic erector spinae muscles. Even one episode of pneumonia can activate trigger points (Aftimos, 1989). Breathing may become chronically shallow, the chest cavity narrowed, the shoulders rounded, and the posture of the neck and upper back distorted. If accessory breathing muscles such as the scalenes are called into play, often the neck can also become stiff. In addition, struggling for breath during asthma attacks, truly a life-threatening situation, can be frightening and emotionally traumatic. Many bodywork techniques can release chronic tension, improve range of motion, and simply help clients feel more at ease (Field, 2002; Witt, 1986; Yilmaz, 2016). Using moist heat can improve the outcome by releasing tension and warming

and loosening both anterior and posterior trunk muscles. This is also an effective treatment for the discomfort of sprained or fractured ribs, sore tight muscles after repeated coughing, and arthritic pain in the upper and mid-back. Contrast treatments of the chest increase local circulation even further and have a more stimulating and less sedating quality. (If you don't have all the items needed for this treatment, a simple steam inhalation on the table can loosen and warms the chest from within.)

TREATMENT

HEAT TO THE CHEST AND UPPER BACK, FOLLOWED BY MASSAGE

Cross-reference

Chapter 4.

Duration and frequency

20 minutes. Perform during a massage session.

Special instructions

1. A warm (not hot) gel pack wrapped in a moist cloth, or a flat plastic hot water bottle, may be substituted for the moist heating pad.

2. Monitor the client carefully for overheating, since a large portion of the body is being warmed.

3. Have the client drink a glass of water since he or she will be sweating.

4. In many cultures, compresses made with vasodilating herbs such as ginger are traditional for chest conditions (Mashadhi, 2013).

Procedure

1. First place a warm flat plastic water bottle on the table and cover it with a cloth, then have the client lie supine so the upper and middle back are being warmed.

2. Next apply a heating pad, hot compress, fomentation, mustard plaster or hot silica gel pack to the chest.

3. Massage another part of the body for 10 minutes; monitor carefully for burning or overheating.

continued

TREATMENT *continued*

4. Remove the heat on the chest and massage that area for 10 minutes (the client still has heat on the back at this stage).

5. Have the client sit up while you remove the warm water bottle, and then turn over so you can massage his or her back.

TREATMENT

CONTRAST TREATMENT OF THE CHEST AND UPPER BACK

Cross-reference

See Chapters 5 and 10.

Duration and frequency

10 minutes. Perform before or during a massage session.

Caution

Clients should never become chilled during or after this treatment.

Procedure

1. Place a flat plastic hot water bottle on the massage table, cover it with a cloth, and have the client lie in the supine position so that the heat is directly on the upper and middle back.

2. Place a fomentation or hydrocollator pack on the chest.

3. After 3 minutes, remove the hydrocollator pack and give a 30-minute cold mitten friction.

4. Repeat steps 1 and 2 twice, for a total of three rounds of hot followed by cold.

5. Have the client sit up and give a 30-second cold mitten friction to the middle and upper back.

6. Remove the flat plastic hot water bottle from the massage table.

7. Begin massage of the chest and upper back.

CHRONIC VENOUS INSUFFICIENCY (CVI)

CVI is a chronic condition that is most common in people aged 50 or older. Obesity, lack of exercise, leg trauma, smoking, and being female all increase the risk of having CVI. When blood doesn't flow back to the heart properly, it pools in the leg veins and the client's legs begin to look puffy and brownish. The condition is most commonly caused when valves in the veins have been stretched by previous blood clots or when the valves themselves are impaired: in both cases, blood leaks back through the damaged valves. Weakness in the leg muscles that squeeze blood forward, or standing for long periods of time, can also contribute to CVI. Sufferers often have leg discomfort, pain, numbness, tingling, a heavy sensation or cramps; even more serious, the pooling of blood may make them more vulnerable to foot or leg ulcers. (As with diabetes, ulcers can be dangerous sites of infections that can harm the extremity or spread through the body.) This condition needs to be managed on an ongoing basis, most often with active exercise, wearing compression stockings, elevating the legs often, and manual lymphatic drainage. Lifestyle changes are also very important in this condition, including losing weight, getting more exercise, and stopping smoking. Herbal preparations and nutrients are sometimes used to strengthen capillaries.

Regular bodywork and hydrotherapy can improve the picture and can help prevent foot or leg ulcers (Carpentier, 2014). Manual lymph drainage is an effective therapy that can decrease foot and lower limb swelling, while gentle circulatory massage on intact skin can be performed around varicose veins to stimulate blood flow (Molski, 2013). Any thermal stimulation— such as contrast footbaths or sprays—is a good pre-massage therapy, and one that clients can also perform at home. The anti-inflammatory leg wrap that follows can be easily incorporated into a session (see Figure 13.4). Neutral baths also help improve venous flow, most likely due to hydrostatic pressure. In 2014, an intense three-week spa regimen for patients with CVI included hands-on leg massage, underwater lymphatic massage, pool-walking and whirlpool baths. This regimen reduced discomfort, tingling/numbness and leg edema, and the therapeutic effect lasted at least one year (Forestier, 2014).

TREATMENT

ANTI-INFLAMMATORY LEG WRAP

This wrap can be used for arthritic pain, chronically cold legs and feet, chronic venous insufficiency, passive swelling in the legs, and peripheral neuropathy.

Cross-reference

See Chapter 6 for the warm footbath, and Chapter 9 for the leg wraps.

Duration

Perform during a massage session.

Caution

This is a warm, not a hot, treatment.

Procedure

1. Layer the table with linens for a leg wrap (Figure 13.4A).

2. Warm the client's legs and feet with a warm, not hot, footbath while you mix the ingredients for the leg wrap solution: add 1½ cups of baking soda, ⅓ cup of lemon juice and ⅓ cup of aloe vera gel to 2¼ quarts of hot water. First mix the baking soda and aloe vera gel with one half of the hot water, stirring well to dissolve the soda completely. Next add the lemon juice and the remaining hot water, and stir again (Figure 13.4B).

3. Have the client lie on the treatment table and cover the pelvic area with a small hand towel. Wring out two large towels in the wrap water (Figure 13.4C).

4. Ask the client to roll onto one hip, then slide one hot towel under the other leg and center it so that the middle of the towel is directly under the back of the leg. Now have the client lie back on it, and wrap it snugly so that the entire leg and foot are entirely covered. Working quickly, repeat the process with the other leg (Figure 13.4D).

5. Cover the towels with the wool or polar fleece blankets, then the space blanket on top (Figure 13.4E).

6. Massage of the upper body can be done during the wrap (Figure 13.4F).

7. After 20–30 minutes, remove the blankets and towels and finish with a cold mitten friction.

8. Begin leg massage.

Constipation

Chronic constipation can result from a variety of medical conditions and habits, ranging from a sedentary lifestyle and constipating medications to chronic dehydration and a low-fiber diet. Clients who spend a great deal of time in bed or in a wheelchair often suffer from constipation. Massage therapists do not treat constipation as such, but it is often the case that abdominal massage has a stimulating effect on intestinal muscles (Sinclair, 2011). A drink of iced water and a contrast treatment before bodywork add stimulation as well. A nightly castor oil pack can be helpful at home.

TREATMENT

CONTRAST TREATMENT TO THE ABDOMEN

Cross-reference

See Chapters 4 and 10.

Duration and frequency

12 minutes. Perform before or during a massage session.

Procedure

1. Have the client drink a glass of very cold water.

2. Apply a moist heating pad, fomentation, castor oil pack, hot compress, warm gel pack wrapped in a moist cloth, or flat plastic hot water bottle over the abdomen. As a home treatment, a nightly castor oil pack may also be used.

3. After 3 minutes, remove the fomentation or compress and give a cold mitten friction for 30 seconds to the abdomen, using ice water if the client can tolerate it.

4. Repeat steps 2 and 3, for a total of three rounds of hot followed by cold.

5. Begin massage.

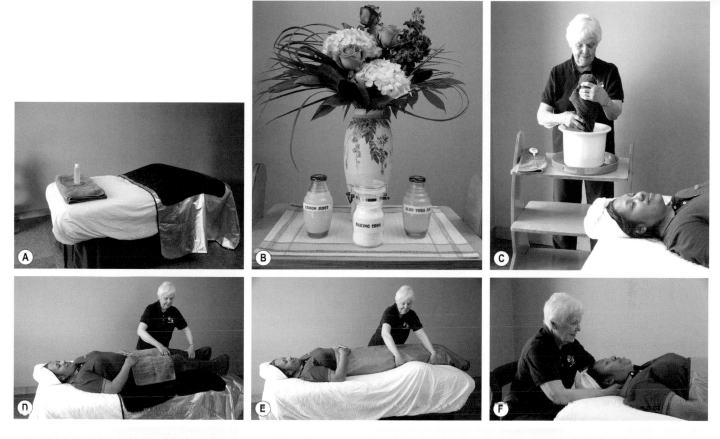

FIGURE 13.4
Anti-inflammatory leg wrap. (**A**) The leg wrap set up. (**B**) Ingredients for the wrap solution. (**C**) Wringing out a leg towel.
(**D**) The legs covered with warm towels. (**E**) The blankets are tucked in so no heat will escape. (**F**) Massage while the legs are absorbing the wrap solution.

DEPRESSION

Those who have this debilitating mood disorder suffer from feelings of hopelessness, sadness, loneliness, despair, low self-esteem, low energy and social isolation. A sizeable percentage of depressed people also complain of physical ailments that are caused by their depression. The mainstream treatment for this condition is antidepressant medication, but it does not always work well and some people cannot tolerate its side-effects.

In 2010, a review of 17 studies on massage for depression confirmed that massage has a powerful positive effect on mood and anxiety and is an excellent complement to other treatments for this difficult problem (Hou, 2010). Some hydrotherapy treatments can also be part of a total program to combat depression, and have been used for centuries. An intense contrast shower is so invigorating and antidepressant that it is an integral part of an all-natural program designed by Neil Nedley, MD; he recommends three showers a day at first (Nedley, 2002). Hot saunas followed by cold dips have the same effect. Molecular biologist Nikolai Shevchuk has proposed a study of using cold exposure therapies as the main treatment for depression, since the simultaneous firing of all our skin's cold receptors at once stimulates the production of noradrenaline and beta-endorphin. He calls for this strategy to be tested by trying a series of daily contrast showers which end with a 2–3 minute cold shower: these should be continued for several weeks or even several months (Shevchuk, 2008). Whole-body heating treatments also help some depressed people: a 2018 *Psychiatric News* article reviewed heat treatment studies which have shown promise for depression, including hot yoga, hot baths and saunas (Karel, 2018). How might this fit into your work with depressed clients? A massage combined with a heat treatment and a brief cold exposure might just double the effect of massage alone.

DIABETES

This common and often devastating metabolic disorder has many complications. For example, damage to blood vessels can lead to kidney disease, peripheral neuropathy, chronic venous insufficiency, depression, and infected foot ulcers which may progress to amputation. Because rates of diabetes in the Western world are rising quickly, it is likely that every massage therapist will be treating clients with this disorder. Many factors have contributed to its increase, including unhealthy diets, a rise in rates of obesity, smoking, sedentary lifestyles, and normal aging. There is also a strong link between air pollution and diabetes (Yang et al., 2020). Today, however, a healthy diet and lifestyle can prevent many of the worst effects of diabetes. Since not everyone has well-controlled blood sugar, diabetics should always receive a doctor's approval before beginning massage and hydrotherapy. Massage can be helpful on two fronts: first, bodywork can improve blood circulation; second, because high stress levels (common in a chronic disease such as diabetes) tend to increase blood sugar to unhealthy levels, massage can have a normalizing effect on blood sugar levels (Thrash, 2015).

Russian medical massage teacher Zhenya Kurashova Wine recommended a massage program for diabetic circulation issues. It began with 30 minutes twice a week for five weeks, and then a maintenance dose of once every two weeks. Her technique consisted of gentle gliding effleurage towards the heart, first in the prone position, stroking the back, then from the thigh upwards to the low back, from the neck downwards, and then finally up the calves. Then the client turned over and the same stroking was done up the front of the leg and arms. Massage was also helpful for scar tissue at frequent insulin injection sites: thickened tissues severely limited mobility, but friction and scar release techniques could help restore it (Wine, 1996).

Hydrotherapy treatments such as neutral baths, salt glows, body wraps, heat-trapping compresses and cold mitten frictions help to promote good circulation and relaxation, just as massage does, so combining them is a natural. Contrast hand or footbaths using warm – *not* hot – water helps to increase circulation without extremes, although the improvement in blood flow will be less dramatic than that in clients without diabetes. Be especially careful to avoid treating limbs with skin wounds unless you have special training in this area and a doctor's approval – these are notoriously slow to heal in diabetics. All these treatments may be performed before or during massage sessions.

Always use mild temperatures, since clients may have less feeling in the hands and feet, and may not be able to tell if water is hot enough to burn. Never give a footbath hotter than 102°F (39°C), and do not apply heat to the feet with heating pads, hot water bottles, heat lamps, fomentations, hydrocollator packs, or even paraffin dips. Steam cabinets of the type where the client is sitting and steam comes up from the bottom of the cabinet should also be avoided. During your initial history-taking, be sure to ask the client how he or she responds to heat, including hot showers or baths. If the client dislikes being warm, this is even more of a reason to avoid heating applications. Endocrinologist and diabetes researcher Phil Hooper conducted a small study of the safety of hot tubs for diabetics and concluded that regular hot tubs at no more than 102°F (39°C) can be beneficial, in part because blood flow to extremities is stimulated (Hooper, 1999; Hooper, 2006). Non-thermal treatments include a daily dry skin brushing or salt glow before a shower, and charcoal packs or baths. For information on treating diabetic complications, see the sections on *Amputations* (page 274), *Chronic venous insufficiency* (page 323), *Depression* (page 325), and *Peripheral neuropathy* (page 352).

DRY SKIN

There are many hydrotherapy treatments that effectively treat dry skin; below are just a few traditional ones you can use before a massage. Massage itself is an excellent treatment for dry skin: not only does it apply massage creams and oils to the skin, but it also stimulates the sebaceous glands.

Whole-body treatments for dry skin

TREATMENT

WHOLE-BODY OIL APPLICATION AFTER A WARM OR HOT SHOWER

Cross-reference

See Chapter 8.

Duration and frequency

5–10 minutes. Perform before or after a massage, and as a daily home treatment.

Procedure

1. Have the client take a warm or hot shower.

2. After the shower, when the client's skin will have absorbed some moisture and is still wet, put five drops of vegetable oil on the palms, and rub them over the entire skin surface, so that the oil is mixed in with the water on the skin.

3. Now dry off: this leaves a very fine film of vegetable oil on the skin.

TREATMENT

WHOLE-BODY HONEY WRAP

Cross-reference

See Chapter 10.

Duration and frequency

20 minutes. Perform before a massage session.

Special instructions

This treatment is a great deal easier to perform using a wet room table.

continued

TREATMENT *continued*

Caution

Contraindicated for diabetics.

Procedure

1. Have the client take a short shower, sauna, or steam bath and blot the skin so it is mostly dry, and then lie down on a wet table (or a regular treatment table covered with towels).

2. Pour one quarter of a cup (60ml) of warmed honey onto your hands and apply it onto the client's still-moist skin, or mix the honey with one quarter of a cup (60 mL) of water and paint it onto the client's body. If honey is applied to the feet, they need to be carefully encased in plastic bags so that the client does not track honey anywhere.

3. Wrap the patient in a dry sheet and send her into a steam bath or sauna for 15 minutes. (A steam canopy can be used, in which case the client remains on the towel-covered table.) After that time, the honey should be completely absorbed into the skin: if it is not, have the client shower before you begin massage.

TREATMENT

WHOLE-BODY HONEY SALT GLOW

Cross-reference

See Chapter 10, Honey–Epsom salts glow in a shower.

Simply mix half honey and half Epsom salts in a non-breakable container, and have the client step into a shower stall and give herself a salt glow with this mixture. The honey should be thoroughly washed off before you begin massage.

TREATMENT

MOISTURIZING WRAP WITH SHEA BUTTER OR A THICK OIL (SUCH AS WHEAT GERM OIL)

Cross-reference

See Chapter 9.

continued

TREATMENT *continued*

Duration and frequency

20 minutes. Perform before a massage session.

Procedure

1. Apply a liberal amount of warmed shea butter or thick oil to the skin and gently massage it in.
2. Using a dry sheet, wrap the client as for a full-body wrap.
3. Wait 20 minutes, during which time the head and neck may be massaged.
4. Unwrap the client and proceed with massage on the rest of the body. The shea butter or thick oil should be sufficient for massage; if not, simply add more.

Partial-body treatments for dry skin

Dry skin on the feet and hands can benefit greatly from applications of paraffin or honey before massage. However, do not risk infection by massaging skin that is so dry and cracked that it is open. Paraffin or honey wraps may be given to the hands or feet, even if you don't massage them during the session. An elderly client with arthritic hands and dry skin will love them.

TREATMENT

PARAFFIN APPLICATIONS ON THE HANDS AND FEET

Cross-reference

See Chapter 6.

Duration and frequency

10–20 minutes. Perform before a massage session or as a daily home treatment.

continued

TREATMENT *continued*

Procedure

1. Briefly soak the client's hands or feet in warm water to cleanse and warm them.
2. Apply a thick layer of emollient cream on the client's hands or feet.
3. Dip the hands or feet in paraffin, wrap them in a plastic bag, and then wrap them in a cloth covering (such as terrycloth gloves for the hands or socks for the feet).
4. After 10–20 minutes, remove the coverings and paraffin and begin massage.

TREATMENT

LOCAL HONEY WRAP

Cross-reference

See the *Whole-body honey wrap* treatment on page 326.

Duration and frequency

10 minutes. Perform before a massage session or as a daily home treatment.

Special instructions

Have a container of warm water available to cleanse your hands of sticky honey, so that it does not get spread around your office!

Procedure

1. Briefly soak the client's hands or feet in warm water to cleanse and warm them.
2. Pour about 2 tablespoons of warmed honey onto your hands and apply it onto the client's still-moist hands or feet, then clean and dry your hands.
3. Wrap the client's hands or feet in plastic bags and a towel.
4. After 10 minutes, remove the towel and clean off the honey with warm wet towels or a brief warm soak.
5. Dry the hands or feet and begin massage.

ECZEMA

Eczema is a generic term for a number of non-contagious, inflammatory skin conditions which may also feature rashes. It is very common and probably related to an overactive immune response to irritating substances. For many years, physicians have observed that emotional stress can contribute to outbreaks of eczema, even in infancy (Rosenthal, 1952). Mainstream medical treatment consists of topical steroid creams and ointments, ultraviolet light therapy, and lifestyle advice. Eczema is often improved by avoiding irritating substances, taking supplements with essential fatty acids, reducing stress, and taking baths with soothing substances. An oatmeal or baking soda bath before a session can soothe and relax the client–but water should not be too hot, and the client should moisturize afterwards. Massage is contraindicated over areas that are red, warm, itchy, puffy, open, or contain blisters, but in other areas of the body it may help the client deal with stress.

TREATMENT

OATMEAL BATH

Cross-reference

See Chapter 6.

Duration and frequency

20 minutes. Perform before or after a massage session. As a home treatment during a flare-up, clients may take oatmeal baths two or three times every day.

Procedure

1. Add oatmeal to the bathwater as the tub begins to fill. Essential oils or herbs appropriate for relaxation can be added as well.
2. Have the client remain in the tub for 20 minutes, then pat the skin dry gently, leaving some of the oat solution on the skin.

TREATMENT

SODIUM BICARBONATE OR BAKING SODA BATH

Cross-reference

See Chapter 6.

Duration and frequency

20 minutes. Perform before or after a massage session. As a home treatment during a flare-up, may be used two or three times daily.

Procedure

1. Add baking soda to bathwater while the tub is filling.
2. Have the client remain in the tub for 20 minutes, then wash all of the soda solution off the skin.

FIBROMYALGIA (FMS)

While achieving high-quality evidence based conclusions is difficult for complex natural therapies such as spa therapy, the existing evidence indicates a positive effect in management of FMS. Whether pain relief is from minerals in the water, hydrostatic pressure or water temperature, or some combination, is unknown … In view of the long history of this modality in the management of pain as well as the inherent difficulties related to use of medications, spa therapy should be recognized as part of a therapeutic program for fibromyalgia.

Fusun Ardic, MD, rheumatologist (Ardic, 2007)

This disorder primarily affects women. Sufferers experience chronic pain, stiffness after rest, low pain tolerance, sensitivity to cold, non-restful sleep, constipation and chronic fatigue. Although its exact cause is unknown, fibromyalgia triggers include physical trauma, depression, magnesium deficiency and viral infections such as the flu. Obesity is also a major risk factor. Standard medical treatment consists of regular physical therapy (stretching and strengthening), medication to improve sleep and reduce pain, and emotional support.

Massage therapy is deeply soothing and pain-relieving and it improves sleep. After receiving massage twice weekly for five weeks, fibromyalgia patients experienced improved mood and sleep along with less tender points, compared to a group receiving relaxation therapy and no massage (Field, 2002). Other studies have found similar results (Harty, 2012). Much research has shown that hydrotherapy is also an effective treatment for fibromyalgia. It can help sufferers feel better and move more comfortably during the day. Hot baths and showers are helpful for morning stiffness and pain; saunas are pain-relieving; and pool therapy can improve muscle function and decrease pain and fatigue. Repeated studies have shown that fibromyalgia sufferers have less pain, less inflammation and less tender points when they are on a regimen of regular mineral water baths for at least three weeks. One study examined the effects of 12 weeks of thermal therapy (sauna and exercising in a heated pool), and between one third and three quarters of the patients reported significant decreases in pain (Ardic, 2007; Evcik, 2002; Matsumoto, 2011). You can combine these two modalities to improve treatment outcomes: during a massage session, moist heat applications such as hydrocollator packs or fomentations can help relieve pain and encourage relaxation, and ice stroking may be used to deactivate trigger points (see page 132 for directions). Clients can use many hydrotherapy treatments at home to make faster progress. Since too much or too deep massage can cause a flare-up of pain, it must be carefully adjusted to how much a client with fibromyalgia can tolerate.

FOOT DEFORMITIES: BUNIONS AND HAMMERTOES

Bunions and hammertoes may seem minor to some, but they can be painful enough to limit walking, cause lameness and postural compensations, and contribute to arthritis.

Bunions

This painful distortion of the foot may begin with very high arches, footwear that squeezes the toes, overpronation, and tension in the muscles of the feet and calves.

High heels are particularly bad for the feet, and perhaps it is no accident that 90% of those with bunions are women. Physical therapy may include toe muscle strengthening and stretching, and orthotics are sometimes used to redistribute body weight and to take pressure off the bunion. Surgery is a last resort if the bunion is extremely painful or if the big toe joint has become arthritic. Some gentle non-invasive strategies that may be used include range of motion exercises and active isolated stretching of the toe, foot and calf muscles. Gentle massage, especially directed to the intrinsic foot muscles and calves, will not reverse a bunion but it will reduce pain. Structural bodywork can address issues of fascial restriction and compensations throughout the entire body that are worsening the bunion. This type of therapy may be uncomfortable, and a paraffin dip or a 20-minute hot foot soak before massage can make stretching and bodywork more tolerable (as a home treatment, clients can do this before stretching). When a bunion is acutely inflamed, ice packs or cold foot soaks can reduce swelling, but once the inflammation has come down, contrast foot soaks are preferable.

Hammertoes

This painful foot distortion is more common in people who have a long second toe– especially if that toe was once broken– and a fallen anterior metatarsal arch. It generally begins when both distal toe flexors and proximal toe extensors are contracted and connective tissues shorten and thicken around them. Footwear that causes the toe to curl forward then exacerbates the problem. Physical therapy may include exercises such as walking on tiptoes to encourage toes to bend and straighten, and stretching the toe tendons and calf muscles. Physicians may prescribe steroid medications, while surgery to move tendons or fuse bones is a last resort.

Bodywork may have little effect if the client's hammertoe is rigid. However, if it is still malleable, massage of the short muscles and tendons of each affected toe joint and of the calf muscles can help to restore the normal balance of tendons and muscles, slow progression, and ease discomfort. This type of therapy might be uncomfortable and a pre-massage paraffin dip or hot foot soak will make stretching and bodywork more tolerable. As a home treatment, clients can do this before stretching. If the hammertoe is acutely inflamed, especially after walking or running, ice packs or cold foot soaks can reduce swelling and inflammation, but once the inflammation has come down, contrast foot soaks are preferable.

HEADACHES
Migraine headache

This headache occurs on one side of the head only and usually includes vertigo, nausea, light sensitivity, and visual changes such as seeing flashing lights. Migraines generally last from 4 to 72 hours, and can be both excruciating and disabling. The exact chain of events that cause them is still unclear, but early in the process there is a strong constriction of brain blood vessels on the affected side of the head. The client may have blurred vision or other sensations that warn that a migraine is starting. That phase ends after 2–4 hours and then the blood vessels dilate strongly. Because the brain cannot expand beyond the cranial bones, the extra blood in the dilated blood vessels puts increased pressure on the structures of the brain itself. This is what causes not only the pain but also the neurological symptoms.

There are many migraine triggers, including cranial bone distortions and trigger points in the temporalis, occipitalis, sternocleidomastoid and posterior cervical muscles (Nerman, 2014). Other triggers include emotional stress, dehydration, magnesium deficiency, fluorescent lights, glare from computer screens, food allergies, altitude changes, fatigue, fluctuations in hormone levels related to menstruation, and low blood sugar. Not all triggers will cause a migraine each time, and sometimes it takes multiple triggers to start one. Before they can confirm that the condition is indeed migraine, doctors must rule out brain tumors, hemangiomas, carotid aneurysms, Ménière's disease, and seizures. The standard medical treatment consists mainly of medication and avoiding of aggravating foods. (If used on a regular basis, many pain-relieving drugs can paradoxically *cause* headaches, in essence converting sporadic migraines to a chronic situation.)

Although it is unlikely that a client will seek out a massage therapist for treatment of a migraine headache, sometimes it happens that a client walks into your office with this complaint. In this case, the classic hydrotherapy treatment for a migraine headache is a hot foot bath, and that can be done during a session. When the feet are immersed in hot water, the blood vessels of the feet dilate and blood flow into congested areas is reduced. The hands may be immersed in hot water at the same time. An ice pack on the back of the neck will stimulate constriction of blood vessels to the brain. (*Do not apply heat to the head* – a client of the author's, who had migraines for thirty years, tried this once and ended up with the most painful and longest-lasting migraine of her life!) In 2006, a head wrap with pockets for frozen gel packs and snug enough to apply pressure to the head was studied: within 25 minutes, it lessened migraine pain by about one third. Combining the wrap with bodywork would give even greater relief (Ucler, 2006). Over time, migraine sufferers have figured out many other ingenious ways to treat migraines with derivation, such as:

1. Taking very hot and very cold contrast showers
2. Taking a hot shower (which causes dilation of capillaries) while rubbing the head with an ice cup (which causes vasoconstriction) or wearing a towel wrapped tightly around the head (which compresses blood vessels)
3. Keeping ice chips at the back of the throat while taking a hot bath
4. Using chilled objects such as stones or gel packs on the head, along with hot compresses on the feet
5. Learning how to dilate the blood vessels in the hands and feet with biofeedback (Rice, 2007).

Some therapists have reported success in relieving migraine headaches with bodywork such as cranial therapy or trigger point treatment, but the longer the migraine has gone on, the less likely it is that bodywork alone will help. The author has had the greatest success in treating full-blown migraines by combining massage with heat to the feet and cold to the head.

All hydrotherapy treatments are more effective at the outset and should be started as soon as possible.

TREATMENT

APPLICATION OF COLD GEL PACKS TO THE HEAD

Cross-reference

See Chapter 5 for the effects of cold.

Duration and frequency

30 minutes or more. Apply the cold gel cap at the first sign of a migraine, or, if the client arrives with one, put it on immediately.

Procedure

1. Apply a cold gel cap by pulling a tension strap and securing it around the client's head, then inserting frozen gel packs into its pockets. Do not put them on the scalp without the wrap, in order to prevent frostbite. You can also use iced compresses or cold (not frozen) gel packs on the skin.
2. Begin massage.
3. After about 30 minutes, remove the cold application and continue massage.

TREATMENT

APPLICATION OF COLD RUNNING WATER TO THE BACK OF THE NECK AND SCALP

Cross-reference

See Chapter 5 for the effects of cold.

Duration and frequency

3 minutes. Perform at the beginning of a massage session; or, as a home treatment, at the first sign of a headache.

Procedure

1. Run tepid water in the sink and have the client place her head under the faucet, being careful to keep the nostrils out of the water so she can still breathe comfortably. Wrap a towel around her to catch drops.

continued

TREATMENT *continued*

2. Gradually make the water as cold as possible, then let the cold water run over the back of the client's head, with as much force as tolerable, for 3 minutes.
3. Dry the client's hair briskly.
4. Begin massage.

TREATMENT

HOT FOOTBATH COMBINED WITH ICE PACK ON THE BACK OF THE NECK

Cross-reference

See Chapters 5 and 6.

Duration and frequency

20 minutes. Perform before or during a massage session.

Special instructions

1. The hot water in the footbath must be kept at 110°F (43°C) for the entire treatment. This means that more hot water must be added as the water cools. The fresh hot water should be added carefully so that it is not poured directly on the client's feet.
2. The footbath may be given with the client in the supine position on the massage table.
3. Massage can be given on other areas of the body during the footbath, and then massage can be given directly to the head and upper body during the rest period afterwards.

Procedure

1. Give the client a hot footbath combined with a cold compress to the forehead and an ice pack to the back of the neck. If desired, add 1 tablespoon of mustard powder per 1–2 gallons (4–8 liters) of water.

continued

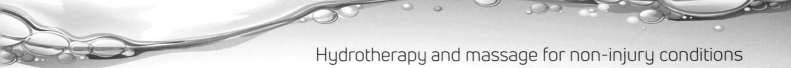

TREATMENT *continued*

2. Change the cold compress every 3 minutes. Another cold compress or cold gel pack may also be placed on the top of the client's head.

3. After 20 minutes, remove both the cold compress and the ice pack from the back of the neck.

4. Pour cold water over the client's feet, dry them off, and then have him lie down and rest for 20 minutes. Massage to the head and neck may begin.

TREATMENT

HOT FOOTBATH COMBINED WITH CONTRAST TREATMENT FOR THE HEAD AND CERVICAL SPINE

Cross-reference

See Chapters 4, 5 and 6.

Duration and frequency

20 minutes. Perform before or during a massage session.

Procedure

1. Give the client a 20-minute hot footbath at 110°F (43°C). See step 1 of the previous hot footbath treatment for further details.

2. Once the client's feet are in the footbath, apply a hot water bottle or hot compress or hot miniature fomentation to the base of the neck and the cervical spine, and at the same time apply ice water compresses or cold gel packs to the upper face (on the forehead, and over the eyes, temples and ears).

3. Wait 3 minutes, then switch the hot and cold applications on the head, so that now you apply ice water compresses on the base of the neck and cervical spine, and hot water compresses to the face, temples, ears and forehead.

4. After 3 minutes, repeat steps 2 and 3 twice more, for a total of three rounds.

continued

TREATMENT *continued*

5. Remove all hot and cold applications from the head.

6. Remove the client's feet from the hot foot soak and dry them well.

7. Begin massage.

TREATMENT

LEG WRAP

Cross-reference

See Chapter 9.

Duration and frequency

15–20 minutes Perform before or during a massage session.

Special instructions

This should be done as soon as possible after the client senses the beginning of a migraine. If desired, you can use a heat lamp to the legs instead of the leg wrap.

Procedure

Follow directions for the *Leg wrap* on page 221 (additives are optional in this case), but add an ice pack on the back of the neck. You may proceed with massage on other areas during the wrap.

Muscle contraction headache

This annoying headache is caused by muscle tightness and/or active trigger points in the face, head, neck or upper back. Tension in the neck and shoulder muscles can have many causes, including eyestrain, poorly aligned teeth or cranial bones, jaw clenching, repetitive strain, poorly healed neck and back injuries, poor posture, and emotional stress. Massage techniques to relieve muscle tension are generally very effective for muscle contraction headaches, and will be more effective if the client is already relaxed and the circulation to neck and shoulder muscles has been increased. In addition, hydrotherapy treatments that are soothing may address the stress component of the "tension" headache.

TREATMENT

APPLICATION OF COLD RUNNING WATER TO THE BACK OF THE NECK AND SCALP

Procedure

Proceed exactly as directed in the previous section, on migraine headache.

TREATMENT

ICE PACK APPLICATION

Cross-reference

See Chapter 5.

Duration and frequency

15 minutes. Perform during a massage session; or, as a home treatment, at the beginning of a headache.

Procedure

1. Apply an ice pack on the back of the client's neck and massage related areas.
2. After 15 minutes, remove the ice pack and begin massage.

TREATMENT

MOIST HEAT APPLICATION

Cross-reference

See Chapter 4.

Duration and frequency

15 minutes. Perform before or during a massage session. A hot shower to the upper body may be substituted.

continued

TREATMENT *continued*

Procedure

1. Place a hot water bottle, moist heating pad, hot gel pad, fomentation or hydrocollator pack on the upper back and neck for 15 minutes.
2. Remove the hot application and begin massage.

Variation: Hot towel treatment

Follow exactly the directions on page 100 for a *Hot towel roll.*

TREATMENT

CONTRAST TREATMENT TO THE UPPER BACK AND NECK

Cross-reference

See Chapters 4 and 5.

Duration and frequency

About 15 minutes. Perform before or during a massage session.

Procedure

1. With the client in a prone position, place a hot water bottle, moist heating pad, fomentation, hot gel pack or hydrocollator pack on the upper back and the back of the neck for 3 minutes.
2. Remove the hot application and place an ice pack, cold gel pack or ice-water compress on the upper back and the back of the neck for 1 minute. Make sure the client is warm, so the ice pack does not cause chilling.
3. Repeat steps 1 and 2 twice, for a total of three rounds of hot followed by cold.
4. Remove the cold application and begin massage.

Post-concussion headache

When the brain is injured by blows to the head, car accidents, sports-related injuries or falls, a "post-concussion

BACKGROUND

Terry was a 45-year-old librarian who had no health problems and received a monthly massage to help relax her tense neck and shoulder muscles. One spring day, however, she began having severe headaches and sinus congestion, which her family doctor diagnosed as due to allergies. She arrived for her massage session with a headache and an uncomfortable feeling of congestion in her upper face; she doubted she would be comfortable lying prone with pressure on her face. The massage therapist asked her if she would like to try a hot foot soak for her headache, plus a contrast treatment over her sinus area to make her more comfortable. She agreed to try this.

TREATMENT

With Terry lying supine, the massage therapist placed her feet directly in a hot footbath, then began massage of her head, neck and shoulders. Within 10 minutes Terry said her sinus area felt more open and her headache was gone. The therapist then removed the footbath, dried Terry's feet, and the massage continued. During the session, the therapist also performed a contrast treatment to Terry's upper face using hot and cold compresses. Terry then lay prone and was pleasantly surprised to find that her face was not uncomfortable after all. After the session, her headache was still gone, her sinus area felt more open, and she was as relaxed as usual after a session.

DISCUSSION QUESTIONS

1. What kind of massage could be used for a headache like Terry's?
2. What other hydrotherapy treatment could have been used instead of the hot footbath?

headache" may result. Brain inflammation and bleeding can create pressure inside the head but the neck is often injured as well, so the cause of the post-concussion headache is not always clear. Involved muscles such as the upper trapezius and semispinalis capitis often spasm to splint and protect the cervical spine. Many but not all post-concussive headaches can be successfully treated with migraine headache medication, indicating that pressure inside the head is a problem. However, other types of headaches, such as tension or cluster headaches, are also common. The majority of post-concussive headaches take place in the initial weeks after an injury and resolve within a few months.

When a client with post-concussive headaches sees you for massage therapy, make sure that he or she is under a doctor's care for the headaches. Then, a hot foot soak combined with an ice pack to the back of the neck (or a head wrap with frozen gel packs) can be performed before or during a massage session. Unfortunately, no research has been done on using this hydrotherapy treatment for post-concussive headaches, but some people claim to have found relief this way. It is safe and easy to use a hot foot bath, so there is certainly no harm in offering one along with your skilled bodywork.

Sinus headache caused by non-infectious sinusitis

See Case history 13.2. Allergies can lead to sinus inflammation and headaches. They often develop during hay fever season or after a cold. A client who has chronic sinusitis may find sinus contrast treatments very invigorating and relieving, and many massage techniques can add to that effect.

TREATMENT

STEAM INHALATION ON THE MASSAGE TABLE
Cross-reference
See Chapter 7.

continued

Chapter thirteen

TREATMENT *continued*

Duration and frequency

15 minutes. Perform before or during a massage session.

Procedure

1. Place a small steam unit on the table underneath the face cradle and place a small towel over the face cradle. Have tissues nearby, as often the client's nose will run. Essential oils may be added to the steam unit water.
2. Have the client lie prone upon the table, with his face in the face cradle.
3. After 15 minutes of steam inhalation, have the client sit up and dry his face with the face towel.
4. Begin face massage.

TREATMENT

SINUS CONTRAST TREATMENT

Cross-reference

See Chapters 4 and 5.

Duration and frequency

10 minutes. Perform before or during a massage session.

Caution

Do not use when the client has a sinus infection, except with a doctor's permission.

Procedure

1. Dip a washcloth in 110°F (43°C) water, then wring it out. Essential oils may be added to the water.
2. Place it across the nose, leaving the nostrils exposed. Fold down the ends 90 degrees from the central point so they lie alongside the nose.
3. After 2 minutes, replace the first washcloth with a different one that has been wrung out in ice water, and leave it on for 1 minute.

continued

TREATMENT *continued*

4. Repeat steps 1 and 2 twice, for a total of three rounds.
5. Begin massage.

INSOMNIA

Insomnia is a common problem—for example, at least one quarter of Americans seldom sleep well, while half of all elderly people have sleep problems (SLEEP, 2019). Emotional stress, chronic pain, and poor sleep habits contribute to this problem, as do many antihistamines, antidepressants, asthma medicines, blood pressure pills, pain relievers, and decongestants. (Graedon, 2008). Strategies that combat insomnia include avoiding caffeine or alcohol late in the day, keeping a regular sleep schedule, trying to relax mentally at night-time, and taking warm baths. Sleeping medications are popular but may have unwanted side-effects.

Modern research has concluded that massage helps reduce insomnia in people of all ages, including people who are hospitalized, have various types of chronic pain, or are under a great deal of stress (AMTA, 2019). At one time back rubs were a standard part of nursing care, known to help anxious or hurting patients to sleep without medications. Hydrotherapy treatments will complement your hands-on work and deepen its effectiveness (if not your client's sleep!). Whole-body baths (neutral or warm temperature) and warm footbaths relieve insomnia in a wide variety of people with health issues (for more on this, see Chapter 6).

Here are some ways to combine hydrotherapy and massage:

1. Have your client take a neutral bath before a session.
2. Use local moist heat during a session, moving it from one area to another as seems appropriate.
3. Combine a warm footbath with hands-on foot massage; then cover the feet warmly, and send the client home to sleep. Some therapists use warming

herbs, essential oils or capsaicin cream along with massage.

4. Heat-trapping compresses can be used at night and, since they present no risk of burns, are far safer than heating pads that a drowsy person might forget to turn off.

5. Towards the end of a session, have the client lie on a warm fomentation or flat plastic hot water bottle that contacts the entire spine, for at least 20 minutes.

6. Encourage your client to use a warm footbath or full body bath at home.

LIFE STRESS

As discussed in Chapter 1, high levels of stress have effects on all aspects of a client's health – emotional, physical and mental. People the world over seek relaxing water treatments combined with the soothing effects of body-work. Some clients will prefer a whole-body treatment such as a sauna, steam bath or tub bath, while others may prefer lying on a bed of warm fomentations or receiving a friction treatment with warm water. Cold treatments are not as conducive to relaxation and are more invigorating than soothing, and many clients don't care for them. Neutral baths reduce stimulation and can be very effective for nervous tension. Numerous studies have found that body heating before bed, using hot footbaths or warm full-body baths, causes a person to fall asleep sooner and sleep more deeply (Sung, 2000; Kanda, 1999; Liao, 2015; Karuchi, 1999; Ebben, 2006; Raymann, 2005). For thousands of years, various herbs and essential oils for relaxation have been added to water treatments.

How would you combine hydrotherapy treatments with massage for stressed-out clients? To give just one example, for a client who is having trouble sleeping, an evening massage session in your office could be followed by a long warm shower, or you could send the client home after the massage session to take a bath and then go directly to bed. (You might also suggest a nightly warm bath as a regular self-care treatment.) For a simple, generally relaxing and nurturing combination, see *"World's best back massage"* on page 235, and also the neutral bath and fomentation treatments here. Better than a sleeping pill!

TREATMENT

NEUTRAL BATH

Cross-reference

See Chapter 6.

Duration and frequency

30 minutes. Perform after a massage session.

Special instructions

The client may also take a neutral bath at home after a massage session and then go directly to bed.

Procedure

1. Help the client into the bath.

2. Maintain the water temperature at 98°F (37°C) so that the client does not become chilled.

3. After 30 minutes, have the client dry off gently, dress, and go home to go directly to bed.

TREATMENT

HOT FOMENTATIONS TO THE BACK AND THIGHS PRIOR TO MASSAGE

Cross-reference

See Chapter 4.

Special instructions

Flat plastic hot water bottles may be substituted for fomentations.

Duration

30 minutes.

Procedure

1. Prepare and heat three fomentations.

2. Place a plastic tub under the massage table.

3. Lay one fomentation on the massage table where the client's back will lie, and one for each thigh. It is important to cover them very carefully so the client will not be burnt, and to check the skin frequently.

4. Have the client lie supine on the fomentations for 30 minutes while massage is being performed on the front of the body.

continued

5. As the client turns over, remove the fomentations and place them in the plastic tub under the table.

6. Dry the skin, if necessary, and cover the client so he or she does not become chilled.

7. If desired, perform tapotement through the sheet from the neck to the soles of the feet, or use a hand-held massager instead.

8. Begin hands-on massage.

LOW BACK PAIN

Lower back pain (LBP) is one of the top ten reasons that American patients visit their doctors. It is also responsible for one third of disability costs in that country, and in one survey was responsible for over 10% of visits to massage therapists (Sherman, 2006). Many disease processes, such as osteoporosis, connective tissue disease, fibromyalgia, cancerous tumors and even infections in the spine, can lead to LBP. Mechanical causes include traumatic injuries to the structures of the back, and strains from heavy or improper lifting. If back muscles, ligaments, discs, bones, and joints are poorly healed, they are likely to continue to hurt. Osteoarthritis, spinal stenosis and magnesium deficiency may be factors. Weak back and abdominal muscles can worsen LBP. And finally, one leading cause is emotional stress. (For more on this topic, see *Acute lower back muscle spasm* on page 346.)

LBP is classified as acute (lasting 6 weeks or less), subacute (lasting 6–12 weeks), or chronic (lasting 12 weeks or more). Acute LBP is typically treated with medications for pain, inflammation and muscle spasm, and heat is generally recommended rather than ice. If low back pain does not improve after a month or two, more tests will be done to look for the source. If no specific cause can be found, standard medical treatment may expand to include physical therapy, other medications, or surgery. Unfortunately, many people are not satisfied with the results of surgery—often their recovery is longer and more painful than expected and there is less relief from chronic pain than they had hoped. Although the majority of lower back pain is either mechanical or stress-related, it is still vital that the client with lower back pain be evaluated by a doctor before receiving massage. How tragic it would be if a client with bone cancer pain was treated with massage rather than the right therapy!

Acute lower back pain

When the structures of the back are involved, hydrotherapy and massage can not only relieve pain but also promote healing. If the client's pain is linked to emotional stress, the nurturing and relaxing qualities of these modalities is also very helpful. Massage performed when the client's tissues are thoroughly warmed and relaxed makes it far more effective. Some doctors who perform spinal manipulation first apply hot silica gel packs, castor oil packs and anti-spasmodic herbs, all to make an adjustment easier and allow it to hold better. Ice massage may help numb the area and give more relief. Agatha Thrash, MD, recommends that during the first 24 hours after an acute back strain (such as from heavy lifting) the client should rest on a heating pad and alternate that with ice massage every 2 hours, and states that this often completely heals the strain (Thrash, 2015). Baths or compresses with Epsom salts may help by warming tissues and encouraging absorption of magnesium.

TREATMENT

MOIST HEAT APPLICATION FOLLOWED BY COLD MITTEN FRICTION

Cross-reference

See Chapters 4 and 10.

Special instructions

Water with added Epsom salts can be used to make a hot compress.

Duration and frequency

20 minutes. Perform before or during a massage session.

continued

TREATMENT *continued*

Procedure

1. Apply moist heat over the lower back, using a moist cloth and a heat lamp, hot compress, hydrocollator pack, castor oil pack, moist heating pad, etc. (Figures 13.5A and 13.5B). If it cools, reheat it or replace with a hotter one.

2. After 20 minutes, remove the moist heat, give a brief cold mitten friction (Figure 13.5C), dry the skin briskly, and begin massage.

TREATMENT

FULL HOT BATH FOLLOWED BY LOCAL MOIST HEAT APPLICATION

Cross-reference

See Chapters 4 and 6.

Duration and frequency

45 minutes. Give the bath before the massage session, then begin the massage session with the moist heat application in place on the lower back.

Procedure

1. Help the client into a hot bath (103–110°F; 40–43°C).

continued

TREATMENT *continued*

2. After 25–30 minutes, help the client out of the bath. Watch for signs of lightheadedness.

3. Have the client dry off and lie prone on the massage table. Apply moist heat to the lower back. Another part of the body may be massaged at this time.

4. After 20 minutes, remove the moist heat over the lower back and perform a brief cold mitten friction over the area.

5. Dry the area briskly and begin massage.

TREATMENT

MUSTARD PLASTER APPLICATION

Cross-reference

See Chapter 4.

Duration and frequency

20 minutes. Perform during a massage session, or as a home treatment before stretching exercises, two or three times daily.

Procedure

1. Apply the mustard plaster over the entire lower back. Monitor carefully to avoid burning.

2. Wait 20 minutes, then remove the plaster and begin massage.

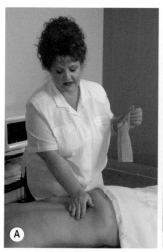 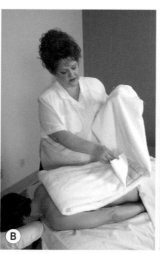 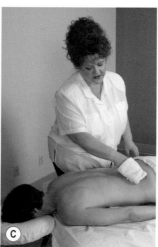

FIGURE 13.5
Moist heat application followed by cold mitten friction for acute lower back pain. (**A**) Checking the area visually. (**B**) Placing a large silica gel pack on the lower back. (**C**) Performing a brief cold mitten friction to the lower back.

TREATMENT

ICE MASSAGE

Cross-reference

See Chapter 5.

Duration and frequency

8–10 minutes. Perform before massage of the lower back or gentle back exercises.

Procedure

1. Perform ice massage on the entire lower back for 8–10 minutes, until the area is thoroughly numb.
2. Dry the skin briskly.
3. Begin massage.

Chronic lower back pain

As during an acute episode, it is vital that the client has been evaluated by a medical doctor and approved for massage treatment. Perpetuating factors are very important in this condition: hydrotherapy and massage can help with symptoms, but factors such as poorly healed injuries, leg-length inequality, postural distortion and muscular imbalance can all be part of the long-term picture. Emotional stress may be the single greatest factor in chronic LBP. Well-known osteopath John Upledger explained the link between his emotions and LBP this way: "I had experienced pain across my low back and into my right sacroiliac area for many years. After much exploration of the pain, it became clear that when I was angry, my back hurt. No amount of physical treatment or manipulation can take away this back pain when I have it, but if I can sit down in a quiet place, identify the anger and resolve it, my back pain automatically goes away" (Upledger, 1997). Someone who has been hurting for a prolonged period of time may also feel worried, discouraged and worn down by pain. In this sense, treating a client with chronic back pain can be quite different from treating someone during an acute pain episode.

Both hydrotherapy treatments and massage are relaxing, nurturing, enhance circulation, ease muscle tension, and may be the best non-drug approach to this problem. Any massage techniques that relieve muscle tension may help with pain as well. A 2011 study of 400 people with chronic low back pain found that 10 massage sessions over 10 weeks gave them more pain relief than their previous care if this had not included bodywork. Relief lasted at least six months (Cherkin, 2011). Of course, if there is an underlying perpetuating factor that is the cause of chronic low back pain, the best approach is to address that. But even as a symptomatic treatment, massage can be tremendously comforting, and hydrotherapy treatments can make massage more effective. Salt glows, contrast showers and ice massage may all help relieve pain and enhance massage. For some clients, both heat and ice may have to be tried to determine which works better.

TREATMENT

MOIST HEAT APPLICATION FOLLOWED BY A SALT GLOW OF THE ENTIRE BACK

Both the moist heat and the salt glow increase circulation to the back.

Cross-reference

See Chapters 4 and 10.

Duration and frequency

25–30 minutes. Perform during a massage session.

Procedure

1. Place a towel on the massage table.
2. With the client prone, apply moist heat in the form of a hydrocollator pack, fomentation, moist heating pad or flat plastic hot water bottle. Keep it hot for the entire time period.
3. After 20 minutes, remove the moist heat and give a brief cold mitten friction.
4. Inform the client that he or she will feel warm water on the back.
5. Gently wash the back with warm water.
6. Apply about 2 tablespoons of moistened Epsom salts to the client's back. Friction the entire back for about 3 minutes, especially in the lower back area.
7. Gently wash the salt off with a wet washcloth, and then dry the client with a dry washcloth.
8. Begin massage.

TREATMENT

CONTRAST SHOWER

This is a modified version of a classic treatment, the hot and cold spray to the back.

Cross-reference

See Chapter 8.

Duration and frequency

About 10 minutes. Perform before a massage session; or, when used as a home treatment, it may be used as often as once an hour.

Procedure

1. Have the client take a 5-minute hot shower (up to 110°F or 43°C). Use the strongest spray that can be tolerated directly on the lower back.
2. Change the water temperature to cold for 30 seconds.
3. Change the water temperature to hot for 2 minutes.
4. Change the water temperature to cold for 30 seconds.
5. Repeat steps 3 and 4.
6. Have the client dry off and lie down for a rest or a massage session.

TREATMENT

ICE MASSAGE

Cross-reference

See Chapter 5.

Duration and frequency

8–10 minutes. Perform before massage of the back, or gentle exercises.

Procedure

1. Perform ice massage on the lower back for 8–10 minutes, until the area is thoroughly numb.
2. Dry the skin briskly.
3. Begin massage or gentle exercises.

LYMPHEDEMA

As a result of surgery, injury, infection, radiation, or some other insult to their lymphatic system, up to 10 million Americans and hundreds of millions of people worldwide suffer from lymphedema. Most cases are caused by scar tissue, which blocks the flow of lymphatic fluid; such tissue is especially common after surgery which removes lymph nodes in the trunk or legs. All cancer surgery survivors need to avoid anything that could bring on lymphedema. As discussed in Chapter 3, this includes hot applications, ice packs over affected areas, and whole-body heating treatments.

Standard treatment for this condition consists of manual lymphatic drainage (MLD), bandaging, various exercises, and skin care. MLD is an important hands-on therapy that can significantly reduce limb volume. (Therapists should obtain training in this modality before treating clients with lymphedema.) What hydrotherapy treatments can you combine with hands-on work to help a client with lymphedema? First and most important is mild cooling of the skin with cold compresses, which makes MLD far more efficient (see Case history 13.3). According to physical therapist and lymphedema specialist Jean Yzer, "Once you begin the treatment session by applying topical skin cooling, you will require less time for lymphatic massage and advance more quickly to hands-on techniques for fibrosis and functional range of motion" (Yzer, 2017A). Cold compresses can reduce skin temperature by about 25°F (13.9°C). They also stimulate vasoconstriction which reduces the movement of fluid out of capillaries and into the interstitium. Cooled tissue is more pliable, underlying scar tissue and fibrotic patches are easier to feel, and pain is reduced. All this makes myofascial lengthening and scar tissue release easier and more comfortable for your client (Yzer, 2017B). Other safe treatments include:

1. Dry skin brushing, which stimulates the lymphatic system and can be done at the beginning of a session or daily by clients.
2. Neutral baths, which can reduce limb volume to some extent, and body wraps, taken to a neutral or warm stage, are safe as well.
3. Aquatic therapy and warm baths up to 102°F (39°C) are safe. In fact, regular participation in water exercise classes helps reduce volume in limbs with lymphedema (Tidhar, 2010).

Chapter thirteen

BACKGROUND

Sylvia was a 69-year-old retired secretary with lymphedema, which developed immediately after axillary lymph nodes were removed during her surgery for breast cancer. Her right arm was hot and swollen from her deltoid to her fingertips and she could not elevate her shoulder or bend her elbow. Her pain was constant and excruciating.

TREATMENT

Massage therapist Harold Packman began a treatment in the hospital physical therapy department by cooling but not freezing the limb. He first wrapped Sylvia's entire right arm in towels wrung from ice water for just 5 minutes, then removed them and waited 5 minutes (this prevented over-cooling of the area). He then used an ice cube to massage from shoulder to fingertip for another 5 minutes, rested 5 minutes, and repeated this four times, for a total of 20 minutes of ice massage. This procedure immediately eliminated Sylvia's pain. Packman repeated his treatment for 5 days in a row, by which time the swelling had diminished dramatically and he was then able to begin massage of Sylvia's entire right arm and hand. After six weeks of treatment she had regained normal range of motion in her shoulder, elbow and hand, and was pain-free (Packman, 2006).

TREATMENT

COLD COMPRESSES BEFORE MANUAL LYMPHATIC DRAINAGE

Cross-reference

See Chapter 5.

Duration and frequency

Apply several cold compresses before each session of manual lymphatic drainage.

Special instructions

Place two small towels in a bowl of ice water. Towels can also be prepared in advance and kept in a refrigerator (not a freezer). Never lay ice or cooling gel packs directly on the skin, as freezing temperatures could occur.

Procedure

1. Wring out one towel and mold it over the affected body part.

2. Once the towel warms up, wring out the other towel and substitute it, applying to the part.

3. Repeat until the skin cools and the towels no longer warm up.

4. Begin lymphatic massage.

MENSTRUAL CRAMPS

Menstrual pain is a very common problem, and in about one in four women leads to pain so severe that it interferes with their activities. Discomfort often begins one or two days before menstrual bleeding starts, and is felt in the lower abdomen, hip, lower back, or inner thighs. It may last from 12 to 72 hours. While pain medication is often used for dysmenorrhea, for thousands of years women have used abdominal heat applications (see Figure 13.6). These have included: animal bladders filled with heated oil or grains; pans of hot water; burning moxa; hot water bottles; warm bricks wrapped in flannel; hot sitz baths; hot herbal compresses; heating pads; castor oil packs; even sea sponges wrung out in hot water. Our clients generally do not seek us out specifically for this problem, but women sometimes arrive for their massage session

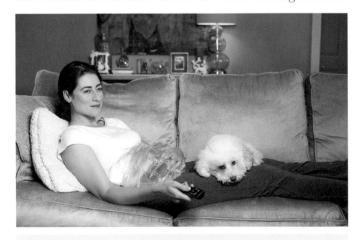

FIGURE 13.6
Flat plastic hot water bottle warming the abdomen. Photo courtesy of Fomentek Company, Fayetteville, AR.

while they are hurting. Many types of bodywork can address menstrual cramps, and combining them with hot and cold treatments will treat the cramps much better than either modality alone. Clients who have no specific pelvic issues are good candidates for tonic treatments between their menstrual periods.

Tonic treatments between menstrual cycles

Discontinue these treatments 12 hours before menstruation is expected to begin.

TREATMENT

DAILY CONTRAST PELVIC SHOWER

Cross-reference

See Chapter 8.

Duration

10 minutes.

Procedure

1. Using a hand shower attachment, spray the pelvic area with water as hot as can be tolerated for 2 minutes.
2. Spray the pelvic area with water as cold as can be tolerated for 1 minute.
3. Repeat steps 1 and 2 twice, for a total of three rounds.

TREATMENT

WEEKLY CONTRAST TREATMENT

Cross-reference

See Chapters 4 and 10.

Caution

Monitor the client's posterior body carefully for burning.

Duration and frequency

45 minutes. Perform during a massage session once a week.

Procedure

1. Give the client water to drink, as she will sweat.

continued

TREATMENT *continued*

2. Place on the massage table two hot fomentations or flat plastic hot water bottles filled with hot water, cover them with a cloth, and have the client lie supine on them; they should be in contact with her body from her scapulae to the top of her thighs.
3. Cover her abdominal and pubic areas with another hot fomentation or moist heating pad.
4. Leave the heat on for 15 minutes, during which time massage may be performed upon another part of the body.
5. Remove the heat from the abdomen.
6. Have the client roll onto one side.
7. Give a 30-second cold mitten friction where the heat was applied—that is, on the abdomen and the posterior of the body from the top of the thighs to mid-scapula. Use water that is as cold as she can tolerate.
8. Have the client roll onto her back; then repeat steps 3–6 twice, for a total of three rounds of hot followed by cold.
9. Begin massage of the abdominal area.

Treatments for pain relief during menses

TREATMENT

MOIST HEAT APPLICATIONS TO THE ABDOMEN

Cross-reference

See Chapter 4.

Duration and frequency

20 minutes. Use during a massage session.

Procedure

1. Have the client lie prone with a flat plastic hot water bottle or fomentation over her low back, and another one underneath her touching the lower abdomen.
2. Remove these after 20 minutes, finish with a brief cold friction, and begin hands-on work.

TREATMENT

HOT FOOTBATH WITH ICE TO ABDOMEN

Cross-reference

See Chapters 5 and 6.

Duration and frequency

20 minutes. Use during a massage session.

Procedure

1. Simply have the client sit in a chair or lie supine on a treatment table with the feet placed in a hot footbath, and add an ice pack over the lower abdomen and pubic bone.

2. After 20 minutes, remove the footbath, dry the feet, and remove the ice pack.

3. Now hands-on work may begin.

MULTIPLE SCLEROSIS

In multiple sclerosis (MS), myelin sheaths around sensory and motor neurons deteriorate, which leads to muscle weakness, stiffness, spasticity, bladder problems, loss of sensation, and decreased motor control. If a person with this disease becomes overheated, he or she can become even weaker. Considered an autoimmune disease, MS may be triggered by environmental factors. Standard medical treatment for this disorder usually consists of medication to reduce symptoms and mild exercise to maintain strength and function. Pool therapy can help patients with multiple sclerosis exercise, but care must be taken that they don't become overheated. Alternating 10 minutes of exercise in a 80°F (27°F) cold pool with 5–10 minutes of exercise in a 94°F (34°C) neutral pool is a typical regimen. Products such as cooling vests and scarves can be purchased to keep MS patients active even in summer heat.

Hydrotherapy and massage may both be used to alleviate some common MS issues, especially muscle stiffness and spasticity, and poor circulation in spastic muscles. Clients in wheelchairs or largely in bed also need support in staying mobile and with keeping healthy tissue healthy; hydrotherapy and massage can alleviate musculoskeletal discomfort and help to maintain breathing capacity. Someone who has stiff extremities and difficulty moving will feel a great deal better after hydrotherapy and massage. Exercises prescribed by a patient's physical therapist may be incorporated into a massage session after a cold application which temporarily decreases spasticity and muscle weakness. In this case, either ice-water compresses or cold-water immersion may be used. For a case history using hydrotherapy treatments for a client with multiple sclerosis, see Case history 6.4.

TREATMENT

WHOLE-BODY SALT GLOW

Cross-reference

Chapter 10.

Duration and frequency

15 minutes. Perform before massage.

Procedure

A whole-body salt glow is an excellent way to stimulate the circulation without using heat. It may be done with the client sitting on a bath chair in a bathtub or shower stall, on a therapy table, or on a bed if the client is bedridden. For house calls to bedridden clients' homes, simply spread a tarp or plastic sheet over the bed, cover that with a cloth sheet, and perform the salt glow there. Then, with the client rolled first to one side and then to the other, the sheet and tarp can be removed and the bed underneath will be dry.

TREATMENT

ICE WATER COMPRESS

Cross-reference

See Chapter 5.

Duration and frequency

8 minutes. Perform during a massage session.

Procedure

1. Prepare a compress by wringing out a towel of the appropriate size in a container that is half ice and half cold water, or by wrapping crushed ice in wet towels and applying that to an entire extremity.

2. Apply the towel to the spastic muscles for 4 minutes.

3. Wring out the towel in the ice water and reapply it, leaving it on for 4 more minutes.

4. Dry the area well.

5. Perform stretching or strengthening exercises, then follow with massage.

TREATMENT

COLD-WATER IMMERSION FOLLOWED BY EXERCISE

Cross-reference

See Chapters 5 and 6.

Duration and frequency

1–5 minutes. Perform before or during a massage session.

Procedure

1. Begin with a large container of water at 35–40°F (2–4°C). Ice cubes will be needed to achieve this temperature. Check to make sure that the client is comfortably warm beforehand.

2. Immerse the body part in the water for 3 seconds.

3. Take the body part out of the water and have the client do isometric contractions or contractions against resistance for 30 seconds. If he or she becomes fatigued, stop the exercises until after the next cold-water immersion.

4. Repeat steps 2 and 3 two to five times.

MUSCLE CRAMPS AND SPASMS

Both **muscle cramps** and **muscle spasms** are involuntary contractions of skeletal muscles. Muscle cramps are generally sudden, strong, and short-lived, which is fortunate as they can be very painful. Muscle spasms, on the other hand, are weaker contractions that last much longer, and a client may ask for your help with these. Many factors contribute to muscle cramps and spasms, including chronic tightness, poor blood flow, various vitamin and mineral deficiencies, inactivity, dehydration, and hyperthyroidism. Acute muscle cramps can begin when a person is sitting or sleeping in a cramped position or begins exercising with cold muscles. Hand muscles sometimes cramp when they are used intensively while writing, playing a musical instrument, sewing, typing, massaging, etc.

Muscle cramps

Sometimes the lower legs or feet of clients, especially elderly people whose local circulation is poor, cramp during a session. Should this occur, immediately apply moist heat or put the part in a hot water bath (see Case history 13.4). Often this helps right away, but if the cramp

---

SPASMODIC MUSCLE CONTRACTION TREATED BY A COMBINATION OF ICE MASSAGE AND MANUAL MASSAGE

CASE HISTORY 13. 4

BACKGROUND

Mrs. Rose, a woman in her early sixties, suffered from a twitch in the muscles around her right eye that could continue for hours at a time and sometimes even woke her from sleep. She was referred to massage therapist Harold Packman by her ophthalmologist, who approved the use of both ice cubes and manual massage.

TREATMENT

Packman began by performing ice massage along the path of the right facial nerve. Using an ice cube, he began at the front of the ear lobe, then moved upward to the temple, then down along the underside of the eye socket, and finally downward along the jaw. The area was treated this way for 5 minutes on, 5 minutes off, and this sequence was repeated three times. After a total of 20 minutes of ice massage, Mrs. Rose rested for 15 minutes and then Packman treated the entire right side of her face with Swedish massage techniques. This concluded her session. Mrs. Rose was treated three times a week for the first two weeks, twice a week for the next two weeks, then once a week for the final two weeks, for a total of 12 sessions. By then her muscle twitch was completely gone and so her treatment concluded. She experienced no muscle twitching at all for two years. After that she felt an occasional twitch, which coincided with periods of high stress (Packman, 2006).

DISCUSSION QUESTIONS:

1. Why was ice applied to the facial nerve?

2. Why was the combination of ice massage and manual massage better than manual massage alone?

persists, try ice next. Sometimes all that is needed is to have the person contract the antagonist muscles, automatically relieving the cramp. Below are instructions for moist heat, ice massage, and contrast treatments. A helpful longer-term strategy is to warm and then stretch the muscle on a regular basis. Podiatrist Myles Schneider recommends moist heat for 10–15 minutes, five or six times a day, until there is no more cramping: this obviously targets the circulation (Goldberg, 1997).

TREATMENT

MOIST HEAT APPLICATION ON AN ACUTELY CRAMPING CALF MUSCLE

Cross-reference

See Chapter 4.

Duration and frequency

30 seconds to a few minutes. Perform during a massage session as soon as the cramp begins.

Special instructions

To be effective, the application must be hot.

Procedure

1. Apply a hot fomentation, moist heating pad or hot compresses to the cramping calf muscle. At the same time, have the client contract the tibialis anterior muscle. Leave the heat on until the cramp has gone away.
2. Begin massage of the calf muscles.

TREATMENT

ICE MASSAGE ON AN ACUTELY CRAMPING MUSCLE IN THE ARCH OF THE FOOT

Cross-reference

See Chapter 5.

Duration and frequency

30 seconds to a few minutes. Perform right when a muscle cramp begins.

continued

TREATMENT *continued*

Procedure

1. Using an ice cup or ice cube, massage directly over the cramping muscle, and continue until the cramp has gone away.
2. Perform brief hands-on massage over the cramping muscle.

TREATMENT

CONTRAST COMPRESS FOR ANY ACUTELY CRAMPING MUSCLE

Cross-reference

See Chapters 4 and 5.

Duration

4 minutes or more.

Special instructions

In a pinch, the client could sit on the side of a bathtub and run alternate hot and cold water over the area while contracting antagonist muscles.

Procedure

1. Apply a hot compress to the cramping muscle for 3 minutes.
2. Apply an ice-water compress to the cramping muscle for 1.
3. Repeat steps 1 and 2 until the muscle stops cramping.

TREATMENT

HOT HAND BATH WITH STRETCHING FOR ACUTE SPASMS IN THE HAND MUSCLES

Cross-reference

See Chapter 6.

Duration and frequency

15 minutes. Perform during a massage session. Also helpful for self-care if hands spasm after doing hand-intensive activities.

TREATMENT *continued*

Procedure

1. Have the client soak the hands in hot water (about 110°F or 43°C), wiggling the fingers and stretching the hand muscles while soaking.

2. After 15 minutes, dry the hands and begin massage.

Acute lower back muscle spasm

As professionals who deal with muscle tension, massage therapists are often called when a person's lower back muscles have gone into spasm. Often, the client's comment is "I just reached over to pick up something" – often as light as a speck of dust – "and then I couldn't even straighten back up." This common affliction can be caused by muscle strain such as can occur with heavy lifting, especially if the person has structural and postural problems. Feelings can also lead to acute spasm: suppressed emotions, particularly anxiety and anger, can cause deep tension in the back muscles (Sarno, 1991). Over a period of thirty years, the author has asked many people with acute spasm about this, and almost without exception, they replied that they were under a great deal of stress. Here are a few examples of events that happened just before clients experienced acute lower back spasm:

1. A college student had just finished his last final examination.

2. A young mother was taking care of a baby with severe asthma attacks.

3. An elderly woman was packing up and moving out of the home where she had lived for 40 years.

4. A 30-year-old man was leaving town to be the best man at a wedding he desperately did not want to attend (as he was in so much pain and had to be carried everywhere on a board, he did not have to be best man after all!).

5. A 50-year-old woman was caring for a severely mentally-ill child.

These were all situations in which the spasm was triggered by the client bending over, but their doctors found no organic problem. A simple movement which results in spasm of back muscles is often simply the final straw for a treacherously tense body.

When a person experiences acute low back spasm, the first step should be a check-in with his or her doctor. With more serious injuries or diseases ruled out, medications to decrease inflammation and spasm are generally prescribed, along with bed rest. Massage therapists may work with clients as soon as they have the doctor's approval. Massage will be helpful in treating the muscle condition. For hydrotherapy treatments, simply use those recommended in the section on acute lower back pain in this chapter.

Acute spasm of neck muscles

This condition, which is sometimes called a "crick in the neck," is usually a strong spasm of the sternocleidomastoid muscle, although the levator scapulae and trapezius muscles may also be involved (Travell, 1999). As with the low back muscles, many factors, including muscle strain, emotional stress, poor work posture, structural problems, postural problems, and poor healing of previous injuries may combine to render the client vulnerable to a "neck attack." On rare occasions, mechanical problems such as herniated discs may also cause neck spasm. This condition may be brought on when an already-tight muscle becomes chilled (for example, by sleeping under an air conditioning vent or by an open window in the dead of winter), or if the client has previously-injured neck ligaments, or when he or she has just had an upper respiratory infection, or when stress finally renders a muscle completely unable to relax. (For a real-life example of an acute neck spasm and its treatment, see Case history 13.5.)

The first step in dealing with this condition should be a thorough examination by a doctor to rule out diseases or other problems. Usually a client with this problem enters your office with a neck that he or she is unable to turn in any direction, and which is painful and sensitive to the touch. A common scenario is the person who "slept wrong" and woke up in the morning with a stiff neck. Osteopath Roland Harris once treated a man who was 6.2 feet (1.9 meter) tall and slept for hours on a 5.7 feet (1.73 meter) sofa with his head jammed forward. In the morning he had pain at the base of his neck, subluxation of the facet joints between the sixth and seventh cervical vertebrae, and marked muscle spasm (Harris, 1961).

Hot applications increase circulation to spasmed muscles and feel comforting to the client, while ice applications slow nerve conduction and relieve pain and muscle spasm. Ice stroking can also be helpful during trigger point treatment, which enables you to stretch the spasmed muscle to its full length. Hands-on massage which treats the sternocleidomastoid and related muscles works beautifully in conjunction with these hot and cold applications. It is important to recognize, however, that if a whiplash or other ligament injury is causing the person's problems, what the client needs most in the long run is ligament healing. Likewise, if emotional stress is a major factor, only dealing with that will address the heart of the problem.

TREATMENT

ICE STROKING (INTERMITTENT COLD WITH STRETCH) OF THE STERNOCLEIDOMASTOID MUSCLE

Cross-reference

See Chapter 5.

Duration and frequency

5 minutes. Perform during a massage session that includes trigger point release.

Special instructions

The sternocleidomastoid muscle on both sides of the neck should be treated, along with any associated trigger points in the levator scapulae, trapezius, splenius cervicis and other posterior neck muscles.

Procedure

1. Use ischemic compression to treat trigger points in the sternocleidomastoid (see Figure 13.7).
2. Gently stretch the muscle to the greatest extent possible without overstretching; then, while you maintain the muscle stretch, stroke the entire length of the muscle three times with the plastic-wrapped ice.
3. Now gently stretch the muscle again, to the greatest extent possible without overstretching it.
4. If the muscle is still not capable of fully lengthening without pain, try applying direct pressure to the trigger point, then gently stretching the muscle again or try having the client contract the antagonist muscle for 30 seconds and then relax completely as you repeat the stretch.

continued

TREATMENT *continued*

5. Repeat steps 2, 3 and 4 until the muscle is pain-free when completely stretched.
6. Apply a heating pad or moist hot pack to the muscle for 5 minutes or more to prevent post-treatment soreness.

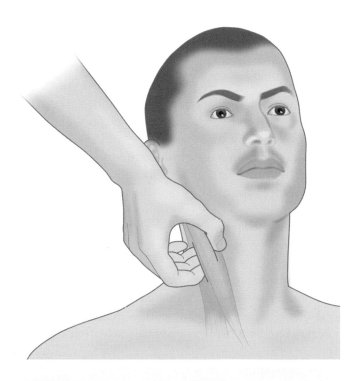

FIGURE 13.7
Trigger point pressure release of the sternocleidomastoid muscle.

TREATMENT

HOT MOIST APPLICATION TO THE NECK

Cross-reference

See Chapters 4 and 5.

Duration and frequency

30 minutes. Perform during a massage session or as a home treatment, two or three times daily.

continued

TREATMENT *continued*

Procedure

1. Apply a hot fomentation, a moist heating pad, or hot compresses to the neck for 30 minutes.
2. Finish with a 1-minute ice application (ice massage or cold mitten friction using ice water) to the client's neck.
3. Begin massage of the neck muscles.

For full instructions and contraindications, see Chapter 4.

TREATMENT

FULL HOT BATH FOLLOWED BY LOCAL MOIST HEAT APPLICATION

Cross-reference

See Chapters 4 and 6.

Duration and frequency

About 40 minutes. Have the client take a hot bath first, then apply the local heat to the neck at the beginning of the session.

Procedure

1. Help the client into a hot bath (103–110°F or 39–43°C). You may need to place a rolled towel or bath pillow under the client's neck for support and comfort.
2. After 20–30 minutes, help the client out of the bath. Watch for signs of lightheadedness.
3. Have the client dry off and lie either supine or prone on the massage table. Apply moist heat to the neck and massage the shoulders, back and upper arms.
4. After 20 minutes, remove the moist heat over the neck, perform a brief cold mitten friction over the area, and dry it.
5. Begin massage of the neck muscles.

TREATMENT

ICE MASSAGE OF THE NECK MUSCLES

Cross-reference

See Chapter 5.

Duration and frequency

5–10 minutes. Perform during a massage session, or as a home treatment, three times daily.

Caution

To avoid pressing on the carotid arteries, do not massage the anterior neck medial to the sternocleidomastoid muscles.

Procedure

Perform ice massage gently on the posterior and lateral neck muscles and the entire length of the sternocleidomastoid muscle. Continue for 5–10 minutes.

MUSCLE SPASTICITY

This condition features continuous contraction of certain muscles. It can occur after a stroke or an injury to the spinal cord or central nervous system. Contracted muscles become stiff and tight, which interferes with normal movement, causes pain, and can lead to contractures. Cold applications are helpful: although the process is not completely understood, the cause is likely to be that when muscle spindles have cooled they no longer help to maintain muscle tone, and spastic muscles can relax.

Massage techniques that increase circulation and decrease tension are helpful; but because spasticity is a really a nervous system issue, massage needs to be given on a regular basis to be effective. Bodywork can also help relieve stress, ease muscle pain, and help maintain joint range of motion. Warm water exercise can help reduce spasticity and retain muscle strength and range of motion.

The following cold applications must be carefully applied, because the core temperature will drop if more than one fifth of the body is covered with a cold compress, or if one part is immersed in cold water long enough.

Chapter thirteen

TREATMENT OF AN ACUTE NECK SPASM BY COMBINING HEAT, ICE, AND HANDS-ON MASSAGE

BACKGROUND

Martin was a 32-year-old student who worked full-time and took college classes at night. A cramped work space for his home computer meant that his body was frequently in an awkward position while he did much of his homework: his head was often twisted far to the left as he read from a stack of papers and typed. One morning, after spending almost an entire weekend at the computer with his head twisted, Martin woke up to find he could not turn his head either to the left or to the right. First he took a hot shower, letting the water beat directly on the muscles on the front and sides of his neck, which loosened them somewhat. Then he called his doctor, who agreed that visiting a massage therapist was a sensible first step.

TREATMENT

Martin's regular massage therapist applied very hot compresses to both sternocleidomastoid muscles for 20 minutes while she massaged his upper back and shoulders. Next she removed the compresses, performed ice massage for 1 minute, used Swedish and trigger point techniques on the muscles, and finished with gentle stretching. Martin left her office feeling much better, but it took three more days before he began to feel completely well again. For those days, he did no typing and took frequent 20-minute hot showers, followed by ice massage and gentle stretching of his sternocleidomastoid muscles. To avoid a recurrence of the same problem, Martin also began to rearrange his workspace so that he didn't have to twist his head when working at his computer.

TREATMENT

ICE-WATER COMPRESS

Cross-reference

See Chapter 5.

Duration and frequency

8 minutes. Use during a massage session.

Procedure

1. Prepare a compress by wringing out a towel of the appropriate size in a container of half ice and half cold water. Crushed ice may be used if it is wrapped in wet towels first.
2. Apply the cold compress to the spastic muscles for 4 minutes.
3. Wring out another towel in the ice water and apply that instead, leaving it on for 4 more minutes.
4. Dry the area well and perform stretching or strengthening exercises.
5. Follow with massage.

TREATMENT

COLD-WATER IMMERSION FOLLOWED BY EXERCISE

Cross-reference

See Chapter 6.

Duration and frequency

5–10 minutes. Perform during a massage session.

Procedure

1. Begin with a large container of ice cubes and water (temperature will be 35–40°F; 2–4°C). Before beginning the cold-water immersion, check to make sure that the client is comfortably warm.
2. Immerse the body part in the water for 3 seconds.
3. Now take it out of the water and have the client perform exercises for 30 seconds.
4. Repeat steps 2 and 3 five times, for a total of six cold-water immersions.
5. Perform other stretching or strengthening exercises.
6. Begin massage.

MUSCLE WEAKNESS

Chronic muscle weakness can stem from many different disabilities, including strokes, muscular dystrophy, spinal cord injuries, post-polio syndrome and cerebral palsy. Not only does muscle weakness make many movements difficult or impossible, but chronic tension and muscle strain can develop when the sufferer overworks a few of their stronger muscles to compensate for the weaker ones. Hydrotherapy can be used in a variety of ways to help clients with muscle weakness.

1. Cold-water immersion can temporarily stimulate muscle strength, and the strengthening exercises that are recommended by the client's physical therapist can be incorporated into a massage session. For example, a weak or paralyzed hand or foot can be immersed in very cold water and then exercised while it is stronger. (Exposure to cold stimulates the action of extensor muscles.) At the moment of immersion, a contraction will be noticed, even if it is weak or inhibited by spasticity. The extensors will be stimulated and the flexors inhibited for about 20 minutes. Exercises and massage strokes can be alternated. If the client can only do a few contractions without becoming fatigued, this is a perfect time for either relaxing or stimulating massage techniques.

2. Another way to combine massage and exercise to build muscle strength is to combine warm water exercise with massage techniques. Dr. Meir Schneider's Self-Healing approach has documented success in building strength in patients with muscular dystrophy: he combines many repetitions of gentle exercise in warm baths or pools with special massage techniques (Schneider, 2004). Watsu has also been combined with exercise for this purpose.

3. For some movement problems caused by brain issues, heat and cold may be of benefit because of their brain-stimulating effect. In 2005, a research study with partially paralyzed stroke survivors placed hot packs followed by cold packs on paralyzed hands and wrists, five times a day for six weeks. Compared to other stroke survivors whose rehabilitation was the same in every other way, the contrast application group improved far more in their ability to flex and extend their wrists. Researchers concluded that the contrast applications were effective because they helped stimulate and reorganize large areas in the brain (Chet, 2005).

TREATMENT

COLD-WATER IMMERSION FOLLOWED BY EXERCISE

Cross-reference

See Chapter 5.

Duration and frequency

1–5 minutes. Perform before or during a massage session.

Procedure

1. Begin with a large container of water at 35–40°F (2–4°C). Ice cubes will be needed to achieve this temperature. Check to make sure that the client is comfortably warm before beginning the cold-water immersion.

2. Immerse the body part in the water for 3 seconds.

3. Take the body part out of the water and have the client do isometric contractions or contractions against resistance for 30 seconds. If he or she becomes fatigued, stop the exercises until after the next cold-water immersion.

4. Repeat steps 2 and 3 two to five times.

NERVE ENTRAPMENT

When a peripheral nerve passes between taut bands in a muscle, or lies between taut trigger point bands and bone, the unrelenting pressure on the nerve can produce pain and loss of function. Chronic compression can affect many peripheral nerves, including the suprascapular, ulnar, radial, peroneal, and sciatic nerves. Here we give examples of two nerve entrapments, thoracic outlet syndrome and piriformis syndrome. In each, combining deep tissue or trigger point massage and hot or cold therapy helps to resolve the problem. According to Travell and Simons (1999) the signs and symptoms may sometimes be relieved within minutes after inactivation of the trigger points and release of the taut bands. Applications of intense moist heat make the tissue that is binding or entrapping the nerve more pliable and easier to treat. Alternately, when the region feels very painful, ice will numb the pain. Ice stroking followed by stretching the muscles helps lengthen them to their fullest extent without pain.

Thoracic outlet syndrome (TOS)

The typical symptoms of TOS include pain, numbness, tingling and muscle wasting, along with possible neck pain, chest pain, headache, vertigo and dizziness. It occurs when tight scalenes or pectorals squeeze the brachial plexus between the clavicle and the first rib. The scalenes can become hard and tight from a forward head posture, scoliosis, trauma such as whiplash or a clavicle fracture, difficult breathing, or hard paroxysms of coughing. The pectoral muscles can become tight through round-shouldered posture, repetitive work tasks or heavy lifting. The standard treatment for TOS is physical therapy and medications for inflammation and pain. Massage can alleviate at least some entrapment symptoms, by treating the tight and shortened muscles using deep tissue myofascial release, deactivating trigger points, then stretching to lengthen the muscles fully. Heat can be used to make the client's muscles more pliable and bodywork more comfortable. Simply use moist heat (warm shower, moist heating pad, hydrocollator pack, etc.) over the upper chest and neck for 15–20 minutes at the beginning of a session. As explained in Chapter 5 (page 132), ice stroking is useful to lengthen muscles after their trigger points have been deactivated.

Piriformis syndrome

Piriformis syndrome usually starts with pain, tingling, or numbness in one or both buttocks. Pain can be severe and may extend down the length of the sciatic nerve: it is caused by compression of the sciatic nerve by taut bands of the piriformis muscle. In many cases, there is a history of trauma such as a muscle tear or fall onto the buttock which led to adhesions and/or trigger points. Sacroiliac joint dysfunction, repetitive activity such as long-distance running, or chronic compression due to prolonged sitting can also lead to this problem. Pain may be triggered by emotional stress, climbing stairs, applying firm pressure directly over the piriformis muscle, or sitting for long periods of time. A tight, contracted or tender piriformis muscle can be easily palpated. A doctor or physical therapist can suggest a program of exercises and stretches to help reduce sciatic nerve compression. Osteopathic manipulative treatment may relieve pain and increase range of motion. Some healthcare providers may recommend anti-inflammatory medications, muscle relaxants, or injections with a corticosteroid or anesthetic.

Massage can reduce the pressure on the sciatic nerve by reducing piriform tightness, first using general warming techniques to soften the gluteals, followed by ischemic compression and cross-fiber friction to treat trigger points. Active-isolated stretching can be incorporated to release the attachments at the anterior sacrum and the trochanter (Lowe, 2015).

Combining simple treatments will assist your work:

1. Heat can make the client's muscles more pliable and bodywork more comfortable. Because there are thick layers of gluteal muscles overlying the piriformis, it is helpful to lower their tone so that they can be worked before the piriformis. Moist heat really helps; have the client lie prone with the area under a heat lamp or covered by a heating pad for 20–30 minutes while you work elsewhere, or have them lie with the painful buttock on top of a flat plastic hot water bottle or fomentation before the hands-on work begins.

2. As explained in Chapter 5, ice stroking helps in lengthening muscles after their trigger points have been deactivated. Simply follow the directions on page 132 to lengthen the piriformis and other related muscles to their full extent.

PARKINSON'S DISEASE

Parkinson's disease (PD) is a complex neurological disorder. It is progressive and often results in severe disability. Some risk factors are unknown, but head injuries, exposure to pesticides, toxic metals and other industrial chemicals are known causes. The two main symptoms of this disorder are muscle stiffness and resting tremors, but frequent complications include cramping, constipation, contractures, sleeping disorders and pain. Mainstream treatment for Parkinson's includes medication (Levadopa), aerobic exercise and physical therapy. Diligent practice of exercises for co-ordination and strength, pool therapy and the Feldenkrais method have all helped patients make great progress. Deep brain stimulation is an approved therapy as well.

Clients with PD often turn to massage seeking relief from pain and rigidity, and at least one type of massage has been shown to be effective. A 2002 study found that when the gentle rocking motion of the Trager Method was given to the upper limbs and bodies of patients for 20 minutes, their muscle rigidity was reduced by one third (Duval, 2002). In another case, a 63-year-old female patient with long-standing PD received five massage sessions in six weeks. Her rigidity and tremors were tested before and after the massage treatments, which consisted of warm silica gel packs and Swedish techniques including passive movement and general relaxation. Massage reduced both resting and postural tremors after each session (Casciaro, 2016). Other sufferers turn to massage for help with constipation and sleep. In a chronic condition of this nature, the sufferers' stress levels are always high, and massage can help with this aspect as well. Stretching, traction and range of motion exercises can slow down weakness and stiffness. Mild hydrotherapy treatments are safe and relaxing, and can be combined with bodywork. For example, a warm bath followed by massage helps reduce pain and bring on sleep; a salt glow and a warm shower are an ideal beginning for a massage, and are also an excellent home treatment; and the *"World's best back massage"* (see page 235) combines mild heat, friction and bodywork techniques to produce deep relaxation. A sensory stimulation footbath (see page 147) is a great technique for a client with very advanced Parkinson's.

PASSIVE SWELLING IN THE LEGS

Fluid retention in the legs can be a symptom of a serious medical condition such as blood clots, kidney disease or heart failure, but in cases where the swelling is mild and there is no underlying health condition, this condition is comparatively benign. Edema or fluid retention occurs when excess fluids build up inside the body and cause swelling in the lower limbs. Sitting or standing for long periods of time, tight clothing that restricts circulation, any injury in the pelvis or lower limbs, pregnancy, peripheral neuropathy, and steroid, antidepressant or hormone medications can all contribute to this condition. Clients who are in wheelchairs often develop this condition. To manage swelling, the standard medical treatment is compression, elevation and lymphatic drainage. Leg muscle stretches, exercises such as ankle pumps and gluteal squeezes, and pool exercise are all helpful. Massage can stimulate circulation and help fluids move through the legs. (Obtain a doctor's approval before performing massage.) In one study, venous blood flow in the lower leg was much faster after friction massage had been performed between the medial and lateral heads of the gastrocnemius muscle (Iwamoto, 2017). Hydrotherapy treatments you may easily combine with bodywork include these:

1. Both contrast baths or contrast leg sprays improve circulation and decrease swelling in patients with varicose veins (Saradeth, 1991; Helal, 2013). The client can perform foot and ankle movements at the same time to further increase blood flow.

2. Neutral baths for 30–60 minutes, before or after a session.

3. Dry skin brushing, followed by an anti-inflammatory leg wrap (see Figure 13.4).

4. Sensory stimulation footbath.

PERIPHERAL NEUROPATHY

Peripheral neuropathy (PN) is an uncomfortable condition in which the sensory nerves below the knees and elbows lose feeling and function. These nerves register sensations such as temperature, pain, touch and vibration, so sufferers experience tingling, numbness and sharp burning pains, and lose movement perception and body balance. PN can be caused by damage to nerves from chemotherapy drugs, sustained high blood-sugar levels in diabetics, chronic venous insufficiency, and poisoning from lead or other toxins. 40% of all PN is caused by diabetes. There is little in the way of effective mainstream treatment for this condition. Doctors may prescribe anticonvulsants, opioids, or antidepressant medications, while physical therapy usually includes aerobic exercise, stretching, and range of motion exercises.

Any techniques which improve blood flow to the extremities are helpful: for example, the biofeedback-assisted relaxation training (called WarmFeet) teaches patients to consciously warm their feet; when done correctly, peripheral blood vessels dilate and blood flow improves. Consistent practice results in less pain and better walking (Rice, 2007). Swedish massage has been shown to be beneficial in PN, beginning with gentle gliding effleurage and eventually progressing to gentle friction and petrissage on the extremities. Foot reflexology is also effective, while Thai foot massage increases sensation and improves balance (Chatchawan, 2015; Thrash, 2015; Wine, 1996; Woods, 2012). Massaged areas are measurably warmer, indicating greater blood flow (Cunningham, 2011). Chronic injection sites may have a build-up of thick scar tissue, and friction and scar release techniques can help restore mobility. Hydrotherapy treatments can also increase circulation, but never use extreme temperatures. One non-thermal treatment for PN is charcoal. (On page 114 we give directions for a charcoal pack.) Adventist doctors at Wildwood Hospital have used charcoal slurry for PN with good success (for more about this hospital, which uses hydrotherapy with all patients, see the "Point of interest" Box 3.4). For example, Marjorie Baldwin, MD, once put a diabetic's severely damaged feet into separate double plastic bags partially filled with a slurry of charcoal and neutral-temperature water. The bags were then tied loosely above the ankles and the patient's feet were propped up and kept in the bags almost round the clock for days. They healed completely (Dinsley, 2005). How exactly charcoal relieves deep tissue pain and draws out toxins when used externally is still a mystery, and more research is needed, but doctors suspect its porous properties may decrease PN by drawing microparticles such as chemicals, toxins and bacteria to the surface of the skin. Charcoal dressings are known to remove fluids and toxins that impair the healing process and reduce inflammation (Kerihuel, 2010; Thrash, 2015).

Hydrotherapy treatments to use with bodywork follow, but heat should be mild because if the client receives a hot footbath, he or she may not be able to sense that the feet are getting too hot, and burning might be a real danger. Below are safe treatments:

1. The leg wrap in Chapter 9 is appropriate, before or after a massage (see Figure 13.4).

2. Contrast footbath (use warm, not hot, water, plus very cold water for the cold portion to create a distinct contrast). Due to the contralateral reflex effect, a contrast footbath can be done on one leg to stimulate blood flow in the other (Shafizadegan, 2016).

3. Warm footbath with Epsom salts, followed by massage.

4. Neutral baths for burning sensations (Thrash, 2015).

5. Heat-trapping compress for the feet, either during a session or as a home treatment for the client (directions in Appendix A, page 372).

6. Charcoal packs, applied at the beginning of a massage session.

PSORIASIS

This chronic, non-contagious autoimmune disorder features itchy patches of skin covered with scaly skin cells. Susceptibility is a combination of genetics and exposure to certain triggers, such as emotional stress, infections, skin injuries, cold dry winter air, and beta-blocker medications. People with psoriasis may wonder if massage is safe for them or feel self-conscious about their skin lesions, but you can reassure them that as long as their skin is intact they can enjoy massage like anyone else. In fact, when skin becomes too dry, it can crack and bleed and become infected, so moisturizing treatments are helpful as long as the skin is not open (for treatments that can be combined with massage, see the *Dry skin section* on page 326). Many baths are beneficial for psoriasis, and for centuries visitors to Dead Sea spas have seen a great improvement (Matz, 2003). In your practice, however, use warm (not hot) oatmeal or Epsom salts baths to reduce itching, warm compresses with baking soda to rehydrate dry skin, and warm castor oil packs to soften it. Baths can be taken during or after a session, and compresses or castor oil packs can be applied during a session. Lotions containing oatmeal can be helpful, as well. Nurse and chiropractor Louella Doub saw great improvement in psoriasis when she gave patients with other immune system problems a series of steam bath fever treatments (see Appendix C for more on this). The condition often went into remission for up to a year (Doub, 1971). About one third of people with psoriasis also develop psoriatic arthritis. It is treated much like rheumatoid arthritis, and the same treatments can be used for both.

RESTLESS LEG SYNDROME (RLS)

RLS is a very uncomfortable condition in which feelings of uneasiness, twitching or restlessness after going to bed interfere with sleep. 10–15% of adult Americans have this underdiagnosed syndrome. While deficiencies of iron and possibly other nutrients are correlated with RLS, most people with this problem are middle aged or older and have cold feet and poor circulation in the legs. One case study found that RLS decreased when a patient was taught thermal biofeedback (Rice, 2007). Standard medical treatment is medications of various types, which work for some, but not everyone. Mineral and vitamin supplements, walking, massage, stretching, hot or cold compresses, or working the legs in a bicycling fashion have worked for some but not all sufferers (Yokum, 2006). Because of their circulation problems, Agatha Thrash, MD, advises patients with restless leg syndrome to keep the legs very warm year-round and to wear compression stockings. Circulatory massage combined with hydrotherapy treatments can help improve leg circulation, and while it is not guaranteed to be successful, it is certainly worth a trial. However, if there is a true deficiency or other underlying cause, this must also be addressed. To combine hydrotherapy treatments with massage, see the section on *Passive swelling in the legs* (page 352). Thrash also suggests to patients that when the unpleasant sensations occur in bed they could try either sponging their legs with very cold water or using a heating pad turned up high. She emphasizes that the pad should not be turned on until the restless feelings occur, should not be used on bare skin, and that no one should ever fall asleep with it turned on (Thrash, 2015).

SCIATICA

This relatively common pain radiates from the lower back along the path of the large sciatic nerve. True sciatica is a compression or inflammation of this nerve, and can be caused by an L5-S1 disc herniation, bone spur, or stenosis (narrowing) which pinches or irritates the nerve root. Symptoms very similar to those caused by a herniated disc can also be caused by trigger points in the gluteus medius that refer pain down the back of the leg along the path of the nerve, or by the piriformis compressing the sciatic nerve. (For more on *Piriformis syndrome*, see page 351.)

Sciatic pain can take different forms and be mild, moderate or severe. The client may feel sharp, burning, tingling or shooting pain, and have weakness, numbness, or difficulty moving the affected leg or foot. Standard medical treatment for sciatica includes medications for inflammation and pain, physical therapy and sometimes surgery. Patients are also encouraged to change their lifestyles by sitting less and doing yoga. Patients with persistent sciatica have no better outcomes with surgery than with a program of physical therapy and exercise (Weinstein, 2006). Both hydrotherapy and massage can increase circulation to painful areas. Heat quiets trigger points and reduces the muscle spasm that comes from the irritation of the sciatic nerve, while ice numbs. However, disc herniation will not be healed by massage, and clients with such a condition should be treated by an orthopedic doctor.

Anti-inflammatory herbs or essential oils are a traditional addition, and can be added to the water used to make ice cups.

TREATMENT

HOT HALF BATH

Cross-reference

See Chapters 5 and 6.

Duration and frequency

20 minutes. Perform before a massage session, or, as a home treatment, two or three times daily.

Procedure

1. Have the client sit in a waist-high hot bath (102–108°F or 39–42°C). Place a towel on the bottom of the tub for comfort if needed. Anti-inflammatory herbs or essential oils can be added.

2. After 20 minutes, finish the half bath with a cold local shower to the area, or have the client lie prone for 2 minutes with a bag of crushed ice or a frozen cold compress over the lower back area.

3. Begin massage.

TREATMENT

ICE MASSAGE FOR SCIATICA

Cross-reference

See Chapter 5.

Duration and frequency

20 minutes. Perform during a massage session.

Procedure

1. Anti-inflammatory herbs or essential oils are a traditional addition and can be added to the water used to make ice cups.

2. Have the client lie prone, with two or three pillows under the pelvis. Using an ice cube or ice cup, perform ice massage over the gluteal muscles, and down the back of the leg, following the path of the sciatic nerve. Continue ice massage for 8–10 minutes until the area is numb.

3. Use no ice for 5 minutes.

4. Repeat steps 1 and 2 three more times, for a total of 20 minutes of ice.

TREATMENT

CONTRAST TREATMENT WITH HOT APPLICATIONS AND ICE PACKS

Cross-reference

See Chapters 5 and 6.

Duration and frequency

25 minutes. Perform during a massage session.

Procedure

1. With the client in a side-lying position, apply moist heat over the painful hip and gluteal muscles in the form of a hot towel roll hydrocollator pack, a heat lamp, a fomentation, a moist heating pad, or a flat plastic hot water bottle. Hands-on massage may be done on another part of the body at this time.

2. After 10 minutes, remove the moist heat and apply an ice pack for 2 minutes.

continued

TREATMENT *continued*

3. Apply the moist heat again.

4. After 5 minutes, remove the moist heat and apply an ice pack for 2 minutes.

5. Repeat steps 3 and 4, for a total of three rounds of hot followed by cold.

6. Begin massage.

STROKE RECOVERY

Stroke is the leading cause of long-term disability in Europe and the United States so massage therapists are likely to see clients with this problem. When the blood supply to the brain is interrupted and brain cells are damaged, many problems may result, depending upon how severe the stroke is and which part of the brain was affected. The person may experience weakness, numbness, paralysis of limbs, facial muscles, or even an entire side of the body. Problems may also occur with chewing, swallowing and speech, vision, walking, co-ordination, balance, and memory. After the initial stroke phase, and once patients are stable, many stroke survivors notice new pain, sometimes severe, in their heads, joints or skin. A sizeable percentage of stroke survivors begin to experience headaches for the first time in their lives. Another unfortunate stroke effect is muscle spasticity, which is characterized by abrupt, choppy movements of weak, tight muscles. Contractures may develop.

Early rehabilitation improves outcomes after a stroke, but improvement often occurs slowly in response to a combination of techniques from a variety of healthcare professionals. Water therapy is one of the best ways to stimulate the brain and build strength, mobility, motor control and aerobic capacity. Massage is helpful on many levels, emotional and physical. For example, one study found slow-stroke back massage eased both anxiety and shoulder pain in post-stroke patients (Mok, 2004). Another found that Thai massage decreased anxiety, depression and spasticity (Thanakiatpinyo, 2014). Various forms of bodywork can reduce muscle pain and headaches, stretch and strengthen muscles, and avoid spasticity, and reducing or ideally eliminating contractures is an important part of keeping quality of life for post-stroke sufferers. When a spastic or paralyzed muscle places an unrelenting pull on the proximal joint, it hurts! Make sure you have a doctor's approval before treating stroke survivors, since they often have other health problems and are taking multiple medications. Hydrotherapy treatments to combine with bodywork include the following:

1. For headaches: use a hot foot soak and massage of the head. Ginger is a traditional additive in both hot water and massage oil.

2. For muscle relaxation: use hot applications during a session.

3. For spasticity: use the cold-water treatment in the section on *Muscle spasticity* (page 349).

4. For brain stimulation, use contrast hot and cold packs followed by massage. For more on how this treatment helps re-develop signals to affected areas, see the section on *Muscle weakness* (page 350).

5. For relaxation, pain, abnormal muscle tone and shallow breathing, perform Watsu. Almost any form of water immersion is helpful for post-stroke patients, but this gentle form of body therapy seems tailor-made for the symptoms of stroke and allows sufferers to drift into a deeper sense of relaxation.

6. For early contractures: use ice packs, massage and stretching.

TREATMENT

ICE PACKS FOR AN EARLY CONTRACTURE (THE JOINT IS OVERLY FLEXED DUE TO SPASTICITY)

Cross-reference

See Chapter 5.

Duration and frequency

Use as soon as there is any sign of a contracture: simply apply the ice pack directly over the shortened tissues for 20 minutes, then begin stretching and massage.

Cautions

Do not overuse ice, and monitor for frostbite.

TEMPOROMANDIBULAR JOINT DISORDER (TMD)

This disorder often features pain in the jaw joint, difficulty opening the mouth, and headaches, ear pain and a stiff neck. Causes of TMD include poor tooth alignment, physical trauma, tension and pain due to tooth grinding, and arthritis in the temporomandibular joint. TMD can also be related to stress, nervous tension or suppressed anger. This condition is generally treated with physical therapy (gentle stretching of involved muscles), anti-inflammatory, muscle relaxant, or pain medications. If TMD is advanced, dental appliances or prolotherapy injections are sometimes used.

Hydrotherapy can be helpful for the person suffering from TMD. Ice packs to the side of the face and temple can be used to relieve muscle spasms; moist heat may be used for increasing blood flow and making tissue more pliable; and ice stroking can be used after trigger points have been treated, for complete lengthening of the jaw muscles. For a real-life example, see Case history 13.6.

For the first 24 hours of an acute flare-up of TMD, apply ice or perform ice massage just above the mandible, until the area is numb, for 10 minutes every hour. (Clients can also do this at home.) After 24 hours, change to moist heat for 15 minutes, applying this five or six times a day. A hot pack applied to the masseter muscle can cause a significant increase in local blood flow and oxygen saturation (Okada, 2005). Contrast treatments can also be used to further increase circulation, ease pain, and decrease inflammation. Massage techniques that decrease muscle tension in the jaw and facial muscles or address misalignment of cranial bones may relieve pain as well.

In one case study, a combination of massage, hydrotherapy, and self-care measures yielded very positive results. The client received two 45-minute massages per week for five weeks: she also had a home-care regimen of stretches, self-massage, postural training, and a contrast treatment that used moist heat for 10 minutes, followed by ice massage until the jaw area was numb. Ultimately, she was able to open her mouth significantly wider, had significantly greater neck range of motion, decreased muscle tone, and a decline in TMD pain from 7/10 to 3/10 (Pierson, 2011).

Chapter thirteen

BACKGROUND

Aminah Salman, a retired schoolteacher, visited a massage therapist due to jaw muscle tightness and pain. When she was 10 years old Aminah received a blow to her left mandible, and has had pain there off and on ever since. Two years ago, she had ten injections into her left mandible before a root canal procedure and from that time on, had pain and muscle spasms in her jaw whenever her mouth was open for even a short time. One month ago she again visited her dentist, and had her mouth open for 45 minutes during dental work: now she was in severe pain and her jaw and neck muscles were incredibly tight. She was taking muscle relaxant medication prescribed by her doctor, but with little relief.

TREATMENT

The massage therapist began the session by wringing out small towels in 104°F (40°C) water and wrapping them around Aminah's jaw and the sides of her face. Aminah felt her muscles start to relax almost immediately. The therapist used hot towels for 20 minutes, replacing each cooled one with a fresh hot one. At the same time she performed cranial holds on Aminah's head, and Swedish techniques on her neck and shoulders. After she removed the last hot compress she performed gentle massage on Aminah's jaw and entire face. Afterwards she finished with two more hot compresses. Aminah felt great relief, and she called the next day to say she had used hot compresses on her face at bedtime and slept much better than she had for many nights. She returned for massage a week later, saying she was still using hot towels at home during the day and before bed, and her tightness and pain had gradually decreased and were now almost gone.

TREATMENT

ICE PACK TO THE SIDE OF THE FACE AND TEMPLES TO RELIEVE SPASM

Cross-reference

See Chapters 4 and 5.

Duration

15 minutes.

Special instructions

It is possible to use a pre-made jaw wrap, with pockets for frozen gel packs and a strap to hold the wrap in place over the jaw. Do not put gel packs directly on the skin.

Procedure:

1. With the client in a side-lying position and the affected side up, place a thin cloth on the client's skin, over the side of the face and the temples, and then place the ice pack on top.

continued

TREATMENT *continued*

2. Remove the ice pack after 10 minutes. Gentle stretching may be performed at this time.

3. After stretching, apply a warm compress to the muscles for 5 minutes to prevent muscle soreness.

TREATMENT

MOIST HEAT APPLICATION TO REDUCE JAW MUSCLE TENSION

Cross-reference

See Chapter 4.

Duration and frequency

20 minutes. Perform during a massage session; or, as a home treatment when the TMD pain is particularly strong, the client may use moist heat as much as once an hour during the day.

TREATMENT *continued*

Procedure

1. Apply moist heat (hot water compresses, a hot gel pack or a mini-fomentation) over the painful area for 20 minutes.

2. Perform stretching and/or massage.

TREATMENT

CONTRAST TREATMENT TO THE JAW MUSCLES

Cross-reference

See Chapters 4 and 5.

Duration and frequency

15 minutes. Perform during a massage session; or as a home treatment the client may use it three or four times during the day.

Procedure

1. Apply moist heat (hot water compresses, baby hot water bottle, mini-fomentation) over the area for 5 minutes.

2. After 1 minute, remove the moist heat and apply an ice-water compress for 1 minute.

3. Apply the moist heat again.

4. After 3 minutes, remove the moist heat and apply an ice-water compress for 1 minute.

5. Repeat steps 3 and 4, for a total of three rounds of hot followed by cold.

6. Begin massage.

TERMINAL ILLNESS

The client who is terminally ill is likely having many unpleasant physical experiences, including pain, fatigue, nausea, difficulty breathing, unpleasant medical procedures and side-effects from medications. Emotional stress is often very high as well. Although many terminally ill people are receiving a great deal of caretaking touch as they are bathed, diapered, fed, dressed, propped up, rolled over, and having oxygen or intravenous lines adjusted, the non-demanding, comforting quality of massage can be the most enjoyable touch of their day. Many types of bodywork can relieve nervous tension as well as physical aches and pains, and in a hospice situation they may reduce the amount of medication that is given for pain and anxiety (Pedersen, 2018). Some forms of hydrotherapy may also be particularly helpful because they soothe, comfort, and relieve pain. They may also be an alternative to medications. For example, patients taking opioids generally become constipated after a short time, and hydrotherapy and massage may relieve the constipation which would otherwise need other medications to alleviate it. Local salt glows, warm compresses and warm hand baths or footbaths gently promote circulation and are nurturing and relaxing. A Japanese study which gave 20 terminally ill cancer patients a series of eight warm foot soaks with lavender oil combined with foot reflexology found that all of the patients were significantly less fatigued afterwards (Kohara, 2004).

Moist heat applications can help relieve different types of pain, from digestive discomfort to the pain of bone metastases. Neutral or warm baths ease the pull of gravity and soothe pain. Simple hydrotherapy treatments may also prove invaluable in cases where massage has been prescribed but the patient has never had a massage before. As a gentle introduction, a warm hand or footbath along with massage can soothe and relax the terminally ill person. The sensory stimulation footbath on page 147 may be the perfect treatment for someone who is ill and in danger of being isolated physically and emotionally. Below are some specific examples of how hydrotherapy was used to improve clients' last days, based upon the author's own experience:

- An 82-year-old woman was living in a nursing home because she required 24-hour care. She suffered from diabetes, dementia, and chronic urinary tract infections, was incontinent and barely conscious, and lay in a fetal position much of the time. Massage was relaxing for her, though challenging to give due to her fetal position. However, every few days staff transported her in a "bath gurney," a chaise-lounge-like contraption, down the corridor to the tub room. They carefully lowered her into a 100°F (38°C) tub and gave her a warm bath, which lasted about 20 minutes. Staff reported that she not only relaxed in the water but clearly enjoyed being there, and when taken back to her bed she slept longer and more deeply than usual. This routine was continued until barely a week before her death, when she became too fragile to move out of bed.

- A 20-year-old man with advanced metastatic cancer had severe pain, seizures, complete loss of vision, and was extremely stressed. His pain was well controlled by medications, but one of them left his skin extremely sensitive to the touch. Massage with this young adult was a challenge due to his skin condition, but using warm foot or arm baths followed by light pressure massage worked very well. Sometimes, simply having warm water poured gently over his hands and feet soothed and relaxed him. He had severe eyestrain due to his vision loss, and warm compresses over the eyes followed by gentle pressure on the acupuncture points around them greatly relieved it.

- A 70-year-old woman had a neurological disorder that caused spasticity in some muscles and weakness in others. Usually warm moist compresses and massage were used just for relaxation. However, a particular problem for this lady was increased tone in her sternocleidomastoid muscles, along with weakness in her hyoid muscles. The tightness in her sternocleidomastoids made it more difficult for her weak hyoid muscles to propel food down into her esophagus, and made it more likely that she would aspirate the food into her lungs. Treating sternocleidomastoid trigger points lowered their tone for a time, but another approach was suggested by an occupational therapist who was part of the hospice team: at mealtimes, warm moist compresses applied directly over the sternocleidomastoids lowered their tone, and at the same time ice applied to her cheeks and inside her mouth stimulated tone in her swallowing muscles.

- An 87-year-old man who lived in a memory care facility had dementia, chronic muscle twitching, and failure to thrive. He was generally awake most of the night and slept during much of the day. Only two interventions would help this frail gentleman to sleep at night: one was a massage at bedtime and the other was a warm shower. For this, staff used a hand sprayer with 106°F (41°C) water while he sat on a shower bench. He relaxed visibly as the warm water poured over him, the staff lathered his body and then rinsed him off with more warm water. When he was dried and put to bed, he would sleep well.

TREATMENT

LOCAL SALT GLOW AND WARM FOOTBATH
Cross-reference
See Chapters 6 and 10.
Duration and frequency
5–10 minutes. Perform during a massage session.
Procedure
1. Have the client sit in a chair, with a towel on the floor. If he cannot sit up, this technique may be performed with him lying in bed with his knees bent and his feet in the container.
2. Place a container of warm water (98–102°F or 37–39°C) on top of the towel and place the client's feet in it.
3. Take one foot out of the water and use a small amount of Epsom salts to perform a salt glow on it. Either hold the client's foot over the footbath while you do this, or lay his foot on the towel next to it.
4. Place the client's foot back in the warm footbath.
5. Repeat steps 4 and 5 with the client's other foot.
6. Holding the client's first foot above the footbath, pour clean water over it and then move the footbath slightly so that the client may put his foot on the towel.
7. Repeat step 6 with the other foot; and after pouring water over it, move the footbath off the towel entirely so there is room for the second foot on the towel.
8. Dry the feet and cover them with the towel to keep them warm.
9. Perform massage of the feet and lower legs while the client remains seated in the chair or is resting on a therapy table. Cover the feet with socks when massage is completed.

TRIGEMINAL NEURALGIA

Trigeminal neuralgia (TN) is a neuropathic disorder characterized by episodes of intense facial pain. It has been called "the worst pain known to mankind" and episodes can last from a few seconds to several minutes or hours. In some cases, it may be a more constant, aching, burning type of pain. The episodes of pain can be triggered by cold winds, chewing, drinking, shaving, even toothbrushing. TN attacks can get progressively worse with time, and the periods of relief from pain can become shorter, while medications to treat it may become less effective over time. TN patients will experience tremendous stress and possibly become depressed. The neck and shoulder muscles can spasm from pain and thus change the way the sufferer holds his or her head. It is not completely clear, but it is thought that TN is caused by compression at the trigeminal root by an enlarged or lengthened artery. Mainstream treatment includes anticonvulsant, muscle relaxant or antidepressant medications. A variety of surgeries are used if medications are no longer helpful, but these often have serious side-effects. The most successful surgery moves the blood vessel off the nerve it is compressing. However, many osteopaths and craniosacral practitioners believe temporal bone distortions, possibly beginning with facial trauma, can squeeze the trigeminal nerve at the root. Some practitioners have reported success with osteopathic or craniosacral therapy and neural mobilization, while lymphatic drainage may address pain by increasing the movement of fluids (Kratz, 2017; Nerman, 2014). Physical therapist D. Khanal used a combination treatment consisting of a TENS unit, neck exercises, moist heat over the trapezius, deep breathing, and advice on managing TN, which significantly reduced pain in sufferers. This was a small pilot study and more research is needed (Khanal, 2014).

How can hydrotherapy and bodywork be combined to help clients suffering from TN? Try one or more of the hot and cold therapies outlined below, along with appropriate hands-on work.

Many people find relief from trigeminal neuralgia pain by applying moist heat to the affected area. Clients can do this by pressing a hot water bottle or hot compress to the painful spot, or breathing steam through the nostril of the painful side; you can try these in your office before hands-on work. Whole-body heat may be helpful: some have tried sitting in hot saunas, while Agatha Thrash, MD, recommends a series of hot baths, while continually sponging the face with cloths wrung out in ice water (Thrash, 2015). Cold may also help relieve the pain, although the client would not enjoy this if she or he is one of the many trigeminal neuralgia sufferers for whom cold triggers symptoms. The client may have to try both heat and cold to find out which works best. A cold pack wrapped in a thin cloth or an ice pack may numb the area.

UNDERSTIMULATION

Sensory stimulation helps ground us by informing the brain of our position in space, our movements, and our relationship to other people and objects in the environment: in short, appropriate sensory stimulation is food for the brain.

Any of us who do not receive enough sensory stimulation or touch can lose the sense of our bodies being whole and strong and may also become bored, isolated or depressed. Those most at risk of understimulation are clients who have chronic illnesses, mobility problems that leave them housebound or bedridden, various developmental disabilities, and brain problems such as dementia. All can benefit greatly from massage and hydrotherapy treatments, which give tremendous information about the body in a soothing and nurturing way. (See Case history 6.1 on page 149, which includes a series of small stimulation techniques.) As long as the therapist is sensitive and does not overload the person, almost any bodywork technique can be helpful. Hydrotherapy treatments can add even more sensory stimulation with the feel of water on the skin, plus different temperatures, textures and pressures. Essential oils added to the treatments give yet another sensory experience.

Simply begin your treatments with milder temperatures, less brisk frictions, and slower, less vigorous strokes. Try the sensory stimulation footbath in Chapter 6 or the *"World's best back massage"* on page 235. A wheelchair-using client of the author who had multiple sclerosis came by special bus to a swimming pool five days a week. He was helped into a flotation vest and was then transferred by sling into a pool. A swimming coach put him through nearly an hour of range of motion, stretching, and other exercises. He then took a shower, read the newspaper and visited with other patrons as he waited for his ride home. This man was getting a full range of sensory stimulation, unlike many other patients in his situation who never left their homes or received therapy.

CHAPTER SUMMARY

In this chapter you have learned how to adapt a wide variety of hydrotherapy techniques to clients with many different conditions. This will allow you to "fine-tune" your work for many different situations and needs, helping to make you a more informed, versatile and creative therapist who creates better outcomes for your clients.

REVIEW QUESTIONS

Essay questions

1. Name three different types of chronic pain, and discuss their treatment with hydrotherapy.
2. Name three conditions that involve difficult movement, and discuss their treatment with hydrotherapy.
3. Name three conditions that involve low back pain.
4. Describe three options for hydrotherapy treatment of a client with acute low back pain who has been referred by his doctor one day after the episode began.
5. Name two muscular conditions which may be affected by ice-water immersion, and discuss how immersion affects them.
6. Describe three conditions for which steam treatments are helpful, and explain why they are effective.
7. List three non-thermal treatments that may be helpful for those who cannot tolerate local heat.
8. Name three helpful treatments that are performed in a shower, and for what conditions.

Fill in the blanks

9. Diabetics must be carefully treated with hydrotherapy due to _____: in particular, _____ to the feet is contraindicated.
10. Name four conditions for which contrast baths may be used: _____, [Four conditions, so: _____, _____, _____, and _____.]
11. Muscle cramps are _____ and _____, while muscle spasms are _____ and _____.

12. Pool therapy is recommended for patients with _____, _____, and _____.
13. Full hot baths can be useful for _____ _____, _____, and _____, but not for patients with _____.

Multiple choice

14. Which one of the following is not a significant risk factor for the development of osteoarthritis?
    A. Joint injury
    B. Depression
    C. Overweight
    D. Hypermobility

15. Which one of the following is a common complaint of patients with osteoarthritis?
    A. Sensitivity to heat
    B. Shock-like pain
    C. Onset of symptoms in teenage years
    D. Stiffness and pain

16. Which type of headache is caused by food allergies?
    A. Sinus headache
    B. Stress headache
    C. Migraine headache
    D. Post-concussion headache

17. Which of these is *not* a helpful strategy for a migraine headache?
    A. Contrast shower
    B. Hot pack to head
    C. Cold stones or ice packs to neck
    D. Hot footbath

REVIEW QUESTIONS *continued*

18. Select the one substance that should not be used for dry skin:

A. Honey

B. Emollient cream

C. Oatmeal

D. Rubbing alcohol

19. Contrast treatments may be used for all but one of the following. Which is the exception?

A. Migraine headache

B. Sciatica

C. Osteoarthritis

D. TMD

E. Adhesive capsulitis

20. Salt glows may be used for all but one of the following. Which is the exception?

A. Eczema

B. Chronic low back pain

C. Multiple sclerosis

D. Terminal illness

Matching

21.

1.	Continuous neutral bath	**A.**	Fibromyalgia
2.	Mustard plaster	**B.**	Muscle weakness
3.	Moist heat	**C.**	Parkinson's disease
4.	Ice-water immersion	**D.**	Rotator cuff tear

22.

1.	Contrast compress	**A.**	Migraine headache
2.	Ice-water immersion	**B.**	Low back spasm
3.	Full hot bath	**C.**	Eyestrain
4.	Hot footbath	**D.**	Muscle spasticity

23.

1.	Salt glow of the feet	**A.**	TMD
2.	Continuous neutral bath	**B.**	Diabetes
3.	Moist heat followed by stretching and ice	**C.**	Rheumatoid arthritis
4.	No hot footbath	**D.**	Terminal illness

24.

1.	Morning stiffness	**A.**	Ice pack
2.	Local rheumatoid arthritis	**B.**	Hot bath or shower
3.	Gouty pain	**C.**	Paraffin bath
4.	Muscle contraction headache	**D.**	Scalp bath

References

AMTA. Massage Therapy and Integrative Care and Pain Management. American Massage Therapy Association, Evanston, IL 2018

AMTA. Massage therapy can help improve sleep. https://www.amtamassage.org/approved_position_statements/Massage-Therapy-Can-Help-Improve-Sleep.html [Accessed July 2019]

Ardic F et al. Effects of balneotherapy on serum IL-1, PGE2 and LTB4 levels in fibromyalgia patients. Rheum Intl, 2007; 27(5): 441–6

Aftimos S. Myofascial pain in children. N Zealand Medical J; 1989: 440–1

Beswick A. What proportion of patients report long-term pain after total knee or replacement for osteoarthritis? BMJ Open 2012; 2(1)

Brown TD et al. Posttraumatic osteoarthritis: a first estimate of incidence, prevalence, and burden of disease. J Orthop Trauma, 2006 Nov-Dec; 20(10): 739–44

Carpentier P. Balneotherapy improves symptoms of chronic venous insufficiency. J Vasc Surg 2014; 59(2): 447–54

Casciaro Y. Massage therapy treatment and outcomes for a patient with Parkinson's Disease: a case report. Int J Ther Massage Bodywork 2016; 9(1): 11–8

Cassileth BR. Massage therapy for symptom control: outcome study at a major cancer center. J Pain Symptom Manage 2004; 28(3): 244–9

CDC: Center for Disease Control and Prevention. https://wonder.cdc.org 2017

Chatchawan U et al. Effects of Thai foot massage on balance performance in diabetic patients with peripheral neuropathy. Med Sci Monit Basic Res 2015; 21: 68–75

Cherkin A. Comparison of massage therapy and usual medical care for chronic low back pain. Ann Int Med 2011; 155(1): 128

Chet J, Liang C, Shaw F. Facilitation of sensory and motor recovery by thermal intervention for the hemiplegic upper limb in acute stroke patients. Stroke 2005; 36: 2665

Cowan T. The Fourfold Path to Healing–Working with the Laws of Nutrition, Therapeutics, Movement and Meditation in the Art of Medicine. Washington, DC: New Trends Pub, 2007

Cunningham JE et al. Case report of a patient with chemotherapy-induced peripheral neuropathy treated with manual therapy (massage). Support Care Cancer 19(9); 2011(1): 473–6

Dahlhamer J et al. Prevalence of chronic pain and high-impact chronic pain among adults – United States, 2016. In MMWR Morb Mortality Weekly Report

D'Ambrosia RD. Epidemiology of osteoarthritis. Orthopedics 2005; 28: 5201–5

Dinsley J. Charcoalremedies.com. Coldwater, MI: Gatekeeper Books, 2005

Doub L. Hydrotherapy. Fresno, CA: self-published manuscript, 1971

Duval C et al. The effect of Trager therapy on the level of evoked stretch responses in patients with Parkinson's disease and rigidity. J Manipulative Physiol Ther 2002; 25(7): 455–64

Ebben MR, Spielman AJ. The effects of distal limb warming on sleep latency. Int J Behav Med 2006; 13(3): 221–8

Evcik D et al. The effect of balneotherapy on fibromyalgia patients. Rheumatology International 2002; 22(2): 56–9

Fagan J. Lipophil-mediated reduction of toxicants in humans: an evaluation of an Ayurvedic detoxification procedure. Alternative Therapies in Health and Medicine 2002; 8(5)

Field T. Children with asthma have improved pulmonary functions after massage therapy. J Pediatr 1998 May; 132(5): 854–8

Field T. Juvenile rheumatoid arthritis: benefits from massage therapy. J Pediatr Psychol 1997; 22(5): 607–17

Field T et al. Fibromyalgia pain and substance P decrease and sleep improves after massage therapy. J Clin Rheumatol 2002; 8: 72–6

Forestier R. Balneotherapy for treatment of chronic venous insufficiency. Vasa 2014; 43: 365–71

Global Asthma Network. The Global Asthma Report 2018. www.globalasthmareport.org/resources

Gok M. The effects of aromatherapy massage and reflexology on pain and fatigue in patients with rheumatoid arthritis: a randomized controlled trial. Pain Manag Nurs 2016; 17(2): 140–9

Goldberg P. Over 1,000 Quick and Easy Pain Remedies. Emmaus, PA Pa: Rodale Press, 1997

Graedon J. Best Choices from the People's Pharmacy. New York: Rodale, 2008

Hardt J, Jacobsen C, Goldberg J et al. Prevalence of chronic pain in a representative sample in the United States. Pain Med 2008; 9: 803–12

Harris R. Subluxation and Distortion of Joints without Fracture. Los Angeles: San Lucas Press, 1961

Harty R. Myofascial release for fibromyalgia. Massage Magazine 191; 2012: 50–4

Helal O. Change in the great saphenous vein diameter in response to contrast baths and exercise: a randomized clinical trial. Journal of American Science, Feb 2013; 9(3): 476–83

Hooper PL. Hot-tub therapy for type 2 diabetes mellitus. N Engl J Med 1999; 341(12): 924–5

Hooper PL. Personal communication with author. 10 August 2006

Hou WH. Treatment effects of massage therapy in depressed people: a meta-analysis. J Clin Psychiatry 2010; 71(7): 894–901

Iwamoto K. Effects of friction massage of the popliteal fossa on blood flow velocity of the popliteal vein. J Phys Ther 2017 Mar: 29(3): 511–14

Jacobs S et al. Pilot study of massage to improve sleep and fatigue in hospitalized adolescents with cancer. Pediatric Blood & Cancer, Jan 2016

Kanda K, Tochihara Y, Ohnaka T. Bathing before sleep in the young and in the elderly. European Journal of Appl Physiol Occup Physiol 1999; 80(2): 71–5

Karel R. Treatments involving heat show promise for alleviating depression. Psychiatric News, 17 May 2018

Karuchi K, Cajochen C, Werth E, Wirz-Justice A. Warm feet promote the rapid onset of sleep. Nature 1999; 401(6748): 36–7

Chapter thirteen

Kerihuel JC. Effect of activated charcoal dressings on healing outcomes of chronic wounds. J Wound Care 2010; 19(5): 208, 210–12, 214–15

Khanal D. Is there any role of physiotherapy in Fothergill's disease? J Yoga Phys Ther 2014; 4: 2

Kohara H. Combined modality treatment of aromatherapy, foot-soak, and reflexology relieves fatigue in patients with cancer. J Palliat Med 2004; 7(6): 791–6

Kratz S. Manual therapies reduce pain associated with trigeminal neuralgia. Journal of Pain Management and Therapy; 2017: 1(1)

Kujala UM et al. Knee osteoarthritis in former runners, soccer players, weight lifters, and shooters. Arthritis Rheum, 1995; 38(4): 539–46

Lawrence C. Estimates of the prevalence of arthritis and other rheumatic conditions in the United States, Part II. Arthritis Rheum 2008; 58(1): 26–35

Liao WC. Effects of passive body heating on body temperature and sleep regulation in the elderly: a systematic review. Int J Nurs Stud 2002; 39(8): 803–19

Lowe W. Orthopedic Massage, 3rd edn. London: Churchill Livingstone, 2015

Malinski M et al. The effect of massage on improving the quality of life for adult chronic asthma patients. Journal of Allergy and Immunology Abstracts 1995; 95(1): 2

Mashadhi N. Anti-oxidative and anti-inflammatory effects of ginger in health and physical activity: review of current evidence. Int J Prev Med 2013; 4(1): S36–S42

Masuda A et al. The effects of repeated thermal therapy for patients with chronic pain. Psychother Psychosom 2005; 74(5): 288–94

Matsumoto G et al. Effects of thermal therapy combining sauna therapy and underwater exercise in patients with fibromyalgia. Complement Ther Clin Pract 2011; 3: 162–6

Matz H. Balneotherapy in dermatology. Dermatol Ther 2003; 16(2): 132–40

McDonald G. Medicine Hands, Massage Therapy for People with Cancer. Forres, Scotland: Findhorn Press, 2014

Mok E. The effects of slow-stroke back massage on anxiety and shoulder pain in elderly stroke patients. Complementary Therapies in Nursing and Midwifery 2004; 10(4): 209–16

Molski P. Manual lymphatic drainage improves the quality of life in patients with chronic venous disease: a randomized controlled trial. Arch Med Sci 2013; 9(3): 452–8

Nedley N. Depression: the Way Out, 2nd edn. Hagerstown, Maryland MD: Review and Herald Pub, 2002

Nerman M. Healing Pain and Injury. Pt. Richmond, CA: Bay Tree Publishing, 2014

Okada K, Yamaguchi T, Minowa K, Inque N. The influence of hot pack therapy on the blood flow in masseter muscles. Journal of Oral Rehabilitation 2005; 32(7): 480–6

Oosterveld FG et al. Infrared sauna in patients with rheumatoid arthritis and ankylosing spondylitis. A pilot study showing good tolerance, short-term improvement of pain and stiffness, and a trend towards long-term beneficial effects. Clin Rheumatol 2009; 28(1): 29–34

Packman, H. Ice Therapy. Victoria, BC; Trafford Publishing, 2006

Patricolo G et al. Beneficial effects of guided imagery or clinical massage on the status of patients in a progressive care unit. Critical Care Nurse 2017; 37(1): 62

Pedersen K. Tactile massage reduces rescue doses for pain and anxiety: an observational study. BMJ Support Palliat Care 2018; 8(1): 30–3

Perez RS. Evidence-based guidelines for complex regional pain syndrome. BMC Neurology 2010; 10: 20

Perlman A, Sabina A et al. Massage therapy for osteoarthritis of the knee; a randomized controlled trial. Arch Intern Med 2006; 166(22): 2533–8

Pierson M. Changes in temporomandibular joint dysfunction symptoms following massage therapy: a case report. Int J Ther Massage Bodywork 2011; 4(4): 37–47

Raymann RJ, Swaab DF, Van Someren EJ. Cutaneous warming promotes sleep onset. AM J Physiol Regul Integ Comp Physio 2005; 288(6): 1589–97

Renner J. The Home Remedies Handbook. Lincolnwood, IL Illinois: Publications International, 1993

Rice BI. Clinical benefits of training patients to voluntarily increase peripheral blood flow: the WarmFeet intervention. Diabetes Educ 2007; 33(3): 44

Roach KE et al. Biomechanical aspects of occupation and osteoarthritis of the hip: a case control study. J Rheumatol 1994; 21(12): 2334–40

Robison JG. Therapeutic massage during chemotherapy and/or biotherapy infusions: patient perceptions of pain, fatigue, nausea, anxiety, and satisfaction. Clin J Oncol Nurs 2016; 20(2): E34–40

Rosenthal M. Psychosomatic study of infantile eczema. Pediatrics 1952; 10: 581–92

Saradeth B et al. A single blind, randomized, controlled trial of hydrotherapy for varicose veins. Vasa 1991; 20(2): 147–52

Sarno J. Healing Back Pain: The Mind-Body Connection. New York, NY: Warner Books, 1991

Schneider M, Larkin M. Movement for Self-Healing. New York: Arcana, 2004

Shafizadegan Z. Comparison of effects of contrast bath in circulation of contralateral lower limb in type 2 diabetic and healthy women. J of Rehab 2016; 3(3): 62–6

Sherman K et al. The diagnosis and treatment of chronic back pain by acupuncturists, chiropractors, and massage therapists. Clinical Journal of Pain 2006; 22: 227–34

Shevchuk NA. Adapted cold shower as a potential treatment for depression. Med Hypotheses 2008; 70(5): 995–1001

Simons DG, Travell JG, Simons LS. Travell and Simons' Myofascial Pain and Dysfunction: the Trigger Point Manual, Vol 1: Upper Half of Body, 2nd edn. Baltimore, MD: Lippincott, Williams and Wilkins, 1999

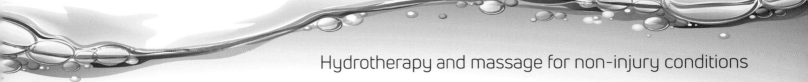
Sinclair M. Environmental costs of pain management pharmaceuticals versus physical therapies. Integrative Medicine 2012; 11(5): 38–44

Sinclair M. Pediatric Massage Therapy, 2nd edn. Baltimore, MD: Lippincott, Williams and Wilkins, 2004

Sinclair M. The use of abdominal massage to treat chronic constipation. J Bodyw Mov Ther 2011; 15(4): 436–45

SLEEP. Sleep in America Polls. https://www.sleepfoundation.org/professionals/sleep-america-polls [Accessed July 2019]

Sung E, Tochihara Y. Effects of bathing and hot footbath on sleep in winter. J Physiol Anthropol Appl Human Sci 2000; Jan 19(1): 21–7

Thanakiatpinyo T. The efficacy of traditional Thai massage in decreasing spasticity in elderly stroke patients. Clin Interv Aging 2014; 9: 1311–14

Thrash A. Nature's Healing Practices. Seale, AL: TEACH Services Publishing, 2015

Tidhar D. Aqua lymphatic therapy in women who suffer from breast cancer treatment-related lymphedema: a randomized controlled study. Support Care Cancer 2010; Mar

Ucler S. Cold therapy in migraine patients: open-label, non-controlled pilot Study. Evid-based Compl and Alt Med 2006; 3(4) 489–93

Upledger J. Your Inner Physician and You: Craniosacral Therapy and SomatoEmotional Release. Berkeley, CA: North Atlantic Books, 1997

Wasserman P. Psychogenic basis for abdominal pain in children and adolescents. Journal of the American Academy of Child and Adolescent Psychiatry 1988; 27(2): 179

Weinstein J. Herniated discs improve with either surgical or non-surgical treatment. JAMA 2006; 296: 2441–50

Wine Z. Massage for diabetes. Massage Magazine, March–April 1996

Witt P. Trager psychophysical integration: a method to improve chest mobility of patients with chronic lung disease. Phys Ther 1986; 66(2): 214

Woods R. A massage protocol for peripheral neuropathy. Massage Today 2012; (12): 2

Yang HL et al. The effects of warm-water footbath on relieving fatigue and insomnia of the gynecologic cancer patients on chemotherapy. Cancer Nurs 2010 Nov–Dec; 33(6): 454–60

Yang, M et al. Effects of long-term exposure to air pollution on the incidence of type 2 diabetes mellitus: a meta-analysis of cohort studies. Environ Sci Pollut Res Int. 2020 Jan; 27(1): 798–811.

Yilmaz Y. Immediate effect of manual therapy on respiratory functions and inspiratory muscle strength in patients with COPD. Int J Chron Obstruct Pulmon Dis 2016; Jun 20

Yokum R. Restless Legs syndrome: Relief and Hope for Sleepless Victims of a Hidden Epidemic. New York: Fireside, 2006

Yzer JA (A). Cooling for Lymphedema. Pembroke Pines, FL: South Florida Breast Cancer Rehab Center, 2017

Yzer JA (B). Local skin cooling as an aid to the management of patients with breast cancer related lymphedema and fibrosis of the arm or breast. Lymphology 2017; 50(2): 56–66

Zhang Y. Epidemiology of osteoarthritis. Clin Geriatr Med 2010; 26(3): 355–69

Recommended resources

Buchman D. The Complete Book of Water Healing. New York: Instant Improvement, Inc., 1994

Moor F et al. Manual of Hydrotherapy and Massage. Hagerstown, MD: Review and Herald Publishers, 1964

Thomas C. Simple Water Treatments for the Home. Loma Linda, CA Ca: Loma Linda University School of Health, 1977

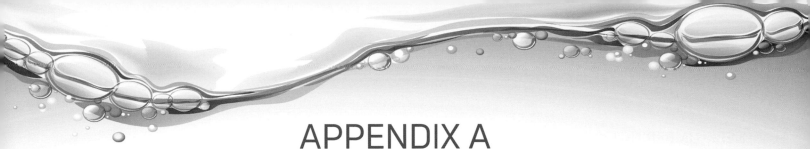

APPENDIX A
Simple hydrotherapy record and self-treatment handouts

TREATMENTS

1. Warm Epsom salts bath.
2. Hot shower and neck-limbering exercises.
3. Contrast treatment with hand-held sprayer.
4. Ice massage.
5. Whole-body contrast shower.
6. Heat-trapping compress.
7. Castor oil pack.

Your home hydrotherapy record

Name of treatment:

How often:

Day of the week	Treatment completed	Treatment completed	Treatment completed	How I felt after the treatment(s)
Monday				
Tuesday				
Wednesday				
Thursday				
Friday				
Saturday				
Sunday				

WARM EPSOM SALTS BATH

Your massage therapist may have recommended an Epsom salts bath for bruises, sprains in the sub-acute stage, soreness after exercise, soreness after massage, nervous tension, arthritis pain, or as a general tonic.

Do not take a warm bath if you have any of the following conditions: seizure disorder, loss of sensation (lack of feeling), multiple sclerosis, inability to tolerate heat, ingestion of alcohol or drugs, or obesity. Do not eat for at least one hour before you take a bath.

You will need a water thermometer, 2–4 cups of Epsom salts for an adult or 1 cup Epsom salts for a child, a bath towel and a bathmat. Grab bars are recommended.

Procedure

1. Pour the Epsom salts directly under the spigot as soon as the tub begins filling with warm water, to make sure they dissolve completely.
2. Get carefully into the tub when it is half full; use a grab bar if you feel unsteady.
3. Adjust the temperature to your tolerance as the bath finishes filling; check with a thermometer to make sure it is 98–102°F (37–39°C).
4. Stay in for 15–20 minutes.
5. At the end of your bath, wash the Epsom salts water off thoroughly.
6. Get out of the tub carefully, so you do not slip.
7. Apply a moisturizing lotion or oil to your skin, then dress.
8. Lie down and rest for 20 minutes or more.

Special tips or instructions

_____

_____

_____

_____

_____

_____

_____

Appendix A

NECK-LIMBERING EXERCISES IN A HOT SHOWER

Your massage therapist may have recommended a hot shower and neck-limbering exercises for tightness in the neck muscles caused by chronically tight muscles, stress, injury, soreness after exercise, muscle spasms or arthritis pain.

Do not stay in a long hot shower if you have any of the following conditions: cardiovascular problems, diabetes, hepatitis, lymphedema, multiple sclerosis, seizure disorders, hypothyroid conditions, loss of sensation (lack of feeling) or any condition that might make you unsteady on your feet, an inability to tolerate heat, or ingestion of alcohol or drugs. However, you may take a short hot shower of about 5 minutes.

You will need a water thermometer, a bath towel and a bathmat. Grab bars are recommended.

Procedure

1. Turn on your shower to hot and get carefully into the shower; use a grab bar if you feel unsteady.

2. Adjust the temperature so it is hot but to your tolerance (about 105–115°F; 40.5–46°C).

3. Let the water beat upon your neck for at least 3 minutes; then, very slowly and with no pain or straining, continue to stand with the hot water beating on the neck muscles while drawing the letters of the alphabet with your nose. This will gently release muscle tension and improve range of motion.

4. Stay in for 5–10 minutes, no longer.

5. Get out of the shower carefully, so you do not slip.

Special tips or instructions

_____
_____
_____
_____
_____
_____
_____

CONTRAST TREATMENT WITH HAND-HELD SPRAYER

Your massage therapist may have recommended a contrast shower over one part of the body, with a hand-held sprayer, for soreness after exercise, muscle spasm, muscle fatigue, arthritis pain, tendonitis, joint swelling from a sprain or after the removal of a cast, or simply to increase local circulation.

Do not perform a contrast shower if you are cold, or if you have any of the following conditions: peripheral vascular disease such as diabetes, Buerger's disease, arteriosclerosis of the lower extremities, Raynaud's syndrome or loss of sensation (lack of feeling).

Never spray water over implanted devices such as cardiac pacemakers, ports, defibrillators or pumps.

You will need a hand-held sprayer, a bath towel and a bathmat. Grab bars are recommended.

Procedure

1. Step carefully into the shower stall or bathtub; if you are going to spray the legs or feet, you may want to sit on the side of the bathtub.

2. Spray the area with water as hot as you can comfortably tolerate for 2 minutes.

3. Spray the area with water as cold as you can comfortably tolerate for 30 seconds.

4. Repeat steps 2 and 3.

5. Repeat steps 2 and 3, for a total of three rounds.

6. Get out of the shower carefully, so you do not slip.

7. Dry the area off and dress quickly to avoid chilling.

Special tips or instructions

_____
_____
_____
_____
_____
_____
_____

ICE MASSAGE

Your massage therapist may have recommended ice massage after a muscle strain, joint sprain, OR bruise, or for acute muscle spasm, arthritis pain, stiff or spastic muscles, bursitis, or muscle weakness.

Do not perform ice massage if you really dislike cold, have Raynaud's syndrome, Buerger's disease, a prior history of frostbite, peripheral vascular disease, a lack of feeling (impaired sensation), marked hypertension, arteriosclerosis or diminished circulation.

Use a chunk of ice made by freezing a paper cup full of water. Perform ice massage for about 5–10 minutes, until the area is numb.

Procedure

1. If necessary, drape towels around the area to be iced.
2. Hold the cup of ice in one hand and gently rub it in a circular motion over the area you are treating, and a few inches above and below the area as well.
3. Continue until the area is numb (about 5–10 minutes). Generally you will feel first a sensation of cold; second, a burning/pricking feeling; third, an aching sensation; and fourth, numbness. When you experience these sensations, they are a good sign that the ice is doing its work. Take the ice away as soon as the area is truly numb.
4. Remove the ice; dry the skin and cover it.
5. If your massage therapist has given you exercises to do, perform them now.

Special tips or instructions

_____
_____
_____
_____
_____
_____

WHOLE-BODY CONTRAST SHOWER

Your massage therapist may have recommended a contrast shower to increase your general wellness, to relieve post-exercise soreness, or to help you tolerate cold better.

Do not take contrast showers if you really dislike cold; have Raynaud's syndrome, cardiovascular problems, diabetes, hepatitis, lymphedema, advanced kidney disease, multiple sclerosis, seizure disorders, hyperthyroid conditions, lack of feeling, or loss of sensation; or if you are cold, very tired, pregnant, or have just eaten a meal.

If you are not accustomed to very hot or cold temperatures, try a warm shower alternated with a cool shower at first, to be sure you can tolerate it.

Procedure

1. Get carefully into the shower. Use a grab bar if you feel unsteady.
2. Adjust the water so it is as hot as you can comfortably tolerate.
3. Stay under the water for 2–5 minutes.
4. Change the water temperature to as cold as you can comfortably tolerate for 30 seconds to 1 minute.
5. Change the water temperature back to hot for 2 minutes.
6. Change the water temperature to cold for 30 seconds to 1 minute.
7. Change the water temperature back to hot for 2 minutes.
8. Change the water temperature to cold for 30 seconds to 1 minute.
9. Get out of the shower carefully, so you do not slip.
10. Towel off, and dress quickly to avoid chilling.
11. Enjoy the feeling of warmth and invigoration.

Special tips or instructions

_____
_____
_____
_____

Appendix A

_____

_____

_____

_____

HEAT-TRAPPING COMPRESS

Your massage therapist may have recommended a heat-trapping compress for joint problems, peripheral neuropathy or pain in any part. A compress for the feet is a traditional naturopathic treatment for nasal congestion. This mild application raises skin temperature by a few degrees over a few hours, and safely increases blood flow to the area. Anti-inflammatory herbs are sometimes added to the compress water.

You will need one or two thicknesses of loosely woven cloth that are wide enough to cover the area and long enough to wrap completely around the part, plus one outer covering of insulating cloth which is somewhat larger than the woven cloth, plus safety pins to secure the compress. Different sizes may be used for various parts: for example, Figures A and B show a heating compress

for the wrist, and cotton socks covered by dry socks may be used for the feet.

Procedure

1. Your body should be warm before you apply the compress.
2. Wet the woven cloth in tap water, and wring it lightly so it does not drip.
3. Wrap the wet inner cloth snugly around the part.
4. Wrap the outer cloth snugly as well, and pin it.
5. Leave the compress in place for several hours or overnight.
6. When you take the compress off, rub the area briefly with a cold washcloth or hold it under cold running water, then dry it briskly.

Special tips or instructions

_____

_____

_____

_____

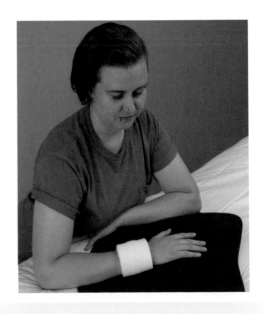

FIGURE A
Therapist applying the wet cloth.

FIGURE B
The finished compress.

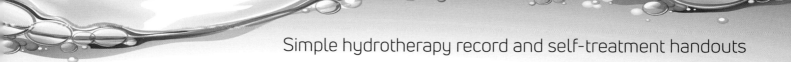

CASTOR OIL PACK

Your massage therapist may have recommended a castor oil pack for muscle or joint pain, tight, fibrous knots, scar tissue, sprains and strains after 24 hours, or to increase blood flow in an area.

You will need a bottle of castor oil, a flannel cloth, a metal pan or tray large enough to hold the flannel, a piece of plastic wrap slightly bigger than the flannel, and a heat source to keep the pack warm, such as a microwave rice bag or hot water bottle. Do not use a heating pad unless it has an automatic shut-off feature. Rice bags and hot water bottles cool off gradually and are safer.

Procedure

1. Cut or fold the flannel to the appropriate size so there will be three layers of cloth (a disposable bed or incontinence pad may be used). Place it on a metal pan or tray.

2. Pour castor oil over the flannel or pad so it is saturated but not dripping.

3. Make sure to check the area before you put it on: how does it look and feel?

4. Put the pack over the area of concern and cover it with the plastic to keep it off clothes or linens.

5. Leave the pack on for 1 hour or more – overnight is ideal.

6. When you remove it, rub any excess castor oil into the skin, especially over knots, adhesions or scars.

Special tips or instructions

_____

_____

_____

_____

_____

APPENDIX B
Pool therapy

Once we are immersed in water, there is a dramatic decrease in the pull of gravity on all our joints. When that effect is combined with water's universally soothing quality, powerful therapy can happen. Most community swimming pools are heated at 80–84°F (27–29°C), ideal for intense aerobic exercise that raises body temperature. Therapeutic pools, however, are heated from 86–90°F (30–32°C) and are ideal for those who suffer from musculoskeletal problems. There are many different approaches to pool therapy, such as *Watsu Aquatic Bodywork,* the *Bad Ragaz* and *Halliwick methods,* and *Cardiaquatics.*

Examples of the therapeutic effects of immersion are given below.

MUSCULOSKELETAL EFFECTS

Musculoskeletal effects include an increased range of motion, increased strength, and decreased pain.

Pool exercise reduces stiffness, weakness and musculoskeletal pain. Those with the following conditions can benefit:

- Chronic spasticity
- Multiple sclerosis
- Parkinson's disease
- Muscular dystrophy
- Cerebral palsy
- Hemiplegia
- Traumatic brain injury
- Osteo- or rheumatoid arthritis
- Poliomyelitis and post-polio syndrome
- Peripheral nerve injuries

- Acute and chronic low back strain
- Muscle contractures
- Recent injuries such as motor vehicle accidents
- Post-operative follow-up for muscle and tendon transplants, dislocations, joint replacements and bone grafts.

Massage therapist Meir Schneider, whose Self-Healing technique has been effective for many people with chronic musculoskeletal problems, combines gentle exercises in a warm bathtub or pool with massage (Schneider, 1994). Osteopathic doctor Maud Nerman believes that the single best exercise for healing an injured or painful neck, such as after a whiplash injury, is swimming with a mask or snorkel: this provides a gentle traction to the neck while buoyancy helps strained muscles and fascia relax (Nerman, 1998). During pregnancy, immersion reduces weightbearing, so exercising and stretching are easier and more effective: this helps prepare the woman's abdominal muscles for birth and speeds post-partum recovery.

IMPROVED CARDIAC AND RESPIRATORY FUNCTION

Even people without musculoskeletal problems can benefit from working out in a pool if they are elderly, frail, or obese, or find it difficult to exercise on land for other reasons. For example, elderly patients with emphysema or bronchial asthma typically find it very challenging to exercise, but when a group of them were put on an aerobic exercise program in 100°F (38°C) water, after two months their respiratory function and blood oxygen levels were greatly improved. These improvements were attributed to stronger respiratory muscles and better ability to clear their airways (Kurabayashi, 1997). While standing in a pool, hydrostatic pressure forces core stabilizers to contract and tighten against the pressure exerted by the water, which helps the person to stand in a more upright position, and can improve muscle strength and balance.

IMPROVEMENT IN SOME MEDICAL CONDITIONS

Some medical conditions will be helped by the compressive effect of hydrostatic pressure, which increases with depth of immersion. A person of average height who is standing immersed in water up to the neck will be under pressure of 1.74lb/in^2 (0.79kg/2cm^2). Since the lower body is deeper in the water, hydrostatic pressure causes fluid to be squeezed upwards. On average 23oz (700ml) of blood moves from the limbs to the thorax. Blood pressure receptors in the trunk register the greater amount of blood and the higher blood pressure that has been caused, and this stimulates the bladder to release fluid and thereby lower the pressure. This is why you feel like you need to urinate when you are swimming in a pool. This effect means that deep-water immersion can be an effective treatment for edema, including lymphedema and toxemia (Root-Bernstein, 1997). For more on immersion to reduce high levels of lead in the bloodstream, see Chapter 11. Scuba divers who have chronic lymphedema have found that the result of hydrostatic pressure has as great an effect as compression bandaging (Chikley, 2001). For pregnant women, the hydrostatic effect reduces varicose veins and swelling in the arms and legs, improves overall body circulation, and stabilizes blood pressure. Because immersion increases urination and excretion of salt, pool therapy has been used as an alternative to prescription medication for **pre-eclampsia** (Harper, 2005). This hydrostatic effect has yet another helpful medical application when cooling a dangerously overheated person: if a tub of ice water which is deep enough to submerge the trunk and limbs is used, blood is squeezed back into the thorax, which helps to maintain normal blood pressure. A cold shower, a cold footbath or spraying a person with cold water is not as effective (Roberts, 1998).

SOOTHING EFFECTS

A mother who gives birth in a warm whirlpool tub is likely to have an easier birth, as the water's soothing and relaxing quality eases the pain of uterine contractions, shortens labor, and helps the mother enjoy greater freedom of movement. As of 2021, hundreds of European and American hospitals offered waterbirths as an option. Also, when they are placed in a warm bath, fussy newborns often quiet remarkably. When Watsu Aquatic Bodywork is performed and the person floats free of gravity and cradled in the therapist's arms, the relaxing effects of massage are greatly enhanced.

SENSORY STIMULATION

People with disabilities can benefit from pool therapy for all the reasons mentioned above, and for one more: sensory stimulation. Children with conditions such as autism are often hypersensitive and benefit from learning to tolerate the sensations of water on the skin, buoyancy and hydrostatic pressure. Over time, as they not only learn a new skill but move better in water than they have ever done on dry land, children become more confident and less hyperactive (Davidson, 2018).

References

Chikly B. Silent Waves: The Theory and Practice of Lymph Drainage Therapy. IHH Publishing, 2001, p. 27

Davidson P. PT and aquatic therapist. Personal communication with the author, April 2018

Harper B. Choosing Waterbirth: A Midwife's Perspective. Rochester, VT: Healing Arts Press, 2005

Kurabayashi H et al. Effective physical therapy for chronic obstructive pulmonary disease: pilot study of exercise in hot spring water. Am J of Phys Med Rahabil 1997; 76(3): 204–7

Nerman M. Healing Pain and Injury. Richmond, CA: Bay Tree Publishing, 2013

Roberts W. Tub cooling for exertional heatstroke. Phys Sportsmed 1998; 26(5): 111–12

Root-Bernstein R, Root-Bernstein M. Honey, Mud, Maggots and Other Medical Marvels: the Science Behind Folk Remedies and Old Wives' Tales. Boston: Houghton Mifflin, 1997

Schneider M, Larkin M. Handbook of Self-Healing. New York: Arcana, 1994

APPENDIX C
Pyrotherapy (treatment of disease with artificial fever)

When we are exposed to infectious organisms such as viruses and bacteria, one of our main defenses is to warm our bodies. We conserve heat by shunting blood from the skin surface to the interior, reducing sweating and beginning to shiver. Now core temperature begins to rise and at the same time, cellular messengers called pyrogens reset the anterior hypothalamus to a new, higher body temperature. This in turn stimulates the release of more white blood cells into the bloodstream and makes them more active against infections. One study found after healthy subjects were immersed in a 103°F (39.4°C) water bath, their macrophages were more active and better able to respond to bacteria (Zellner, 2002), while another researcher found subjects had more white blood cells in their bloodstream after a single sauna (Pilch, 2013). Modern scientific evidence does not support routine use of anti-fever medications, which may worsen outcomes by interfering with the body's natural defense mechanisms (Ludwig, 2019). In fact, because bacteria and viruses do not replicate as well at higher temperatures, infected people who are not running high temperatures tend to shed more virus or bacteria: thus, reducing fevers is likely to increase transmission of infections during a pandemic such as influenza (Earn, 2014).

In addition to their effect on white blood cells, higher temperatures also inactivate or kill many viruses and bacteria, including the viruses that cause warts, common colds, AIDS, polio, and herpes, and the bacteria that cause gonorrhea and syphilis. HIV can be significantly inactivated by prolonged core temperatures of 102°F (39°C), while gonorrhea bacteria die at 104°F (40°C) and cancer cells are selectively destroyed at temperatures of 106–110°F (41–43°C) (Standish, 2002; Palazzi, 2019; LoCriccho, 1962; Schuller-Lewis, 2014).

Many coronaviruses that have infected humans – SARS, MERS, EBOLA and SARS-COV-2, the virus involved in the 2020 worldwide pandemic of COVID-19 – can be traced back to bats. Because these animals run unusually high body temperatures when flying, viruses that afflict them can tolerate higher temperatures than most other mammalian viruses (Brook, 2015). However, although it takes temperatures as high as 132–140°F to completely inactivate it, the SARS coronavirus begins to be inactivated at 100.4°F (Chan, 2011; Darnell, 2004). The main concern that originally led to trying to keep fevers down is that brain damage can occur when temperatures reach 106–107°F.

How was the connection between higher temperature and recovery from infectious illness discovered? Perhaps someone with an infectious illness accidentally became very hot, then got better; or perhaps a person with one immune system illness, such as syphilis or cancer, improved after having a fever due to a second illness. Observant folk may have noticed that someone who took regular saunas had fewer colds than other people. In 1990, the first systematic study of this phenomenon confirmed that this was true (Ernst, 1990). It may have even have been observation of sick animals. Holistic veterinarian Martin Goldstein once treated an eight-year-old boxer dog with leukemia and lymph cancer who ran an untreated fever of 102–107°F (39–42°C) for a week, and then was found to be completely cured, as confirmed by blood tests and clinical findings (Goldstein, 2000).

Cultures around the world treat infectious illnesses with hot baths, steam baths, sweat lodges and other heating hydrotherapy treatments. (Air temperatures inside steam rooms are typically higher than 109°F (43°C), the temperature at which the common cold virus begins

Appendix C

to weaken.) The ancient Greeks used body heating for syphilis and tuberculosis; Native Americans used the sweat lodge to treat many infectious illnesses; Sebastian Kneipp used steam baths for influenza, while wet sheet packs were widely used for pneumonia during the 1918 influenza epidemic. At Battle Creek Sanitarium, hot baths, electric light boxes or sweating packs were used for influenza, laryngitis, acute bronchitis, scarlet fever, and many other infectious illnesses. Such treatments were mainstream medicine until the introduction of penicillin in 1943, when more labor-intensive treatments for many illnesses were quickly abandoned.

Since then, a few holistically oriented physicians have continued to use whole-body heating to strengthen the immune system and inactivate viruses and cancer cells (Thrash, 2015; Boyle, 1988; Weil, 2000). Seventh Day Adventist nurse and chiropractor Louella Doub used artificial fever for over 30 years to stop the progression of diseases such as hepatitis, mononeucleosis, lupus, multiple sclerosis, and rheumatoid arthritis. Doub used Russian steam baths to raise patients' core temperature to 103°F (39°C) and keep it there for 30 minutes (Doub, 1971). At Uchee Pines Institute in Seale, Alabama, a typical regimen for cancer patients is to give them repeated full-body hot baths designed to raise core temperatures to 102–104°F (39–40°C) To prevent the brain from getting too hot, cold is applied to the head and around the neck during the baths.

Therapeutic hyperthermia is better known in Europe than in the United States, and there are European hyperthermia centers that treat patients with cancer and immune system conditions. As discussed in Chapter 10, whole-body heating may be combined with chemotherapy as a more effective treatment than either alone. According to oncologist Sungmin Lee, "Hyperthermia is a cancer treatment where tumor tissue is heated to around 40°C [104°F]. Hyperthermia shows both cancer cell cytotoxicity [cell-inactivating effect] and activation of macrophages, natural killer cells, dendritic cells, and T cells. Moreover, hyperthermia is commonly used in combination with different treatment modalities, such as radiotherapy and chemotherapy, for better clinical outcomes" (Lee, 2018). Many heating techniques, from the traditional full-body hot bath to hot wax, saunas, warming blankets, infrared lamps, and whole-body ultrasound, are now being used to raise patients' temperatures. A newer technique is a machine which extracts small amounts of blood from the bloodstream, warms it to nearly 108°F, then puts the heated blood back into the body (Alonso, 1994; Palazzi, 2019).

Recently scientists have realized that some hyperthermia treatments that involve breathing very moist air (hot showers, steam rooms, sweat lodges) can pack a "double punch": they not only warm the body, but can decrease transmission of viruses such as influenza, rhinovirus (common cold), and SARS-Co-v-2, the virus that causes COVID-19. Influenza cases rise in the winter partly because the air inside our houses is very dry, and then when an infected person coughs, mucus droplets carrying viruses evaporate in the dry air; rather than falling to the ground, virus particles then circulate high in the air where they are more likely to be inhaled (Noti, 2013). In addition, the mucus in our upper respiratory systems, which normally traps viruses before they can contact skin cells, dries out when we breathe dry air and then does not trap viruses as well. And finally, the cilia in the lungs which are normally capable of getting rid of inhaled virus particles, do not function as well in dry air (Kudo, 2019; Yale University, 2019). Therefore, some scientists recommend the preventative measure of inhaling very moist air by taking long hot showers, steam baths or local steam inhalations (Iwasaki, 2019; Sajadi, 2020).

References

Alonso K et al. Systemic hyperthermia in the treatment of HIV-related disseminated Kaposi's sarcoma. Long-term follow-up of patients treated with low-flow extracorporeal perfusion hyperthermia. AM J Clin Oncol 1994; 17(4)

Boyle W, Saine A. Lectures in Naturopathic Hydrotherapy. Sandy, OR: Eclectic Medical Publications, 1988

Brook CE, Dobson AP. Bats as "special" reservoirs for emerging zoonotic pathogens. Trends Microbiol 2015; 23(3): 172–80

Chan KH et al. The effects of temperature and relative humidity on the viability of the SARS coronavirus. Advances in Virology 2011; Oct 2011

Darnell M et al. Inactivation of the coronavirus that induces severe acute respiratory syndrome, SARS-Co. J Virol Methods 2004 Oct; 121(1): 85–91

Doub L. Hydrotherapy. Self-published manuscript. Fresno, CA, 1971

Duan S et al. Stability of SARS coronavirus in human specimens and environment and its sensitivity to heating and UV irradiation. Biomed Environ Sci 2003; 16(3): 246–55

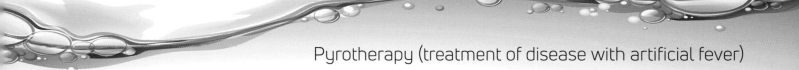

Earn D et al. Population-level effects of suppressing fever. Proc Biol Sci 2014; 28 (1778): 20132570

Ernst E et al. Regular sauna bathing and the incidence of common colds. Ann Med 1990; 22(4)

Goldstein M. The Nature of Animal Healing. Ballantine/Random House, 2000

Iwasaki A. Why is flu more serious in the winter? Yale University. YouTube video, May 15, 2019 (https://www.youtube.com/watch?v=Rfb_TtlbuNM)

Kudo E et al. Low ambient humidity impairs barrier function and innate resistance against influenza infection. Proceedings of the National Academy of Sciences May 13, 2019; DOI: 10.1073/pnas.1902840116

Lee S. Immunogenic effect of hyperthermia on enhancing radiotherapeutic efficacy. Int J Mol Sci 2018; Sep 17; 19(9)

LoCriccho L. Hot water treatment for warts. Cleveland Clinic Quarterly 1962; July: 29

Ludwig J. Antipyretic drugs in patients with fever and infection: literature review. British J Nurs 2019; May 23; (28(10): 610–18

Noti J et al. High humidity leads to loss of infectious influenza virus from simulated coughs. PLOS ONE Feb 27, 2013

Palazzi M. Role of hyperthermia in the battle against cancer. Tumori 2019; 96(2)

Pilch W et al. Effect of a single Finnish sauna session on white blood cell profile and cortisol levels in athletes and non-athletes. Int J of Hyperthermia 2013; Dec 31: 39

Sajadi M et al. Temperature, humidity and latitude analysis to predict potential spread and seasonality for COVID-19. March 9, 2020. Available at SSRN: https://ssrn.com/abstract=3550308 or http://dx.doi.org/10.2139/ssrn.3550308

Schuller-Lewis G et al. Treatment of recalcitrant warts with occlusive warming patches. J Drugs Dermatol Oct 2014; 13(10)

Standish L. AIDS and Complementary Medicine. Edinburgh: Churchill Livingstone, 2002

Thrash A. Nature's Healing Practices. Seale, AL: TEACH Services Publishing, 2015

Weil A. Spontaneous Healing: How to discover and embrace your body's natural ability to maintain and heal itself. New York: Ballantine, 2000

Yale University. Flu virus' best friend: low humidity. ScienceDaily, 13 May 2019. Available at: www.sciencedaily.com/releases/2019/05/190513155635.htm

Zellner M et al. Human monocyte stimulation by experimental whole body hyperthermia. Wein Klin Wochenehr 2002 Feb 15; 114(3)

APPENDIX D
Answers to review questions

Chapter 1
Short answer

1. Any five from the following list:
   a. Achieve same therapeutic goals as massage.
   b. Relaxing and stress-reducing.
   c. Help adjust client's body temperature.
   d. Provide a variety of skin sensations.
   e. Reduce stress on the massage therapist's hands.
   f. Make the massage therapist more versatile.
   g. Provide home self-treatment suggestions for clients.
   h. Helpful as part of a rehabilitation program.
   i. Part of a health-promoting lifestyle

2. Any two from the following list:
   a. Spiritual power of deity is in water, heals ailment.
   b. Water helps balance humors in the body.
   c. Applications of hot and cold strengthen the body.
   d. Water is a chemical compound with scientific effects.
   e. Warm applications trigger unconscious response and feelings of safety.

3. Bather would begin exercising in a gymnasium, proceed to a heated room (sauna), then plunge in a cold pool before receiving a massage.

4. Any Students can choose from:
   a. Flotation therapy for chronic pain.
   b. Watsu for relaxation.
   c. New products that apply heat and cold.
   d. Water exercise baths for hospitalized premies.
   e. Hyperthermia treatments for depression.

Multiple choice
5 = B; 6 = D; 7 = B; 4 = B; 8 = D

True/False
9 = False; 10 = True; 11 = True; 12 = False

Matching
13: 1 = D; 2 = C; 3 = A; 4= B
14: 1 = D; 2 = C; 3 = B; 4=A
15: 1 = B; 2 = C; 3 = D; 4 = A
16: 1 = E; 2 = D; 3 = A; 4 = C; 5 = B
17: 1 = E; 2 = D; 3 = C; 4 = A; 5 = B

Chapter 2
Short answer

Here are some key elements which you may have mentioned

1. Any six from: heat; cold; heat-pain; cold-pain; light touch; deep pressure; vibration; proprioception.
2. Any one of these: gag reflex; blushing; corneal reflex; withdrawal reflex; patellar reflex; cutaneous vasodilation reflex; sneeze reflex.
3. See Tables 2.1 and 2.4.
4. See Tables 2.2 and 2.3.

Fill in the blanks
5. Dilation; reflex areas.
6. Metabolic, glucose.
7. Stimulation.

Multiple choice
8 = D; 9 = C; 10 = D; 11 = C

Appendix D

Matching

12: 1 = C; 2 = D; 3 = E; 4 = A; 5 = B

13. 1 = C; 2 = E; 3 = A; 4 = D; 5 = B

14. 1 = B; 2 = D; 3 = C; 4 = A

Chapter 3

Short answer

1. You may choose from the following list:
    a. Abundant and affordable.
    b. Weight and hydrostatic pressure.
    c. Versatility.
    d. Ease of use.
    e. Provides a variety of tactile sensations.
    f. Buoyancy.
    g. Mind-body effects.
    h. Ability to dissolve many substances.
    i. Absorbs and holds heat or cold.
    j. Conducts both heat and cold.

2. When heated to 212°F (100°C), water molecules fly apart and become a gas. Cooling reverses the process. When cooled to about 32°F (0°C), water molecules crystallise as a solid. Heating reverses the process.

3. Conduction is the transfer of heat by direct contact of one heated or cooled substance with another; convection is the giving off of heat by moving currents of liquid or gas; condensation is the process which changes water vapor (a gas) into water (a liquid); evaporation, the reverse of condensation, is the process of changing water (a liquid), into water vapor (a gas); radiation is the transfer of heat through space, without two objects touching, through the emission of heat.

4. Any six of: body composition; genetics; season; physical condition; skin temperature; core temperature; part of body treated; treatment temperature; abruptness of temperature; duration of temperature; proportion of the body exposed; use of friction or pressure; body temperature after the treatment; aversion to heat or cold.

5. Have you ever had a whole-body wrap? If so, how did you like it? Some people love being wrapped up in blankets, and find it warm and cozy, but some people may feel too confining. Do you ever feel claustrophobic? (If the person is claustrophobic, another treatment should be used instead of a wrap.) Do you know of any medical reason why you shouldn't have hot or cold treatments on your skin? Do you know of any medical reason why you shouldn't have hot or cold treatments on your whole body at once, such as a hot tub or a cold shower?

Multiple choice

6 = C; 7 = C; 8 = D; 9 = F; 10 = D; 11 = C; 12 = B

Matching

13. 1 = C; 2 = D; 3 = A; 4 = B

14. 1 = D; 2 = C; 3 = B; 4 = A

15. 1 = F; 2 = D; 3 = E; 4 = B; 5 = A; 6 = C

16. 1 = E; 2 = G; 3 = D; 4 = C; 5 = B; 6 = A; 7 = E

17. 1 = C; 2 = E; 3 = D; 4 = B; 5 = A

18. 1 = D; 2 = E; 3 = C; 4 = B; 5 = A

Discussion questions

19. The derivative effect caused by dilation of skin blood vessels shifts blood flow away from the brain and internal organs.

20. The goal of the treatment, such as stress relief, treatment of an injury, derivation or nurturing touch.

True/False

21 = True; 22 = False; 23 = True; 24 = True; 25 = True

Chapter 4

Short answer

1. Burns.

2. Any five from: lack of feeling (numbness) in a specific area; rashes or other skin conditions that could be worsened by heat; inflammation; swelling; broken skin; cancerous tumor, unless approved by client's doctor; implanted devices; peripheral vascular disease; diabetes; sensitivity to heat.

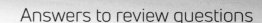

3. Any three from: nervous tension; muscle spasm; poor local circulation; musculoskeletal pain (muscle soreness, chronic pain, stiff, sore or arthritis joints); muscle tightness; tissue that needs to become more pliable and stretchable; possible post-treatment soreness; menstrual cramps; active trigger points; when a derivative or fluid-shifting effect is desired; chilled area; chilled client.

4. Hot stones and dry heating pad use dry heat; and silica pack and fomentations use moist heat.

5. Local heat makes myofascial trigger points less painful to pressure while they are treated, and less sore after treatment.

6. Charcoal pack.

Multiple choice

7 = E; 8 = D; 9 = C; 10 = D; 11 = C

True/False

12 = False; 13 = False; 14 = True; 15 = True; 16 = False

Chapter 5

Multiple choice

1 = B; 2 = A; 3 = E; 4 = A; 5 = D

True/False

6 = True; 7 = False; 8 = True; 9 = True; 10 = False

Chapter 6

Short answer

1. Any two of: paraffin bath; hot local bath or hot full bath; contrast local bath; contrast whole bath; paraffin bath; continuous bath.

2. Hot footbath; hot leg bath; hot arm bath; hot half bath; hot full bath; cold scalp bath.

3. Baking soda neutralizes toxins; Epsom salts draw water and toxins and provide magnesium and sulfate needed for detoxification; sea salts draw water and

toxins; and the warm water encourages a moderate amount of sweating.

4. Any two of: hot footbath; hot leg bath; neutral bath; powdered mustard bath; hot full bath; warm full bath.

5. Water completely surrounds an area, so its temperature can be conducted to the entire surface area.

6. Any four of: migraine headache; foot or body warming; foot problems such as arthritis; fatigue; insomnia; sleep disturbances; improving blood or lymphatic flow.

7. Any two of: when the therapist wishes to help stimulate blood flow; when the client is overheated; to give the client a feeling of invigoration; after a hard workout.

Fill in the blank

8. Burns; pressure sores; cuts; any area of open skin.

9. Hot footbath; paraffin bath.

10. Poor choice or bad choice.

11. Irritation.

12. Any three of: bruises; subacute sprains; soreness after exercise; nervous tension; arthritis pain; general tonic; detoxification.

13. Perform active movements.

14. Make scars softer and/or easier to stretch.

15. "fall" ... because they are (all the following are correct): obese; lightheaded; too weak to get out of tub; clumsy; too stiff to get out of tub.

Chapter 7

Short answer

1. Sauna uses dry air; steam bath uses wet air.

2. Wet heat penetrates more deeply, so then muscles are more relaxed.

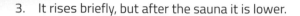

3. It rises briefly, but after the sauna it is lower.

4. Explain that her heart and circulatory system have to work harder than normally in the steam bath, so doctors do not recommend it for anyone who has had strokes in the past.

5. Steam liquefies congestion in the nose and chest; steam warms the respiratory tract; steam warms and relaxes muscles.

6. The heart has to pump harder to move blood, and the heart of someone with congestive heart failure may be too weak to do this.

7. Any three of: to prevent muscle soreness after a workout; when you want to expose the client's skin to herbal or essential oils added to steam water; if the client prefers the sensation of a steam bath over that of a sauna; when your client is getting over a cold but still has a lot of nasal congestion.

Multiple choice

8 = C; 9 = B; 10 = B; 11 = C; 12 = B; 13 = A

Chapter 8

Short answer

1. By adding a friction treatment such as a salt glow.

2. It should be set as high as the client can tolerate to desensitize the area, but not so high that it causes pain or discomfort.

3. A hot shower causes generalized vasodilation; a cold shower causes generalized vasoconstriction; and a contrast shower combines vasodilation and vasoconstriction, ultimately increasing blood flow in peripheral vessels even more than a hot shower.

4. A hot chest shower increases local blood flow and relaxes the chest muscles.

5. When cold is applied to the arms and hands of someone with Raynaud's syndrome, it can cause prolonged vasospasm.

6. A salt glow made with Epsom salts and other ingredients; shower tablets containing essential oils; herbal teabags contained in a special showerhead.

True/False

7 = False; 8 = True; 9 = True; 10 = False; 11 = True; 12 = False; 13 = False

Chapter 9

Multiple choice

1 = A; 2 = B; 3 = B; 4 = A; 5 = C

Fill in the blank

6. Stimulate; cancer cells.

7. Moist blanket; wet sheet.

8. Tonic; muscle; joint.

9. Cooling.

10. Sedative.

Short answer

11. Cold to head for migraine during a leg wrap; cold cloth to forehead when the client is sweating in a wrap.

12. Essential oils; herbs; powdered foods.

Chapter 10

Short answer

1. Cold mitten friction.

2. Weaker patients who could not tolerate cold could handle the salt glow.

3. Friction stimulates nerve endings and leads to skin vasodilation as a defense against injury; cold stimulates cold receptors and leads to a burst of heat in the area.

4. Change the water temperature, or add herbs or essential oils to the water.

5. A contrast shower stimulates cold receptors.

6. Neutral bath from previous chapter; dry brushing from this chapter.

Multiple choice

7 = A; 8 = D; 9 = B; 10 = B; 11 = C

Chapter 11
Multiple choice

1 = C; 2 = D; 3 = C; 4 = D; 5 = C

Fill in the blanks

6. Gently; pain.

7. Faster; more forcefully.

8. Muscles; trained.

9. Retained; illness; poor.

10. Cold; cuts; wounds.

11. Water; hydrostatic.

Chapter 12
Fill in the blanks

1. Rotator cuff tears; muscle strains; and sub-acute bursitis.

2. Contrast.

3. Peripheral blood vessels, deeper vessels.

4. Ligaments; muscles.

5. Muscle contraction.

Essay

6. First the blood vessels contract to avoid blood loss; then they open more widely to send white blood cells and nutrients to the area.

7. Any three from: contrast treatment over the dislocated shoulder; warm tub or whirlpool; castor oil pack; heat-trapping compress; contrast treatment over the non-injured shoulder.

8. Any two from the following (if injuries are not properly healed): carpal tunnel syndrome can lead to nerve damage; torn cartilage can lead to arthritis; torn rotator cuff can lead to frozen shoulder; shin splints can lead to stress fracture; shin splints can lead to lower leg compartment syndrome; sprains can lead to osteoarthritis; spinal cord injury can lead to scoliosis; poorly healed scar tissue can lead to adhesions; whiplash can lead to neck pain; injury to quadratus lumborum can lead to leg-length inequality; hematoma can lead to scar tissue.

Multiple choice

9 = C; 10 = B; 11 = B; 12 = D; 13 = B

Chapter 13
Essay questions

1. Any three of: arthritis; fibromyalgia; migraine headache; low back pain; post-stroke pain.

2. Any three of: arthritis; fibromyalgia; muscle weakness; muscle spasticity; Parkinson's disease; multiple sclerosis; stroke.

3. Any three of: arthritis; fibromyalgia; piriformis syndrome; low back spasm; sciatica; insomnia; nervous tension.

4. Hot moist application to the lower back; full hot bath followed by local moist heat application; or ice massage of the lower back.

5. Muscle weakness and muscle spasticity.

6. Any three of: arthritis; asthma; cancer detox; sinus headache; trigeminal neuralgia.

7. Any three of: dry skin brushing; neutral bath; charcoal pack; salt glow; wet sheet pack to neutral stage.

8. Any three of: honey–Epsom salts glow, for dry skin; low back contrast treatment, for low back pain; whole-body hot shower, used to relieve arthritic pain; whole-body cold shower, used to combat depression; whole-body hot shower, for deepening respiration, relaxing and

warming trunk muscles in asthma; whole-body hot shower, for relieving the pain of trigeminal neuralgia.

Fill in blanks

9. Arterial disease, heat.

10. Any four of: arthritis; constipation; menstrual cramps, varicose veins; migraine headache; sinus headache; muscle spasms; sciatica; TMD.

11. Short-lived and strong; longer-lasting, not as strong.

12. Any three of: Parkinson's disease; MS; arthritis; fibromyalgia; lymphedema; post-stroke.

13. Arthritis; fibromyalgia; low back pain; nervous tension. Not for (any one of) multiple sclerosis; diabetes; Parkinson's disease.

Multiple choice

14 = B; 15 = D; 16 = C; 17 = B; 18 = D; 19 = E; 20 = A

Matching

21. 1 = C; 2 = D; 3 = A; 4 = B
22. 1 = C; 2 = D; 3 = B; 4 = A
23. 1 = D; 2 = C; 3 = A; 4 = B
24. 1 = B; 2 = C; 3 = A; 4 = D

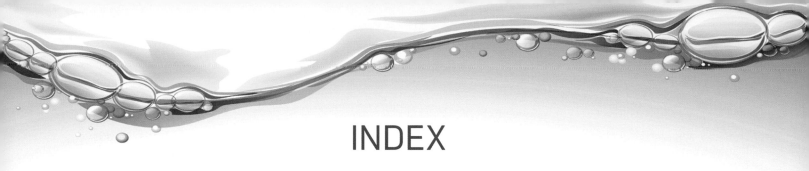

INDEX

Page number followed by f indicates figures, t indicates tables, and b indicates box respectively

A

Abdominal shower, 200–201, 200f
Acute bursitis, 275–277
Acute local inflammation, hydrotherapy in, 65
Acute lower back muscle spasm, 347
Acute lower back pain, 338–340
Acute spasm of neck muscles, 347
Adhesive capsulitis, 275, 290, 313–314
Amputations, 274
Anti-inflammatory leg wrap, 221, 325f
Aquatic therapy, 341
Arm and leg whirlpools, 144b
Arm baths, 155, 155f
Arm shower, 201–203, 201f
Aromatherapy wraps, 218b
Arteriosclerosis, of the feet and legs, 65
Arthritis, 314–315
    chronic, 316
Artificial devices, hydrotherapy in, 65
Asthma, 319
Asthma patient, hydrotherapy in, 65
Athletic injuries
    football injury, 270
    mountain-biking injury, 270–271
Attention deficit disorder patient, hydrotherapy in, 62
Autonomic nervous system, 35–37
    parasympathetic, 36
    sympathetic, 36

B

Baking soda baths, 168–169. *See also* Whole-body baths
Bath, England, 2, 3f, 6, 8, 8f, 14b
Baths of Diocletian, 5
Battle Creek Sanitarium, 13
Bell's palsy, 319
Biceps stretch, 260f
Bladder stones, 5
Blood pressure receptors, 376
Body areas
    chronic tension in the facial muscles, 320–321
Body wraps, 217
    additives, 218b

cold wet sheet, 224–226
dry sheet, 222–224, 223f
moist blanket, 219–222, 220f
Bronchospasm, 169
Buerger's disease, 89
    hydrotherapy in, 65
Bunions, 330
Bursitis, 275
    acute, 275–277
    sub-acute, 277

C

Cancer, 319–320
Cancer patient, hydrotherapy in, 64
Capsaicin, 49
Carpal tunnel syndrome, 277–278
Cartilage tears, 279
Case study
    fibromyalgia, 222
    releasing muscle tension, 321
Castor oil packs, 110–113, 113f
Central nervous system, 34–35
Charcoal packs, 113–114, 114f
    for inflammation and pain, 114
Chemical treatments, physiological effects of, 49
Chest showers, 199–200, 199f
Chronic arthritis, 316
Chronic constipation, 324
Chronic lower back pain, 340
Chronic venous insufficiency, 323
Circulatory system, 26–29
    arteries and veins of, 27f
    conditions, hydrotherapy in, 65
    plan of, 28f
    responses, 29b–30b
Cold applications
    cautions, 124
    contraindications, 122–124
    indications, 122
    primary effects of, 120b–121b
Cold arm baths, 156. *See also* Partial-body baths
Cold compresses, 134–135, 135f. *See also* Compresses
Cold footbaths, 142, 149–151

Cold hand baths, 153–154. *See also* Partial-body baths
Cold mitten friction, 219–222, 220f, 232–234, 233f
Cold showers, 211
Cold treatments, 1. *See also* Hydrotherapy
Cold wet sheet wraps, 224–227
Complex regional pain syndrome, 313
Compresses, 133–134
    cold, 134–135, 135f
    contrast, 136–138, 137f
    iced, 135–136, 136f
Condensation, 57b
Conduction, 57b
Constipation
    chronic, 324
Continuous baths, 163b
Contralateral reflex, 44
    effect, 42
Contralateral reflex effect, 280, 282
Contrast arm baths, 156
    half baths, 156–157
    leg baths, 157
Contrast baths, 166–167. *See also* Whole-body baths
Contrast compresses, 136–138, 137f. *See also* Compresses
Contrast footbaths, 151
Contrast hand baths, 154–155, 154f. *See also* Partial-body baths
Contrast showers, 212–213
Contrast treatments, 46–47
Cool footbaths, 149
    for hot burning feet, 150
Cranial nerves, 34
Cryokinetics, 122

D

Depletion, 39, 44
Depression, 325–326
Derivation, 39
Detoxification baths, 171. *See also* Whole-body baths
Detoxification treatments, 243–249
    charcoal bath for, 248
    hydrotherapy sweating treatment for detoxification, 245–246b, 246f

Index

Diabetes, 326
Diabetes patient, hydrotherapy in, 66
Diastole, 26
Dislocations, 279–280
  cold gel pack to knee, 280f
  subglenoid shoulder dislocation, 280f
Doctrine of humors, 4–5. *See also*
    Western hydrotherapy
Dry brushing, 238–240, 239f
Dry electric heating pads, 102
Dry sheet wrap, 222–224, 223f
Dry skin, 327–328
Dry skin brushing, 341

E

Eczema, 329
Elders, hydrotherapy in, 63
Electric heating pads, 102
  dry, 102
  moist, 102
Epidermis, 31
Epsom salts, 59
  baths, 169–170 (*see also*
    Whole-body baths)
Epsom salts bath, 288–289
Evaporation, 57b
Extreme sports injuries, 270
Eye baths, 143b

F

Fibromyalgia, 222, 329–330
  moist blanket wraps, 219–222, 220f
Flat plastic water bottles, 128, 129f
Fluid-shifting effect, to leg, 48
Fomentation, 56, 87f, 92–95, 97f
  how to make, 96b
  for a painful muscle spasm, 94–95
  for polio, 94f
Fomentek flat hot water bottle, 59
Football injury, 270
Footbaths, 142–143, 145f. *See also*
    Partial-body baths
  charcoal, 147
  with client lying down, 146
  cold, 142, 149–151
  contrast, 151
  cool, 149
  epsom salts, 147
  hot, 145–147
  sensory stimulation, 147–148, 148f
  sweating, 147
  vasodilating, 147
  warm, 147–148
Foot deformities, 329–330
  bunions, 330
  hammertoes, 330–331

Foot showers, 204–205, 204f
Foot-strenuous activities, 301
Fractures, 282–285, 284f
Friction treatments, 231–240
  cold mitten friction, 219–222, 220f,
    232–234, 233f
  dry brushing, 238–240, 239f
  salt glows, 234–238, 236f, 237f
  Swedish massage, 198, 250

G

Gel packs, 125, 125f
  to reduce pain, 126
Graduated showers, 210–211
Greece, hydrotherapy in ancient, 2–3.
    See also Western hydrotherapy

H

Hammertoes, 330–331
Hand bath, 142f, 151–152, 152f.
    See also Partial-body baths
Headaches
  migraine, 331–333
  muscle contraction headache,
    333–334
  post-concussion headache, 334–335
  sinus, 335–336
Head-out steam baths, 187. *See also*
    Hot wet air baths
Head showers, 196–199, 197f
Heat and cold
  to and from the body, 57b
  physiological effects of, 37–39, 39f
    contrast treatments, 46–47
    local cold treatments, 44–46
    local heat, 42–43, 42f
    neutral treatments, 47
    whole body cold, 43, 44f
    whole body heat, 39–41
Heat lamps, 106–109, 108f
Heat-trapping compress, 134b, 372
Heat-trapping compresses, 295
Herbal tea wraps, 218b
High blood pressure and stress, 41
HIV/AIDS patient, hydrotherapy in, 64
Homeostatic, 23
Hot and cold, local applications of, 45t
Hot arm baths, 155–156. *See also*
    Partial-body baths
Hot baths, 162–165, 164f. *See also*
    Whole-body baths
Hot compresses, 98–100, 99f
  disadvantage of, 98
Hot dry air bath, 180–184, 180f
  medical uses of, 181b
Hot footbaths, 145–147, 146b

Hot hand baths, 152–153. *See also*
    Partial-body baths
Hot shower, 259
  stretching and range of motion
    exercises, 259–262
Hot showers, 206–210, 209f
Hot towels, 100–101, 100f
  individual, 101
  rolls, 100, 101f
Hot water bottles, 103–106
  flat plastic, 105–106, 107f
  rubber, 103
Hot wet air baths, 184–186
  head-out steam baths, 187
  local steam baths, 184–186
  steam cabinets, 189–190, 189f
  steam canopies, 187–189, 187f
  steam rooms, 190–192, 190f, 191f
  whole-body steam baths, 186–187
Hubbard tank, 144b, 144f
Hunting reaction, 44
Hydropathy, 8, 9f
Hydrostatic pressure, 55
Hydrotherapy
  benefits of, 1
  equipment for treatment, 57f
  herbs used for injuries, 306b–307b
  and inflammation, 271–272, 271f
  and pain, 311–312
  partial-body, 3
  principles of, 25b–26b
  and scar tissue, 272–274
  for soldiers, 14b–15b
  somato-emotional issues and, 6b
  treatments for psychiatric problems, 13b
  Western, history of, 2–18.
    See also Western hydrotherapy
Hydrotherapy treatments
  cautions and contraindications, 62–68
  client health history, 72, 73f
  to cool the client, 70b
  different settings, 76–80
  equipment, 54, 56–60
    factors, 60–61
    sanitation protocols, 61–62
    water and its characteristics, 54–56
  guidelines for, 72–74
  heat and cold
    body composition and genetics, 69
    body temperature after a whole-
      body treatment, 72
    client's hydration status, 68–69
    client's physical condition, 69
    client's skin and core temperature, 70
    dislike of heat or cold, 72
    friction or percussion, 72
    length of temperature, 71
    part of the body treated, 71
    proportion of the body, 71–72

seasonal considerations, 69
treatment temperature, 71
water temperature is switched, 71
massage in a hospital setting, 77b–78b
post-operative discomfort, 76
session design, 74–76
to warm the client, 71b
Hyperthermia, therapeutic, 378
Hypothalamus, 36

I

Ice bags, 127, 127f, 128f
Iced compresses, 135–136, 136f. *See also*
Compresses
Ice massage, 119, 128–130, 130f, 294, 371
for chronic inflammation, 131
for muscle spasm, acute inflammation,
and pain, 130–132
Ice packs, 126
home made, 127
Ice stroking, 132–133, 133f
Iliotibial band disorders, 285
Indian herbal steams, 1
Industrial revolution, hydrotherapy
in, 7–8. *See also* Western
hydrotherapy
Inflamed plantar fascia, 289
Inflammation, 300
Inflammatory arthritis
gout, 314–315
Injuries
sports, 268–270
traumatic, 267–268
Insomnia, 336–337
Intermittent claudication, 254

J

Jacuzzis, 171
Japanese hot springs, 1
Japanese soaking tub, 60
Jetted hydrotherapy tub, 58b
Jetted tubs, 171–172. *See also*
Whole-body baths

K

Knee injuries, 285

L

Latent heat, 56
Leg baths, 157
cold, 159
contrast, 159–160
hot, 157–158

Leg shower, 203–204, 203f
Life stress, 337–338
Local cold treatments, long versus
short, 46t
Local heat applications, 89
cautions, 89
contraindications, 89
indications, 89
primary effects of, 88b
special safety note, 89
Lower back pain (LBP), 338–340
acute lower back pain, 338–340
chronic lower back pain, 340
Lower leg compartment syndrome,
294
Lower-leg whirlpools, 288
Lymph, 27
Lymphedema, 72, 341–342
patient, hydrotherapy in, 66

M

Manual lymphatic drainage (MLD),
342–344
Massage therapist and modern
hydrotherapy, 16–17
Mechanical treatments, physiological
effects of, 47–49
Menstrual pain, 342–344
tonic treatments, 342
Metabolic wastes, 244
Middle ages, hydrotherapy in, 5–7, 7f.
See also Western hydrotherapy
Moist blanket wraps, 219–222, 220f
Moist heat application, 297
Moist heating pads, 102, 104f
Molecular sponge, 243
Mountain-biking injury, 270–271
Mud baths, 58b
Multiple sclerosis (MS), 172, 344
hydrotherapy in, 66–67
Muscle contraction headache, 333–334
Muscle cramps, 345
Muscle fibers absorb, 294
Muscle soreness, 289
Muscle spasms, 345
Muscle strains, 286
Muscle weakness, 351
Mustard plasters, 109–110, 111f
for rib muscle pain, 110

N

Neck-limbering exercises, 370
Neck stretch, 260f
Nerve entrapment, 351–352
Nerve or crush injuries, hydrotherapy
in, 67

Nervous system, 33–34, 36f
autonomic, 35–37
central, 34–35
peripheral, 35
Neuropathy, 196
Neutral baths, 4, 165–166, 341. *See also*
Whole-body baths
Neutral shower, 211
Neutral treatments, 47

O

Oatmeal baths, 167–168, 168f. *See also*
Whole-body baths
Opioid medications, 312
Osteoarthritis (OA), 315–317, 316f
partial-body treatments for, 317
whole-body treatments for, 317
Overweight clients, hydrotherapy
in, 64

P

Paraffin baths, 160–161, 160f
history of, 161b
Parkinson's disease (PD), 352–353
hydrotherapy in, 64
Partial-body baths, 141–142
cold arm baths, 156
cold footbaths, 149–151
cold hand baths, 153–154
cold leg baths, 159
contrast arm baths, 156
half baths, 156–157
leg baths, 157
contrast footbaths, 151
hand baths, 151–152, 152f
contrast hand baths, 154–155, 154f
contrast leg baths, 159–160
paraffin baths, 160–161, 160f
cool footbaths, 149
footbaths, 142–143
hot arm baths, 155–156
hot footbaths, 145–147
hot hand baths, 152–153
hot leg baths, 157–158
sanitation, 142
warm footbaths, 147–148
Partial-body hydrotherapy, 3
Pectoral muscle stretch, 260f
Pediluvia, 142
Percussion douche, 58b
Peripheral nervous system, 35
Peripheral neuropathy (PN),
353–354
Phlebitis patient, hydrotherapy in, 65
Piriformis syndrome, 352
Plantar fasciitis, 289

Index

Polio
    fomentations and stretching
        treatment, 94f
Pollutants, 244
Polychlorinated biphenyls (PCBs), 244
Pool therapy
    improved cardiac and respiratory
        function, 375–376
    musculoskeletal effects, 375
    sensory stimulation, 376
    soothing effects, 376
Post-concussion headache,
    334–335
Powdered mustard, 170, 170f. *See also*
    Whole-body baths
Precordium, 43
Pre-eclampsia, 169
Pregnancy, hydrotherapy in, 64
Prolotherapy, 316
Psoriasis, 354–355
Psychiatric problems treatment,
    hydrotherapy for, 13b
Pyrogens, 377

R

Radiation, 57b
Raynaud's syndrome, 23
    hydrotherapy in, 65
Reflexes, 36–37, 37f, 38f
Repetitive strain injury (RSI) in
    therapists, 257
Repetitive stress injuries, 270
Restless leg syndrome (RLS), 355
Rheumatism, 3
Rheumatoid arthritis (RA), 318, 318f
    partial-body treatments for, 318
    whole-body treatments for, 318
Roman baths, 1, 2f
Roman Empire, hydrotherapy in, 5
    See also Western hydrotherapy
Rotator cuff tears, 290–291
Rubber hot water bottles, 103, 105f
Russian saunas, 1
Russian steam bath, 187

S

Salt glows, 234–238, 236f, 237f
    whole-body, 235–238, 237f
Sauna, 180–184, 180f, 247
    and footbath, 7f
    medical uses of, 181b, 183
Scalp baths, 143b
Scar tissue, 292
Sciatica, 355–356
Scotch hose, 58b
Scrofulous tumors, 5

Sea salt baths, 170. *See also* Whole-body
    baths
Seizure disorders patient, hydrotherapy
    in, 67
Sensation and movement, 296
Sensory stimulation, 361–362
Shiatsu massage therapy, 174
Shin splints, 294
Short cold baths, 166. *See also* Whole-
    body baths
Showers
    abdominal, 200–201, 200f
    arm, 201–203, 201f
    chest, 199–200, 199f
    cold, 211–212
    contrast, 212–213
    disadvantage to, 196
    foot, 204–205, 204f
    graduated, 210–211
    head, 196–199, 197f
    higher-end spas, 195
    hot, 206–210, 209f
    leg, 203–204, 203f
    neutral, 211
    partial-body, 196
    safety, 196
    skin-stimulating effect of, 195
    treatment, 196
    underwater, 205
    whole-body, 206–208
Silica gel cold packs, 124–125
Silica gel hot packs, 91–92, 93f
Sinus baths, 143b
Sinus headache, 335–336
Sitz baths, 143b
Skeletal muscle, 27
    pump, 29f
Skin, 29–33
    anatomy of, 31f
    blood supply to, 32f
    conditions and hydrotherapy, 67
    role of, 31
Solvents, 247
Spa
    bathtubs, 173 (*see also* Whole-body
        baths)
    level equipment, 58b
Spinal cord injuries, 296–297
Sports injuries, 268–270, 269t
    extreme, 270
Sprains, 294–295
Stainless steel whole-body whirlpools,
    173–174. *See also* Whole-body
    baths
Standard baths, 162. *See also* Whole-body
    baths
Steam Bath chair, 7f
Steam cabinets, 189–190, 189f. *See also*
    Hot wet air baths

Steam canopies, 60, 187–189, 187f. *See
    also* Hot wet air baths
Steam rooms, 190–192, 190f, 191f. *See
    also* Hot wet air baths
Stratum corneum, 31
Strenuous exercise, 288
Stretching treatment
    for polio, 94f
Stroke, 356–357
Sub-acute bursitis, 277
Subglenoid shoulder dislocation, 280f
Sulphur springs, 5
Swiss shower, 58b

T

Tailbone trauma, 298–299
Temporomandibular joint disorder (TMD),
    357–359
Tendonitis, 299–300
Terminal illness, 359–360
Thermal baths, 4
Thermal sensation, 62t
Thermic impression, 56
Thoracic outlet syndrome (TOS), 352
Throat baths, 143b
Throat ice bag, 257f
Thyroid disorders, hydrotherapy in, 67
Tired, aching feet, 301–302
Toasted skin syndrome, 90b, 90f
Tonic hydrotherapy treatments,
    250–254
    for anterior cervical muscles and
        throat, 256
    for the digestive system, 255
    for the eyes, 255
    for the massage therapist, 257–259
    for poor local circulation, 254
    for respiratory system, 256
    for self-care treatments, 257
    for skeletal muscles, 255
    for the skin, 257
Tonic treatments, 243
    for the anterior cervical muscles and
        throat, 256
Toxins, 243–244
Trapezius stretch, 260f
Traumatic brain injuries, 302–303
Traumatic injuries, 267–268
Trigeminal neuralgia (TN), 361
Turkish baths, 1

U

Underwater showers, 205
United States, hydrotherapy in, 10
    See also Western hydrotherapy
Universal solvent, 56

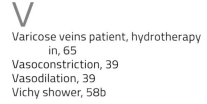

V

Varicose veins patient, hydrotherapy in, 65
Vasoconstriction, 39
Vasodilation, 39
Vichy shower, 58b

W

Warm baths, 165
Warm epsom salts bath, 369
Warm footbaths, 147–148
Warm Springs Institute for Rehabilitation, 12
Warm-water whirlpools, 274
Water
  cure, decline of, 11–12
  cycle, 54
  forms of, 54t
  spiritual and religious function of, 3–4
Watsu, 17, 171, 174–175. *See also* Whole-body baths
  pool, 58b, 60

Western hydrotherapy, history of, 2–18
  decline of, 11–12
  doctrine of humors, 4–5
  European spas, resurgence of, 10–11
  humoral pathology, 5
  in ancient Greece, 2–3
  in the middle ages, 5–7, 7f
  in 19th century, 8
    Preissnitz, Vincent, 8–10, 9f
    Kneipp, Sebastian,10, 10f
  in the renaissance and industrial revolution, 7–8
  in Roman Empire, 5
  in 20th century, 12–16, 15f
  in United States, 10, 11f
  modern, 16–17
  Native American, 4b
  spiritual and religious function of water, 3–4
Whiplash, 303–305
Whole-body baths
  baking soda baths, 168–169
  contrast baths, 166–167

  detoxification baths, 171
  epsom salts baths, 169–170
  hot baths, 162–165
  jetted tubs, 171–172
  neutral baths, 165–166
  oatmeal baths, 167–168
  powdered mustard, 170
  sea salt baths, 170
  short cold baths, 166
  spa bathtubs, 173
  stainless steel whole-body whirlpools, 173–174
  standard baths, 162
  warm baths, 165
  watsu, 174–175
Whole-body cold treatments, effects of, 45t
Whole-body contrast shower, 371
Whole body heat, 39–41
  treatments, effects of, 41t
Whole-body heating, 244–247
Whole-body showers, 206–208
Whole-body steam baths, 186–187. *See also* Hot wet air baths
Wilbarger brushing therapy, 239